CANCER 3

A COMPREHENSIVE TREATISE

BIOLOGY OF TUMORS: Cellular Biology and Growth

Volume 1 • ETIOLOGY: Chemical and Physical Carcinogenesis

Volume 2 • ETIOLOGY: Viral Carcinogenesis

Volume 3 • BIOLOGY OF TUMORS: Cellular Biology and Growth

Volume 4 • BIOLOGY OF TUMORS: Surfaces, Immunology, and Comparative Pathology

Therapies will be covered in subsequent volumes.

CANCER 3

A COMPREHENSIVE TREATISE

BIOLOGY OF TUMORS: Cellular Biology and Growth

FREDERICK F. BECKER, EDITOR
New York University School of Medicine

PLENUM PRESS • NEW YORK AND LONDON

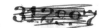

Library of Congress Cataloging in Publication Data

Becker, Frederick F
  Biology of tumors.

  (*His* Cancer, a comprehensive treatise; 3)
  Includes bibliographies and index.
  1. Tumors. 2. Cancer cells. 3. Carcinogenesis.
4. Growth regulators. I. Title. [DNLM: 1. Neoplasms. QZ200
C2143]
RC261.B42   vol. 3   [RC262]   616.9'94'008s   [619.9'94'07]
ISBN 0-306-35203-6   75-22290

© 1975 Plenum Press, New York
A Division of Plenum Publishing Corporation
227 West 17th Street, New York, N.Y. 10011

United Kingdom edition published by Plenum Press, London
A Division of Plenum Publishing Company, Ltd.
Davis House (4th Floor), 8 Scrubs Lane, Harlesden, London, NW10 6SE, England

Printed in the United States of America

Preface

As was shown in the first two volumes of this series, great strides have been made in identifying many of the agents or classes of substances responsible for carcinogenesis and in delineating their interactions with the cell. Clearly, the aim of such studies is that, once identified, these agents can be eliminated from the environment. Yet, despite these advances and the elimination of some important carcinogenic agents, one major problem exists. It is a constant monitor of all oncologic study and diminishes the importance of every experiment and of every clinical observation. *As we noted earlier, that problem is our inability to define the malignant cell.* It is through studies of the fundamental biology of tumors that we seek this definition.

A vast amount of information has been gathered which describes *what* this cell does and—to a lesser extent—*how* it does it. But the *why* evades us. We have been unable to define the malignant cell, save in broad terms by comparing it to its normal counterpart. The major problem appears to be that the malignant cell does so much. It is a chimera, mystifyingly composed of normal activities and structures, of phenotypic schizophrenia with embryonic, fetal, and adult charac- teristics and, occasionally, a hint of an unclassifiable capacity unique to malignant cells.

The clues as to the *why* of cancer function must be derived directly or by induction from the *what* and *how*. Malignant cells replicate when replication is not required. Whether by escaping the normal inhibitory controls of the host, or by suprasensitivity to stimulation, or by some defect other than these, the tumor grows. The growth is noncompensatory and nonfunctional. The malignant cell also lives beyond its normal span. Together, growth and increased life span result in disruptive cellular accumulation. And what is more, malignant cells compete rather than participate with their normal neighbors and then competitively invade and destroy. The malignant cell itself evades destruction by humoral, immunological, and cellular defense mechanisms. It is therefore characterized by autonomous behavior, living off the host rather than with it. Are these abnormal activities the result of a single alteration or many? One integrated pattern or many? And what genetic or epigenetic or genetic–epigenetic alteration is respon- sible for this successful, this deadly capacity? An examination of the biology of

v

tumors presented in Volumes 3 and 4 serves many purposes. It may enable us to better understand normal cell biology. It may suggest crucial cellular alterations induced by carcinogenic agents. And, by understanding its aberrations of control and the advantages thus gained by the malignant cell, we may be better able to find a means of reversing them and halting their destructive processes.

New York   Frederick F. Becker

Contributors

to Volume 3

A. M. ATTALLAH, Research Foundation, Children's Hospital, Washington, D.C.

ARMIN C. BRAUN, Department of Plant Biology, The Rockefeller University New York, New York

KELLY H. CLIFTON, Departments of Radiology and Pathology, University of Wisconsin Hospitals, Radiotherapy Center, Madison, Wisconsin

WILLIAM H. FISHMAN, Tufts Cancer Research Center, Tufts University School of Medicine, Boston, Massachusetts

JUDAH FOLKMAN, Children's Hospital Medical Center, Boston, Massachusetts

A. CLARK GRIFFIN, Department of Biochemistry, M. D. Anderson Hospital, University of Texas, Houston, Texas

M. PIETRO GULLINO, Division of Experimental Pathology, National Cancer Institute, Bethesda, Maryland

A. ALLAN HORLAND, Department of Pathology, New York University Medical Center, New York, New York

JOHN C. HOUCK, Research Foundation, Children's Hospital, Washington, D.C.

CHARLES LIGHTDALE, Memorial Sloan-Kettering Cancer Center, New York, New York

MARTIN LIPKIN, Memorial Sloan-Kettering Cancer Center, New York, New York

JOSEPH LOBUE, Department of Biology, Laboratory of Experimental Hematology, Graduate School of Arts and Sciences, New York University, New York, New York

DANIEL MEDINA, Department of Cell Biology, Baylor College of Medicine, Houston, Texas

WILLIAM D. ODELL, Department of Medicine, Harbor General Hospital, Torrance, California

HENRY C. PITOT, McArdle Memorial Laboratory, University of Wisconsin Medical Center, Madison, Wisconsin

viii

MILAN POTMESIL, Department of Biology, Laboratory of Experimental Hematology, Graduate School of Arts and Sciences, New York University, New York, New York

GIOVANNI, ROVERA, Department of Pathology, Temple University, School of Medicine, Philadelphia, Pennsylvania

ROBERT M. SINGER, Cancer Research Center, Tufts University School of Medicine, Boston, Massachusetts

BHAVANI N. SRIDHARAN, Departments of Radiology and Pathology, University of Wisconsin Hospitals, Madison, Wisconsin

JOSÉ URIEL, Institut de Recherches Scientifiques sur le Cancer, Villejuif, France

CHARLES E. WENNER, Department of Health, Roswell Park Memorial Institute, Buffalo, New York

ADA WOLFSEN, Department of Medicine, Harbor General Hospital, Torrance, California

SANDRA, R. WOLMAN, Department of Pathology, New York University Medical Center, New York, New York

Contents

General Concepts

Differentiation and Dedifferentiation   1

ARMIN C. BRAUN

Fetal Characteristics of Cancer   2

JOSÉ URIEL

Ectopic Isoenzymes: Expression of Embryonic Genes in Neoplasia　　　3

WILLIAM H. FISHMAN AND ROBERT M. SINGER

Ectopic Hormone Secretion by Tumors   4

WILLIAM D. ODELL AND ADA WOLFSEN

Tumor Progression   5

DANIEL MEDINA

Metabolic Controls and Neoplasia 6

HENRY C. PITOT

Genetics of Tumor Cells 7

SANDRA R. WOLMAN AND ALLAN A. HORLAND

Growth of Tumors

Cell Division and Tumor Growth   8

CHARLES LIGHTDALE AND MARTIN LIPKIN

Stimulation   9

JOSEPH LoBUE AND MILAN POTMESIL

Extracellular Compartments of Solid Tumors 12

Pietro M. Gullino

Tumor Angiogenesis 13

Judah Folkman

Regulation of Energy Metabolism in Normal and Tumor Tissues 14

Charles E. Wenner

DNA-Nucleoproteins 15

Giovanni Rovera

Protein Synthesis   16

A. CLARK GRIFFIN

General Concepts

Differentiation and Dedifferentiation

ARMIN C. BRAUN

1. Introduction

The tumor problem has been viewed by certain investigators as being essentially one of anomalous differentiation, in which the basic cellular mechanisms that underlie the neoplastic state are similar to those involved in the cellular differentiation that occurs during the normal course of development in all multicellular organisms (Braun, 1969, 1970, 1974; Markert, 1968; Pierce, 1970). A distinction between this type of heritable cellular change, which is epigenetic in nature and is concerned merely with persistent alterations in the *expression* of the genetic determinants present in the nucleus of a cell, and changes of a mutational type, which involves changes in the integrity of that information, would appear to be of more than academic interest. If changes of a mutational type are involved, irreversibility is implied, and control in the foreseeable future would be limited essentially to the methods presently being used. If, on the other hand, epigenetic mechanisms underlie the neoplastic state, then the state is potentially reversible; if this is true, it could open, in principle at least, entirely new avenues of approach to the tumor problem. What, then, is the experimental evidence that can be marshalled in support of the suggestion that epigenetic mechanisms underlie the tumorous state generally?

2. Normal Cell Differentiation: Epigenetic Control Mechanisms

During the normal course of development, the many billions of cells of which higher organisms are composed arise from mitotic divisions and are the progeny

ARMIN C. BRAUN • The Rockefeller University, New York, N.Y.

of a single activated egg cell. These mitotic divisions give rise to genetically identical cells which, following induction and determination during early development, differentiate in a highly predictable manner into the many morphologically, physiologically, and biochemically diverse cell types found in higher organisms. An abundance of evidence derived from a variety of experimental approaches indicates that cellular differentiation does not, in most instances at least, involve a change in the integrity of the genetic determinants present in the diverse differentiated cell types. The available evidence also indicates that more than 90% of the genetic information present in nuclei of cells is repressed and hence nonfunctional and that different genes or constellations of genes are responsive to different specific signals that derepress them and regulate their activities (Braun, 1969; Davidson, 1968; Markert and Ursprung, 1971). Thus differences among cells with an identical complement of genes are believed to be due to the action of different genes in the diverse differentiated cell types. Certain genes—for example, those coding for the respiratory enzymes—are functional in most if not all cells, while those concerned with differentiated function are selectively activated or repressed, different ones for the histologically distinct, differentiated cell types. With a conceptual model such as this, it is easy to understand why, for example, nucleated red blood cells synthesize hemoglobin while lymphocytes and leukocytes do not, why liver cells produce serum albumin while kidney cells do not but instead synthesize as a product of their differentiation an enzyme such as L-amino oxidase. Nuclei found in essentially undifferentiated cells such as the basal cells of the skin and stem cells of various tissues are also programmed specifically and stably for the cellular phenotype into which they are destined to differentiate. The specific pattern of synthesis for which such cells are programmed is not expressed, however, until differentiation occurs. An abundance of experimental evidence indicates, moreover, that the specific programming of the genetic information present in the nucleus of a cell is largely determined by the cytoplasmic environment in which a nucleus is found (Braun, 1969; Davidson, 1968; Markert and Ursprung, 1971).

Embryonic induction leading to determination and ultimately to the differentiation of a cell clearly involves profound and persistent switches in metabolic patterns which are different for histologically distinct cell types and which lead to the persistent synthesis by such cells of the specific products that characterize the differentiated state in each instance. Cell division, like cell differentiation, also involves a profound switch in metabolic pattern, and a persistently dividing cell, such as a tumor cell, produces significant amounts of a specialized protein in the form of microtubular protein which has a highly specialized function to perform during the mitotic phase of the cell cycle. Thus cell division, like cell differentiation, appears to be an inductive process with a resulting synthesis in either case of specialized products that have specialized functions to perform. We can maintain with confidence that the key mechanisms involved in the production of these new and specialized products required for both cell differentiation and cell division act through the processes and components of the gene action system, which is ubiquitous in its fundamental aspects and is thus common to all cells. Variable gene activity against a constant cellular genome is, then, the guiding concept on which much of the current research in the field of cell differentiation and cell division is based.

3. The Tumor Problem as a Problem of Anomalous Differentiation

3.1. Criteria That Must Be Satisfied to Establish the Concept

If epigenetic mechanisms similar to those involved in normal cellular differentiation are also concerned in the establishment and maintenance of the tumorous state, then it would appear necessary to demonstrate that nuclei of normal cells and tumor cells are genetically equivalent and that, therefore, all of the genetic information required to account for the cancer phenotype is present in normal cells and needs only to be persistently activated and thus expressed. This could perhaps be demonstrated most convincingly by showing that the neoplastic state is reversible and thus depends for its expression on active and inactive gene states within a constant cellular genome. It would also appear necessary to demonstrate experimentally that all of the essential properties that characterize the malignant state (e.g., unrestrained growth and ability to spread by invasion and metastasis) are inherently present in normal cells and that one or more or all of these properties may be expressed in the absence of neoplasia. A capacity of certain normal cell types to invade tissues and migrate freely through an organism is, of course, commonly recognized. Morphogenetic cell movements play an important part in the structural molding of a developing embryo. Melanoblasts, for example, migrate actively through many tissues of an embryo before finally localizing at specific sites and then differentiating into nonmigrating and nondividing melanocytes. Certain normal cells of adult organisms such as the macrophages, leukocytes, and lymphocytes may invade tissues extensively and move freely through an organism, and thus they show certain fundamental attributes of cancer cells. Those cells do not develop into malignant growths, however, because their division mechanisms are precisely regulated. That epithelial cells may show all of the phenotypic attributes of cancer cells in the absence of neoplasia can perhaps be illustrated by citing the early studies of Bernard Fischer. In 1906 Fischer injected substances of many different kinds beneath the skin of rabbits in an attempt to find some that were carcinogenic. Of the substances tested, the fat-soluble dye Scharlach R (scarlet red) caused epithelial cells directly exposed to it to behave for the time being precisely as though they had been transformed to the malignant state. These cells multiplied actively, invaded underlying tissues deeply, and even entered the blood vessels and lymph channels. The stimulated cells, which mimicked the malignant state perfectly, reverted completely to normal when the Scharlach R (scarlet red) disappeared from the site of injection. Although Scharlach R has, since Fischer's report, been shown to be weakly carcinogenic, it was clearly not acting as a carcinogen in Fischer's studies because the stimulated epithelial cells reverted again to normal. Since one would hardly expect a compound such as Scharlach R to be the carrier of new genetic information, the conclusion seems unmistakable that the dye was causing a temporary change in the expression of the genetic determinants present in the nucleus of the epithelial cells, resulting in the development of the cancer phenotype. These observations suggest then that all of the genetic information necessary to establish the cancer phenotype is present in normal epithelial cells and that the maintenance of that state is merely a question of determining how the information is regulated so that it is persistently expressed.

The ultimate proof that normal cells contain all of the genetic information required for the establishment and maintenance of the neoplastic state would require a demonstration that it can be achieved in the absence of the addition, deletion, or permanent rearrangement of genetic information normally present in a cell and that once it is firmly fixed as a heritable cellular trait it is completely reversible, leading to a normalization of the neoplastic cells. An unequivocal example of this is now available in the plant literature (Binns and Meins, 1973; Lutz, 1971). When normal plant cells are grown under defined conditions of culture, they may acquire, as do animal cells, neoplastic properties. When this occurs, the phenomenon is known as habituation. In plant tumor systems, this results from a persistent activation of a series of quite distinct but well-defined biosynthetic systems whose products are concerned with cell growth and division. Those same biosynthetic systems are repressed and hence nonfunctional in normal cell types, as described in detail in Volume 4, Chapter 12, of this series. Once the biosynthetic systems responsible for the production of the essential growth-regulating substances and metabolites have become persistently activated in the cultured cells, the heritable cellular alteration is highly stable and may persist indefinitely. Such habituated tissues are transplantable (Limasset and Gautheret, 1950). That habituation is a completely reversible process has now been demonstrated with the use of a significant number of cloned lines of habituated tissues (Binns and Meins, 1973; Lutz, 1971). A demonstration of the reversibility of the neoplastic state in this instance was possible only because of certain unique properties of higher plant species, as described in Volume 4, Chapter 12, of this series. These studies with the use of habituated plant tissues provide the ultimate proof that the neoplastic state, in plants at least, may arise and be perpetuated indefinitely as a result of persistent changes in gene expression. Since all of the genetic information required for the establishment and maintenance of the neoplastic state is present in the normal cell genome and since this process is regularly reversible under special experimental conditions, one does not need to postulate drastic changes of a mutational type to account for the continued abnormal and autonomous proliferation of a tumor cell. If mutations should ultimately be found to be etiologically involved in tumorigenesis, their action would probably be via epigenetic pathways to alter the expression of other parts of the host cell genome. Any new genetic information added to a cell as a result of infection by an oncogenic virus might perhaps be looked on as persistently activating that segment of the host cell genome concerned with continued cell growth and division rather than coding specifically for one or more substances required for the autonomous proliferation of tumor cells.

During the transition from a normal cell to a tumor cell, there is, as indicated above, a profound and persistent reorientation of patterns of metabolism, going from the precisely regulated metabolism concerned with differentiated function that is characteristic of a mature normal resting cell to one involving the persistent synthesis of the nucleic acids, the mitotic and enzymatic proteins, and other substances concerned specifically with continued cell growth and division that characterizes a persistently dividing cell such as a tumor cell. At one extreme we find the very rapidly growing, fully autonomous tumor cells, which may show such a pronounced deterioration of form and function that it is difficult for a pathologist to determine the precise cell type from which the tumor was derived. In such instances, the pattern of metabolism concerned with differentiated function appears to be completely overwhelmed and hence not expressed. This leads to a dedifferentiation of such cells with an accompanying loss of characteristic form and function. When, on the other hand, essentially undifferentiated but determined stem cells of various tissues are converted into tumor cells of a very rapidly growing type, the potentials for differentiation present in those cells are often simply not expressed. In both instances, this is probably true because fully autonomous, rapidly growing tumor cells are highly efficient proliferating systems whose energy is directed largely toward a synthesis of substances required for cell growth and division to the exclusion of the production of substances concerned with differentiated function. In the vast majority of tumors, however, the neoplastic cells show a sufficient capacity for differentiated function that they are readily recognizable as to the cell type of their origin and yet possess a capacity for autonomous growth.

3.3. Evidence for Selective Gene Activation in Tumor Cells

In tumors such as certain of the more slowly growing transplantable and malignant Morris hepatomas, a high degree of differentiation is achieved and cells of the tumors deviate minimally from their normal counterparts in their capacity for differentiation and function. There are in addition certain hormone-secreting endocrine tumors such as the islet cell carcinomas of the pancreas, which may produce huge amounts of insulin even when microscopic in size. Similarly, tumors of the thyroid may give rise to extreme hyperthyroidism, while pituitary tumors may synthesize large quantities of trophic hormones, resulting in gigantism or acromegaly from growth hormone excess and in Cushing's syndrome from an excess of ACTH. More interesting perhaps are instances of inappropriate hormone synthesis: for example, an ACTH-like substance was found to be produced by a primary carcinoma of the lung (Marks *et al.*, 1963), while gonadotropin was found to be secreted by a bronchogenic carcinoma (Faiman *et al.*, 1967). Numerous other examples of this type have been extensively reviewed in the literature (Gellhorn, 1969; Lipsett *et al.*, 1964; see Chapter 4). There are in addition examples of embryonic or fetal antigen contained in liver tumor cells; the antigen is identical to one present in embryonic tissue but is not found in normal adult liver cells (Abelev *et al.*, 1963). Similar findings have been reported for certain gastrointestinal tumors (Gold and Freedman, 1965*a,b*; see Chapter 2).

These observations can perhaps best be interpreted by assuming that the genetic information required for inappropriate hormone synthesis as well as for production of the fetal antigens is inherently present in all cells but the information is not expressed until those cells are.converted to the tumorous state. All of these studies suggest then that two areas of metabolism—one involved with differentiated function, which is characteristic of a normal mature resting cell, and the other concerned with persistent cell growth and division, which characterizes the tumorous state—compete with one another for ascendancy. The degree to which a cell is transformed would appear to determine the extent to which either pattern is expressed.

3.4. Evidence for the Reversibility of the Cancerous State

The question that arises next is how the pattern of metabolism required for continued cell growth and division as well as for an ability of a cell to spread by invasion and metastasis is established and maintained in a persistently dividing population of cells in the absence of a change in the integrity of the genetic information present in the nucleus of a cell. In order to approach problems of this kind experimentally, it would appear necessary to demonstrate that the nuclei of comparable normal and tumor cells are genetically equivalent. This could perhaps be accomplished most convincingly by demonstrating that the tumorous state is a reversible process, thus showing that a persistent genetic change is not an essential prerequisite for the neoplastic state.

Before consideration of this matter, it should be noted that cellular differentiation, like the neoplastic transformation, represents a stable heritable change and that extreme cases of terminal differentiation are clearly irreversible. Even the histologically undifferentiated stem cells of various tissues are strongly determined for the cell type into which they will ultimately differentiate. Thus, although such cells may contain a complete complement of genes, they are programmed for particular patterns of metabolism and hence are not easily manipulated. Therefore, only in the more favorable situations would a reversal of the neoplastic state be expected to be demonstrable experimentally even though the potential for reversibility might be present in cells of many different tumors. It should also be recalled that many secondary changes such as chromosomal abnormalities, alterations in respiration, and deletion of enzymes may and commonly do occur in certain tumors. Thus even if those properties of a cell that lead to autonomous growth were potentially reversible the result would not necessarily be a normal cell, since the recovered cell might retain certain of the secondarily acquired properties originally possessed by the tumor cell. Even though such a reverted cell might be abnormal, it would nevertheless be nontumorous and thus fulfill the criterion for the reversion of a cell from the malignant to the nonmalignant state.

3.4.1. Lucké Adenocarcinoma of the Leopard Frog

That a normalization of the neoplastic state may, in fact, occur has now been well documented in a wide spectrum of organisms ranging from higher plant species to man. A number of selected examples that appear to illustrate particularly well the biological principles underlying this phenomenon have therefore been selected for discussion. The first example to be considered is the Lucké adenocarcinoma of the leopard frog. This is a particularly malignant tumor that is caused by a herpes-type virus (Naegele *et al.*, 1974) and is commonly found to develop in frogs in the New England states. The virus in this instance transforms rather specifically cells of the convoluted tubules of the kidney. In studying this disease an attempt was made to determine the developmental potentialities of a cancer nucleus (McKinnell *et al.*, 1969). In order to have a nuclear marker to distinguish the cancer nuclei from normal nuclei, adenocarcinomas were induced in a triploid line of frogs and the nuclei of the resulting cancer cells had a triploid complement of chromosomes. Triploid nuclei were then isolated from the cancer cells and injected into activated but enucleated normal frog eggs. Not only did the cancer nuclei participate in normal cleavage, but also a significant number of apparently normal, fully functional, triploid, swimming-stage larvae, or tadpoles, were produced. Such remarkable results are of considerable significance as far as the biology of cancer is concerned. It is clear, first of all, that the genetic information present in a cancer cell nucleus was effectively reprogrammed by those cytoplasmic factors and mechanisms present in the frog egg that regulate nuclear gene activity during the normal course of development. The tadpoles that developed from a cancer nucleus possessed all of the diverse differentiated cell types, tissues, and organs found in control tadpoles of the same age. There was, moreover, a complete absence of any evidence of malignancy in tadpoles derived from a cancer nucleus. This study provides excellent evidence then that the genetic information present in a cancer nucleus is not irreversibly programmed, as was believed for so many years, but can, in fact, be manipulated experimentally in such a way that it behaves as an essentially normal nucleus.

The demonstration described above was possible only because of the truly unique characteristics of the experimental test system employed, and it seems not unlikely that the generality of cancer nuclei would behave similarly if it were possible to subject them to the same type of experimental approach.

3.4.2. Influence of Inductively Active Embryonic Tissues and Regenerating Tissues on Tumor Development

A limited number of attempts have been made to study the effects of inductively active embryonic tissues (Crocker and Vernier, 1972; DeCosse *et al.*, 1973; Ellison *et al.*, 1969; Lustig *et al.*, 1968; Mathis and Seilern-Aspang, 1962; Seilern-Aspang *et al.*, 1963) and of regenerating tissues (Seilern-Aspang and Kratochwil, 1962, 1963) on changes in the growth and development of tumors of various types. One such study was carried out with the European newt, an animal well known for its pronounced regenerative capacities (Seilern-Aspang and Kratochwil, 1962,

1963). Carcinogenic hydrocarbons (a mixture of 2% dibenzanthracene and 0.2% benzpyrene in olive oil was most effective) were introduced subcutaneously, and following the injections tumors arose in multicentric fashion from the basal cells of the mucous glands of the skin. These coalesced to form expansively growing tumors that infiltrated and destroyed normal tissues and metastasized freely to all parts of the animals. That somewhat more than half of the animals which developed the expansively growing tumors died is evidence of the malignant quality of the new growths. In many other instances, a most remarkable thing happened. After the tumors had reached large size, had infiltrated and metastasized, the neoplastic process ended with a spontaneous regression of the tumors. The basis of the regressions was not death of the tumor cells but the maturation and differentiation of those cells into cells with nontumorous properties. Within the expansively growing tumor, the neoplastic elements differentiated into typical integumental epithelium, pigment cells, cornified layers, and mucous glands, while the infiltrating portions of such tumors developed into fibrous connective tissue. When maturation of the tumor cells was complete, the animals recovered from the disease. Recovery from the neoplastic state was most readily achieved by inducing a tumor at a site close to the base of the tail of the newts and then removing part of the tail to stimulate regenerative processes in the animals. Although the inductive factors or other mechnisms through which such morphogenetic transformations occur are not yet known, the results obtained in these studies appear to be strikingly similar to those reported for the neuroblastomas of humans, which will be discussed later.

3.4.3. The Teratocarcinoma of the Mouse

Although the examples of reversibility of the neoplastic state that have thus far been described were concerned with plants and with the lower vertebrates, there is now an abundance of evidence to suggest that this same sort of thing occurs in mammalian tumor systems as well. A well-documented example is the teratocarcinoma of the mouse. This is a malignant tumor thought to arise from primitive germ cells or from misplaced blastomeres. The teratocarcinoma typically contains derivatives of all three embryonic germ layers and presents a wide variety of cell types, including bone, muscle, nodules of cartilage, nerve tissue, glands, tooth buds, and hair follicles. These well-differentiated cells are scattered in completely disorganized array within the tumor. Interspersed among the differentiated cells are groups of essentially undifferentiated cells known as embryonal carcinoma cells, which represent the malignant component of the tumor. The pertinent question in studying the population dynamics of this complex tumor was whether the several well-differentiated cell types found in the tumor developed independently of one another or were all derived from a common precursor or stem cell, which would in this case be the embryonal carcinoma cell. In order to test the second possibility, Kleinsmith and Pierce (1964) injected single embryonal carcinoma cells into peritoneal cavities of mice. Of the somewhat more than 40 of the single cancer cells that established themselves and grew, all developed into malignant tumors that killed the mice in a few weeks' time. A histological examination of the resulting tumors showed, however, that they were commonly composed of the same eight to 14 different, well-differentiated cell types found in the original tumor together with embryonal carcinoma cells. It was demonstrated, moreover, that the differentiated derivatives that were present in the tumor had lost their tumorous properties. It seems perfectly clear from these studies, then, that the embryonal carcinoma cell is a multipotential cell that is highly malignant in the undifferentiated state but is capable of giving rise to a number of different and quite distinct differentiated derivatives that have lost their neoplastic properties. It should be noted, however, that the acquisition by tumor cells of the differentiated state does not necessarily terminate malignancy. It has been found, for example, that parietal yolk sac carcinomas and choriocarcinomas, which are both derived by differentiation from stem cells of teratocarcinomas, remain malignant.

3.4.4. The Epidermoid (Squamous) Carcinoma of Animals and Man

Another experimentally well-documented example of the reversal of the cancerous state in mammals is found in the common epidermoid (squamous) carcinoma. This tumor is derived from the basal cells of the skin of or the hair follicles. The basal cells are undifferentiated cells that are, however, strongly determined and thus specifically programmed for the cell type into which they are destined to differentiate. It is well known that when a normal basal cell divides it gives rise to one derivative that differentiates and becomes heavily keratinized while the other member of the dividing pair retains the potentialities of the basal cell from which it was derived. The epidermoid carcinoma consists structurally of an agglomeration of epidermal cell pegs that are embedded in a matrix of connective tissue. It is only the cancer cells found at the extreme rim of each peg that divide actively, while the entire core of such pegs is composed of heavily keratinized cells that may show pycnotic nuclei, do not divide, and thus appear to have become terminally differentiated. Pierce and Wallace (1971) studied the origin of the differentiated cells at the center of the peg and found that they were derived from the dividing cancer cells at the rim of the peg. When the dividing cancer cells were implanted into appropriate hosts, they commonly developed into typical epidermoid (squamous) carcinomas; however, when the differentiated keratinized cells were similarly implanted, tumors did not develop. The dividing cancer cells found at the rim of a peg thus behave like the normal basal cells in that when they divide they give rise to one derivative that differentiates and, in this instance, loses its neoplastic properties, while the other member of the dividing pair retains the potentialities of the cancer cell from which it is derived. It is clear, therefore, that these cancer cells, like those of the teratocarcinoma, retain a capacity for differentiation with the loss of neoplastic properties, and the problem of control would thus appear to resolve itself into learning how to bring about the controlled expression of these potentialities in all cells of the tumor.

The partial or even the occasional complete spontaneous self-healing of squamous cell carcinomas and prickle-cell epitheliomas in humans is not an uncommon observation in general pathology (Charteris, 1951; Dunn and Smith, 1934; Grzybowski, 1950; Smith, 1934; Sommerville and Milne, 1950; Witten and Zak, 1952). At least some of these instances appear to result from the differentiation of all of the cells of the new growth with a concomitant loss of malignancy.

3.4.5. The Neuroblastomas of Man

Evidence for the spontaneous regression of malignant tumors in humans is now considerable (Everson and Cole, 1966) and by no means are all such regressions due to immune responses, endocrine influences, unusual sensitivity to usually inadequate therapy, or interference with the nutrition of a tumor. In some instances, which are particularly well illustrated in the neuroblastomas, regressions may involve a maturation and differentiation of neuroblastoma cells into ganglion cells that have lost their malignant properties. The first well-documented example of that type recorded in the literature is the study of Cushing and Wolbach (1927), who presented a detailed case report covering many years in which all of the cells of an advanced metastasizing paravertebral sympathicoblastoma were converted spontaneously into ganglion cells, resulting in the development of benign ganglioneuromas which could be easily dealt with. More recently, a number of other similar and equally well-documented examples have been recorded (Dyke and Mulkey, 1967; Everson and Cole, 1966; Visfeldt, 1963). Patients in whom such regressions occurred lived for more than 20 years without recurrence of the malignant tumor. If the maturation and differentiation of neuroblastoma cells into ganglion cells can occur spontaneously, as clearly happens in these instances, there must be an underlying cause, and one approach to the problem of control of this disease would appear to depend on identifying the nature of that cause.

3.5. Naturally Occurring Substances That Influence the Cancer Phenotype

Attempts have been made to cause neuroblastoma cells to mature and differentiate into ganglion cells under defined conditions of cell culture. It has been found that all neuroblastoma cells explanted from humans and grown in culture tend to differentiate. When the tumor cells are first isolated they have no processes, but eventually neurites sprout from the cell bodies if the tumor cells attach to the substrate. More dramatic results were reported when relatively high levels of purified nerve growth factor were incorporated into the culture medium. The response of the neuroblastoma cells to this protein was observed between 10 and 20 days after it was applied to the medium and it resulted in a large increase in the number of processes found on the neuroblastoma cells and the differentiation of those cells into types resembling the perikarya of ganglion cells (Goldstein, 1972). An as yet uncharacterized substance(s) that is secreted into a culture medium by glial cells has also been found to induce a high degree of morphological differentiation of neuroblastoma cells cultured *in vitro* (Monard *et al.*, 1973). Here,

then, is a striking example of a highly malignant tumor whose cells have the potential to, and occasionally do, mature and differentiate into ganglion cells with the loss of neoplastic properties *in situ.*

There are other recorded examples in which neoplastic cells could be made to mature and differentiate with the use of specific naturally occurring substances. An interesting example of this is found in the case of acute myelogenous leukemia. It had been found that cells of various types including spleen cells and fibroblasts secrete an inducer which causes normal undifferentiated hematopoietic cells to mature and differentiate into macrophages and granulocytes (Fibach *et al.*, 1973). The purified inducer, known as the MGI protein (mol wt about 65,000), required an adenine-containing cofactor to effectively promote differentiation in the normal immature cells. When this same differentiation-inducing protein was applied to acute myeloid leukemic cells, they could be made to mature and differentiate into macrophages and granulocytes (Fibach *et al.*, 1972). Cellular differentiation in this instance did not require an exogenous source of the cofactor, as did the normal hematopoietic cells, because the leukemic cells themselves synthesized the cofactor. Of particular interest in these studies was the finding that differentiation could be induced in cloned lines of leukemic cells that no longer contained the normal diploid complement of chromosomes. The fact that the induction of differentiation could be accomplished *in vitro* in leukemic cells obtained from patients with acute myeloid leukemia led to the suggestion that the MGI protein might be of therapeutic value in that leukemia (Fibach *et al.*, 1972).

The chalones are a diverse group of naturally occurring tissue-specific substances synthesized by cells that appear to be importantly involved in the regulation of both cell division and cell differentiation (Bullough, 1965). Chalones have now been isolated from about ten different cell types. The liver chalone was found to be a polypeptide of low molecular weight (Verly *et al.*, 1971), while the epidermal chalone is a basic glycoprotein having a molecular weight of about 35,000 (Hondius Boldingh and Laurence, 1968). Since the antimitotic effect of these substances is tissue specific and since they are essentially nontoxic, they would appear to be almost ideal candidates for use in the suppression of growth with a restoration of differentiated function in tumors that have lost the ability to synthesize their own chalones but remain sensitive to their inhibitory effects (see Chapter 11).

Experimental evidence obtained from many different studies indicates that cellular properties including some of the most important ones that distinguish cancer cells from normal cells, such as a capacity of the former to invade and metastasize, may be expressed as surface properties. A factor has been isolated from cells transformed by Rous sarcoma virus that can cause normal cells in culture to mimic the appearance and growth habit of tumor cells (Rubin, 1970). Studies have suggested that two proteins—one a protease secreted by the transformed cells and the other, plasminogen, present in serum—interact to give rise to the biologically active substance (Ossowski *et al.*, 1973; Unkeless *et al.*, 1973).

As well as being a growth-promoting factor, this substance may contribute to or be responsible for the invasiveness of the tumor cells. A migration factor that could contribute importantly to malignancy has, moreover, been found to be released in culture by SV40-transformed BALB/c3T3 cells. This factor is as yet uncharacterized chemically (Bürk, 1973).

Recently it has been reported that a contact-inhibited melanocyte culture produces a protein-containing substance capable of restoring contact inhibition of growth to a highly malignant hamster melanocyte cell line (Lipkin and Knecht, 1974). Thus the capacities for invasion and migration as well as for contact inhibition of growth, in these instances at least, appear to be controlled by specific substances.

3.6. Non-Naturally Occurring Substances That Influence the Cancer Phenotype

In addition to such naturally occurring differentiation-inducing substances as the nerve growth factor, the glial cell factor, and the MGI protein, such rather unlikely non-naturally-occurring substances as dimethylsulfoxide and 5-bromodeoxyuridine can profoundly influence the cancer phenotype. It has been reported by Friend *et al.* (1971), for example, that cells of an erythroid leukemia of the mouse can be made to differentiate fully in culture and appear in every respect to be normal when they are treated with dimethylsulfoxide. Silagi and Bruce (1970) have reported, moreover, that highly malignant melanoma cells of the mouse can be made to show the normal phenotype when exposed to appropriate concentrations of 5-bromodeoxyuridine. The melanoma cells, instead of piling up in random fashion characteristic of tumor cells, grow as do normal cells in monolayer culture and they are largely contact inhibited. The treated cells do not synthesize melanin and when implanted into appropriate hosts are significantly less tumorigenic than are the untreated cells. Essentially two points of interest emerge from this and subsequent studies (Christman *et al.*, 1975). The first is that the tumorous state is completely and repeatedly reversible and whether the cells show the cancer phenotype or the normal phenotype is determined by whether or not 5-bromodeoxyuridine is present in the culture medium. The second point of interest is the finding that the decrease in melanoma cell tumorigenicity in the presence of 5-bromodeoxyuridine is correlated with a decrease in detectable cellular plasminogen activator. The results of this study support the suggestion made by others that synthesis by tumor cells of cellular plasminogen activator is associated with the malignant state and that the suppression of tumorigenicity by 5-bromodeoxyuridine in the melanoma system reflects the capacity of that base analogue to inhibit the expression of a specialized function closely correlated with malignancy.

If, as seems likely, 5-bromodeoxyuridine replaces specifically thymidine in the chromosomal DNA, and thus brings about a change in the DNA's integrity, then this system provides a beautiful model for studying the effects of specific changes in the DNA on the development of the tumorous state and on its reversal. The

capacity of 5-bromodeoxyuridine to reversibly inhibit both synthesis of the
plasminogen activator and tumorigenicity in the melanoma cells suggests that the
development of the tumorous state, in this instance as in certain others, reflects
the persistent activation of one or more previously unexpressed genes. 5-
Bromodeoxyuridine has also been found to influence differentiation in certain
specific ways in a number of different normal cell systems (Abbott and Holtzer,
1968; Bischoff and Holtzer, 1968, 1970; Coleman *et al.*, 1968, 1969; Lasher and
Cahn, 1969).

3.7. Evidence That Viral Genetic Information Can Be Manipulated

The results reported thus far suggest that at least some tumor cells are subject to
many of the same regulatory mechanisms that control the growth and development of their normal counterparts. It does not appear necessary to postulate
drastic changes of a mutational type involving the deletion or permanent
rearrangement of the genetic information to account for the cancer phenotype.
What about the addition of new genetic information accompanying cellular
transformation by the oncogenic viruses? The evidence now appears clear that in
the case of both the DNA- and the RNA-containing oncogenic viruses the viral
genetic information may either be integrated directly by covalent linkages into the
chromosomal DNA of the host cell (Sambrook *et al.*, 1968) or, in the case of the
RNA viruses, give rise to a DNA provirus which is similarly integrated (Varmus *et
al.*, 1973). Thus there is in both instances a persistent change in the integrity of the
genetic information present in a host cell. The pertinent question that arises,
therefore, is whether this new genetic information is coding specifically for one or
more substances required to establish and maintain the tumorous state or whether
it is acting in such a way as to persistently activate that part of the normal cell
genome that is concerned with the development of the cancer phenotype. The
study of Macpherson (1965) clearly demonstrates that the continued presence of
the viral genome in a derepressed form is required for the continued expression
of the neoplastic phenotype, at least in the Rous system. This study moreover
demonstrates that virus infection leading to transformation need not necessarily
cause any permanent changes of a mutational type involving, for example,
chromosome breaks that may be etiologically involved in transformation, as
suggested by Nichols *et al.* (1967), since following loss or persistent repression of
the viral genome the hamster cells revert again to the normal phenotype.

   That the expression of new viral genetic information integrated into the
genome of a cell can be readily manipulated experimentally is evidenced from
studies carried out with the temperature-sensitive mutants of the Rous sarcoma
virus (Stephenson *et al.*, 1973; Toyoshima and Vogt, 1969; Warren *et al.*, 1972;
Wickus and Robbins, 1973). In those studies it was found that cells transformed by
the mutant, when incubated at a temperature of 36°C (permissive temperature),
showed the neoplastic phenotype while when the same transformed cells were
incubated at 41°C (nonpermissive temperature) they appeared normal by all

criteria. Infectious virus is produced by the cells equally well at both temperatures. The temperature-sensitive process is completely and repeatedly reversible in both directions, indicating that the genetic information required for expression of the neoplastic state can be turned on or off at will in these systems. There is, moreover, now an abundance of evidence to show that clonal lines of mouse, hamster, and rat cells, which to not commonly produce the complete virus, can be made to do so and become transformed into tumor cells when treated with radiation or carcinogenic chemicals. It is perfectly clear in these instances that the viral genetic information is present in cryptic form in the untransformed cells but is not expressed. The oncogene theory of cancer postulates, moreover, that all adult vertebrates carry within their cells an unexpressed viral genome, and it has been suggested that the difference between individuals who develop cancer and those who do not resides in whether the viral oncogene present in the host cell genome is expressed or repressed (Huebner and Todaro, 1969; Todaro and Huebner, 1972). Since the viral oncogene is assumed to be present in cryptic form in all vertebrate cells and since it is transmitted as a characteristic Mendelian trait, it must be considered to be an intrinsic part of the normal cell genome. The heritable cellular mechanism underlying this postulated type of cellular change would therefore be epigenetic in nature.

In the case of the DNA-containing oncogenic viruses, we have reviewed a dramatic instance of the developmental potential of a cancer nucleus derived from the Lucké adenocarcinoma of the leopard frog. This disease, it will be recalled, is caused by a herpes-type virus and when a cancer nucleus was isolated and implanted into an activated but enucleated frog egg the genetic information present in the nucleus was reprogrammed in such a way as to permit normal development to proceed at least to the tadpole stage. These studies suggest then that the genetic information present in a cancer nucleus is not irreversibly fixed but can, in fact, be manipulated experimentally.

3.8. Chromosomal Imbalance and the Reversibility of the Tumorous State

3.8.1. DNA-Containing Oncogenic Viruses

It was found that cells transformed in culture by either one of the two very small DNA-containing viruses, SV40 or polyoma, may give rise to a high percentage of cells that revert to the normal phenotype (Pollack *et al.*, 1968; Rabinowitz and Sachs, 1968). This reversion was commonly accompanied by either somewhat greater or somewhat fewer than the normal diploid complement of chromosomes in the reverted cells (Bloch-Shtacher *et al.*, 1972). This finding led to the suggestion that the malignant transformation and its reversion are controlled by the balance between genes for expression of malignancy and those for its suppression. It was suggested further that conditions that stabilize the reverted state produce the right type of stable aneuploid cells required for reversion.

It might be profitable in this connection to digress to a brief description of a plant tumor system that appears to bear directly on this matter of chromosomal imbalance and tumor development. When two plant species such as *Nicotiana glauca* ($2n = 24$) and *N. langsdorffii* ($2n = 18$) are crossed and the seed of the F_1 hybrid ($2n = 21$) is sown, the resulting plants commonly grow normally until they reach maturity, at which time a profusion of tumors invariably arise spontaneously from all parts of the plants. These hybrid tumors have their counterparts in animal pathology (Gordon, 1958; Little, 1939). In studies dealing with plant tumors, fully differentiated leaf cells from both parent plant species were isolated, grown in culture, and mixed together to permit fusion of cells of the two parent species to occur (Carlson *et al.*, 1972). The resulting amphiploid ($2n = 42$) hybrids were isolated and grown separately in culture under conditions that permitted the development of shoots. These shoots were excised and grafted to appropriate stock plants, where they grew in an organized manner and some not only ultimately flowered and set fertile seed but also developed spontaneous tumors at the graft union. This experimental test system appears to be particularly illuminating because it clearly demonstrates that, despite serious chromosomal imbalance in all cells of the hybrid plant, the same abnormal karyotype can give rise to morphologically perfectly normal-appearing plants all of whose cells are beautifully differentiated and fully functional. That same abnormal karyotype can, on the other hand, give rise to neoplastic growths. These two metastable states are readily reversible in both directions. The results of this study demonstrate then that despite serious chromosomal imbalance the tumorous state in this instance is completely reversible. These findings would appear to provide strong support for the concept that the neoplastic state, like normal developmental processes, may stem from persistent changes in the expression of a genetically equivalent although, in this instance, abnormal karyotype.

4. Conclusions

It seems clear from the discussion presented herein that tumor cells of many different kinds found in a broad spectrum of organisms may retain the potentialities for differentiation with the loss of neoplastic properties. One approach to the problem of control would thus appear to resolve itself into learning how to bring about the controlled expression of those potentialities in all cells of a tumor. There is certainly no longer any good reason for believing that nuclear gene function in a cancer cell is beyond hope of correction, and we now appear to be at the very beginning of an understanding of the factors and mechanisms required to achieve that end. This is an area of cancer biology that has until quite recently been largely neglected. It is, nevertheless, one that will have to be explored in depth if we are really to understand the cancer problem.

5. References

ARMIN C. BRAUN

ABBOTT, J., AND HOLTZER, H., 1968, The loss of phenotypic traits by differentiated cells. V. The effect of 5-bromodeoxyuridine on cloned chondrocytes, *Proc. Natl. Acad. Sci. U.S.A.* **59**:1144.

ABELEV, G. I., PEROVA, S. D., KHRAMKOVA, N. I., POSTNIKOVA, Z. A., AND IRLIN, I. S., 1963, Embryonic serum alpha-globulin and its synthesis by transplantable mouse hepatomas, *Biokhimiya* **28**:625.

BINNS, A., AND MEINS, F., JR., 1973, Habituation of tobacco pith cells for factors promoting cell division is heritable and potentially reversible, *Proc. Natl. Acad. Sci. U.S.A.* **70**:2660.

BISCHOFF, R., AND HOLTZER, H., 1968, Inhibition of hyaluronic acid synthesis by BUdR in cultures of chick amnion cells, *Anat. Rec.* **160**:317 (abst.).

BISCHOFF, R., AND HOLTZER, H., 1970, Inhibition of myoblast fusion after one round of DNA synthesis in 5-bromodeoxyuridine, *J. Cell Biol.* **44**:134.

BLOCH-SHTACHER, N., RABINOWITZ, Z., AND SACHS, L., 1972, Chromosomal mechanism for the induction of reversion in transformed cells, *Int. J. Cancer* **9**:632.

BRAUN, A. C., 1969, *The Cancer Problem: A Critical Analysis and Modern Synthesis*, Chap. 5, Columbia University Press, New York.

BRAUN, A. C., 1970, On the origin of the cancer cell, *Am. Sci.* **58**:307.

BRAUN, A. C., 1974, *The Biology of Cancer*, 169 pp., Addison-Wesley, Reading, Mass.

BULLOUGH, W. S., 1965, Mitotic and functional homeostasis: A speculative review, *Cancer Res.* **25**:1683.

BÜRK, R. R., 1973, A factor from a transformed cell line that affects cell migration, *Proc. Natl. Acad. Sci. U.S.A.* **70**:369.

CARLSON, P. S., SMITH, H. H., AND DEARING, R. D., 1972, Parasexual interspecific plant hybridization, *Proc. Natl. Acad. Sci. U.S.A.* **69**:2292.

CHARTERIS, A. A., 1951, Self-healing epithelioma of the skin, *Am. J. Roentgenol.* **65**:459.

CHRISTMAN, J. K., SILAGI, S., NEWCOMB, E. W., SILVERSTEIN, S. C., AND ACS, G., 1975, Correlated suppression by 5-bromodeoxyuridine of tumorigenicity and plasminogen activator in mouse melanoma cells, *Proc. Natl. Acad. Sci. U.S.A.* **72**:47.

COLEMAN, A. W., KUNKEL, D., WERENER, I., and COLEMAN, J. R., 1968, Cellular differentiation *in vitro*: Perturbation by halogenated deoxyribonucleosides, *J. Cell Biol.* **39**:27a.

COLEMAN, J. R., COLEMAN, A. W., AND HARTLINE, E. J. H., 1969, A clonal study of the reversible inhibition of muscle differentiation by the halogenated thymidine analog 5-bromodeoxyuridine, *Dev. Biol.* **19**:527.

CROCKER, J. F., AND VERNIER, R. L., 1972, Congenital nephroma of infancy: Induction of renal structures by organ culture, *J. Pediat.* **80**:69.

CUSHING, H., AND WOLBACH, S. B., 1927, The transformation of a malignant paravertebral sym-pathicoblastoma into a benign ganglioneuroma, *Am. J. Pathol.* **3**:203.

DAVIDSON, E. H., 1968, *Gene Activity in Early Development*, 375 pp., Academic Press, New York.

DeCOSSE, J. J., GOSSENS, C. L., KUZMA, J. F., AND UNSWORTH, B. R., 1973, Breast cancer: Induction of differentiation by embryonic tissue, *Science* **181**:1057.

DUNN, J. S., and SMITH, J. F., 1934, Self-healing primary squamous carcinoma of the skin, *Br. J. Dermatol.* **46**:519.

DYKE, P. C., AND MULKEY, D. A., 1967, Maturation of ganglioneuroblastoma to ganglioneuroma, *Cancer* **20**:1343.

ELLISON, M. L., AMBROSE, E. J., AND EASTY, G. C., 1969, Differentiation in a transplantable rat tumour maintained in organ culture, *Exp. Cell Res.* **55**:198.

EVERSON, T. C., AND COLE, W. H., 1966, *Spontaneous Regression of Cancer*, 560 pp., Saunders, Philadelphia.

FAIMAN, C., COLWELL, J. A., RYAN, R. J., HERSHMAN, J. M., AND SHIELDS, T. W., 1967, Gonadotropin secretion from a bronchogenic carcinoma: Demonstration by radioimmunoassay, *New Engl. J. Med.* **277**:1395.

FIBACH, E., LANDAU, T., AND SACHS, L., 1972, Normal differentiation of myeloid leukaemic cells induced by a differentiation-inducing protein, *Nature New Biol.* **237**:276.

FIBACH, E., HAYASHI, M., AND SACHS, L., 1973, Control of normal differentiation of myeloid leukemic cells to macrophages and granulocytes, *Proc. Natl. Acad. Sci. U.S.A.* **70**:343.

FISCHER, B., 1906, Die experimentelle Erzeugung atypischer Epithelwucherungen und die Ent-stehung bösartiger Geschwulste, *Muench. Med. Wochenschr.* **53**:2041.

FRIEND, C., SCHER, W., HOLLAND, J. G., AND SATO, T., 1971, Hemoglobin synthesis in murine virus-induced leukemic cells *in vitro*: Stimulation of erythroid differentiation by dimethyl sulfoxide, *Proc. Natl. Acad. Sci. U.S.A.* **68**:378.

GELLHORN, A., 1969, Ectopic hormone production in cancer and its implication for basic research on abnormal growth, *Advan. Intern. Med.* **15**:299.

GOLD, P., AND FREEDMAN, S. O., 1965*a*, Demonstration of tumor-specific antigens in human colonic carcinomata by immunological tolerance and absorption techniques, *J. Exp. Med.* **121**:439.

GOLD, P., AND FREEDMAN, S. O., 1965*b*, Specific carcinoembryonic antigens of the human digestive system, *J. Exp. Med.* **122**:467.

GOLDSTEIN, M. N., 1972, Growth and differentiation of normal and malignant sympathetic neurons *in vitro*, in: *Cell Differentiation* (R. Harris, P. Allin, and D. Viza, eds.), pp. 131–137, Munksgaard, Copenhagen.

GORDON, M., 1958, A genetic concept for the origin of melanomas, *Ann. N.Y. Acad. Sci.* **71**:1213.

GRZYBOWSKI, M., 1950, A case of peculiar generalized epithelial tumours of the skin, *Br. J. Dermatol.* **62**:310.

HONDIUS BOLDINGH, W., AND LAURENCE, E. B., 1968, Extraction, purification and preliminary characterisation of the epidermal chalone: A tissue specific mitotic inhibitor obtained from vertebrate skin, *Eur. J. Biochem.* **5**:191.

HUEBNER, R.J., AND TODARO, G. J., 1969, Oncogenes of RNA tumor viruses as determinants of cancer, *Proc. Natl. Acad. Sci. U.S.A.* **64**:1087.

KLEINSMITH, L. J., AND PIERCE, G. B., JR., 1964, Multipotentiality of single embryonal carcinoma cells, *Cancer Res.* **24**:1544.

LASHER, R., AND CAHN, R. D., 1969, The effects of 5-bromodeoxyuridine on the differentiation of chondrocytes *in vitro*, *Dev. Biol.* **19**:415.

LIMASSET, P., AND GAUTHERET, R., 1950, Sur le caractère tumoral des tissus de tabac ayant subi le phénomène d'accoutumance aux hétéro-auxines, *C. R. Acad. Sci. Paris* **230**:2043.

LIPKIN, G., AND KNECHT, M. E., 1974, A diffusible factor restoring contact inhibition of growth to malignant melanocytes, *Proc. Natl. Acad. Sci. U.S.A.* **71**:849.

LIPSETT, M. B., ODELL, W. D., ROSENBERG, L. E., AND WALDMANN, T. A., 1964, Humoral syndromes associated with nonendocrine tumors, *Ann. Intern. Med.* **61**:733.

LITTLE, C. C., 1939, Hybridization and tumor formation in mice, *Proc. Natl. Acad. Sci. U.S.A.* **25**:452.

LUSTIG, E. S., LUSTIG, L., AND JAUREGUI, H., 1968, Action *in vitro* of the embryonic inducers on experimental and human tumours, in: *Cancer Cells in Culture* (H. Katsuta, ed.), pp. 135–142, University Park Press, Baltimore.

LUTZ, A., 1971, Morphogenetic aptitudes of tissue cultures of unicellular origin, *Colloq. Int. C.N.R.S.* **193**:163–168.

MACPHERSON, I., 1965, Reversion in hamster cells transformed by Rous sarcoma virus, *Science* **148**:1731.

MARKERT, C. L., 1968, Neoplasia: A disease of cell differentiation, *Cancer Res.* **28**:1908.

MARKERT, C. L., AND URSPRUNG, H., 1971, *Developmental Genetics*, 214 pp., Prentice-Hall, Englewood Cliffs, N.J.

MARKS, L. J., RUSSFIELD, A. B., AND ROSENBAUM, D. L., 1963, Corticotropin-secreting carcinoma, *J. Am. Med. Assoc.* **183(2)**:115.

MATHIS, G., AND SEILERN-ASPANG, F., 1962, Die Beeinflussung des Embryonalfeldes des Hühnchens durch Cancerogene, *Naturwissenschaften* **49**:110.

MCKINNELL, R. G., DEGGINS, B. A., AND LABAT, D. D., 1969, Transplantation of pluripotential nuclei from triploid frog tumors, *Science* **165**:394.

MONARD, D., SOLOMON, F., RENTSCH, M., AND GYSIN, R., 1973, Glia-induced morphological differentiation in neuroblastoma cells, *Proc. Natl. Acad. Sci. U.S.A.* **70**:1894.

NAEGELE, R. F., GRANOFF, A., AND DARLINGTON, R. W., 1974, The presence of the Lucké herpesvirus genome in induced tadpole tumors and its oncogenicity: Koch-Henle postulates fulfilled, *Proc. Natl. Acad. Sci. U.S.A.* **71**:830.

NICHOLS, W. W., LEVAN, A., AND HENEEN, W. K., 1967, Studies on the role of viruses in somatic mutation, *Hereditas* **57**:365.

OSSOWSKI, L., UNKELESS, J. C., TOBIA, A., QUIGLEY, J. P., RIFKIN, D. B., AND REICH, E., 1973, An enzymatic function associated with transformation of fibroblasts by oncogenic viruses. II. Mammalian fibroblast cultures transformed by DNA and RNA tumor viruses, *J. Exp. Med.* **137**:112.

PIERCE, G. B., 1970, Differentiation of normal and malignant cells, *Fed. Proc.* **29**:1248.

PIERCE, G. B., AND WALLACE, C., 1971, Differentiation of malignant to benign cells, *Cancer Res.* **31**:127.

POLLACK, R. E., GREEN, H., AND TODARO, G. J., 1968, Growth control in cultured cells: Selection of sublines with increased sensitivity to contact inhibition and decreased tumor-producing ability, *Proc. Natl. Acad. Sci. U.S.A.* **60**:126.

RABINOWITZ, Z., AND SACHS, L., 1968, Reversion of properties in cells transformed by polyoma virus, *Nature (London)* **220:**1203.

RUBIN, H., 1970, Overgrowth stimulating factor released from Rous sarcoma cells, *Science* **167:**1271.

SAMBROOK, J., WESTPHAL, H., SRINIVASAN, P. R., AND DULBECCO, R., 1968, The integrated state of viral DNA in SV40-transformed cells, *Proc. Natl. Acad. Sci. U.S.A.* **60:**1288.

SEILERN-ASPANG, F., AND KRATOCHWIL, K., 1962, Induction and differentiation of an epithelial tumour in the newt *(Triturus cristatus), J. Embryol. Exp. Morphol.* **10:**337.

SEILERN-ASPANG, F., AND KRATOCHWIL, K., 1963, Die experimentelle Aktivierung der Differenzierungspotenzen entarteter Zellen, *Wien. Klin. Wochenschr.* **75:**337.

SEILERN-ASPANG, F., HONUS, E., AND KRATOCHWIL, K., 1963, Cartilage induction in a fowl sarcoma *in vitro* by the addition of chorda from chick embryos, *Acta Biol. Med. Ger.* **10:**447.

SILAGI, S., AND BRUCE, S. A., 1970, Suppression of malignancy and differentiation in melanotic melanoma cells, *Proc. Natl. Acad. Sci. U.S.A.* **66:**72.

SMITH, J. F., 1934, A case of multiple primary squamous-celled carcinomata of the skin in a young man, with spontaneous healing, *Br. J. Dermatol.* **46:**267.

SOMMERVILLE, J., AND MILNE, J. A., 1950, Familial primary self-healing squamous epithelioma of the skin (Ferguson Smith type), *Br. J. Dermatol.* **62:**485.

STEPHENSON, J. R., REYNOLDS, R. K., AND AARONSON, S. A., 1973, Characterization of morphologic revertants of murine and avian sarcoma virus-transformed cells, *J. Virol.* **11:**218.

TODARO, G. J., AND HUEBNER, R. J., 1972, The viral oncogene hypothesis: New evidence, *Proc. Natl. Acad. Sci. U.S.A.* **69:**1009.

TOYOSHIMA, K., AND VOGT, P. K., 1969, Temperature sensitive mutants of an avian sarcoma virus, *Virology* **39:**930.

UNKELESS, J. C., TOBIA, A., OSSOWSKI, L., QUIGLEY, J. P., RIFKIN, D. B., AND REICH, E., 1973, An enzymatic function associated with transformation of fibroblasts by oncogenic viruses. I. Chick embryo fibroblast cultures transformed by avian RNA tumor viruses, *J. Exp. Med.* **137:**85.

VARMUS, H. E., VOGT, P. K., AND BISHOP, J. M., 1973, Integration of deoxyribonucleic acid specific for Rous sarcoma virus after infection of permissive and nonpermissive hosts, *Proc. Natl. Acad. Sci. U.S.A.* **70:**3067.

VERLY, W. G., DESCHAMPS, Y., PUSHPATHADAM, J., AND DESROSIERS, M., 1971, The hepatic chalone. I. Assay method for the hormone and purification of the rabbit liver chalone, *Can. J. Biochem.* **49:**1376.

VISFELDT, J., 1963, Transformation of sympathicoblastoma into ganglioneuroma: With a case report, *Acta Pathol. Microbiol. Scand.* **58:**414.

WARREN, L., CRITCHLEY, D., AND MACPHERSON, I., 1972, Surface glycoproteins and glycolipids of chicken embryo cells transformed by a temperature-sensitive mutant of Rous sarcoma virus, *Nature (London)* **235:**275.

WICKUS, G. G., AND ROBBINS, P. W., 1973, Plasma membrane proteins of normal and Rous sarcoma virus-transformed chick-embryo fibroblasts, *Nature New Biol.* **245:**65.

WITTEN, V. H., AND ZAK, F. G., 1952, Multiple, primary, self-healing prickle-cell epithelioma of the skin, *Cancer* **5:**539.

2

Fetal Characteristics of Cancer

José Uriel

1. Introduction

The resemblance between neoplastic and embryonic tissues has attracted the attention of biologists for more than a century because of its apparent physiopathological implications. This resemblance is highly significant since it stems from the convergence of a series of observations on the behavior and properties of cancerous and embryonic cells.

Embryos and neoplasms first appear as cellular populations which grow at a rapid rate and with a certain autonomy compared to the cellular dynamics and organization of the host. Both ontogenic and neoplastic development progress in a stepwise fashion, probably by alternating periods of cell differentiation and division. A characteristic property of malignant cells, but also of numerous embryonic cells, is their ability to migrate, which permits them to invade and colonize tissues or organs at considerable distances from their place of origin. At the optical and ultrastructural level, many neoplastic cells can be distinguished by the more or less significant loss of morphological characters common to their normal adult counterparts. This is equally characteristic of embryonic cells, especially at early stages of ontogenic development.

Analogies also exist in the metabolic patterns of the two cellular populations. About 30 years ago, Greenstein (1945) concluded from his studies on the enzymatic activities of tumoral and nontumoral tissues that "tumors tend to converge to common enzymatic patterns" and that in certain cases these patterns resemble those of fetal tissues. The question was brought up again more recently

José Uriel ● Institut de Recherches Scientifiques sur le Cancer, Villejuif, France.

by the observations of Schapira *et al.* (1963) concerning the presence of aldolase A (muscle-type aldolase) in a soluble extract of rat hepatomas. This isozyme, although absent from normal adult liver, is normally associated with aldolase B (liver-type aldolase) in fetal liver. A new impetus to the whole problem was given at the same time by the discovery of Abelev *et al.* (1963) of the reappearance of a fetospecific protein, α-fetoprotein, in the sera of adult mice bearing chemically induced hepatomas, thus opening a new field of research on fetal antigens associated with neoplasia.

Numerous cellular constituents normally present during embryonic or fetal development, but absent or not detectable in tissues and organs of mature individuals, are present in spontaneous or experimentally induced tumors. In this chapter, we shall first present the essential results obtained during the last 10 years from the search for cellular constituents of fetal origin in tumors and then try to incorporate this knowledge into the general problem of carcinogenesis and its relation to cellular differentiation and ontogenic development.

2. Immunological Findings

2.1. Fetal Antigens in Experimental Tumors

Cell or serum constituents, most of them of unknown biological activity, are generally designated as tumor-associated antigens when demonstrated in tumor-bearing animals by virtue of their immunological properties: they elicit cell- or humoral-mediated immune responses in the host and/or they are immunogenic in heterologous species. The tumor-associated fetal antigens belong to this group of substances. We shall consider as embryospecific or fetospecific any antigen expressed during intrauterine or early postnatal life but completely or almost completely repressed in the mature state. This less restrictive meaning of fetospecificity seems necessary in view of the recent evidence of residual synthesis of this type of antigen in adults (see also Section 2.3).

Some of the known tumor-associated fetal antigens have been isolated and their physicochemical properties are well defined. They can be detected and quantified by serological methods using specific heterologous antisera. Gel immunodiffusion techniques (e.g., immunoelectrophoresis, counterelectrophoresis, Ouchterlony tests, electroimmunodiffusion) are most frequently employed; more sensitive techniques such as radioimmunoassays are being increasingly utilized for antigens that exist at very low concentrations (e.g., in the ng/ml range). Other fetal antigens must be defined in rather operational terms, i.e., by the evaluation with appropriate techniques of the humoral- and cell-mediated immune reactions that they evoke in the host or in appropriate target cells (e.g., tumor rejection, cell growth inhibition, and cytotoxicity).

2.1.1. In Chemically Induced Tumors

a. α-Fetoprotein. The first α-globulin to appear in mammalian sera during ontogenic development is α-fetoprotein (αFP); it is the dominant serum protein in

early intrauterine life. The principal sites of synthesis are the liver and, to a much
lesser extent, the yolk sac and the gastrointestinal tract. αFPs from several species,
including man, have been isolated and their similar physicochemical properties
and antigenic cross-reactivity are now well established, Homologous proteins to
mammalian αFP have been demonstrated in birds and fish, which indicates that
this protein is widely distributed in the animal kingdom (see Gitlin, 1974).
Although the exact biological activity of αFP is unknown, the recent discovery of
its estrogen-binding properties in rat, mouse, and man under certain conditions
(Nunez *et al.*, 1971; Uriel *et al.*, 1972) throws some light on the possible function of
αFP in the prenatal state. Several reviews summarize the bulk of work published
on the biochemistry and physiopathology of rat, mouse, and human αFP (Abelev,
1971; Masseyeff, 1972; Uriel, 1969; Uriel and de Néchaud, 1973; Hirai *et al.*,
1973; Wepsic and Sell, 1974).

Since the work of Abelev and his coworkers on the reappearance of αFP in the
blood of adult mice bearing transplanted hepatomas, most effort has been
devoted to determining the significance of the association between αFP and
primary liver cancer. The key questions that must be answered are whether the
reappearance of αFP could be due to the derepression in malignant parenchymal
cells of a gene silent in the adult stage and whether that derepression is specifically
linked to malignant transformation.

Studies on the kinetics of αFP secretion during hepatocarcinogenesis in rats by
Watabe (1971), Kroes *et al.* (1972, 1973), Kitagawa *et al.* (1972), and de Néchaud
and Uriel (1973) established the following points:

1. When rats are fed a basal diet supplemented with an appropriate chemical
   (e.g., azo dye or nitrosamine derivative, or aflatoxin B), a characteristic
   kinetic pattern of serum αFP is observed. It begins with the transient
   appearance of αFP in a high proportion of animals, as early as 2–5 wk after
   feeding the carcinogenic diet, and in the absence of any histological sign of
   neoplastic transformation. However, Becker and Sell (1974), utilizing a
   sensitive radioimmunoassay, have demonstrated an even earlier increase in
   αFP in rats receiving *N*-2-fluorenylacetamide.
2. As a rule, the precociousness and the frequency of αFP appearance increase
   with the dose of hepatocarcinogen and diminish with the age of the rats,
   young animals being more susceptible than older ones.
3. In addition to some individual and strain pecularities, the response is
   influenced by the type of hepatocarcinogen used and its mode of administration.
4. Several waves of αFP secretion can follow the initial one, and even if the
   carcinogen is discontinued serum αFP persists and increases in concentration in many animals.
5. Animals whose serum αFP appears early and persists later have a high
   probability of developing or already having hepatocellular carcinoma.
   Nevertheless, αFP may be undetectable (up to 30% frequency in certain
   experimental series) in the serum of animals with developed hepatomas.

6. Administration of the basal diet either alone or supplemented with a noncarcinogenic analogue (e.g., 4'-methyl-4-dimethylaminoazobenzene) can result in αFP appearance, although after a longer delay and lower frequency than in experiments with hepatocarcinogens.

7. Histological observations during chemical induction of hepatomas have resulted in some correlation between the early phase of αFP appearance and the presence of hyperplastic nodules of a special type of liver cell designated as "oval cells" by Farber (1956) and "transitional cells" by Inaoka (1967).

In these studies, αFP was evaluated by immunoprecipitation techniques with sensitivity limit between 400 and 1000 ng/ml. The kinetics of αFP secretion appears different when more sensitive techniques are used but without critically changing the profile outlined here.

Studies using transplantable rat hepatomas as experimental models have supplied additional information on αFP production and liver cancer. Working with a series of Morris hepatomas and a sensitive radioimmunoassay for αFP quantitation, Sell and Morris (1974) found some correlation between elevated αFP production and various factors such as growth rate, degree of differentiation, and chromosomal composition. Serum αFP concentrations were high in rats grafted with fast-growing, poorly differentiated tumors, while slow-growing, well-differentiated hepatomas gave moderate or normal levels. Significant exceptions to this rule were nevertheless noticed. The same was the case for the inverse relationship, first reported by Becker et al. (1973), between karyotype and αFP production: aneuploid, but not diploid or near-diploid tumors were more frequently found to secrete elevated quantities of αFP. The serum αFP levels in rats bearing different transplanted hepatomas varied across an extremely large range (Sell and Morris, 1974), with some animals showing as much as 18×10^6 ng/ml, while others (six out of 39) had normal values (less than 60 ng/ml). On the other hand, Tsukada et al. (1974) found that 26 out of 78 (33%) cell lines derived from rat ascites hepatomas did not produce αFP when established by intraperitoneal transplantation, suggesting the existence of mixed cell populations, αFP(+) and αFP(−), in the original tumor nodules. The suggestion was confirmed by clonal experiments in vitro.

Research was conducted to explore the association of elevated levels of αFP with pathological situations other than hepatomas. These studies show that liver cell injuries provoked in mice or rats by either partial hepatectomy (Perova et al., 1971; Sell et al., 1974; Uriel et al., 1975) or acute liver poisoning with hepatotoxics (Bakirov, 1968; de Néchaud and Uriel, 1971, 1972; Pihko and Ruoslahti, 1973) are followed by a transient production of αFP which starts 24–48 h after the initial intervention and returns to normal values about 6–8 days later. The frequency and the intensity of the response are age dependent, young animals being more sensitive than older ones to both hepatectomy and acute liver injury.

The above results lead to the conclusion that the derepression or, more exactly, the enhanced activity of the gene coding for αFP is not specific for malignant

transformation in rats since significant levels of serum αFP occur during liver
regeneration in the absence of neoplastic features. Nevertheless, the high
frequency of the association of hepatoma with persistently elevated serum αFP
concentrations remains an outstanding fact.

Whether tumoral hepatocytes are αFP producers is still unknown since the exact type of liver cell which synthesizes αFP has not been determined. The existence of primary and transplantable rat hepatomas growing with normal levels of host serum αFP demonstrates that malignancy does not necessarily imply enhanced αFP synthesis and/or serum release. The possibility that liver cells of a transitional type, probably immature precursors of hepatocytes and cholangiocytes, could be the site of αFP synthesis has been advanced by Watabe (1971) and Iwasaki et al. (1972) on the basis of the dynamics of liver cell populations during carcinogenesis, and by Uriel et al. (1973) from the estrogen-binding properties of both αFP and transitional liver cells (Fig. 1). If this hypothesis is confirmed, the serum αFP increase would be initially linked to the hyperplastic growth associated with liver regeneration and repair.

b. Rat α_M-Fetoprotein. Another fetospecific constituent of rat serum, already detectable in 12- to 13-day rat embryos (Stanislawski-Birencwajg, 1965, 1967), is α_M-fetoprotein (α_MFP). The serum concentration is maximal between days 17 and 20 of gestation, decreases slowly during the first week of extrauterine life, and becomes undetectable by immunodiffusion techniques (<400 ng/ml) about 1 month later and in normal adult animals (Perova and Abelev, 1967; de Néchaud and Uriel, 1972). Rat α_MFP had been assigned different names by different authors: α_2-acute phase globulin (Weimer and Benjamin, 1965), α_2-glycoprotein (Stanislawski-Birencwajg, 1965), and α_2-macroglobulin (Boffa et al., 1964). But once the immunological identity of these proteins was established (Uriel et al., 1969) the term "α_M-fetoprotein" was recommended[1].

The hepatic origin of α_MFP was first demonstrated by immunological methods in isolated livers from rats bearing Walker 256 carcinosarcoma (Sarcione, 1967). In contrast to rat α-fetoprotein (αFP), the synthesis of α_MFP can be easily induced or enhanced by different types of experimental manipulations. Weimer and Benjamin (1965) demonstrated the reappearance of α_MFP in the serum of adult rats during the acute phase of the inflammatory states following injection of turpentine. Release of α_MFP into the serum was also provoked in young and adult animals by either short-term hepatic injuries (single injections of $CdSO_4$, dimethylnitrosamine, partial hepatectomy) or chronic hepatic lesions of neoplastic or nonneoplastic character following long-term oral ingestion of hepatocarcinogens (Stanislawski-Birencwajg et al., 1967). By use of immunoautoradiographic methods, the specific incorporation of [^{14}C]leucine into α_MFP and its inhibition by cycloheximide have been observed in young and adult animals subjected to acute liver injury, which is evidence for the de novo synthesis of this

---

[1] The terminology used in this chapter to designate fetospecific serum protein is that proposed in the course of the Meeting of Investigators for Evaluation of a Serological Test for Liver Cancer, Lyon, France, 1969, and published in the Bulletin of the World Health Organization 43:309–310, 1970.

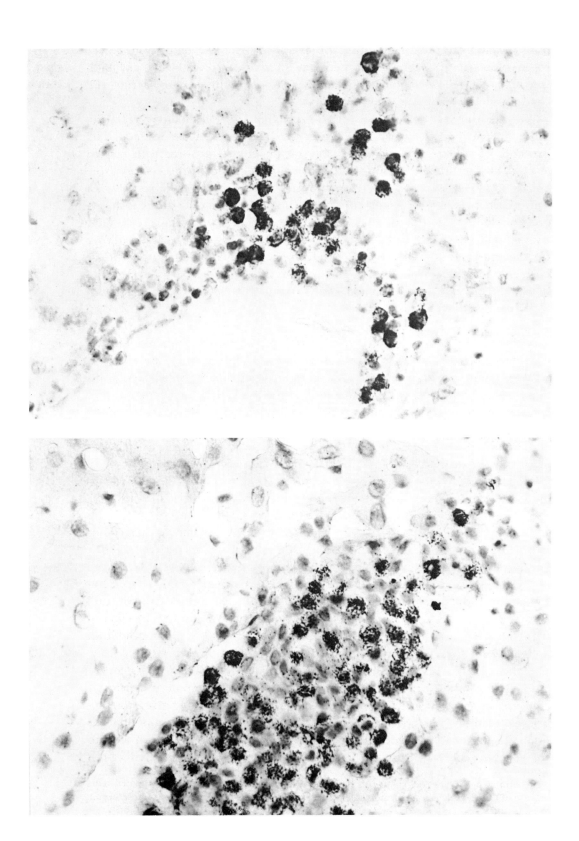

protein associated with reparative liver regeneration (de Néchaud and Uriel, 1972). Although α_MFP exists at high levels in animals bearing hepatomas, it is clearly not a tumor-specific antigen.

c. *Cell-Surface-Associated Fetal Antigens.* Previous evidence that chemically induced tumors express membrane-associated antigens of embryonic origin was provided by Brawn (1970), who, working with murine sarcomas induced by 3-methylcholanthrene (MC), showed that colony formation of tumor cells was significantly inhibited after exposure to lymph node cells from multiparous mice. The finding was confirmed and extended to DBA-induced hepatomas[2] and CM-induced sarcomas in rats by Baldwin *et al.* (1971, 1972). Microtoxicity tests with cultured tumor cells show the sensitization of multiparous rats against embryonic antigens on both hepatoma and sarcoma cells. Also, membrane immunofluorescence techniques demonstrate that tumor cells from a large variety of chemically induced hepatomas and sarcomas and cells from developing embryos are stained by individual sera from multiparous rats. The reaction can be inhibited by adsorption of the sera with target cells derived from a single tumor, which is conclusive proof that these membrane-associated fetal antigens are common to tumor types of different origin. Such cross-reactivity and the small role which they appear to play in tumor rejection reactions (Baldwin *et al.*, 1974) clearly distinguish them from other tumor-associated antigens on chemically induced neoplasms, called "tumor rejection antigens," which have been extensively studied in the past two decades and reviewed by Baldwin (1973).

2.1.2. In Viral Tumorogenesis

a. *In DNA-Virus-Induced Tumors.* Tumors induced by certain DNA-viruses contain transplantation antigens that elicit both humoral- and cell-mediated immune responses in the host. There is now good evidence that some of the antigens shared by these tumors are fetal antigens common to cells of widely different origin. Studies on SV40-induced tumors have demonstrated that hamster and mouse fetal cells contain antigen(s) that cross-reacts with hamster cells transformed by SV40. This finding is supported by the induction in adult hamsters immunized with X-irradiated hamster fetal cells of cytostatic antibodies that inhibit tumor cell growth and of cell-mediated immune responses that protect against tumor transplants (Coggin *et al.*, 1970). In addition, Duff and Rapp (1970) observed that normal pregnant hamsters develop antibodies against SV40 hamster tumor cell S antigen.

Adenovirus-31 tumorigenesis was also inhibited in neonatally infected hamsters by a single injection of fetal hamster cells 3 wk after birth and before the

---

[2] Hepatomas induced by dimethylbenzanthracene.

FIGURE 1. Cell affinity labeling with [^{3}H]estrone of an 18-day rat fetal liver (top) and of the liver of an adult rat bearing a mixed hepatoma-cholangiocarcinoma induced by 3'-Me-DAB (bottom). In both cases, radiolabeled cells of similar morphology accumulate at the border of a blood vessel. Magnification ×400 (reduced 28% for reproduction). See also Uriel *et al.* (1973).

appearance of the tumor (Coggin *et al.*, 1971). It is noteworthy that (1) the antigens seem to be expressed mostly during a short, transient period of the overall process of ontogenic development, (9- to 12-day fetuses) and (2) the immunological response is displayed only after previous irradiation of the fetal cells.

Further confirmation of the main features revealed by these studies was provided by several authors. Thus antisera obtained from guinea pigs immunized with unfertilized C37BL/6 mouse eggs were cytotoxic for SV40-transformed cells (Baranska *et al.*, 1970). Moreover, hamster antisera to purified SV40 preparations reacted, as shown by cell membrane immunofluorescence, with SV40-transformed cells and also with several tumor cell lines induced spontaneously (BHK-21) or arising from cells transformed by heterologous oncogenic DNA and RNA viruses. Cells from hamster embryos at early gestation periods were also labeled by the same antisera (Berman, 1972). Finally, the results reported by Pearson and Freeman (1968) suggest a relationship between embryonic antigen(s) and transplantation antigens induced in hamster fibroblasts by polyoma virus. Spleen cells from hamsters immunized with X-irradiated hamster embryonic fibroblasts were cytotoxic to polyoma-virus-transformed fibroblasts and provided some protection against growth. However, no protection was obtained after direct immunization of adult hamsters with normal embryonic fibroblasts, which supports the statement that fetal cell irradiation is a requirement for efficient immunization.

b. In Murine and Avian RNA-Virus-Induced Leukemias. Fetal antigens in RNA-virus-induced tumors have received less attention than those in DNA-virus-induced neoplasms. Using a rabbit antiserum to mouse embryo extracts adsorbed with adult organ homogenates, Stonehill and Bendich (1970) showed that tumors induced by RNA viral agents (i.e., Bittner, Gross, Rauscher, and Friend) contained antigens that cross-reacted in immunodiffusion tests with soluble antigens extracted from the mouse embryos. More conclusive evidence was provided by Hanna *et al.* (1971), who observed that immunization of BALB/c mice with mouse irradiated fetal cells suppressed growth in Millipore diffusion chambers of mouse spleen cells infected with Rauscher leukemia virus (RLV). The immunization had also a repressive effect on the development of RLV-induced splenomegaly. Teplitz *et al.* (1974) demonstrated a membrane-associated antigen on the red blood cells (RBCs) of chickens with leukemia induced by avian myeloblastosis virus. The same antigen is present in RBCs at the time of hatching but disappears after development. As expected, the antigen can be localized in tissues involved in RBC renewal, particularly in bone marrow of normal adult animals.

2.1.3. In Experimental Teratocarcinomas

Mouse transplantable teratocarcinomas, arising from abnormally proliferating germ cells in male embryos, can express other fetal antigens of the membrane-associated type in addition to αFP which are present at the very early stages of embryonic development.

Working with antisera obtained from young rabbits immunized with packed 29
embryoid bodies from an ascites subline of strain 129 teratocarcinoma, Edidin *et* FETAL
al. (1971) demonstrated the cross-reactivity of these antisera with tumoral cells CHARACTERISTICS
and endodermal cells from early normal embryos up to 6 days of age. Antitumor OF CANCER
antisera also reacted with unfertilized mouse eggs. It was interesting to note that
the antigen(s) were present in embryos lacking the major histocompatibility
antigen system of the adult, but disappeared when *H-2* antigens and other surface
antigens pertinent to differentiated cells were expressed. Edidin *et al.* used
immunoadsorption procedures that did not assure complete removal of undesira-
ble nonspecific antibodies. Nevertheless, their findings were, for the most part,
confirmed and extended by Artzt *et al.* (1973), who provided better sustained
proofs employing syngeneic instead of xenogeneic antisera produced in mouse
strain 129 males by hyperimmunization with irradiated cells from a cultured cell
line of teratocarcinoma. The specific antiserum reacted with primitive
teratocarcinoma cells and with cleavage-stage embryos but not with unfertilized
eggs. Proof of the specificity of the antiserum was the finding that it did not
react either with differentiated cells derived from the primitive tumor cell
line or with cells or tissues of adult mice, except male germinal cells. Also highly
significant was the short transient period when the antigen(s) was detectable
since it seemed to be restricted to the morula stage. The conclusive demonstration in the adult of the immunogenic properties of antigens which pertain
to the very early stages of embryonic development is the most relevant part of
these studies.

2.2. Fetal Antigens in Human Neoplasms

Soon after Abelev and his coworkers discovered that αFP reappeared in the sera
of mice bearing hepatomas, Tatarinov (1964) extended the same observation to
primary liver cancer in man. Later, Gold and Freeman (1965) described a
perchlorosoluble glycoprotein which they designated "carcinoembryonic
antigen" (CEA) because of its presence in adenocarcinomas of the human
digestive tract and in homologous fetal tissues.

Preliminary reports on elevated serum levels of αFP and CEA in clinical tumor
pathology suggested the specific character of their association with malignancies
and raised the possibility of developing large-scale serological tests for diagnostic
purposes. The importance of this eventuality greatly stimulated further studies
on these substances and the search in humans for other fetal antigens with
analogous properties.

2.2.1. Carcinoembryonic Antigen

CEA is a human glycoprotein made of a single polypeptide chain with an
approximate molecular weight of 200,000; it is soluble in perchloric acid and
strong salt solutions. It possesses the electrophoretic mobility of a serum β-
globulin and some degree of molecular microheterogeneity, as demonstrated, for

instance, by isoelectric focusing. CEA is preferentially found associated with cell membranes in fetal and tumoral tissues of the digestive tract, from where it is released by an unknown mechanism into the serum and other body fluids (urine, feces, saliva, meconium, etc.). It belongs to a family of immunologically cross-reactive antigens widely distributed in normal and neoplastic tissues of both fetuses and adults. Reviews with complete bibliographic lists of studies on CEA have been published by several authors (Laurence and Neville, 1972; Kupchik *et al.*, 1973; Neville and Laurence, 1974).

Although rigorous standardization of CEA, preparation of homologous antisera, and methods of quantitative evaluation have not yet been achieved, cumulative information has led to some general agreements. A comparative study of CEA levels in tissue extracts by Khoo *et al.* (1973) has clearly established the following: (1) CEA content in normal organs is very low or undetectable, except in the pancreas and gastrointestinal tract, where the amounts found range from 65 to 200 ng per gram of wet tissue in fetuses and from 28 to 86 ng/g in adults. (2) Much higher average amounts are found in a variety of malignant tumors, including carcinomas, sarcomas and their metastases, and Hodgkin's disease, with the highest contents in rectocolonic neoplasms (up to almost 3000 ng/g) and lung carcinomas (up to 500 ng/g). (3) Moderate or slightly raised levels are observed in several pathological, albeit nonmalignant tissues, which confirms previous work (Martin and Martin, 1970; Kupchik and Zamchek, 1972; Burtin *et al.*, 1972).

Normal plasma concentrations of CEA are even lower than in tissues (2.5–10 ng/ml, according to different standards and assays). Raised levels of serum CEA have been reported in a high proportion of patients with cancer of the gastrointestinal, pulmonary, and genitourinary systems, but also in cases of benign tumors and nonmalignant diseases (colitis, diverticulitis, alcoholic pancreatitis, and liver cirrhosis). However, persistently elevated or increasing values of serum CEA are not usually associated with benign tumors.

From these observations, it appears that CEA would not be considered as a tumor-specific antigen. Moreover, search for its presence in sera would seem inadequate for cancer screening and only of limited value for the differential diagnosis between neoplastic and nonneoplastic diseases. On the other hand, serial determinations of serum CEA are useful in clinical prognostic assessment, or to detect residual and recurrent tumors and to monitor therapeutic interventions (Fig. 2).

A point of physiopathological interest is the existence of a family of per-chlorosoluble glycoproteins related to CEA by their antigenic properties and similar serum and tissue distribution. These CEA-like substances, first characterized by Mach and Pusztaszeri (1972) and von Kleist *et al.* (1972), were described under a variety of names by different authors. Some of these substances are identical to each other in immunodiffusion tests and all of them cross-react with CEA antibodies but possess a molecular weight about one-fourth that of CEA. By immunofluorescence labeling, CEA and CEA-like substances were localized at the apical pole of epithelial cells lining the lumen of cancerous and noncancerous glands (von Kleist and Burtin, 1969; Burtin *et al.*, 1973).

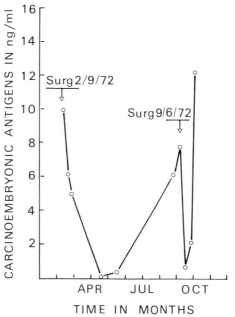

FIGURE 2. Carcinoembryonic antigen (CEA) vs. clinical course following surgery. Reproduced with permission from Min Chu (1973).

A current interpretation of these findings is not feasible since little is known about the structure and antigenic profile of CEA and related substances, their synthetic and catabolic routes, and also the mechanisms of their release from cell membranes. They may be a group of macromolecules whose polypeptide and/or carbohydrate moieties differ slightly in structure and composition but which share a common core of antigenic determinants (Khoo *et al.*, 1973).

2.2.2. α-Fetoprotein

As reported in Section 2.1.1, human αFP possesses physicochemical properties very close to those of rat and mouse αFP: similar molecular weight, electrophoretic mobility, and molecular microheterogeneity. Fetal liver, which is the principal source of αFP, secretes the protein into the blood, from where it probably equilibrates between the intra- and extravascular compartments of both fetus and mother. The serum concentration drops rapidly at birth, and after 1 month αFP is no longer detectable by immunodiffusion techniques.

The first two reports describing the statistically significant high incidence of αFP in the sera of patients bearing primary liver cancer raised the possibility that elevated levels of serum αFP could be clinically useful as pathognomic of hepatoma (Abelev *et al.*, 1967; Uriel *et al.*, 1967). Until 1971, when Ruoslahti and Seppala introduced a radioimmunoassay for the quantitation of αFP in the nanogram range, most studies on serum αFP levels were conducted with immunodiffusion techniques. In spite of their lesser sensitivity (see Table 1), they did permit the following major observations, discussed in detail by Abelev (1971, 1974), Uriel and de Néchaud (1972), Masseyeff (1972, 1974), Hirai *et al.* (1973),

TABLE 1
Human Serum αFP in Liver Diseases[a]

Diagnosis	Double diffusion (500–1000 ng/ml)[b]		Double antibody autoradiography (50–100 ng/ml)[b]		Radioimmunoassay (<5 ng/ml)[b]	
	αFP (+)/ number of cases	% αFP (+)	αFP (+)/ number of cases	% αFP (+)	αFP (+)/ number of cases	% αFP (+)
Hepatoma	35/53	64	44/53	83	19/24	79[c]
Secondary liver cancer	2/334	0.6	3/21	14	7/79	10[c]
Hepatitis	2/176	1.1	23/176	13	5/25	20[c]
Cirrhosis	0/172	0	0/[d]	0	9/61	15[c]
Miscellaneous (nonneoplastic)	15/5984	0.25	1/08	1	8/100	8[c]

[a] Compiled from data of Abelev (1971), Ruoslahti *et al.* (1974), and Uriel and de Néchaud (1972).
[b] Claimed minimum range of sensitivity.
[c] αFP (+): sera containing more than 25 ng/ml.
[d] Total number of cases unknown.

and Wepsic and Sell (1974):

1. Positive levels of serum αFP are found with high frequency (mean rate 50–60%) in primary hepatomas and embryonal carcinomas of ovarian or testicular origin, but also, though at a much lesser rate, in cases of secondary liver cancer and of nonneoplastic liver diseases such as viral hepatitis (Abelev, 1971), congenital tyrosinemia (Buffe and Rimbaut, 1973), Indian juvenile cirrhosis (Nayak *et al.*, 1972), and acute liver atrophy (Opolon *et al.*, 1973).
2. The proportion of cases with positive αFP levels in both hepatomas and embryonal carcinomas decreases inversely with the age of the patients.
3. Rates of positive αFP levels in primary hepatomas appear related to geographical and ethnic factors (50–60% rates for white and 80% for nonwhite patients), even though such differences may be due to variations in the mean age of the patients (Mawas *et al.*, 1970).
4. Tumor therapy and recurrent evolution are reflected by detectable changes in αFP serum concentrations.

The more recent use of radioimmunoassay or other sensitive techniques for αFP detection and quantitation had confirmed most of the findings listed above, particularly the existence of hepatomas that developed with persistent normal values of serum αFP. In addition, the αFP in sera of healthy adults (<5–20 ng/ml) could be demonstrated with these techniques, which also led to a better knowledge of the distribution of αFP levels among neoplastic and nonneoplastic liver diseases. As shown in Table 1, the number of hepatoma-bearing patients recorded increases with the sensitivity of the technique employed for αFP detection, but, at the same time, the tumor specificity of the test decreases because pathological levels of αFP are then revealed in a greater proportion of nonneoplastic diseases.

Moreover, the presence of abnormal αFP levels has also been observed in
association with other pathological disorders that had escaped previous αFP
search by less sensitive methods. These include, among others, alcoholic cirrhosis
(Abelev, 1971; Hirai *et al.*, 1972) and ataxia-telangiectasia (Waldmann and
McIntire, 1972).

At present, one may conclude that αFP, like the carcinoembryonic antigen
(CEA), does not seem to be pathognomic of neoplasia, although persistently high
or increasing levels of serum αFP are strongly indicative of primary liver cancer if
embryonal carcinoma can be excluded. Alternatively, periodic determinations of
αFP are of clinical interest in monitoring therapeutic effects on tumor evolution
(Fig. 3) or of prognostic value in the surveillance of diseases where the appearance
of elevated values of serum αFP would be transient (hepatitis, acute liver atrophy)
or where increases in αFP levels reflect the incidence of malignant transformation
(cirrhosis).

The cumulative information on the relationship between αFP and hepatocarcinogenesis led to the opinion that the enhanced synthesis and secretion of αFP
associated with liver pathology may be dependent on two distinct but not mutually
exclusive factors. One is the reparative hyperplasia which follows liver injury of
varied etiology (e.g., hepatectomy, chemical poisoning, or viral infection) and the
other is malignant transformation itself. Liver regeneration usually accompanies
tumor development but it seems unlikely that it alone is responsible for the high
and persistent αFP serum levels characteristic of hepatomas. Since elevated serum
αFP is also found in embryonal carcinomas, it seems more plausible that the
enhanced synthesis of αFP may be preferentially due to the development of a
population of immature liver cells. Obviously, the crucial point is to know whether
such a population is the neoplastic population itself or whether it is composed of
normal hepatocyte precursors—oval or transitional cells—indistinguishable from
those associated with reparative liver processes. Unfortunately, as pointed out in
Section 2.1.1, the exact type of cell which synthesizes αFP has not been clearly
determined.

2.2.3. α₂H-Ferroprotein

α₂H-Ferroprotein (α₂H) is a glycoferroprotein isolated from fetal liver and
hepatomas, where it is present in high amounts (Buffe *et al.*, 1972). Fetal serum
levels of α₂H range between 200 and 500 ng/ml, according to the period of
gestation, whereas values around 100 ng/ml are found in infant and adult sera. By
contrast, elevated concentrations (>200 to >5000 ng/ml) were demonstrated in a
high proportion of sera (about 80%) from subjects (adult and infants) suffering
from neoplastic diseases (Buffe *et al.*, 1968, 1970, 1972; Wada *et al.*, 1970; Martin *et
al.*, 1972). Like other tumor-associated fetal antigens, α₂H is not specific to the
neoplastic state since elevated levels can be demonstrated in almost 20% of
patients with nonneoplastic diseases of varied origin.

Although immunodiffusion methods reveal no differences between α₂H and
adult liver ferritin, both proteins differ in several physicochemical and chemical

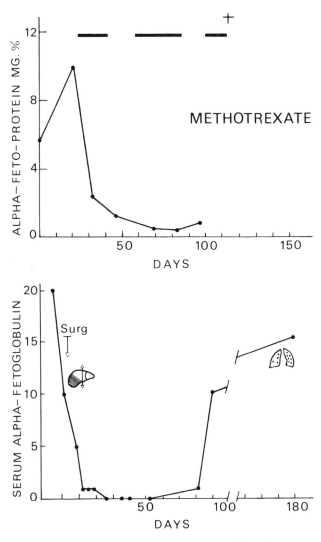

FIGURE 3. Top: αFP levels during treatment with methotrexate infused into the hepatic artery. Despite the fall of αFP, no useful clinical response was observed. Reproduced with permission from Purves *et al.* (1970). Bottom: Effect of hepatic lobectomy on αFP levels and clinical course in a case of primary liver cancer. Reproduced with permission from Lin *et al.* (1972).

properties. α_2H-Ferroprotein, for example, is insoluble in low-ionic aqueous solutions and possesses a much higher glucide content and a stronger tendency to polymerize. Very probably, α_2H, like ferritin, belongs to a family of membrane-bound ferroproteins widely distributed among different tissues.

2.2.4. Others

All the human fetal antigens discussed above have been isolated and their properties extensively studied. Another well-characterized tumor-associated antigen is the Regan isozyme, a placental type of alkaline phosphatase (Fishman *et al.*, 1968). A detailed account of this antigen is given in Chapter 3.

Several other human antigens have been described in association with tumoral and fetal tissues. Most of them are of a membrane-bound type, lack organ specificity, and reappear in the serum of patients with neoplasms of different origins and localization. They are not pathognomic of neoplastic transformation since they are also found in either benign tumors or nonneoplastic diseases. Most of these antigens are still poorly characterized by other than immunological methods; their biological significance and clinical usefulness need to be supported by more conclusive data. The increasing number of reports on new tumor-associated antigens attests to the interest in this field and the very general character of such association. The reader will find detailed accounts and references to original work in reviews by Laurence and Neville (1972) and Alexander (1972).

2.3. Conclusions

Since the beginning of this century, when the rejection of tumor transplants by mice immunized with fetal tissues was reported for the first time (Schöne, 1908), many fetal antigens present in malignant diseases of varied origin have been described. Claims on the specific character of their reappearance in neoplasia have often been advanced. However, no confirmation has been obtained in any case where the antigen could be isolated and characterized as well as rigorously explored. One wonders whether fetal antigens with such specificity actually exist.

As we have seen, tumor-associated fetal antigens are either slightly or not immunogenic in the tumor-bearing host (e.g., CEA, αFP, α_2H) or poorly effective as tumor rejection or tumor growth-inhibition antigens (e.g., fetal antigens in DAB- and MC-induced tumors). Only virus-induced fetal antigens seem to escape this rule. It is unclear whether this inadequacy to display competent immune responses is a characteristic which distinguishes them from other tumor-associated rejection antigens or whether it results from their insufficient concentration or mislocation on the cell surface.

The great variety and number of cancerous tissues containing fetal antigens have evoked the possibility that most, if not all, tumor-associated antigens are in fact of embryonic or fetal origin. Although this eventuality appears rather unlikely at first sight, it nevertheless deserves some comment. The term "fetal antigens" would seem to include cell substances synthesized only during intrauterine life. As used in tumor immunology, the term is somewhat ambiguous because antigens of this type were not only demonstrated in embryos and fetuses but also in newborns and in renewing tissues of adult animals (e.g., bone marrow, germinal cells, and endodermal epithelium). There is also increasing evidence that these "fetal antigens" are related to the molecular events of cell differentiation, a process which is operative beyond intrauterine life. Several years ago, the more general term of "transitory cell antigens" was proposed to designate normal biosynthetic products of the cellular genome whose expression is restricted to a *transient* period of the overall process of cell differentiation irrespective of whether they are expressed during intrauterine or adult life (Uriel, 1969). The "fetal antigens" outlined in this section enter under such a designation because all of them possess the common property of being transiently produced sometime during the developmental history of cells and tissues. Certain types of these antigens appear only at the very early cleavage stage of embryonic development. Other transitory cell antigens such as the membrane antigens in DAB- and MC-induced tumors are maximally synthesized around the middle of gestation, while antigens like αFP are produced during relatively long periods covering intrauterine and early postnatal life. Another group is associated with physiological renewal of adult cells and tissues (e.g., endodermal epithelium, red and white blood cells, and germinal cells of the gonads). It has been postulated that neoplasms emerging from adult, fully differentiated cells undergo a process of "stepwise retrodifferentiation" (Uriel, 1969) or "retrogenic expression" (Stonehill and Bendich, 1970) leading to the reappearance of biosynthetic patterns characteristic of immature or incompletely differentiated cells.

If we now reformulate the question as to whether all tumor-associated antigens (virus-coded cell products obviously excepted) are transitory cell antigens, a positive answer becomes more plausible. To test this possibility, however, more information is needed on the turnover and dynamics of cell populations implicated in the synthesis of these transient antigens and also on the immunogenicity of cells undergoing differentiation.

For several decades, immunologists searching for specific antigens of malignant tumors were in fact laying the groundwork for the field of transplantation immunity. Modern studies on tumor-associated antigens may actually be developing the immunology of cell differentiation.

3. Biochemical Findings

The classical work of Warburg on the glycolysis and respiration of human and experimental tumors provided deep insight into the field of cancer biochemistry. Warburg observed that most tumors, when metabolizing glucose under aerobic or anaerobic conditions, produce lactate at a higher rate than do normal tissues. He thus concluded that damage to the respiratory mechanism of growing cells was the cause of cancer.

The early experiments of Warburg and his contemporaries also showed that, in addition to a few normal resting and renewing tissues (e.g., brain, retina, and bone marrow), whole embryos and fetal lung and liver display high rates of anaerobic glycolysis. One can easily understand, however, that the enthusiastic search for what was then considered the biochemical clue to neoplastic transformation did not prompt biochemists to carry out a systematic and more careful exploration of glycolysis in tissues during ontogenic development. Only much later did Villee (1954) demonstrate a significantly high aerobic glycolysis in all the human embryonic tissues of the gestational period studied.

The relationship between cancer and immature cells was reinvestigated in 1945 by Greenstein on the basis of individual enzymatic activities. Analyzing data from his own work and that of others, Greenstein (1945) formulated a series of remarkable observations which can be summarized as follows: enzymatic activities of tumors of different origin tend "to converge to a common pattern" because the specific functional enzymes of the corresponding normal tissues are deleted during neoplastic progression. In the particular case of hepatomas, Greenstein noted the homology of their enzymatic pattern with that of fetal liver and concluded that "neoplasms may revert to a more primitive and less differentiated metabolism." This was probably the first time the old concept of embryonic reversion of malignant tumors was postulated from experimental findings.

Greenstein's observations, however, did not awake excessive interest at the time. Although immunologists were actively engaged in searching for tumor antigens, they neglected to explore fetal tissues, which would provide, 20 years later, a fruitful area of research in tumor immunology.

Most of the subsequent work on individual enzyme activity has been done with rat hepatomas and with adult, immature, and regenerating liver as normal controls or resting and growing tissues. This choice was determined by the availability of a large spectrum of transplantable rat hepatomas of varied growth rate, morphological differentiation, and karyotype composition (Morris, 1965).

Whatever the model and techniques used, studies on individual tissue enzymes yielded information which must be taken only as an approximation. Most tissues, such as liver, represent heterogeneous cell populations whose dynamics change during ontogenic development, experimental manipulation, and tumor induction and progression. The relative contribution of these cellular species to the average values of enzyme activities is still unknown.

3.1. Enzyme Activities and Metabolic Changes in Liver During Ontogenic Development, Regeneration, and Malignant Transformation

Assuming a specific pattern in the metabolism of the cancer cell, Weber and his colleagues have, since 1957, explored the possibility that the development of a metabolic imbalance together with the emergence of a given enzymatic pattern could be characteristic of neoplastic transformation (Weber and Cantero, 1957). They used transplantable rat hepatomas which ranged from slowly to rapidly growing. Among the numerous enzymes of carbohydrate, lipid, protein, and nucleic acid metabolism whose activities were evaluated, those showing a correlation with the growth rate were selected and integrated in separate but ordered patterns of metabolic behavior. The integrated data led to a "molecular correlation concept" (Weber, 1966) which stipulates that the increasing growth rate of hepatomas parallels a progressive loss of metabolic equilibrium of the cancer cell evidenced by (1) gradual predominance of catabolic pathways over anabolic ones in carbohydrate metabolism (glycolytic activity rises whereas gluconeogenesis decreases) and (2) a reverse behavior of protein and nucleic acid metabolism, where synthetic routes become preponderant. Weber (1966, 1972) has insistently concluded that this metabolic imbalance is a specific characteristic of neoplasia since no similar patterns are found in normal growing tissues (developing and regenerating liver).

Although the great interest of the work of Weber's group should be stressed, the assertion that such metabolic changes are intrinsically specific to neoplasia no longer appears tenable. The body of information provided by studies on fetal-type antigens and isozymes, as well as the presence of fetal forms of tRNA in various experimental and human cancers (Yang, 1971; Mittelman, 1971; Gonano et al., 1973), points conclusively toward the striking analogies between developmental and malignant tissues and, as far as we know, weakens claims on specific patterns of gene expression in cancer.

Another conclusion advanced by Weber (1972)—namely, that at no time during postnatal development does metabolic imbalance "even remotely" resemble that observed in hepatomas—is contradicted by recent work. The shift from high to low K_m isozymes associated with well and poorly differentiated hepatomas is also observed in both fetal and neonatal livers: glucokinase and liver-type pyruvate kinase—high K_m isozymes—decrease, whereas hexokinase and muscle-type pyruvate kinase increase (Jamdar and Greengard, 1970; Walker and Potter, 1972; Weinhouse et al., 1972). On the other hand, the activity of ribonucleotide reductase, an enzyme which plays a critical role in the biosynthetic processes of nucleic acids, increases greatly not only in rat hepatomas and fetal and regenerating liver but also in livers from newborn animals up to 7 days of age (Elford, 1972, 1974; Larsson, 1969).

Table 2 is a compilation of enzyme activities, most of them involved in carbohydrate and nucleic acid metabolism, which were selected from studies including comparative data on adult, immature, regenerating, and neoplastic rat liver. The table illustrates again what has been repeatedly pointed out in the preceding pages: the biochemical resemblance among tissues of the same origin growing under either physiological or pathological stimuli including cancer. Quantitative differences in enzymatic activities are certainly found between very rapidly growing hepatomas and immature liver, but such differences greatly lessen when the latter is compared to hepatomas of moderate growth rate. Moreover, highly differentiated, slowly growing hepatomas may show metabolic and antigenic patterns almost indistinguishable from those of normal adult liver.

The values of enzymatic activity in regenerating rat liver appear also to approximate those in hepatomas with moderate growth rates more closely than those in rapidly growing tumors. Regenerating liver is often compared to rapidly growing hepatomas on the basis of DNA incorporation rates of [^{14}C]thymidine (Lea et al., 1966). However, this method is not the most adequate evaluation of liver growth after partial hepatectomy because a significant proportion of labeled cells do not necessarily divide. In fact, hyperplastic growth of hepatocytes—the only cells that should be used in the calculation of cell replication rates—contributes only partially to the restoration of the initial liver mass, which is also provided by cellular hypertrophy.

TABLE 2

39

FETAL
CHARACTERISTICS
OF CANCER

TABLE 2

Comparative Data of Enzyme Activities in Rat Liver[a]

Enzyme	Immature liver	Regenerating liver	Hepatomas[b]	Reference
Glucokinase	Fetal (17–21 day) N.M.[c]	(24 h) 0.3	(9618A):0.3 (7800):N.M. (5123C):N.M.	Walker and Potter (1972)
Hexokinase	Fetal (17–21 day) 3	(24 h) 1.5	(9618A):1.8 (7800):2.2 (5123C):1.2	Walker and Potter (1972)
Pyruvate kinase	Fetal (19–21 day) 0.4	(24–72 h) 0.5	(9611B):0.4 (5123A):0.2	Farina *et al.* (1974)
Thymidine kinase	Fetal (21 day) 23	(23 h) 25	(5123) 24	Klemperer and Haynes (1968), Bresnick *et al.* (1964)
Deoxycytidylate deaminase	Fetal (18 day) 40	(48 h) 17	(5123B) 6	Malcy and Maley (1961)
Thymidylate synthetase	Fetal (18 day) N.M.	(48 h) 1000	(5123) 960	Maley and Maley (1961)
Ribonucleotide reductase	Newborns (7 days) 5000	(24 h) 18,000	(5123C) 18,000	Elford (1972)

[a] Activities in arbitrary units. Normal adult liver activity taken as 1.
[b] Numbers in parentheses represent Morris hepatomas of medium growth rate.
[c] N.M., Not measurable.

3.2. Fetal Patterns of Isozymes in Cancer

Since the work of Markert and Moller (1959), considerable evidence has shown that enzymes exist in multimolecular forms which differ from each other in some physiochemical, chemical, immunological, and/or kinetic properties. In spite of several attempts to define and classify isozymes on a conceptual basis (Markert, 1968; Uriel, 1969; Commission on Biochemical Nomenclature, 1965, 1971; Schapira, 1973), no general agreement has been reached. The term as it prevails today has an operational sense: molecular forms of enzymes are distinguished by their electrophoretic, chromatographic, and/or kinetic behavior.

There is an ever-growing literature, started in 1963 (Schapira *et al.*, 1963), pointing to profound alterations of isozymic patterns in neoplastic tissues, namely, the progressive loss of specific tissue forms and their replacement by isozymic counterparts preponderant in other adult or fetal tissues. Biochemical transitions of this type can occur without significant modifications in total enzymatic activities, thereby providing a means of revealing fine changes in enzymatic patterns that would otherwise escape notice. The subject has been extensively reviewed on several occasions (Criss, 1971; Knox, 1972; Ono and Weinhouse, 1972; Schapira, 1973).

Since the isozymes are treated in more detail in Chapter 3, we shall limit this discussion to studies where tumor isozymic patterns were correlated with those characteristic of both fetal tissues and adult nonneoplastic growing tissues (i.e., liver regeneration subsequent to physical or chemical injury).

3.2.1. Isozymes Involved in the Catabolic Pathway of Glucose

a. Glucose-ATP Phosphotransferase. Isozymic analysis has revealed in most mammalian tissues four molecular forms of glucose-ATP phosphotransferase, a key enzyme of glucose utilization. Three of them (types I, II, and III), with a low K_m for glucose, are collectively referred to as "hexokinases" and the fourth (type IV), possessing a high K_m for glucose, is designated as "glucokinase." Hexokinase type I and, particularly, glucokinase are the predominant forms in adult liver, whereas in fetal liver glucokinase is barely detectable, hexokinase type II (Sato *et al.*, 1969) or type I (Weinhouse *et al.*, 1972) being preponderant.

The general picture of these isozymes in well and poorly differentiated hepatomas and in most primary hepatomas induced by chemical carcinogens is of a fetal type, with very low levels of glucokinase and rather high values of hexokinase isozymes, which, according to Sato *et al.* (1969), shift from type I to type II. In contrast, highly differentiated hepatomas with very slow growth rates were found to have an almost adult liver pattern of both hexokinase and glucokinase (Weinhouse, 1973). Liver regeneration after partial hepatectomy gave controversial results as obtained by kinetics assays. On the other hand, electrophoretic patterns of the fetal type were reported for hexokinase and glucokinase (Sato *et al.*, 1969).

Early hyperplastic and reparative growth of liver in response to the administration of hepatocarcinogens (3'-Me-DAB) was concomitant in rats with an isozymic transition of the fetal type: progressive lowering of glucokinase during the first 6–8 wk of diet, followed by a gradual increase of hexokinase activity (Walker and Potter, 1972). This transition parallels the enhancement of α-fetoprotein synthesis and secretion (see Section 2) which is observed in rats under similar circumstances.

Hexokinase isozymes of uterine tumors have been investigated by Sato *et al.* (1972) using analytical electrophoresis. Here again, fetal type II hexokinase was strongly predominant in cervical and corpus carcinomas, while in control tissues, cervical epithelium, and endometrium only type I isozyme was revealed.

b. Phosphofructokinase. Chromatographic separation has revealed at least four molecular forms of phosphofructokinase (Tanaka *et al.*, 1971). Their distribution in adult rat tissues led to the proposal of three main tissue groups. The first is composed of muscle, heart, and brain, where isozyme I (muscle type) is the only form present. A second group, including liver, kidney, and red blood cells, contains isozyme IV (liver type) as the preponderant constituent. To the third group, where isozymes II and/or III predominate, belong the majority of tissues not included in the other two groups. Isozyme IV was found to be the major constituent in both regenerating liver and liver from newborns. A series of rat and human tumors, including three of nonhepatic origin (Walker carcinosarcoma and two gastric cancers), were examined and all showed isozyme IV as the preponderant form. Tanaka *et al.* (1972) studied isozyme patterns of phosphofructokinase in neonatal but not in fetal tissues. Nevertheless, if isozyme IV (liver type), which is preponderant in newborns, also represents the fetal-type form, then it would appear that tumors from other than liver shift to a common fetal or neonatal molecular form of phosphofructokinase. The same isozyme form (isozyme IV) was preponderant in both normal and neoplastic liver, probably because adult and fetal liver possess the same isozymic pattern.

c. Pyruvate Kinase. Early work on the isozymic pattern of pyruvate kinase provided somewhat confusing results. We will limit the discussion to more recent studies whose results are in close agreement (Inamura and Tanaka, 1972; Tanaka *et al.*, 1972; Weinhouse *et al.*, 1972; Walker and Potter, 1972; Farina *et al.*, 1974).

By chromatographic and electrophoretic methods, pyruvate kinase can be resolved into three major, noninterconvertible molecular forms: isozymes I, II, and III, also referred to as liver, muscle, and kidney type, respectively. Isozyme I predominates in adult liver, where isozyme III appears only as a minor constituent. By contrast, a completely inverted pattern is observed in fetal liver. In transplantable hepatomas, a transition to the fetal pattern occurs in parallel with the increasing growth rate and low differentiation of the tumors. The fetal transition is also characteristic of primary hepatomas induced by chemical carcinogens and of Walker carcinosarcoma, a tumor of nonhepatic origin. Only highly differentiated hepatomas showed an isozymic pattern virtually identical to that of adult liver.

Through the 24- to 72-h period of rapid liver regeneration after partial hepatectomy, isozyme III (fetal type) increased to more than twice the normal value, with a concomitant drop in the type I/type III ratio to below 3 (normal ratio is 11) (Walker and Potter, 1972; Farina *et al.*, 1974). Moreover, an analogous shift from type I to type III isozyme was demonstrated in homogenates of isolated parenchymal liver cells of adult rats during 2–15 days after partial hepatectomy (Bonney *et al.*, 1973; Garnett *et al.*, 1974).

As in the case of glucokinase, when rats were fed the hepatocarcinogen 3′-Me-DAB, a similar change toward the fetal pattern of pyruvate kinase was observed. The activity of isozyme I gradually decreased, while the reverse was true for the type III isozyme. By the sixth week of the hepatocarcinogen diet, the activity of isozyme I fell to less than 10% of the initial value and correspondingly that of enzyme III increased almost sixfold (Walker and Potter, 1972).

d. Aldolase. Aldolase exists in multimolecular forms of tetrametric structure designated as muscle type (isozyme A), liver type (isozyme B), and brain type (isozyme C) according to the tissue where each form prevails. Isozyme A is the most widely distributed among fetal tissues and is the preponderant form in all of them (Farron *et al.*, 1972).

There is now evidence that aldolase isozymes revert to the fetal pattern (see review by Schapira, 1973) in rat, mouse, and human hepatocellular carcinomas, in rat transplantable hepatomas, and also in tumors of different origin, such as spleen reticulosarcoma, rhabdomyosarcoma, kidney carcinomas, and mammary carcinoma (Farron *et al.*, 1972). More recently, isozyme C (brain type), which is also present in fetal liver although to a lesser extent than isozyme A, was found associated with ascites hepatomas (Sugimura *et al.*, 1970; Schapira and Josipowicz, 1970).

No significant deviations from normal adult patterns were reported for aldolase in regenerating liver after partial hepatectomy. Nevertheless, Bergès *et al.* (1974) recently demonstrated by electrophoretic and immunological methods the reappearance of isozymes A and C and their hybrids 24–72 h after one-third or two-thirds partial hepatectomy. They pointed out that the inclusion of a nonionic detergent in the buffers used to prepare liver homogenates was necessary for the complete solubilization of these isozymes, and its absence should explain previous failure to demonstrate their presence in regenerating liver.

In the precancerous liver of rats fed hepatocarcinogens, the isozymic changes of aldolase were characterized, as in the case of glucokinase and pyruvate kinase, by a progressive loss of the adult pattern and an increase in the muscle-type form proper to fetal and neonatal liver (Endo *et al.*, 1972; Walker and Potter, 1972).

3.2.2. Others

The enzymes described above are probably the most representative examples of isozymic reversion to fetal and neonatal patterns in malignant tumors. Others such as the isozymes of glutaminase (Katunuma *et al.*, 1972), branched-chain amino acid transferase (Ichihara and Ogawa, 1972), lactate dehydrogenase (Uriel, 1969; Farron *et al.*, 1972), and carboxylic esterases (Kaneko *et al.*, 1974) can also be added. The list is, obviously, incomplete and ever-growing.

3.3. Conclusions

In the preceding section, we presented experimental facts showing that some metabolic and biochemical patterns specific to immature, incompletely differentiated tissues are found in malignant tumors. Even though the body of evidence may be convincing, it would be dangerous to make any generalization, chiefly because the data obtained result from the analysis of an extremely complex material.

Tumors, like normal developing and renewing tissues, are made up of heterogeneous cell populations undergoing phase-associated changes as growth progresses. The extent to which either cancerous cells or other nonmalignant elements contribute to the biochemical changes observed is unknown. Farber (1968) emphasized the need for "cellular purity" in molecular analysis of biological phenomena associated with neoplastic development. It is hoped that in the near future the finding of new experimental models and the improvement of tissue fractionation techniques will provide the means to surmount the problem.

Some general conclusions can, however, be drawn from the data outlined in this section:

1. Metabolic pathways and isozyme patterns characteristic of the functional activity of adult tissues tend to vanish when they enter malignant transformation and to be replaced by the rather common pathways and patterns proper to tissues undergoing developmental growth. Therefore, when the isozymic pattern of a tissue differs from that of its fetal or neonatal counterpart (liver aldolase and glutaminase, kidney lactate dehydrogenase, etc.), the tumor expresses the fetal-type isozyme. However, if the same isozyme is predominant in both adult and fetal tissue (kidney aldolase and pyruvate kinase, muscle aldolase, etc.), the pattern does not change in the corresponding tumor. These observations confirm, at the level of isozyme patterns, Greenstein's views on enzyme behavior during neoplastic development. The isozymic distribution in fetal tissues has not been explored in a systematic way, but one can anticipate that the molecular forms of a given enzyme should converge to a common pattern in most, if not all, the tissues of an individual in the early stages of ontogenic development. If "tumors possess a more uniform and less diverse pattern of enzymatic activity than normal tissues" (Greenstein, 1945), it is probably because of their reversion toward early phases of cell differentiation.

2. The reversion of neoplasms toward immature tissues is accentuated to a certain extent as the tumor's growth rate increases and/or as differentiation lessens. It is unclear whether this reflects the differentiated state of the cell or its metabolic adaptation to a higher growth rate. Probably both processes are implicated.

3. While widely common among tumors, the biochemical transitions discussed here seem to be neither essential nor unique to malignancy: highly differentiated, slowly growing hepatomas show enzyme patterns very close to those of normal resting tissues, and, in contrast, patterns of the fetal or neonatal type can be observed in adult tissues undergoing noncancerous growth. There are several undeniable examples of fetal-type transitions associated with liver repair after partial hepatectomy (pyruvate kinase, aldolase, hexokinase, glucokinase, glutaminase, etc.). These transitions were, nevertheless, reported absent for other enzymes. Liver regeneration is a very complex phenomenon at the morphological, biochemical, and molecular levels and still is obscure because of the diversity and rapidity of the sequential events that occur in a relatively short period of time. If the model is not carefully explored, fine changes can escape experimental observation and this perhaps may explain some controversial results.

Another example of fetal-type transitions associated with noncancerous growth in adult individuals is provided by the hyperplastic development in livers subjected to chemical injury. In Section 2.1.1, we described the early reappearance of serum α-fetoprotein in rats fed hepatotoxics or hepatocarcinogens, and this in the absence of any morphological signs of neoplastic transformation. Similarly, the gradual reversion to the immature type of several isozymic patterns (glucose-ATP phosphotransferases and aldolase) was observed during the pre-cancerous phase of liver carcinogenesis. The observation is especially interesting because this phase is morphologically characterized by the appearance of a considerable population of oval and transitional liver cells and of hyperplastic nodules considered as noncancerous precursors of hepatocellular carcinomas (Farber, 1956).

4. Speculative Approaches

The hypothesis that malignant transformation of cells may be concomitant with mutational changes induced by physical, chemical, or biological stimuli has long received wide acceptance as a causal explanation of cancer. However, the extensive immunological and biochemical studies over the last 15 years have failed to demonstrate new antigens, enzymes, or molecules which logically would be expressed by the progeny of the mutated cells. More recently, an alternative, although not mutually exclusive, hypothesis of neoplastic development has been advanced which focuses on abnormal cell differentiation due to the mispro-grammed expression of normal genes (Pierce, 1967, 1970; Markert, 1968; Potter, 1969; Uriel, 1969).

4.1. Misprogrammed Gene Function

After careful examination of the basic characteristics of cancer cells—rate of cell division, migration, and biochemical activity—and of the best-established etiologi-cal factors of neoplasia, Markert (1968) concluded that malignancy is a disease of cell differentiation, fundamentally ascribable to an "aberrant programming of gene function" which can occur at any step of cell differentiation from primordial to fully differentiated adult cells. Thus in the case of human retinoblastoma, a tumor imputable to a single dominant autosomal mutation, he noted that although each cell of an affected individual bears the mutated gene, it becomes operational as a carcinogenic stimulus in only a few retinal cells and only in those having attained a relatively advanced stage of differentiation. Tumors induced by viruses, chemical carcinogens, or pharmacologically active molecules (e.g., hor-mones and antihormones) may also be viewed in terms of normal cell differentia-tion if one assumes that such agents can force cells to metabolic adaptations which in turn provoke new patterns of gene expression leading to neoplastic transfor-mation. Markert concludes that the shift from a normal to a neoplastic cell probably does not differ from a step in normal cell differentiation and that the genetic basis of neoplasia rather depends on the abnormal programming of normal gene function.

Sugimura et al. (1972) proposed the term "disdifferentiation" to define any abnormality of differentiation associated with phenotypic patterns of cancer cells. Contrary to Markert's views, Sugimura and his coworkers consider gene expression of cancer cells (i.e., tumor isozyme patterns) as distinct from that of normal or

embryonic tissues. We discussed this problem in Section 3 and presented data
which seem to disprove Sugimura's conclusion. While it is likely that the normal
unfolding of the program for cell maturation may be disturbed during neoplastic
development, the existence of new and specific antigen and enzyme patterns of
gene activity in cancer cells has not been demonstrated.

4.2. Arrested Differentiation

Testicular teratocarcinoma is a tumor arising from abnormal growth of male
germ cells and is composed of many somatic or trophoblastic tissues in addition to
a highly malignant tissue called embryonal carcinoma. Studies on the developmental behavior of the tumor demonstrated that embryonal carcinoma cells are
the stem cells of teratocarcinoma and that they can differentiate into benign tissue
(see Pierce, 1967). Further experimental confirmation of the possibility of
malignant to benign reversion in neoplasms was obtained from a malignant
squamous cell carcinoma of rats (Pierce, 1970). Histologically, the tumor
was a mixture of undifferentiated cancer cells and of squamous pearls containing keratotic centers, the latter being morphologically comparable with
normal squamous differentiation. Isotope tracer techniques showed that the
undifferentiated malignant stem cells differentiated into benign mature
squamous cells.

Pierce (1970) therefore concluded that in carcinogenesis the target cell is
actually the stem cell normally present in tissues. According to the etiological
factor involved, the result could be either some mutational change or an alteration
in the control of nuclear activity, both leading, if the stem cell survives, "to a block
in differentiation or to an unbalance between proliferation and differentiation."
This hypothesis brings up again on an experimental basis and in terms of cell
differentiation the old concept of the embryonal origin of cancer advanced late in
the nineteenth century by Cohnheim and Durante (see Triolo, 1965). It excludes
adult or mature cells as possible targets for neoplastic transformation since "what
has been interpreted as dedifferentiation is in reality an abortive attempt of
differentiation" (Pierce, 1970).

Somewhat different views, although along the same line of reasoning, were
developed by Potter (1969) and Potter *et al.* (1972) under the concept of
"oncogeny as blocked ontogeny," which proposes that cancer arises from the
arrested development of a population of stem cells. This population may be
already present in the normal tissue or may be generated by the reversion of adult
cells to the immature state. As the progeny of such stem cells undergoing
ontogeny or reontogeny (Walker and Potter, 1972) pass through a variety of
differentiation stages, and as the blockage can occur at any of these stages, there is
a strong possibility for considerable diversification in tumor phenotypes. The
same possibility is inferred from Pierce's hypothesis.

Potter and his coworkers derived these conclusions from their own and
corresponding work on biochemical transitions (discussed in Section 3) and

particularly on the changes observed in isozymic patterns associated with fetal, regenerating, precancerous, and cancerous liver.

4.3. Unbalanced Retrodifferentiation

While the arrested differentiation of stem cells seems to meet with general agreement as a possible explanation of neoplastic development, the concept of cell reversion and neoplasia has received less detailed analysis. We have suggested that "unbalanced retrodifferentiation" may be implicated in the carcinogenesis of tumors emerging from adult tissues (Uriel, 1969).

A variety of connotations, sometimes without clear definition, are associated with the process of cell differentiation, whereas the term "dedifferentiation" is even more loosely used to describe a loss in morphological differentiation. We shall consider differentiation as a time and space sequence of biosynthetic patterns that reflects the diversified activity of the genome during developmental growth, and retrodifferentiation as an ordered sequence of cytogenetic events opposite to those of differentiation.

In contrast to bacteria and, to a lesser extent, plants, where differentiation reversibility occurs under physiological conditions, retrodifferentiation is infrequent in animals because of the high stability of their fully differentiated cells. However, several examples of reversibility can be mentioned. One is illustrated by the experiments of Gurdon (1962a,b) with the nuclei from gut epithelial cells of *Xenopus* tadpoles. When nuclei from these differentiated cells were transplanted into enucleated eggs of the same species, normal development into feeding tadpoles could be promoted in 24% of the transplants. This experiment apparently implies the complete reversion of the donor nuclei to a primordial stage before the reconstituted egg is able to resume the whole program of tadpole ontogenesis. Another example of reversibility is provided by the epimorphic regeneration of amputated parts of many amphibians. There is now conclusive evidence that the blastema cells which accumulate at the site of transection emerge from retrodifferentiated mature tissues and not from a reserve of stem cells (see Burgess, 1974). The Wolffian lens regeneration system of urodeles (see Yamada, 1967) probably is the most significant example of sequenced retrodifferentiation in lower animals. After removal of the lens, the organ is completely regenerated by a cell population derived from the dorsal part of the iris epithelium. The fully differentiated iris cells convert into lens cells following an ordered stepwise sequence of morphological and biosynthetic patterns which starts by a retrodifferentiating pathway of iris cells: nuclear activation, replication, and depigmentation. Afterward, lens regeneration begins with the synthesis of lens-specific antigens (γ-crystallins) and progresses by morphological changes until complete lens organogenesis. As pointed out by Yamada, "the convergence of regenerative and ontogenic lens formation implies that Wolffian lens regeneration involves recovery of an embryonic condition by the iris epithelial cell." The example is particularly interesting for our discussion because it shows that in metaplastic transitions the shift from one cell species to another also does not occur by a direct or aberrant change in gene expression but rather following an ordered program. The metaplastic phenomena which are sometimes observed in experimental and human tumors (e.g., ectopic production of hormones) may also develop according to a similar program: reversion to a stem cell and then redifferentiation in another direction.

Most adult tissues susceptible to hyperplastic growth contain a population of fully differentiated cells and a reserve of stem cells. Both may be considered as resting cells until, in response to adequate signals, their programs for growth are unfolded (Fig. 4). We have postulated that when the adult cell retrodifferentiates and the stem cell differentiates they probably travel through similar stages albeit sequenced in opposite order. Thus in a cell entering retrodifferentiation the synthesis of one or another fetospecific antigen and/or the transition to a given pattern of enzymatic activity may depend on how far the reversion proceeds and how it modulates between the stages of the sequence.

The analysis of fetal-type biological transitions accompanying hepatomas and liver regeneration after partial hepatectomy or chemical injury led us to envisage them as demonstrative examples of retrodifferentiation in mammalian tissues. While stepwise reversion toward immature cell phenotypes probably accounts for the antigenic and biochemical analogies observed between hepatoma and regenerating rat liver, the dynamics of both processes are clearly distinct. In regenerating liver the change is a cyclic one: initial retrodifferentiation of parenchymal cells is "counterbalanced" after a short period of active growth by a process of reontogeny which restores the phenotypic properties of the adult tissues. During the preneoplastic phase of liver carcinogenesis, cells also retrodifferentiate, but at a given moment and by an unknown mechanism the system escapes compensatory redifferentiation and becomes malignant. Thus "unbalanced retrodifferentiation" may characterize neoplastic development arising in adult tissues.

The purpose of this hypothetical scheme of neoplastic development, outlined in Fig. 4, is to emphasize, as has been done by others, that the biological behavior and properties of cancer cells can be largely explained in terms of normal differentiation and that the existence, as often claimed, of specific patterns intrinsically associated with them remains to be demonstrated. Terms like "aberrant," "spurious," "abnormal," and "misprogrammed" have frequently been applied to define malignant cells *per se* but their adequacy seems questionable because they are derived by comparing the malignant cells (or tissues) with their normal adult counterparts. When the malignant tumors are compared with immature or incompletely differentiated tissues, the "abnormality" of the former becomes much less apparent. Indeed, the critical difference that should distinguish neoplastic from normally growing tissues is not known.

Cell lineages emerging from primordial elements diversify as differentiation progresses and become distinct when each lineage attains full maturity and acquires its own functional specialization. Antigens, enzymes, and other macromolecular products of gene activity form phase-specific patterns of this

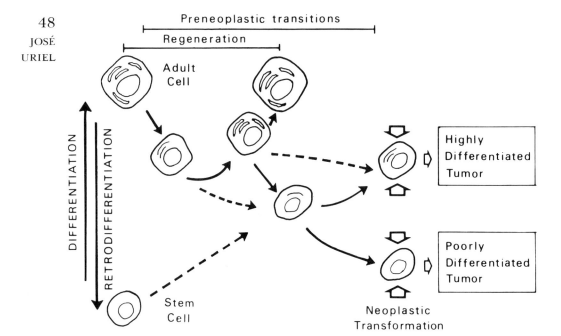

FIGURE 4. Schematic representation of hypothetical neoplastic development arising in adult tissues. A mature liver parenchymal cell enters retrodifferentiation under hepatic injury. The initial transition follows distinct pathways: either it can be "counterbalanced" by a process of reontogeny which restores the phenotypic properties of the mature cell (regeneration) or it can persist "unbalanced" and even progress, the cell traveling through various stages of development until the neoplastic transformation takes place. The antigenic and enzymatic patterns of the tumor will reflect the level of differentiation where the transformation occurs. Dashed arrows indicate alternative routes which emphasize the plasticity of the hypothetic model. Several phenotypes of malignant clones may coexist in the same tumor.

programmed sequence of multiple events. The whole developmental history of cells and tissues resembles an intricately branched tree whose precise delineation presently constitutes a discouraging and almost impossible task. However, studies on transitory cell antigens and enzymes of the type outlined in this chapter represent an accessible way to a better knowledge of developmental changes in neoplastic and nonneoplastic cells. These transient constituents, probably of limited number, are molecular markers of gene expression and when correctly sequenced in the overall process of cell differentiation they should contribute to characterization of the dynamics of growing cell populations. If the populations involved are made of malignant cells, there is a chance that a careful and comparative study of these transitory patterns will throw some light on the intrinsic events associated with the neoplastic transformation.

5. Final Remarks

We have stressed in the preceding pages the convergence of many spontaneous and experimental malignant tumors toward stages of incomplete forms of cell differentiation. The noncoincidental character of the biological transitions involved seems to be sustained by several fundamental observations. Thus certain types of transitory cell antigens reappear in association with a given class of tumors—e.g., αFP and hepatomas and embryonal carcinomas; CEA and tumors of the digestive, pulmonary, and genitourinary tracts. Fetal-type antigens can be demonstrated in a great variety of tumors of different etiology (viral, chemical, biological). The biochemical phenotypes of different tumors show analogous changes in enzyme activity and isozymic patterns.

The bulk of information acquired strongly suggests that, in order to ascertain intrinsic qualitative differences, the eventual findings with respect to the biochemical and antigenic phenotypes of cancer should henceforth be carefully compared with those for growing populations of nonneoplastic cells in fetal, neonatal, and adult tissues. Much effort must then be devoted to discovering new transitory cell antigens or other markers of cell differentiation. Developmental patterns of isozymes in neoplastic and normal growing tissues should also be actively explored.

While the arrest of cell differentiation appears as a possible explanation of neoplastic development, the direction of the events—differentiation from a stem cell or retrodifferentiation from a mature element—has not been clarified, at least in cancers starting from adult cells. The question is of importance because the elucidation of the nature of the target cells from which neoplastic growth emerges has obvious physiopathological and therapeutic implications. For the same reason, research on the immunogenicity of cells undergoing differentiation and on the factors controlling the immune responses which they can elicit in the host must be greatly stimulated. Last but not least, studies on transitory cell antigens and enzymes are contributing to a better knowledge of the developmental differentiation of multicellular organisms, which remains one of the major subjects of biological research.

ACKNOWLEDGMENTS

I wish to thank Professor R. Monier (I.R.S.C., Villejuif, France) and Professor F. Grande (Fundacion Cuenca Villoro, Zaragoza, Spain) as well as my colleagues at the I.R.S.C., and particularly Drs. S. von Kleist, D. Buffe, J. Jami and M. Stanislawski, for their helpful and critical comments.

The author's work was supported in part by grants from the Centre National de la Recherche Scientifique, Délégation Générale à la Recherche Scientifique et Technique and Foundation pour la Recherche Médicale Française.

6. References

ABELEV, G. I., 1971, Alpha-fetoprotein in ontogenesis and its association with malignant tumors, *Adv. Cancer Res.* **14**:295.

ABELEV, G. I., 1974, α-Fetoprotein as a marker of embryo-specific differentiation in normal and tumor tissues, *Transplant. Rev.* **20**:3.

ABELEV, G. I., PEROVA, S. D., KHRAMKOVA, N. I., POSTNIKOVA, Z. A., AND IRLIN, I. S., 1963, Production of embryonal α-globulin by transplantable mouse hepatomas, *Transplantation* **1**:174.

ABELEV, G. I., ASSECRITOVA, I. V., KRAEVSKY, N. A., PEROVA, S. D., AND PEREVODNIKOVA, N. I., 1967, Embryonal serum alpha-globulin in cancer patients: Diagnostic value, *Int. J. Cancer* **2**:551.

ALEXANDER, P., 1972, Foetal "antigens" in cancer, *Nature (London)* **235**:137.

ARTZT, K., DUBOIS, P., BENNETT, D., CONDAMINE, H., BABINET, C., AND JACOB, F., 1973, Surface antigens common to mouse cleavage embryos and primitive teratocarcinoma cells in culture, *Proc. Natl. Acad. Sci. U.S.A.* **70**:2988.

BAKIROV, R. D., 1968, Appearance of embryonal serum alpha-globulin in adult mice after inhalation of carbon tetrachloride, *Byull. Eksp. Biol. Med.* **65**:45.

BALDWIN, R. W., 1973, Immunological aspects of chemical carcinogenesis, *Adv. Cancer Res.* **18**:1.

BALDWIN, R. W., GLAVES, D., AND PIMM, M. V., 1971, Tumor-associated antigens as expressions of chemically-induced neoplasia and their involvement in tumor–host interactions, in: *Progress in Immunology* (B. Amos, ed.), pp. 907–920, Academic Press, New York.

BALDWIN, R. W., GLAVES, D., AND VOSE, B. M., 1972, Embryonic antigen expression in chemically induced rat hepatomas and sarcomas, *Int. J. Cancer* **10**:233.

BALDWIN, R. W., GLAVES, D., AND VOSE, B. M., 1974, Immunogenicity of embryonic antigens associated with chemically-induced rat tumor, *Int. J. Cancer* **13**:135.

BARANSKA, W., KOLDOVSKY, P., AND KOPROWSKI, H., 1970, Antigenic study of unfertilized mouse eggs: Cross-reactivity with SV40-induced antigens, *Proc. Natl. Acad. Sci. U.S.A.* **67**:193.

BECKER, F. F., AND SELL, S., 1974, Early elevation of α_1-fetoprotein in N-2-fluorenylacetamide hepatocarcinogenesis, *Cancer Res.* **34**:2489.

BECKER, F. F., KLEIN, K. M., WOLMAN, S. R., ASOFSKY, R., AND SELL, S., 1973, Characterization of primary hepatocellular carcinomas and initial transplant generations, *Cancer Res.* **33**:3330.

BERGÈS, J., DE NÉCHAUD, B., AND URIEL, J., 1974, Reappearance of aldolase C in rat liver during compensatory regeneration after partial hepatectomy, *FEBS Letters* (in press).

BERMAN, L. D., 1972, The SV40 antigen: A carcinoembryonic-type antigen of the hamster, *Int. J. Cancer* **10**:326.

BOFFA, G. A., NADAL, C., ZADJELA, F., AND FINE, J. M., 1964, Slow alpha-globulin of rat serum, *Nature (London)* **203**:1182.

BONNEY, R., WALKER, P., AND POTTER, V. R., 1973, Isoenzyme patterns in parenchymal and non-parenchymal cells isolated from regenerating and regenerated rat liver, *Biochem. J.* **136**:947.

BRAWN, R. J., 1970, Possible association of embryonal antigen(s) with several primary 3-methyl-cholanthrene-induced murine sarcomas, *Int. J. Cancer* **6**:245.

BRESNICK, E., THOMPSON, U. S., MORRIS, H. P., AND LIEBELT, A. G., 1964, Inhibition of thymidine kinase activity in liver and hepatomas by TTP and d-CTP, *Biochem. Biophys. Res. Commun.* **16**:276.

BUFFE, D., AND RIMBAUT, C. 1973, L'α_1-foetoprotéine dans les atteintes hépatiques et les maladies métaboliques de l'enfant, *Biomedicine* **19**:172.

BUFFE, D., RIMBAUT, C., AND BURTIN, P., 1968, Présence d'une protéine d'origine tissulaire, l'α_2H-globuline, dans le sérum des sujets atteints d'affections malignes, *Int. J. Cancer* **3**:850.

BUFFE, D., RIMBAUT, C., LEMERLE, J., SCHWEISGUTH, O., AND BURTIN, P., 1970, Présence d'une protéine d'origine tissulaire, l'α_2H-globuline, dans le sérum des enfants porteurs de tumeurs, *Int. J. Cancer* **5**:85.

BUFFE, D., RIMBAUT, C., FUCCARO, C., AND BURTIN, P., 1972, Isolement et caractérisation d'une ferroprotéine tissulaire: l'α_2H-Globuline, *Ann. Inst. Pasteur* **123**:129.

BURGESS, A. M. C., 1974, Genome control and the genetic potentialities of the nuclei of dedifferentiated regeneration blastema cells, in: *Neoplasia and Cell Differentiation* (Sherbert, ed.), pp. 106–148, Karger, Basel.

BURTIN, P., MARTIN, E., SABINE, M. C., AND VON KLEIST, S., 1972, Immunological study of polyps of the colon, *J. Natl. Cancer Inst.* **48**:25.

BURTIN, P., VON KLEIST, S., SABINE, M. C., AND KING, M., 1973, Immunohistochemical localization of carcinoembryonic antigen and non-specific cross-reacting antigen in gastrointestinal normal and tumoral tissues, *Cancer Res.* **33**:3296.

COGGIN, J. H., AMBROSE, K. R., AND ANDERSON, N. G., 1970, Fetal antigen capable of inducing transplantation immunity against SV40 hamster tumor cells, *J. Immunol.* **105**:524.

COGGIN, J. H., AMBROSE, K. R., BELLAMY, B. B., AND ANDERSON, N. G., 1971, Tumor immunity in hamsters immunized with fetal tissues, *J. Immunol.* **107**:526.

COMMISSION ON BIOLOGICAL NOMENCLATURE, 1965, *Recommendations (1964) of the IUB on the Nomenclature and Classification of Enzymes.* Elsevier, Amsterdam.

COMMISSION ON BIOLOGICAL NOMENCLATURE, 1971, The nomenclature of multiple forms of enzymes. Recommendations, *Biochim. Biophys. Acta* **258:**1.

CRISS, W. E., 1971, A review of isozymes and cancer, *Cancer Res.* **31:**1523.

DE NÉCHAUD, B., AND URIEL, J., 1971, Antigènes cellulaires transitoires du foie de rat. I. Sécrétion et synthèse des protéines sériques foetospécifiques au cours du développement et de la régénération hépatique, *Int. J. Cancer* **8:**71.

DE NÉCHAUD, B., AND URIEL, J., 1972, Antigènes cellulaires transitoires du foie de rat. II. Effet des inhibiteurs de synthèse sur les foetoprotéines sériques à la fin du premier mois de vie et après intoxication hépatique aiguë, *Int. J. Cancer* **10:**58.

DE NÉCHAUD, B., AND URIEL, J., 1973, Antigènes cellulaires transitoires du foie de rat. III. Mode de réapparition de l'α-foetoprotéine au cours de l'hépatocarcinogénèse chimique, *Int. J. Cancer* **11:**104.

DUFF, R. J., AND RAPP, F., 1970, Reaction of serum from pregnant hamsters with surface of cell transformed by SV40, *J. Immunol.* **105:**521.

EDIDIN, M., PATTHEY, H. L., MCGUIRE, E. J., AND SHEFFIELD, W. D., 1971, An antiserum to "embryoid body" tumor cells that reacts with normal mouse embryos, in: *Proceedings of the First Conference and Workshops on Embryonic and Fetal Antigens in Cancer* (N. G. Anderson and J. H. Coggin, eds.), pp. 239–248, Oak Ridge National Laboratory, Oak Ridge, Tenn.

ELFORD, H. L., 1972, Mammalian ribonucleotide reductase and cell proliferation, *Gann Monogr.* **13:**205.

ELFORD, H. L., 1974, Subcellular localization of ribonucleotide reductase in Novikoff hepatoma and regenerating rat liver, *Arch. Biochem. Biophys.* **163:**537.

ENDO, M., EGUCHI, M., YANAGI, S., TORISU, T., IKEHARA, Y., AND KAMIYA, T., 1972, Biochemical studies on the preneoplastic state, *Gann Monogr.* **13:**235.

FARBER, E., 1956, Similarities in the sequence of early histological changes induced in the liver of the rat by ethionine, 2-acetylaminofluorene, and 3'-methyl-4-dimethylaminoazobenzene, *Cancer Res.* **16:**142.

FARBER, E., 1968, Biochemistry of carcinogenesis, *Cancer Res.* **28:**1859.

FARBER, E., 1973, Carcinogenesis—Cellular evolution as a unifying thread: Presidential address, *Cancer Res.* **33:**2537.

FARINA, F. A., SHATTON, J. B., MORRIS, H. P., AND WEINHOUSE, S., 1974, Isozymes of pyruvate kinase in liver and hepatomas of the rat, *Cancer Res.* **34:**1439.

FARRON, F., HSU, H. H. T., AND KNOX, W. E., 1972, Fetal-type isozymes in hepatic and non-hepatic rat tumors, *Cancer Res.* **32:**302.

FISHMAN, W. H., INGLIS, N. I., STOLBACH, L. L., AND KRANT, M. J., 1968, A serum alkaline phosphatase isoenzyme of human neoplastic origin, *Cancer Res.* **28:**150.

GARNETT, M. E., DYSON, R. D., AND DOST, F. N., 1974, Pyruvate kinase isozyme changes in parenchymal cells of regenerating rat liver, *J. Biol. Chem.* **249:**5222.

GITLIN, D., 1974, Phylogeny and ontogeny in the evolution of αFP compared to the emergence of immunoglobulins, in: *Colloque sur l'Alpha-Foetoprotéine* (R. Masseyeff, ed.), pp. 393–401, INSERM, Paris.

GOLD, P., AND FREEMAN, S. O., 1965, Specific carcinoembryonic antigens of the human digestive system, *J. Exp. Med.* **122:**467.

GONANO, F., PIRRO, G., AND SILVETTI, S., 1973, Foetal liver tRNA^phe in rat hepatoma, *Nature New Biol.* **242:**236.

GREENSTEIN, J. P., 1945, Enzymes in normal and neoplastic tissues, in: *AAAS Research Conference on Cancer* (F. R. Moulton, ed.), pp. 191–215, AAAS, Washington, D.C.

GURDON, J. B., 1962a, The developmental capacity of nuclei taken from intestinal epithelial cells of feeding tadpoles, *J. Embryol. Exp. Morphol.* **10:**622.

GURDON, J. B., 1962b, Adult frogs from single somatic cell nuclei, *Dev. Biol.* **4:**256.

HANNA, M. G., TENNANT, R. W., AND COGGIN, J. H., 1971, Suppressive effect of immunization with mouse fetal antigens on growth of cells infected with Rausher leukemia virus and on plasma-cell tumors, *Proc. Natl. Acad. Sci. U.S.A.* **68:**1748.

HIRAI, H., NISHI, S., AND WATABE, H., 1972, Radioimmunoassay of α-fetoprotein, in: *Protides of the Biological Fluids*, Vol. 20 (Peeters, H., ed.), pp. 579–587, Pergamon Press, Oxford.

HIRAI, M., NISHI, S., WATABE, M., AND TSUKADA, Y., 1973, Some chemical, experimental and clinical investigations of α-fetoprotein, *Gann Monogr.* **14:**19.

52

JOSÉ
URIEL

ICHIHARA, A., AND OGAWA, K., 1972, Isozymes of branched chain amino transaminase in normal rat tissues and hepatomas, *Gann Monogr.* **13**:181.

INAMURA, K., AND TANAKA, T., 1972, Multimolecular forms of pyruvate kinase from rat and other mammalian tissues. I. Electrophoretic studies, *J. Biochem.* (*Tokyo*) **71**:1043.

INAOKA, Z. Y., 1967, Significance of the so-called oval cell proliferation during azo-dye hepatocarcinogenesis, *Gann* **58**:355.

IWASAKI, T., DEMPO, K., KANEKO, A., AND ONOE, T., 1972, Fluctuations of various cell populations and their characteristics during azo-dye carcinogenesis, *Gann Monogr.* **63**:21.

JAMDAR, S. C., AND GREENGARD, O., 1970, Premature formation of glucokinase in developing rat liver, *J. Biol. Chem.* **245**:2779.

KANEKO, A., DEMPO, K., YOSHIDA, Y., CHISAKA, N., AND ONOE, T., 1974, Deviation in esterase isozyme pattern during early stage of hepatocarcinogenesis by 3'-methyl-4-dimethyl-aminoazobenzene, *Cancer Res.* **34**:1816.

KATUNUMA, N., KUTODA, Y., YOSHIDA, T., SANADA, Y., AND MORRIS, H. P., 1972, Relationship between degree of differentiation and growth rate of minimal deviation hepatomas and kidney cortex tumors studied with glutaminase isozymes, *Gann Monogr.* **13**:143.

KHOO, S. K., WAENER, N. L., LIE, J. T., AND MACKAY, I. R., 1973, Carcinoembryonic antigenic activity of tissue extracts: A quantitative study of malignant and benign neoplasms, cirrhotic liver, normal, adult and fetal organs, *Int. J. Cancer* **11**:681.

KITAGAWA, T., YOKOCHI, T., AND SUGANO, H., 1972, α-Fetoprotein and hepatocarcinogenesis in rats fed 3'-methyl-4-(dimethylamino)-azobenzene or N-2-fluoroenyl-acetamide, *Int. J. Cancer* **10**:368.

KLEMPERER, H. G., AND HAYNES, G. R., 1968, Thymidine kinase in rat liver during development, *Biochem. J.* **108**:541.

KNOX, W. E., 1972, *Enzyme Patterns in Fetal, Adult and Neoplastic Tissues*, Karger, Basel.

KROES, R., WILLIAMS, G. M., AND WEISBURGER, J. H., 1972, Early appearance of serum α-fetoprotein during hepatocarcinogenesis as a function of age of rats and extent of treatment with 3'-methyl-4-dimethylaminoazobenzene, *Cancer Res.* **32**:1526.

KROES, R., WILLIAMS, G. M., AND WEISBURGER, J. H., 1973, Early appearance of serum α-fetoprotein as a function of dosage of various hepatocarcinogens, *Cancer Res.* **33**:613.

KUPCHIK, H. Z., AND ZAMCHECK, W., 1972, Carcinoembryonic antigen(s) in liver disease. II. Isolation from human cirrhotic liver and serum and from normal liver, *Gastroenterology* **63**:101.

KUPCHIK, H. Z., ZAMCHECK, N., AND SARAVIS, C. A., 1973, Immunochemical studies on carcinoembryonic antigens: Methodologic considerations and some clinical implications, *J. Natl. Cancer Inst.* **50**:1741.

LARSSON, A., 1969, Ribonucleotide reductase from regenerating rat liver, *Eur. J. Biochem.* **11**:113.

LAURENCE, D. J. R., AND NEVILLE, M., 1972, Foetal antigens and their role in the diagnosis and clinical management of human neoplasms: A review, *Br. J. Cancer* **26**:335.

LEA, M. A., MORRIS, M. P., AND WEBER, G., Comparative biochemistry of hepatomas. VI. Thymidine incorporation into DNA as a measure of hepatoma growth rate, *Cancer Res.* **26**:465.

LIN, T., CHU, S., CHEN, M., AND CHEN, C., 1972, Serum alpha-fetoglobulin and primary cancer of the liver in Taiwan, *Cancer* **30**:435.

MACH, J. P., AND PUSZTASZERI, G., 1972, Carcinoembryonic antigen (CEA): Demonstration of partial identity between CEA and normal glycoprotein, *Immunochemistry* **9**:1031.

MALEY, F., AND MALEY, G. F., 1961, Activities of deoxycytidylate deaminase and thymidylate synthetase in normal rat livers and hepatomas, *Cancer Res.* **21**:1421.

MARKERT, C. I., 1968, Neoplasia: A disease of cell differentiation, *Cancer Res.* **28**:1908.

MARKERT, C. I., AND MOLLER, F., 1959, Multiple forms of enzymes: Tissues, ontogenetic and species specific patterns, *Proc. Natl. Acad. Sci. U.S.A.* **45**:753.

MARTIN, F., AND MARTIN, M. S., 1970, Demonstration of antigens related to colonic cancer in the human digestive system, *Int. J. Cancer* **6**:352.

MARTIN, J. P., CHARLIONNET, R., AND ROPARTZ, C., 1971, L'α₂-H sérigne au cours des hémopathies malignes et des cirrhoses. Valeur évolutive. *Presse méd.* **79**:2313.

MASSEYEFF, R., 1972, Human alpha-fetoprotein, *Pathol. Biol.* **20**:703.

MASSEYEFF, R., (ed.), 1974, *Colloquium on α-Fetoprotein*, INSERM, Paris.

MAWAS, C., BUFFE, D., AND BURTIN, P., 1970, Influence of age on α-fetoprotein incidence, *Lancet* **1**:1292.

MIN CHU, T., 1973, The clinical studies of CEA, presented at First Biological Marker Meeting (CEA) UICC, Chester Beatty Research Institute, London.

MITTELMAN, A., 1971, Patterns of isoaccepting phenylalanine transfer RNA in human leukemia and lymphoma, *Cancer Res.* **31**:647.

MORRIS, H. P., 1965, Studies on the development, biochemistry and biology of experimental hepatomas, *Adv. Cancer Res.* **9**:227.

NAYAK, W. C., CHEWLA, V., MALAVIYA, A. N., AND CHANDRA, R. K., 1972, α-Fetoprotein in Indian children's cirrhosis, *Lancet* **1**:68.

NEVILLE, A. M., AND LAURENCE, D. J. R., 1974, Report of the workshop on the carcinoembryonic antigen (CEA); the present position and proposals for future investigations, *Int. J. Cancer* **14**:1.

NUNEZ, E., SAVU, L., ENGELMAN, F., BENASSAYAG, C., CREPY, O., AND JAYLE, M. F., 1971, Identification et purification préliminaire de la foetoprotéine liant les oestrogènes dans le sérum des rats nouveau-nés, *C. R. Acad. Sci. (Paris)* **273**:245.

ONO, T., AND WEINHOUSE, S., (eds.), 1972, Isozyme and enzyme regulation in cancer, *Gann Monogr.* **13**, University of Tokyo Press.

OPOLON, P., HIRSCH-MARIE, H., GATEAU, P., AND CAROLI, J., 1973, Apparition de l'alpha-1-foetoprotéine circulante au cours de l'atrophie aiguë du foie, *Ann. Med. Interne* **124**:883.

PEARSON, G., AND FREEMAN, G., 1968, Evidence suggesting a relationship between polyoma virus-induced transplantation antigen and normal embryonic antigen, *Cancer Res.* **28**:1665.

PEROVA, S. D., AND ABELEV, G. I., 1967, Embryonal antigens in the serum of the rats, *Vop. Med. Khim.* **13**:369.

PEROVA, S. D., ELGORT, D. A., AND ABELEV, G. I., 1971, Alpha-fetoprotein in the sera of rat after partial hepatectomy, *Byull. Eksp. Biol. Med.* **3**:45.

PIERCE, G. B., 1967, Teratocarcinoma; model for a developmental concept of cancer, in: *Current Topics in Developmental Biology*, Vol. 2 (A. Monroy and A. A. Moscona, eds.), pp. 223–246, Academic Press, New York.

PIERCE, G. B., 1970, Differentiation of normal and malignant cells, *Fed. Proc.* **29**:1248.

PIHKO, M., AND RUOSLAHTI, E., 1973, High level of alpha-fetoprotein in sera of adult mice, *Int. J. Cancer* **12**:354.

POTTER, V. R., 1969, Recent trends in cancer biochemistry: The importance of studies on fetal tissue, *Can. Cancer Conf.* **8**:9.

POTTER, V. R., WALKER, P. R., AND GOODMAN, J. I., 1972, Survey of current studies on oncogeny as blocked ontogeny: Isozyme changes in livers of rats fed 3'-methyl-4-dimethylaminoazobenzene with collateral studies on DNA stability, *Gann Monogr.* **13**:121.

PURVES, L. R., BERSOHN, I., PATH, F. C., AND GEDDES, E. W., 1970, Serum alpha-fetoprotein and primary cancer of the liver in man, *Cancer* **25**:1261.

RUOSLAHTI, E., AND SEPPALA, M., 1971, Studies on carcino-fetal proteins. III. Development of a radioimmunoassay for alpha-fetoprotein in serum of healthy human adults, *Int. J. Cancer* **8**:374.

RUOSLAHTI, E., SALASPURO, M., PIHKO, H., ANDERSSON, L., AND SEPPALA, M., 1974, Serum α-fetoprotein: Diagnostic significance in liver disease, *Br. Med. J.* **393**:527.

SARCIONE, E. J., 1967, Hepatic synthesis and secretory release of plasma α$_2$ (acute phase)-globulin appearing in malignancy, *Cancer Res.* **27**:2025.

SATO, S., MATSUSHIMA, T., AND SUGIMURA, T., 1969, Hexokinase isozyme pattern of experimental hepatomas of rats, *Cancer Res.* **29**:1437.

SATO, S., KIRUCHI, Y., TAKAKURA, K., CHIEN, T. C., AND SUGIMURA, T., 1972, Diagnostic value of aldolase and hexokinase isoenzymes for human brain and uterine tumors, *Gann Monogr.* **13**:279.

SCHAPIRA, F., 1973, Isozymes and cancer, *Adv. Cancer Res.* **18**:77.

SCHAPIRA, F., AND GREGORI, C., 1971, Pyruvate kinase de l'hépatome, du placenta et du foie foetal de rat, *C. R. Acad. Sci. (Paris)* **272**:1169.

SCHAPIRA, F., AND JOSIPOWICZ, A., 1970, Anomalies de type foetal des isozymes de l'aldolase et de la lactico-deshydrogénase dans des hépatomes ascitiques, *C. R. Soc. Biol.* **164**:37.

SCHAPIRA, F., DREYFUS, J. C., AND SCHAPIRA, G., 1963, Aldolase in primary liver cancer, *Nature (London)* **200**:995.

SCHÖNE, G., 1908, cited by Alexander (1972).

SELL, S., AND MORRIS, P., 1974, Relationship of rat α$_1$-fetoprotein to growth rate and chromosome composition of Morris hepatomas, *Cancer Res.* **34**:1413.

SELL, S., NICHOLS, M., BECKER, F. F., AND LEFFERT, L., 1974, Hepatocyte proliferation and α$_1$-fetoprotein in pregnant, neonatal and partially hepatectomized rats, *Cancer Res.* **34**:865.

STANISLAWSKI-BIRENCWAJG, M., 1965, Etude immunochimique d'antigènes embryonnaires du rat, *C. R. Acad. Sci. (Paris)* **260**:364.

STANISLAWSKI-BIRENCWAJG, M., 1967, Specific antigens of rat embryonic serum, *Cancer Res.* **27**:1982.

STANISLAWSKI-BIRENCWAJG, M., URIEL, J., AND GRABAR, P., 1967, Association of embryonic antigens with experimentally induced hepatic lesions in rat, *Cancer Res.* **27**:1900.

STONEHILL, E. H., AND BENDICH, A., 1970, Retrogenic expression: The reappearance of embryonal antigens in cancer cells, *Nature (London)* **228**:370.

SUDA, M., TANAKA, T., YANACI, S., HAYASHI, S., INAMURA, K., AND TANIUCHI, K., 1972, Dedifferentiation of enzymes in the liver of tumor-bearing animals, *Gann Monogr.* **13**:79.

SUGIMURA, T., SATO, S., AND KAWABE, S., 1970, The presence of aldolase C in rat hepatoma, *Biochem. Biophys. Res. Comm.* **39**:626.

SUGIMURA, T., MATSUSHIMA, T., KAWACHI, J., KOGURE, K., TANAKA, N., MIYAKE, S., HOZUMI, M., SATO, S., AND SATO, H., 1972, Disdifferentiation and discarcinogenesis, *Gann Monogr.* **13**:31.

TANAKA, T., ANN, T., AND SAKUE, Y., 1971, Studies on multimolecular forms of phosphofructokinase in rat tissues, *J. Biochem. (Tokyo)* **69**:609.

TANAKA, T., INAMURA, K., ANN, T., AND TANIUCHI, K., 1972, Multimolecular forms of pyruvate kinase and phosphofructokinase in normal and cancer tissues, *Gann Monogr.* **13**:219.

TATARINOV, Y. S., 1964, Detection of embryo-specific α-globulin in the blood sera of patients with primary liver tumors, *Vop. Med. Khim.* **10**:90.

TEPLITZ, R. L., SANDER, B. G., BRODETZKY, A. M., FUNG, H., AND WILEY, K. L., 1974, Fetal leukemic antigen of chicken blood cells, *Cancer Res.* **34**:1049.

TRIOLO, V. A. 1965, Nineteenth century foundation of cancer research—Advances in tumor pathology: Nomenclature and theories of oncogenesis, *Cancer Res.* **25**:75.

TSUKADA, Y., WATABE, H., ISAKA, H., AND HIRAI, M., 1974, AFP production by rat ascites hepatoma cells: Cloning and cell cycle, in: *Colloque sur l'alpha-Foetoprotéine* (R. Masseyeff, ed.), pp. 521–524, INSERM, Paris.

URIEL, J., 1969, Transitory liver antigens and primary hepatoma in man and rat, *Pathol. Biol.* **17**:877.

URIEL, J., AND DE NÉCHAUD, B., 1972, La recherche d'alpha-foetoprotéine en pathologie humaine: Etat actuel de la question, *Ann. Inst. Pasteur* **122**:829.

URIEL, J., AND DE NÉCHAUD, B., 1973, An outline of the physiopathology of rat alpha-fetoprotein, *Gann Monogr.* **14**:35.

URIEL, J., DE NÉCHAUD, B., STANISLAWSKI-BIRENCWAJG, M., MASSEYEFF, R., LEBLANC, L., QUENUM, C., LOISILLIER, F., AND GRABAR, P., 1967, Antigènes embryonnaires et cancer du foie chez l'homme: Association de l'α₁-foetoprotéine sérique avec l'hépatome primaire, *C. R. Acad. Sci. (Paris)* **265**:75.

URIEL, J., DE NÉCHAUD, B., AND DUPIERS, M., 1972, Estrogen-binding properties of rat, mouse and man fetospecific serum proteins: Demonstration by immuno-autoradiographic methods, *Biochem. Biophys. Res. Comun.* **46**:1175.

URIEL, J., AUSSEL, C., BOUILLON, D., DE NÉCHAUD, B., AND LOISILLIER, F., 1973, Localization of rat liver α-foetoprotein by cell affinity labelling with tritiated oestrogens, *Nature New Biol.* **244**:190.

VILLEE, C. A., 1954, The intermediary metabolism of human fetal tissues, *Cold Spring Harbor Symp. Quant. Biol.* **19**:186.

VON KLEIST, S., AND BURTIN, P., 1969, Localisation cellulaire d'un antigène embryonnaire de tumeurs coliques humaines, *Int. J. Cancer* **4**:874.

VON KLEIST, S., CHAVANEL, G., AND BURTIN, P. 1972, Identification of an antigen from normal human tissue that cross-reacts with the carcinoembryonic antigen, *Proc. Natl. Acad. Sci. U.S.A.* **69**:2492.

WADA, T., ANZAI, T., YACHI, A., TAKAHASHI, A., AND SAKAMOTO, S., 1970, Incidences of three different fetal proteins in sera of patients with primary hepatoma, in. *Protides of the Biological Fluids*, Vol. 18 (Peeters, H., ed.), pp. 221-226, Pergamon Press, Oxford.

WALDMAN, T. A., AND MCINTIRE, K. R., 1972, Serum-alpha-fetoprotein levels in patients with ataxia-telangiectasia, *Lancet* **2**:1112.

WALKER, P. R., AND POTTER, V. R., 1972, Isozyme studies on adult, regenerating, precancerous and developing liver in relation to findings in hepatomas, *Adv. Enzyme Regul.* **10**:339.

WATABE, H., 1971, Early appearance of embryonic α-globulin in rat serum during carcinogenesis with 4-dimethylaminoazobenzene, *Cancer Res.* **31**:1192.

WEBER, G., 1966, The molecular correlation concept: Studies on the metabolic pattern of hepatomas, *Gann Monogr.* **1**:151.

WEBER, G., 1972, Molecular correlation concept: Ordered expression of gene expression in neoplasia, *Gann Monogr.* **13**:47.

WEBER, G., AND CANTERO, A., 1957, Glucose-6-phosphatase utilization in hepatoma, regenerating and newborn rat liver, and in the liver of fed and fasted normal rats, *Cancer Res.* **17:**995.

WEIMER, H. E., AND BENJAMIN, D. C., 1965, Immunochemical detection of an acute-phase protein in rat serum, *Ann. J. Physiol.* **209:**736.

WEINHOUSE, S., 1973, Metabolism and isozyme alterations in experimental hepatomas, *Fed. Proc.* **32:**2162.

WEINHOUSE, S., SHATTON, J. B., WAYNE, E. C., FARINA, F. A., AND MORRIS, H. P., 1972, Isozymes in relation to differentiation in transplantable hepatomas, *Gann Monogr.* **13:**1.

WEPSIC, H. T., AND SELL, S., 1974, α-Fetoprotein in human disease and in rat experimental models, *Oncology* (in press).

YAMADA, T., 1967, Cellular and subcellular events in Wolffian lens regeneration, in: *Current Topics in Developmental Biology*, Vol. 2 (A. Monroy and A. A. Moscona, eds.), pp. 267–283, Academic Press, New York.

YANG, W. K., 1971, Isoaccepting transfer RNA's in mammalian differentiated cells and tumor tissues, *Cancer Res.* **31:**639.

3

Ectopic Isoenzymes: Expression of Embryonic Genes in Neoplasia

WILLIAM H. FISHMAN AND ROBERT M. SINGER

1. Introduction

The emergence of the phenomenon of ectopic polypeptide hormone production by tumors as described in the next chapter has coincided with the recognition of ectopic isoenzymes in the serum and tumor tissues of human cancer patients and in experimental rodent tumors. The two phenomena are related in their significance, which is the reason for the juxtaposition of this chapter and the subsequent one.

In contrast to the recognition in 1959 of polymorphic species of enzymes termed "isozymes," only recently has there been the observation that polypeptide hormones may consist of families of isohormones. The most interesting of these to us is the case of chorionic gonadotropin, which can be distinguished from pituitary gonadotropin by virtue of its β-subunits. This distinction has made possible a radioimmunoassay technique which is specific for chorionic gonadotropin (Vaitukaitis *et al.*, 1972).

WILLIAM H. FISHMAN and ROBERT M. SINGER ● Tufts Cancer Research Center and the Department of Pathology, Tufts University School of Medicine, Boston, Massachusetts. Work was supported by Grants-in-Aid (CA-13332 and CA-12924) from the National Cancer Institute, National Institutes of Health, Bethesda, Md. W. H. F. is the recipient of Career Research Award K6-CA-18453. The support of the Tobacco Research Council is gratefully acknowledged (935-M).

WILLIAM H.
FISHMAN AND
ROBERT M. SINGER

By "ectopic isoenzymes," we principally mean those isoenzymes found in the course of embryonic development which are present in tumor tissues but not in the tissue of tumor origin.

Historically, it appears that an aldolase with the substrate specificity of muscle aldolase (fructose-1,6-diphosphate and not fructose-1-phosphate) was found in primary liver cancer by Schapira *et al.* (1963). This muscle-type aldolase is the one present in fetal liver tissues (Nordmann and Schapira, 1966). This finding was attributed to the resurgence of the fetal aldolase proteins in cancer cells at the expense of the adult liver aldolase.

Subsequent workers (Brox *et al.*, 1969; Gracey *et al.*, 1970) crystallized aldolase from Novikoff ascites hepatoma and from normal rat liver and muscle, and found identity between muscle and tumor aldolase with regard to amino acid composition and tryptic fingerprints. These and other findings (e.g., Kawabe *et al.*, 1969) have supported the original results and interpretation of the Schapira laboratory. Finally, it was recognized rather early in these studies that the reappearance of fetal forms of enzymes in cells is not necessarily specific to tumors.

The widespread adoption of electrophoretic and chromatographic techniques has brought into view isozyme species of a large number of enzymes, which do become redistributed during development and in oncogenesis. Three reviews (Criss, 1971; Schapira, 1973; Weinhouse, 1973) list these isozymes, which include oxidoreductases, such as enzymes of the glycogen cycle and of glycolysis, and a variety of hydrolases and transferases.

An example of the manner by which a key mechanism in intermediary metabolism can be seriously affected by the activation of fetal genes occurs in the glycolysis and respiration of tumor cells. Thus Weinhouse (1973) reviewed a comprehensive study of the isozymes operating during glycolysis and respiration in a series of experimental transplantable hepatomas. A common pattern was observed in the key enzymes, glucose-ATP phosphotransferases, aldolases, pyruvate kinases, and glycogen phosphorylases. In the most undifferentiated fast-growing tumors, these isozymes, characteristic of adult liver which are under host dietary and hormonal control, practically disappear. They are replaced by their fetal counterparts, which are suited for efficient utilization of metabolic fuel but are no longer subject to host regulation. At the other end of the spectrum are the minimal-deviation hepatomas, which possess an adult liver isoenzyme pattern. It is this conversion to the fetal glycolytic mechanism which mainly accounts for the high glycolytic rate of tumors first discovered by Warburg in 1930.

Aside from fetal isozymes of the glycolytic cycle, hepatomas have evidenced non-liver-type isozymes, e.g., fetal glutaminase (Katanuma *et al.*, 1972), glutamine-fructose-6-phosphate aminotransferase (Tsuiki *et al.*, 1972), fetal branched-chain aminotransferases (Ichihara and Ogawa, 1972), phosphofructokinase isozyme (Tanaka *et al.*, 1967), and ferritins (Linder *et al.*, 1970).

In terms of human cancer, fetal forms of (placental) alkaline phosphatase (Fishman *et al.*, 1968*a,b*, 1971) (Regan isoenzyme), aldolases (Schapira *et al.*, 1963;

Schapira, 1973), ferritins (Alpert *et al.*, 1973), thymidine kinase (Taylor *et al.*, 1972), and possibly histaminase (Lin *et al.*, unpublished) have been recognized. In addition, nonenzyme proteins such as α-fetoprotein (Abelev, 1971), carcinoembryonic antigen (Gold and Freedman, 1965), human chorionic gonadotropin (Braunstein *et al.*, 1973), and placental somatomammotropin (Weintraub and Rosen, 1971) are members of a rapidly lengthening list of embryonic protein phenotypes which are receiving wide attention as "markers" of malignancy.

A number of other properties both enzymic and nonenzymic are shared by embryonic and neoplastic cells. These include agglutination by plant lectins (Moscona, 1971) and presence of unique tRNA forms (Manes and Sharma, 1973; Rennert, 1971) and tRNA methyltransferases (Kerr and Borek, 1973).

The ever-increasing accumulation of findings of embryonic gene products in neoplasia coming from the areas of isoenzymes, hormones, and protein antigens is causing a reevaluation of our viewpoint on the nature of cancer. The aim in this chapter is to examine our recent experiences with the carcinoplacental antigen, Regan isoenzyme, as a model system for studying the regulation of embryonic gene expression in cancer cells, the relevance of the cell cycle, and the nature of the gene product in membranes. From such an examination, we will attempt to fit these facts with current information and to construct a perspective on the nature of cancer from the point of view of ectopic isoenzymes.

3. Regan Isoenzyme

Regan isoenzyme is a placental type of alkaline phosphatase first discovered in a patient (Mr. Regan) with metastatic bronchogenic cancer whose primary and metastatic tumor tissues contained a heat-stable, L-phenylalanine-sensitive, neuraminidase-cleavable alkaline phosphatase whose migration on starch gel electrophoresis matched that of placental alkaline phosphatase (Fishman *et al.*, 1968*a*,*b*; Kang *et al.*, 1972). Studies have appeared on the clinical significance of this Regan isoenzyme (Stolbach *et al.*, 1969; Nathanson and Fishman, 1971; Cadeau *et al.*, 1974).

The Nagao isoenzyme is another form of the Regan isoenzyme discovered in Japan by Nakayama *et al.* (1970). It has all the properties of the Regan isoenzyme with the added features of the ability to be inhibited by L-leucine and by 4.0 mM EDTA.

It now appears that the Nagao isoenzyme corresponds to the rare D-variant phenotype of human placental alkaline phosphatase, according to Inglis *et al.* (1973). They exhibit similar rates of migration on starch gel electrophoresis and both are inhibited by L-leucine. Surprisingly, the D-variant phenotype is expressed much more frequently in cancer cells exhibiting placental alkaline phosphatase, close to 50%, as compared to the incidence of this phenotype in placentas.

A hepatoma Regan variant discovered by Warnock and Reisman (1969) has been thoroughly characterized by Higashino *et al.* (1972). It has the same antigenic determinants as the placental alkaline phosphatase as well as the properties of being inhibited by L-phenylalanine but not by L-homoarginine. However, like the liver enzyme, it is more heat labile than the placental isoenzyme. The question of whether this hepatoma Regan variant is possibly composed of subunits of placenta and liver isozymes has been raised.

Human tumors frequently express non-Regan isoenzyme of alkaline phosphatase (Timperley, 1968). No evidence has yet appeared as to the possible fetal origin of this tumor isoenzyme. Also, other cancer tissues may exhibit only very low levels of alkaline phosphatase.

In ultrastructural and histochemical studies of the alkaline phosphatase isoenzymes of ovarian cancer cells, sites of enzyme activity were demonstrated in the plasma membrane, perimitochondrial endoplasmic reticulum, and lysosomes. Examples were found of cancer cells which exhibited only Regan isoenzyme, non-Regan isoenzyme, or a mixture of both (Sasaki and Fishman, 1973).

Regan isoenzyme can be detected with current methodology in the serum of one of seven cancer patients (Stolbach *et al.*, 1969; Nathanson and Fishman, 1971), with respect to a large variety of tumors. The highest incidence continues to be in ovarian and other gynecological cancers (Cadeau *et al.*, 1974). It is of interest that proliferative conditions predisposing to or accompanying cancer are associated on occasion with elevated serum Regan isoenzyme and that trace amounts of the isoenzyme occur in the nondiseased population (Inglis *et al.*, 1971; Usategui-Gomez *et al.*, 1973).

4. Model System for the Study of Gene Expression in Cancer Cells

Systematic study of the factors which control the expression of Regan isoenzyme was initiated with the finding that HeLa cells produce the placental form of alkaline phosphatase (Fishman *et al.*, 1968a; Elson and Cox, 1969; Bottomley *et al.*, 1969). Since HeLa cells are derived from cervical cancer, the placental-type Regan isoenzyme is considered ectopic in that population.

It has been shown that HeLa cells (Portelius *et al.*, 1960) and other human and animal cell lines (Maio and DeCarli, 1962) demonstrate heterogeneity with respect to alkaline phosphatase. This heterogeneity is apparent as variation in the levels of alkaline phosphatase activity as well as the isoenzymic forms produced by different cells of a given population, as will now be described.

To investigate the nature of gene expression of the Regan isoenzyme in culture, HeLa cells were cloned and a subline (TCRC-1) was selected which produced only the Regan isoenzyme (Singer and Fishman, 1974). Another cell line cloned by Dr. Rustigian (TCRC-2) (Rustigian *et al.*, 1974) was shown to produce only non-Regan alkaline phosphatase.

These cells were found to be distinct from each other in several other properties. Prednisolone in the culture medium was found to enhance the alkaline phosphatase activity in the HeLa TCRC-1 cells, but had no effect on HeLa TCRC-2. Additionally, β-glucuronidase, an enzyme whose existence in neoplastic tissue is well known (Fishman *et al.*, 1959; Watta and Goldberg, 1969), is fivefold higher in HeLa TCRC-1 than in TCRC-2.

A property exclusively found in HeLa TCRC-1 is the ability to synthesize ferritin when grown in the presence of iron. HeLa TCRC-2 is unable to grow in the presence of iron (unpublished findings). Further study using isoelectric focusing revealed that the ferritin produced by HeLa TCRC-1 is made up of variant isoferritins which are similar to those of the placenta, hepatoma, and fetal liver cells (Drysdale and Singer, 1974). It was thus shown that this isoferritin in HeLa cells is a carcinofetal form.

It is apparent that although HeLa TCRC-1 was selected for high levels of the Regan isoenzyme there appear to be several other cancer-related gene products associated with this cell line. Using this cell line as our model, we are studying the regulation of the expression of the Regan isoenzyme, as well as other cancer-related proteins.

5. Regulation of Carcinoembryonic Isoenzymes of Alkaline Phosphatase

Corticoid-hormone-induced alterations of isoenzyme profiles of alkaline phosphatase have been observed by several investigators. Beckman and Regan (1964), using RA human amnion cells, found an alteration in the zymogram pattern on starch gel electrophoresis in cells grown in the presence of cortisone. These investigators found that the synthesis of a fast-moving enzyme form was prevented, while that of a slower enzyme form was increased. Griffin and Bottomley (1969) found using acrylamide gel electrophoresis that growth in medium containing hydrocortisone caused the appearance of a new isozyme form. Later studies revealed that this new enzyme form was a function of the degree of confluency of the culture rather than of the effect of hormone treatment. Hormone-mediated alterations in isozymes of alkaline phosphatase have also been demonstrated by Spencer (1970), which were most apparent when cells were grown in calf serum rather than fetal calf serum.

A study by Herz (1973) attempted to further characterize the differential effect of hyperosmolarity and prednisolone on the isozymic forms of alkaline phosphatase in KB cells. Although both treatments caused a decease in enzyme activity, a transition of activity occurred whereby the predominantly heat-labile form present diminished while a relatively heat-stable form was elevated.

In these previous studies, the identity of the various isozyme bands was not established. The first characterization of the isozyme alteration in prednisolone-treated cultures was undertaken by Singer and Fishman (1975). Using disc gel electrophoresis (L. Fishman, 1974), they examined the isozyme profile of alkaline phosphatase in four human cell lines treated with prednisolone. The cell lines included HeLa TCRC-1, a cell line monophenotypic for the Regan isozyme, HeLa TCRC-2, monophenotypic for the non-Regan alkaline phosphatase, and FL amnion and HEp-2 cell lines. The HeLa TCRC-1 alkaline phosphatase is inducible by prednisolone, and its single-band isozyme profile is unaltered,

TABLE 1
Properties of Cell Lines

Cell line	Specific activity[a] (μmol/min/mg)	Percent inhibition by L-phenylalanine	Percent residual enzyme activity after 5 min at 65°C
HeLa TCRC-1	0.83	76.7	91.5
+ prednisolone	1.53	76.5	94.2
HeLa TCRC-2	1.4	0	0
+ prednisolone	1.7	—	2.6
HEp-2	3.47	70.5	80.7
+ prednisolone	3.61	68.7	80.8
FL amnion	1.59	77.6	51.6
+ prednisolone	2.04	79.1	57.4

[a] Values after 96 h in culture, hormone having been introduced after 24 h.

whereas the HeLa TCRC-2 enzyme is unaffected by prednisolone in levels of activity or its single-band isozyme profile (see Table 1).

The FL amnion and HEp-2 cell lines were shown to have an altered isoenzyme profile after hormone treatment (see Fig. 1). As shown in Fig. 2, each of these cell lines had an intestinal alkaline phosphatase component, as determined by biochemical and immunological criteria, which was found to be diminished by hormone treatment. Additionally, the HEp-2 cell line had a Regan band which was increased in activity by treatment. The FL amnion cell prior to hormone treatment had no enzyme activity at the Regan position; however, hormone treatment caused the appearance of an enzyme band at the Regan position, which was shown to be the Regan isoenzyme. From these data, we conclude that the regulation of alkaline phosphatase in these cell lines results from specific inverse alteration of the relative activities of the various isozyme forms.

In examining the possible explanations for the totally different responsiveness of TCRC-1 and TCRC-2 cells to prednisolone, we offer the speculation that perhaps TCRC-1 possesses corticoid hormone cell surface receptors which TCRC-2 lacks, the two lines differing in the length of compartments of the cell cycle (see below). The dependence of the expression of hormone receptors on cell cycle has been reported for melanocyte-stimulating hormone (Varga *et al.*, 1974). Additionally, the admission of prednisolone to the cell may alter the cell cycle in such a way that there is prolongation of the interval during which Regan isoenzyme is expressed.

6. Membrane-Derived Multienzyme Complexes

The ectopic Regan isoenzyme has been associated with the plasma membrane of HeLa cells (Fig. 3) and with the microsomal fraction in homogenates of these cells (Singer *et al.*, 1974). The possibility that membrane-derived aggregates of such

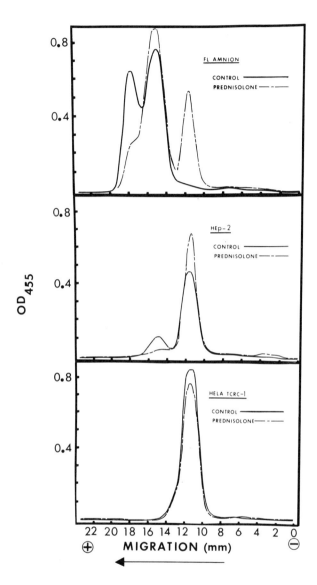

FIGURE 1. Gel scans of polyacrylamide electrophoresis of FL amnion, HEp-2, and HeLa TCRC-1 showing the alteration in isoenzyme profiles after growth in prednisolone (72 h). Reproduced from *Isozymes; Developmental Biology,* Academic Press, with the permission of Dr. C. L. Markert, Editor.

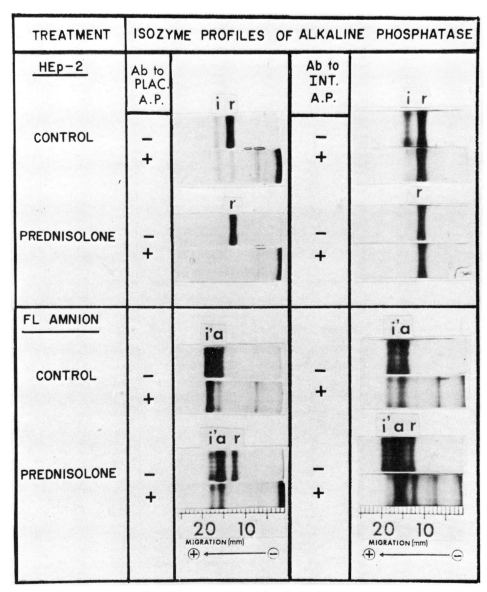

TREATMENT	ISOZYME PROFILES OF ALKALINE PHOSPHATASE			

FIGURE 2. Polyacrylamide disc gel isozyme profiles. Specific antisera to placental and to intestinal alkaline phosphatase were mixed separately with the specimen prior to application to the gel. The test of immunological reaction is the retardation of migration of the antigen–antibody complex, which usually exhibits enzyme activity. The anodal fast band of the HEp-2 control (*i*) is prevented from entering the gel or from migrating to the expected band position in the presence of antisera prepared against intestinal alkaline phosphatase. The slower band of activity (*r*) is not affected by this antisera; however, it is completely and specifically immobilized by antisera against placental alkaline phosphatase. After hormone treatment, the fast band disappears and only the slow-moving Regan band (*r*) is present. The double-banded isozyme profile of the FL amnion control (*i'* and *a*) is converted by hormone treatment ot a triple-banded profile due to the appearance of a slower band (*r*) whose migration distance is identical to that of the slower band of the HEp-2 cell line (*r*). The hormone caused the disappearance of the fastest band of activity (*i'*). This band cross-reacted with the antisera to intestinal alkaline phosphatase and did not enter the gel. The newly appearing slow band (*r*) cross-reacted with antisera to placental alkaline phosphatase. The intermediate band (*a*) of the hormone-treated FL amnion cell line partially cross-reacted with both intestinal and placental antisera.

plasma membrane enzymes are shed into the circulation has been suggested in recent publications.

Thus an observation by Dymling (1966) of an alkaline phosphatase which is excluded from Sephadex G200 in the serum of a patient with biliary occlusion has been pursued as a possible indicator of disease states. Further studies by Dunne *et al.* (1967) using gel filtration revealed elevated levels of a macromolecular alkaline phosphatase in the serum of patients with malignant bone conditions, metastatic malignant liver disease, and nonmalignant liver disease. It was suggested that this

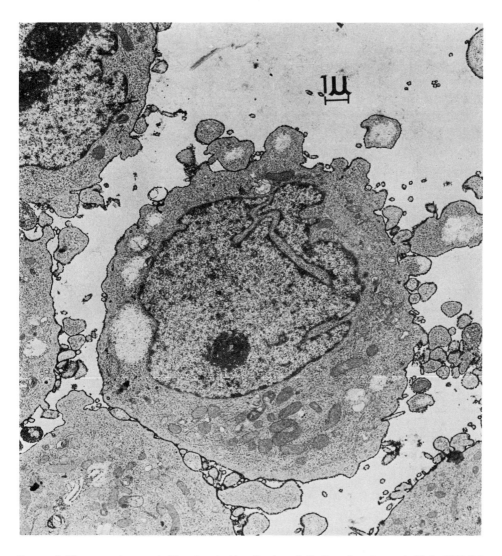

FIGURE 3. Electron microscopic histochemical localization of alkaline phosphatase in HeLa TCRC-1 using the method of Hugon and Borgers (1966). Enzyme activity is found to be associated with the plasma membrane.

enzyme form was a lipoprotein complex, a view supported by Jennings *et al.* (1970), who found that *n*-butanol extraction of the 19 S macromolecular enzyme form resulted in the movement of the enzyme activity to the 7 S position on starch gel electrophoresis (Jennings *et al.*, 1970).

Shinkai and Akedo (1972) discovered a lipid–protein complex in the serum of hepatic cancer patients that contains five marker enzymes of the plasma membrane. The enzymes in this multienzyme complex include alkaline phosphatase, Mg^{2+}:adenosinetriphosphatase, Na^+:K^+:Mg^{2+}:adenosinetriphosphatase, L-leucyl-β-naphthylamidase, and 5′-nucleotidase. This complex was found to have antigenic determinants similar to those of the liver plasma membrane, and is believed to be a plasma membrane fragment released from the liver of patients with hepatobiliary disease, including hepatic cancer. Later studies by Fritsche and Adams-Park (1974) revealed in the serum of patients with neoplastic or obstructive liver disease the presence of isoenzymic forms of alkaline phosphatase whose molecular weights were higher than those present in liver, bone, and intestine. They believe that isoenzyme analysis of these high molecular weight enzymes will be helpful in the differential diagnosis of liver and hepatobiliary disease.

A similar form of macromolecular alkaline phosphatase has been identified in ascites fluids from ovarian cancer patients (Doellgast and Fishman, 1975). It has been shown that the amount of this form of the enzyme increases during the course of the disease.

It seems clear that this high molecular weight multienzyme complex with some properties of plasma membrane may be released during a disease state by injured or dying cells. Singer *et al.* (unpublished data) recently examined the medium of human cancer cells grown in culture for the presence of a macromolecular alkaline phosphatase. Using exclusion from a Sepharose 4B column as the criterion to define this enzyme form, they discovered that it is released along with leucine aminopeptidase, a plasma membrane enzyme (Coleman and Fineman, 1966) into cultured human cell medium. The release of this heavy molecular weight form of alkaline phosphatase appears to be dependent on high cell density and lowered calcium in the medium. Additionally, the amount of this enzyme form in the medium increased directly as the number of nonviable floating cells increased. It is hoped that further study of this phenomenon may result in the development of a model system for the study of the clinical significance of this high molecular weight alkaline phosphatase.

7. The Cell Cycle

7.1. Synthesis of DNA, RNA, Protein, and Enzymes

The concept of the cell cycle as we now understand it is due to the work and interpretation by Howard and Pelc (1951), who illustrated the significance of the interphase nucleus, which was previously thought of as a resting step. They determined that nuclear DNA replication was accomplished during a discrete period of interphase, which was denoted as the S period. The postmitotic interval before S was called the G_1 period, and the interval after S and before mitosis the G_2 period. The cell cycle was thus defined on the basis of nuclear DNA replication.

Since the work of Howard and Pelc, many techniques have been developed which refine the experimental approach. For example, Quastler and Sherman (1959) determined duration of the compartments of the cell cycle by use of a single pulse of tritiated thymidine and subsequent observation of labeled mitoses. The pattern of appearance and disappearance of labeled mitoses was used to estimate the duration of the compartments of the cell cycle.

Variable rates of protein and RNA synthesis occur throughout the cell, not being confined to any single interval as has been found for DNA replication. Protein synthesis has been shown to vary during the cell cycle, and comparisons have been made between different stages of the cycle (Kolodny, 1969; Kolodny and Gross, 1969). Study of RNA has revealed that levels of synthesis of these macromolecules also fluctuate throughout the cell cycle (Rusch, 1969; Donnelly and Sisken, 1967; Killander and Zetterberg, 1965; Cummins, 1968).

As a consequence of RNA and protein synthesis, it is not surprising that the activity of many enzymes also fluctuates during the cell cycle. These include lactate dehydrogenase (Klevecz, 1969), thymidine kinase (Brent *et al.*, 1965; Littlefield, 1966), ornithine transaminase (Volpe, 1969), tyrosine aminotransferase, glucose-6-phosphate dehydrogenase, alcohol dehydrogenase (Martin *et al.*, 1969), and acid phosphatase (Kapp and Okada, 1972).

7.2. Role of Cell Cycle in Gene Expression

Therefore, it seems apparent that to the extent that alterations in growth kinetics occur in tumors one can expect to observe cell-cycle-dependent changes in levels and activities of certain tumor enzymes. This view is one of the tenets of this chapter.

A possible role the cell cycle may play is in the control of the opportunity for gene expression depending on the duration of each phase of the cycle. For example, it has been shown that α_1-fetoprotein, an oncofetal protein associated with malignancy of the liver (Abelev, 1971) is synthesized and secreted into the medium by cultured fetal rat hepatocytes as a function of the growth rate as well as of the position of the hepatocyte in the cell cycle (Leffert and Sell, 1974). Since normal cells may demonstrate an orderly sequence of enzyme synthesis and activity, it would also be expected that a stable population of malignant cells would also have an orderly sequence which, if it were delayed in the α-fetoprotein-producing compartment, would result in the production of abnormal amounts of this embryonic protein.

The relationship of the cell cycle to hormone induction of alkaline phosphatase has been demonstrated by Griffin and Ber (1969). These investigators discovered that glucocorticoid induction is initiated during the S phase of the cell cycle. They postulate the presence of a hormone receptor site during DNA replication (mention may again be made of the studies of Varga et al., 1974, on the MSH receptors appearing in the G_2 phase of melanocytes). This phenomenon is believed to be responsible for the extensive lag periods between addition of hormones and induction of alkaline phosphatase.

Since Singer and Fishman (1975) have shown that hormone induction of alkaline phosphatase is specific for the Regan isoenzyme, and Griffin and Ber (1969) have shown that hormone induction is cell cycle dependent, it is clear that the hormonal regulation of this carcinoplacental Regan isoenzyme may be a cell-cycle related event. Using our monophenotypic cell lines, we are presently pursuing this question.

Finally, an interesting correlation of enzymic phosphorylation of histones with the events of cell replication and tumor growth has been recently reported. Thus Balhorn et al. (1972) demonstrated a correlation between phosphorylation of the lysine-rich F1 histone fraction and growth rates of tumors. Further studies by Gurley et al. (1974) indicated that phosphorylation of histone F1 is the earliest biochemical event observed when nondividing cells in G_1 arrest are allowed to divide. This occurs during the late G_1 period of the cell cycle of cells traversing into the S phase. Also, the F3 and a subfraction of F1 histone were found to be rapidly phosphorylated at the time when cells were crossing the G_2/M boundary. Of particular interst to us is the finding by Lake (1973) of two classes of phosphokinase which apparently differ in activity during the cell cycle. Using Chinese hamster cells, he identified the histone phosphokinases KI and KII. These two major phosphokinase activities differ biochemically by several criteria. Phosphokinase KII was found to be the predominating activity in cells arrested at mitosis. It is concluded that the histone phosphorylation occurring in mitotic arrested cells is qualitatively and quantitatively distinct from that which occurs throughout interphase of the cell cycle.

7.3. Comments on Cell Cycle and Growth Rate of Tumors

The growth rate of tumors in general is not unique and distinct compared to normal tissue. High levels of proliferation associated with fast-growing tumors are also found in rapidly renewing normal tissue (i.e., lung, cornea, duodenal crypt epithelium). Similarly, slow-growing tumors may have growth characteristics which are comparable to those of slowly expanding normal tissue (i.e., liver, kidney). In a previous review by Baserga (1965), it was pointed out that the cell cycle time of fast-growing experimental tumors may in fact be longer than the cycle time of some normal tissues. Thus there does not appear to be a tumor-specific cell cycle kinetic pattern, and other additional parameters are important in tumor growth.

Although there are exceptions (Killmann et al., 1963), certain populations of tumor cells usually demonstrate a shorter cell cycle than the cells from which they originated (Bresciani, 1968). This phenomenon indicates that tumor cells are progressing through the biochemical pathways involved in cell division faster than their surrounding normal counterparts.

Other factors which play a role in tumor growth include the size of the proliferation fraction and the degree of cell loss. The proliferation fraction, originally named by Mendelsohn (1962), is the fraction of proliferating cells in a given cell population. Several investigations have attempted to determine the kinetics of tumor growth in humans (Bennington, 1969; Young and DeVita, 1970; Muggia and DeVita, 1972). The problem which was encountered was the variety of growth patterns throughout the tumors. In squamous carcinoma of the human cervix, for example, the majority of cells synthesizing DNA are at the periphery of the nodule (Bennington, 1969). The rationale of these types of studies is to predict the usefulness of chemotherapy, and to follow the effectiveness of treatment.

8. Discussion

This chapter has given us an opportunity to critically evaluate present and previous concepts of the significance of ectopic isoenzymes, hormones, and antigens with their potential importance in cancer etiology. These concepts will be discussed in relation to the question "Is the selective activation of embryonic genes a necessary step in neoplastic transformation?"—which is defined as the central question of our interdisciplinary research effort.

What is meant by "activation of embryonic genes"? The product of any gene is thought of as a specific protein which may be recognizable as an isoenzyme, polypeptide hormone, binding protein, or antigen. The detection in any cell or secretion of the product of genes which function in embryonic life would be evidence of embryonic gene activation. By "embryonic life," we mean the period beginning with the union of the gametes and ending with parturition of a full-term viable individual. *In this meaning, "embryonic" is used in a generic sense to include all gestational tissues such as blastocyst, embryo, fetus, placenta, amniotic membranes and fluid, and cord blood.* If it is not possible to distinguish an adult gene product from an embryonic gene product, then such a protein albeit in the adult is designated embryonic. An example of persistence of cells with certain embryonic phenotypes in the adult is the case of the calcitonin-producing C-cells of the APUD system.

What is the reason for using the term "activation" rather than "derepression"? Admittedly, there is a tendency to accept the Jacob–Monod negative-control model of gene expression worked out for prokaryotic organisms as the mechanism which operates in the regulation of genes in mammalian cells. In this conception, gene expression follows the removal of a specific repressor protein from the DNA locus in a sequence termed "derepression." In the absence of convincing evidence for derepression in eukaryotic cells and in the presence of known complicated nuclear and cytoplasmic sequences of transmission of genetic information to the ribosomal site of specific protein synthesis, it is more appropriate to employ the term "activation" in describing the event of gene expression.

How does one define "selective activation"? In this connection, one should consider the possibility not only of the activation of single genes but also of *sets of genes* during neoplastic transformation. Evidence for phase-specific gene activation during early embryonic development has been reviewed by Manes (1974), and the identification of phase-related patterns of CEA in colon cancer has been made by Rule and Goleski-Reilly (1974). It is entirely possible that in anaplastic cancer cells both single genes and multiple sets of genes are activated simultaneously.

What is "a necessary step"? Here, we are trying to distinguish a simple manifestation of neoplasia from one that includes an etiological role in neoplasia of one or several of its constituent components. An example of a simple manifestation is pleomorphism. It is a visible characteristic of malignant cells; yet, in itself, this condition is not understood to be "a necessary step" in neoplastic transformation. Likewise, an invisible neoplastic phenomenon, anaerobic glycolysis, may represent only the product of the metabolic machinery of the cancer cell and not be the instrument for maintaining its autonomy of growth. However, because of the predominant role of fetal isoenzymes in the glycolytic cycle of cancer cells, anaerobic glycolysis may be due in large measure to the activation of embryonic genes. It is also reasonable to suggest that, because of their independence of host control mechanisms, embryonic forms of such enzymes may be fitted best for sustaining the rapid growth of embryos, and so the appearance of fetal glycolytic isoenzymes in neoplasia may constitute an essential step in tumor maintenance.

We are also considering the possibilities that (1) the activation of certain embryonic genes, individually or in sets, may constitute one of the necessary steps, but that these steps may have to be evidenced in a certain sequence to lead to an *irreversible* state of neoplasia; (2) the activation of embryonic genes unrelated to those required for the essential steps could well have a controlling or permissive role in furthering malignant change; and (3) the transforming genes of virus may be identical to certain genes of embryogenesis, as suggested by Comings (1973).

How does one define "neoplastic transformation"? This is not difficult to observe in the natural history of a number of spontaneous tumors in animals and in humans such as the cellular events which precede the recognition of carcinoma *in situ* of the skin or cervix. Also, the hyperplastic C cells in the thyroid may be considered the precursors of medullary thyroid carcinoma. One also must be aware of the clinical and laboratory experiences of reversibility of neoplastic transformation, phenomena which have been reported, for example, in hormone-induced neoplasms and in virus-transformed cells growing in culture (revertants).

It is in the realm of the *in vitro* cell culture systems that neoplastic transformation may have several end points depending on the purpose of the experiment. For example, loss of contact inhibition and change in cell morphology are convenient properties of transformed cells for the investigator, provided that it is recognized that these cells may or may not be able to grow into autonomous tumors in animals. If one knows of particular gene products unique to the neoplastic cell which will grow in experimental animals, then their appearance in cells growing in culture could constitute direct evidence of complete transformation. A transformed cell is defined as one which will grow into a tumor when injected into a suitable animal.

Our attention must extend beyond the study of transformation to the mechanisms which control the *reversibility* of transformation and then to the examination of embryonic phenotypes in the spontaneous cancer of humans and of experimental animals. It is entirely possible that certain of the embryonic genes will be expressed during transformation, but will be inactive in neoplasia and *vice versa*.

8.1. Relationship Between Embryology and Oncology

Anomalous developmental differentiation and neoplasia have long been regarded by some as two extremes of the same spectrum with teratocarcinoma somewhere in the middle (Schwalbe, 1907; Witschi, 1952). Thus the stage at which the developmental mishap occurs will determine the abnormality, ranging from identical twins and conjoined twins on the one hand to teratomas, mixed tumors, and benign or malignant tumors on the other hand.

Embryonic and neoplastic cells share the characteristics of repeatedly undergoing cell divisions and of the ability to migrate to tissue sites other than their origin.

Aside from cell division and cell migration, the products of embryonic genes do have other profound biological consequences. For example, low molecular weight inducers have a role in the development of metanephric mesenchyme in mammals and birds, and individual proteins have been observed (Witschi, 1952; Toivonen, 1950; Toivonen *et al.*, 1961; Tiedemann, 1959) to either induct muscle and connective tissue or to direct presumptive ectoderm to develop the anterior brain. Maternal steroid hormones act as inducers in the embryonic differentiation of gonads (Wolff and Ginglinger, 1935). Also, evidence has been reported linking the injection of natural and synthetic estrogens into pregnant mothers with the later appearance of adenocarcinomas of vagina and endometrium of their young female offspring (Tiedemann and Tiedemann, 1964).

With regard to the biological potency of embryonic gene products, Lasfargues *et al.* (1974) reported that the spent medium collected from cultures of human embryonic cells contains mitogenic factors which stimulate rapid multiplication of human breast carcinoma cells *in vitro*.

Aside from embryonic mitogenic factors, it appears that a single embryonic gene product can be responsible for a multitude of alterations in the cell in which it appears and in neighbouring cells.

Thus a tumor-specific plasminogen activator produced by transformed chicken embryo fibroblasts (Unkeless *et al.*, 1974) has been shown to cause morphological changes in normal untransformed cells cocultivated with these transformed cells (Ossowski *et al.*, 1974). This plasminogen-activator factor has been observed in a human cancer patient (Davidson *et al.*, 1969) and its production has been shown to be associated with transformation *in vitro* by either DNA or RNA viruses (Reich, 1973).

8.2. Are Viral Transforming Genes Embryonic in Origin?

Viral transforming genes are defined (Comings, 1973) as the genes that code for factors that bring about neoplastic cell transformation. If it can be shown that these genes are identical to the normal ones which are responsible for the specific events of embryogenesis, then oncogenic viruses can be easily fitted into the view of loss of regulatory control of expression of normal genes in relation to neoplasia.

Some circumstantial evidence in favor of the embryonic origin of virus is as follows. Kang and Temin (1972) detected reverse transcriptase activity in chicken embryos which has a great specificity for a particular cellular RNA. Later, Temin and Mizutani (1972) demonstrated a close serological relation between normal chick embryo DNA polymerase and a new avian oncornavirus, reticuloendotheliosis virus. (These data have led Temin to postulate that perhaps all oncornaviruses originated from normal cellular components. Could these be embryonic?) Baluda (1972) demonstrated homology of DNA segments between normal chick cells and tumor virus. Subak-Scharpe (1969) observed that the dinucleotide profile of tumor viruses resembles that of mammalian DNA. Finally, C-type virus particles have been demonstrated in placental and fetal tissues (Schidlovsky and Ahmed, 1973; Vernon *et al.*, 1973; Chase and Pikó, 1973) and these are not expressed in adult life, suggesting a turning-off of the virus genes in adult tissues.

Most recently, Ahmed *et al.* (1974) developed a rhesus placental cell line which produces two kinds of virus, Mason-Pfizer and C type. These viruses contain a reverse transcriptase that can utilize endogenous template or poly $\cdot$ rA $\cdot$ (dT) in the presence of Mg^{2+} ion. Does this mean that these viruses are products of normal embryonic development and does it follow that the activation of virus production and the activation of embryonic genes are equivalent in biological terms?

8.3. Normal Host Genes

As a rule, products of many normal host nonembryonic genes are persistently expressed in neoplasia—for example, acid phosphatase in prostatic carcinoma and melanin in melanoma.

However, there are a number of tumors which express the phenotype of tissues other than the one from which the tumor developed. For example, carcinoma of the lung has been reported to exhibit on occasion a variety of polypeptide hormones such as ACTH, ADH, erythropoietin, MSH, chorionic gonadotropin, and placental somatomammotropin. The last two phenotypes have been proven to be embryonic ones, a fact which suggests the possibility that the others may be, also.

Accordingly, we see an equilibrium in the expression of embryonic and adult host genes which can move in the direction of neoplastic transformation or can operate in the direction of the normal cell phenotypes.

Neoplastic transformation may then be regarded as an anomaly of gene expression, with the turning-off of genes coding for proteins of adult differentiated tissue simultaneously with the turning-on of embryonic genes which are normally inactivated. These gene products may, in turn, exert profound influences on the cells' cycle of division and replication just as in embryonic cells, and, in particular combinations, lead to a persistent state of malignancy.

8.4. Oncogenic Mechanisms

Current oncogenic mechanisms will now be reviewed briefly in order to place into perspective the possible role of embryonic genes in neoplastic transformation.

Both of the mechanisms based on *deletion or change in DNA* are developments of the concept of somatic cell mutation, and *the acquisition of new genetic information* is a view stemming from studies on oncogenic viruses.

It must be admitted that the somatic cell mutation theory (Boveri, 1929) appears to have reached the limit of its ability to advance our understanding of cancer much further. Thus the three types of evidence on which the theory is based each have an underlying uncertainty.

For example, chromosomal anomalies are supposed to be frequently associated with malignancy, yet no consistent karyotypic patterns are common to cancer cells. In fact, in cancer one observes the usual aneuploidy and karyotypic variability as well as a significant number of normal diploid karyotypes (Hauschka, 1961; Banerjee and DeOme, 1963). Chromosome breakage induced by chemicals, X-irradiation, and viruses has been suggested (Nichols *et al.*, 1967) as a common etiological event in oncogenesis, but these breaks may well be the consequence of neoplasia. An exception to karyotypic variability in cancer is the G-group Philadelphia chromosome, which is a specific marker for chronic myelocytic leukemia (Tjio *et al.*, 1966), the etiological significance of which still remains in doubt.

Also, the correlations described earlier between mutagenicity and carcinogenicity are now found to be less convincing (Burdett, 1955) and a lack of parallelism is often observed even with X-irradiation (Brues, 1954). Moreover, it has been proposed (Nordling, 1953) that at least seven successive mutations are necessary for a fully autonomous cancer to develop, a process that would require a highly specific targeting of the mutational agents. Such an ordered process is out of character with the great variability in phenotype which characterizes cancer cells.

That mutations may result in the deletion of specific proteins or enzymes essential for the control of growth has been an idea popular with cancer biochemists (Miller and Miller, 1966; Potter, 1958; Pitot and Heidelberger, 1963). The consequence would be unregulated cell growth. However, when a complement of chromosomes of a normal cell is introduced into a cancer cell by somatic cell hybridization, supposedly correcting the deletion, the resulting hybrid still produces a tumor in animals (Davidson and Ephrussi, 1965). Alternatively, other investigators postulate that these tumors appear in the host only when the portion of genome carrying information preventing the development of the malignant state is lost from such hybrids (Defendi *et al.*, 1967). Also, the fact that so many examples now exist of tumor cells which progress in experimental and clinical situations to a completely normal benign phenotype militates against accepting somatic cell mutation as the *sine qua non* of neoplasia, a view which is emphasized by Braun (1969). Finally, one would expect to find many proteins which were the product of neoplastic (mutated?) cell genes to be chemically and physically different from their counterparts derived from nonmutated genes. No evidence of such major differences is known to us. However, the only course left is to assume that mutation of *regulatory genes* rather than structural genes could be the event of significance.

The acquisition of new genetic information is a concept associated with the role of both DNA and RNA oncogenic viruses in neoplastic transformation.

In the case of DNA virus, neoplastic transformation has been accomplished with purified viral DNA (DiMayorca *et al.*, 1959), and the continued presence of the viral genome has been demonstrated in the form of T antigen and TSTA cell-surface antigen (Sjogren *et al.*, 1961; Habel, 1961). SV40 contains enough genetic information to code for six to eight polypeptides. One-half to two-thirds of this information is required to specify virion proteins. The remainder may specify the cell-surface TSTA and intranuclear T antigen among other proteins.

With regard to RNA viruses, the Rous sarcoma virus (RSV) genome is believed to code for the production of at least 25 new proteins (Braun, 1969). That the viral genome may be integrated into host cell chromosomal DNA is an interesting interpretation of Temin's work (1963, 1964), in which he showed that a small region of a DNA chain from RSV-infected cells is complementary to RSV RNA.

From the knowledge that DNA and RNA viruses are capable of producing such a small fraction of the proteins of the cancer cell, it follows that quantitatively the manifestations of cancer can be attributed to host nonviral gene products. Does the viral genome function as a template for the synthesis of *new* products which produce and maintain neoplasia? This is the central question of the oncogene hypothesis, which is still being examined, a corollary of which is that the new products cause a persistent activation of the host genome directing cell growth and division. One may also ask in what sense are the products *new*? Are they new in the sense that embryonic proteins are new to an adult host cell?

The loss of regulatory control of expression of host genes is the third possible oncogenic mechanism which deserves attention. This does not imply necessarily that the nuclear DNA is the sole site of regulatory control, but the idea can include extrachromosomal epigenetic loci. In any case, it is widely accepted that the bulk of the normal cell's genetic information is not expressed and that cellular differentiation endows each cell type with a set of activated genes which code for the products which characterize that cell type.

In cancer, the expression in cancer cells of embryonic genes in the form of specific fetal proteins is evidence of a loss of regulatory control. To some investigators, however, this appearance of embryonic gene products is an event of vital importance with regard to the etiology of cancer.

According to Beard (1902) and Manes (1974), the trophoblast cell possesses the important specifications of the neoplastic cell—for example, its ability to invade the endometrium, to resist immune rejection by the host, to evoke an angiogenesis response, and to share common surface antigens. Moreover, A- and C-type particles have been demonstrated in the rabbit blastocyst, with a concentration of C-type particles in the trophoblast cells. If it is assumed that such viral particles are normal gene products of the earliest events of embryogenesis, then there is no need to consider a separate theory for virus etiology of cancer. All oncogenic agents such as viruses, chemicals, and X-irradiation are thus considered to interrupt the controls of gene regulation to an extent which permits the expression of the genetic information usually required for normal placentation. In this connection, the recognition of three placental proteins associated with human lung carcinoma is suggestive (Charles *et al.*, 1973).

It is perhaps too early to rule out a role for the embryoblast which might be synergistic to that of the trophoblast, particularly since the two are so interdependent.

The most attractive feature of the view that cancer may be a disease of loss of control of embryonic gene activation is the prospect it offers for the design and execution of pertinent experiments.

9. Conclusions

Ectopic isoenzymes, present in tumor tissues but not in the tissue of tumor origin, are predominantly embryonic in type. The Regan- and non-Regan-isoenzyme-producing HeLa cells provide a suitable model system for the study of a variety of factors which are involved in the expression of ectopic isoenzymes of the carcinoembryonic category. Information on cell cycle and hormonal regulation of embryonic gene expression in cancer cells may contribute to our understanding of the role of this phenomenon in the process of neoplastic transformation which may reflect a disorder of gene regulation with the reappearance of properties of the trophoblast. Such traits evidenced by transforming cells may be a consequence of whatever oncogenic agent (chemicals, radiation, viruses) produces a specific loss of regulatory control of embryonic genes.

10. References

ABELEV, C. I., 1971, Alpha-fetoprotein in ontogenesis and its association with malignant tumors, *Adv. Cancer Res.* **14**:295.

AHMED, M., MARTIN, D., YEH, J., SCHIDLOVSKI, G., KOROL, W., AND MAYYASI, S., 1974, Biological characterization of oncornaviruses present in rhesus placental cultures, *Proc. 65th Ann. Meet. Am. Assoc. Cancer Res.* **15**:44.

ALPERT, E., COSTON, R. C., AND DRYSDALE, J. E., 1973, Carcino-foetal human liver ferritins, *Nature (London)* **242**:194.

BALHORN, R., BALHORN, M., MORRIS, H. P., AND CHALKLEY, R., 1972, Comparative high resolution eletrophoresis of tumor histones: Variation in phosphorylation as a function of cell replication rate, *Cancer Res.* **32:**1775.

BALUDA, M. A., 1972, Widespread presence, in chickens, of DNA complementary to the RNA genome of avian leukosis viruses, *Proc. Natl. Acad. Sci. U.S.A.* **69:**576.

BANERJEE, M. R., AND DEOME, K. B., 1963, Chromosomes in normal, preneoplastic, and neoplastic tissues of the mammary glands of C3H/CRgl female mice, *Cancer Res.* **23:**546.

BASERGA, R., 1965, The relationship of the cell cycle to tumor growth and control of cell division: A review, *Cancer Res.* **25:**581.

BEARD, J., 1902, Embryological aspects and etiology of carcinoma, *Lancet* **1:**1758.

BECKMAN, L., AND REGAN, J. D., 1964, Isozyme studies of some human cell lines, *Acta Pathol. Microbiol. Scand.* **62:**567.

BENNINGTON, J. L., 1967, Cellular kinetics of invasive squamous carcinoma of the human cervix, *Cancer Res.* **29:**1082.

BOTTOMLEY, R. H., TRAINER, A. L., AND GRIFFIN, M. J., 1969, Enzymatic and chromosomal characterization of HeLa variants, *J. Cell Biol.* **41:**806.

BOVERI, T., 1929, *The Origin of Malignant Tumors,* Williams and Wilkins, Baltimore.

BRAUN, A. C., 1969, *The Cancer Problem: A Critical Analysis and Modern Synthesis,* p. 160, Columbia University Press, New York.

BRAUNSTEIN, G. D., VAITUKAITIS, J. L., CARBONE, P. P., AND ROSS, G. T., 1973, Ectopic production of human chorionic gonadotrophin by neoplasms, *Ann. Int. Med.* **78:**39.

BRENT, T. P., BUTLER, J. A. V., AND CRATHORN, A. V., 1965, Variations in phosphokinase activities during the cell cycle in synchronous populations of HeLa cells, *Nature (London)* **207:**176.

BRESCIANI, F., 1968, Cell proliferation in cancer, *Eur. J. Cancer* **4:**343.

BROX, L. W., LACKO, A. G., GRACY, R. W., ADELMAN, R. C., AND HORECKER, B. C., 1969, Muscle type aldolase isolated from a liver tumor, *Biochem. Biophys. Res. Commun.* **36:**994.

BRUES, A. M., 1954, Ionizing radiation and cancer, *Adv. Cancer Res.* **2:**177.

BURDETTE, W. J., 1955, The significance of mutation in relation to the origin of tumors, *Cancer Res.* **15(4):**201.

CADEAU, B. J., BLACKSTEIN, M. E., AND MALKIN, A., 1974, Increased incidence of placenta-like alkaline phosphatase activity in breast and genitourinary cancer, *Cancer Res.* **34:**729.

CHARLES, M. A., CLAYPOOL, R., SHAAF, M., ROSEN, S. W., AND WEINTRAUB, B. D., 1973, Lung carcinoma associated with production of three placental proteins, *Arch. Int. Med.* **132:**427.

CHASE, D. G., AND PIKÓ, L., 1973, Expression of A- and C-type particles in early mouse embryos, *J. Natl. Cancer Inst.* **51:**1971.

COLEMAN, R., AND FINEMAN, J. B., 1966, Preparation and properties of isolated plasma membranes from guinea pig tissues, *Biochim. Biophys. Acta* **125:**197.

COMINGS, D. E., 1973, General theory of carcinogenesis, *Proc. Natl. Acad. Sci. U.S.A.* **70:**3324.

CRISS, W. E., 1971, A review of isozymes in cancer, *Cancer Res.* **31:**1523.

CUMMINS, J. E., 1968, in: *The Cell Cycle* (G. Padilla, G. Whitson, G. and I. Cameron, eds.), Academic Press, New York.

DAVIDSON, J. F., MCNICOL, G. P., FRANK, G. L., ANDERSON, T. J., and DOUGLAS, A. S., 1969, Plasminogen-activator-producing tumour, *Br. Med. J.* **1:**88.

DAVIDSON, R. L., and EPHRUSSI, B., 1965, A selective system for the isolation of hybrids between "L" cells and normal cells, *Nature (London)* **205:**1170.

DEFENDI, V., EPHRUSSI, B., KOPROWSKI, H., AND YOSHIDA, M. C., 1967, Properties of hybrids between polyoma-transformed and normal mouse cells, *Proc. Natl. Acad. Sci. U.S.A.* **57:**299.

DIMAYORCA, G. A., EDDY, B. E., STEWART, S. E., HUNTER, W. S., FRIEND, C., and BENDICH, A., 1959, Isolation of infectious deoxyribonucleic acid from SE polyoma-infected tissue cultures, *Proc. Natl. Acad. Sci. U.S.A.* **45:**1805.

DOELLGAST, G. W., AND FISHMAN, W. H., 1975, New chromatographic approaches to the separation of human alkaline phosphatase isozymes, in: *Isozymes; Molecular Structure* (C. L. Markert, ed.), Academic Press, New York, Volume 1, p. 293.

DONNELLY, G. M., AND SISKEN J. E., 1967, RNA and protein synthesis required for entry of cells into mitosis and during the mitotic cycle, *Exp. Cell Res.* **46:**93.

DRYSDALE, J. W., AND SINGER, R. M., 1974, Carcinofetal human isoferritins in placenta and HeLa cells, *Cancer Res.* **34:**3352.

DUNNE, J., FENNELLY, J. J., AND MCGEENEY, K., 1967, Separation of alkaline phosphatase enzymes in human serum gel-filtration (Sephadex G-200) techniques, *Cancer* **20:**71.

DYMLING, J. F., 1966, Separation of serum and placental alkaline phosphatase by agarose gel electrophoresis and Sephadex chromatography, *Scand. J. Clin. Lab. Invest.* **18:**129.

ELSON, N. A., AND COX, R. P., 1969, Production of fetal-like alkaline phosphatase by HeLa cells, *Biochem. Genet.* **3:**549.

FISHMAN, L., 1974, Acrylamide disc gel electrophoresis of alkaline phosphatase of human tissues, serum and ascites fluid using Triton X-100 in the sample and gel matrix, *Biochem. Med.* **9:**309.

FISHMAN, W. H., BAKER, J. R., AND BORGES, P. R. F., 1959, Localization of β-glucuronidase in some human tumors, *Cancer* **12:**240.

FISHMAN, W. H., INGLIS, N. R., GREEN, S., ANSTISS, C. L., GHOSH, N. K., REIF, A. E., RUSTIGIAN, R., KRANT, M. J., AND STOLBACH, L. L., 1968a, Immunology and biochemistry of Regan isoenzyme of alkaline phosphatase in human cancer, *Nature (London)* **219:**697.

FISHMAN, W. H., INGLIS, N. R., STOLBACH, L. L., AND KRANT, M. J., 1968b, A serum alkaline phosphatase isoenzyme of human neoplastic cell origin, *Cancer Res.* **28:**150.

FISHMAN, W. H., INGLIS, N. R., AND GREEN, S., 1971, Regan isoenzyme: A carcinoplacental antigen, *Cancer Res.* **31:**1054.

FRITSCHE, H. A., AND ADAMS-PARK, H. R., 1974, High molecular weight isoenzymes of alkaline phosphatase in human serum-demonstration by cellulose acetate electrophoresis and physico-chemical characterization, *Clin. Chim. Acta* **52:**81.

GOLD, P., AND FREEDMAN, S. O., 1965, Specific carcinoembryonic antigens of the digestive system, *J. Exp. Med.* **122:**467.

GRACEY, R. W., LACKO, A. G., BROX, L. W., ADELMAN, R. C., AND HORECKER, B. L., 1970, Structural relations in aldolases purified from rat liver and muscle and Novikoff hepatoma, *Arch. Biochem. Biophys.* **136:**480.

GRIFFIN, M. J., AND BER, R., 1969, Cell cycle events in the hydrocortisone regulation of alkaline phosphatase in HeLa S₃ cells, *J. Cell Biol.* **40:**297.

GRIFFIN, M. J., AND BOTTOMLEY, R. H., 1969, Regulation of alkaline phosphatase in HeLa₃ clones of differing modal chromosome number, *Ann. N.Y. Acad. Sci.* **166:**417.

GURLEY, L. R., WALTERS, R. A., AND TOBEY, R. A., 1974, Cell cycle-specific changes in histone phosphorylation associated with cell proliferation and chromosome condensation, *J. Cell Biol.* **60:**356.

HABEL, K., 1961, Resistance of polyoma virus immune animals to transplanted polyoma tumors, *Proc. Soc. Exp. Biol. Med.* **106:**722.

HAUSCHKA, T. S., 1961, The chromosomes in ontogeny and oncogeny, *Cancer Res.* **21:**957.

HERZ, F., 1973, Alkaline phosphatase in KB cells: Influences of hyperosmolarity and prednisolone on enzyme activity and thermostability, *Arch. Biochem. Biophys.* **158:**225.

HIGASHINO, K., HASHINOTSUME, M., KANG, K. Y., TAKAHASHI, Y., AND YAMAMURA, Y., 1972, Studies on a variant alkaline phosphatase in sera of patients with hepatocellular carcinoma, *Clin. Chim. Acta* **40:**67.

HOWARD, A., AND PELC, S. R., 1951, Nuclear incorporation of P³² as demonstrated by autoradiographs, *Exp. Cell Res.* **2:**178.

HUGON, J., AND BORGERS, M., 1966, Ultrastructural localization of alkaline phosphatase activity in the absorbing cells of the duodenum of mouse, *J. Histochem. Cytochem.* **14:**629.

ICHIHARA, A., AND OGAWA, K., 1972, Isozymes of branched chain amino acid transaminase in normal rat tissues and hepatomas, in: *Isozymes and Enzyme Regulation in Cancer* (T. Ono and S. Weinhouse, eds.), pp. 181–190, Gann Monograph No. 13, University of Tokyo Press, Tokyo.

INGLIS, N. R., GUZEK, D. I., KIRLEY, S., GREEN, S., AND FISHMAN, W. H., 1971, Rapid electrophoretic membrane techniques for Regan isoenzyme (placental type alkaline phosphatase) using a fluorogenic substrate, *Clin. Chim. Acta* **33:**287.

INGLIS, N. R., KIRLEY, S., STOLBACH, L. L., AND FISHMAN, W. H., 1973, Phenotypes of the Regan isoenzyme and identity between the placental D-variant and the Nagao isoenzyme, *Cancer Res.* **33:**1657.

JENNINGS, R. C., BROCKLEHURST, D., AND HIRST, M., 1970, A comparative study of alkaline phosphatase enzymes using starch gel electrophoresis and Sephadex gel-filtration with special reference to high molecular weight enzymes, *Clin. Chim. Acta* **30:**509.

KANG, K.-Y., HIGASHINO, K., HASHINOTSUME, M., TAKAHASHI, Y., AND YAMAMURA, Y., 1972, Production of the placental type alkaline phosphatase isoenzyme by lung cancer tissue. *GANN* **63:**217.

KAPP, L. N., AND OKADA, S., 1972, Factors affecting acid phosphatase activity in exponentially and synchronized L5178Y mouse leukemia cells, *Exp. Cell Res.* **72:**465.

KATANUMA, N., KURODA, Y., YOSHIDA, T., SANADA, Y., AND MORRIS, H. P., 1972, Relationship between degree of differentiation and growth rate of minimal deviation hepatomas and kidney cortex tumors studied with glutaminase isozymes, in: *Isozymes and Enzyme Regulation in Cancer* (T. Ono and S. Weinhouse, eds.), pp. 151, Gann Monograph No. 13, University of Tokyo Press, Tokyo.

KAWABE, S., MATSUSHIMA, T., AND SUGIMURA, T., 1969, Crystallization and properties of aldolase from a transplantable rat sarcoma, *Cancer Res.* **29:**2075.

KERR, S. J., AND BOREK, E., 1973, Regulation of the tRNA methyltransferases in normal and neoplastic tissues, *Adv. Enzyme Regul.* **11:**63.

KILLANDER, D., AND ZETTERBERG, A., 1965, Quantitative cytochemical studies on interphase growth. I. Determination of DNA, RNA and mass content of age determined mouse fibroblasts *in vitro* and of intercellular variation in generation time, *Exp. Cell Res.* **38:**272.

KILLMANN, S. A., CRONKITE, E. P., ROBERTSON, J. D., FLEIDNER, T. M., AND BOND, V. P., 1963, Estimation of phases of the life cycle of leukemic cells from labelling in human beings *in vivo* with tritiated thymidine, *Lab. Invest.* **12:**671.

KLEVECZ, R. R., 1969, Temporal order in mammalian cells. I. The periodic synthesis of lactate dehydrogenase in the cell cycle, *J. Cell Biol.* **43:**207.

KOLODNY, G. M., 1969, Patterns of protein synthesis in the HeLa cell, *Am. J. Roentgenol. Radium Ther. Nucl. Med.* **105:**746.

KOLODNY, G. M., AND GROSS, P. R., 1969, Changes in patterns of protein synthesis during the mammalian cell cycle, *Exp. Cell Res.* **56:**117.

LAKE, R. S., 1973, Further characterization of the F1-histone phosphokinase of metaphase arrested animal cells, *J. Cell Biol.* **58:**317.

LASFARGUES, E. Y., COUTINHO, W. G., AND MOORE, D. H., 1974, Cell-mediated factors that stimulate growth of human breast carcinoma cells in tissue culture, *Proc. 65th Ann. Meet. Am. Assoc. Cancer Res.* **15:**67.

LEFFERT, H. L., AND SELL, S., 1974, Alpha-fetoprotein biosynthesis during the growth cycle of differentiated fetal rat hepatocytes in primary monolayer culture, *J. Cell Biol.* **61:**823.

LINDER, M., MUNRO, H. N., AND MORRIS, H. P., 1970, Rat ferritin isoproteins and their response to iron administration in a series of hepatic tumors and in normal and regenerating liver, *Cancer Res.* **30:**2231.

LITTLEFIELD, J. W., 1966, The periodic synthesis of thymidine kinase in mouse fibroblasts, *Biochim. Biophys. Acta* **114:**398.

MAIO, J. J., AND DECARLI, L. L., 1962, Distribution of alkaline phosphatase variants in a heteroploid strain of human cells in tissue culture, *Nature (London)* **196:**600.

MANES, C., 1974, Phasing of gene products during development, *Cancer Res.* **34:**2044.

MANES, C., AND SHARMA, O. K., 1973, Hypermethylated tRNA in cleaving rabbit embryos, *Nature (London)* **244:**283.

MARTIN, D., TOMKINS, G. M., AND GRANNER, D., 1969, Synthesis and induction of tyrosine aminotransferase in synchronized hepatoma cells in culture, *Proc. Natl. Acad. Sci.* **62:**248.

MENDELSOHN, M. L., 1962, Autoradiographic analysis of cell proliferation in spontaneous breast cancer of C3H mouse. III. Growth fraction, *J. Natl. Cancer Inst.* **28:**1015.

MILLER, E. C., AND MILLER, J. A., 1966, Mechanisms of chemical carcinogenesis: Nature of proximate carcinogens and interactions with macromolecules, *Pharmacol. Rev.* **18:**805.

MOSCONA, A. A., 1971, Embryonic and neoplastic cell surfaces: Availability of receptors for concanavalin A and wheat germ agglutinin, *Science* **171:**905.

MUGGIA, F. M., AND DEVITA, V. T., 1972, *In vivo* tumor cell kinetic studies: Use of local thymidine injection followed by fine-needle aspiration, *J. Lab. Clin. Med.* **80:**297.

NAKAYAMA, T., YOSHIDA, M., AND KITAMURA, M., 1970, L-Leucine sensitive, heat-stable alkaline phosphatase isoenzyme detected in a patient with pleuritis carcinomatosa, *Clin. Chim. Acta* **30:**546.

NATHANSON, L., AND FISHMAN, W. H., 1971, New observations on the Regan isoenzyme of alkaline phosphatase in cancer patients, *Cancer* **27:**1388.

NICHOLS, W. W., LEVAN, A., AND HENEEN, W. K., 1967, Studies on the role of viruses in somatic mutation, *Hereditas* **57:**365.

Nordling, C. O., 1953, A new theory on the cancer-inducing mechanism, *Br. J. Cancer* **7**:68.

Nordmann, Y., and Schapira, F., 1966, Action inhibitrice de l'adenosine triphosphate sur l'aldolase de l'hépatome humain, *C. R. Acad. Sci. Ser. D* **262**:1896.

Ossowski, L., Quigley, J. P., and Reich, E., 1974, Fibrinolysis associated with oncogenic transformation, *J. Biol. Chem.* **249**:13, 4312.

Pitot, H. C., and Heidelberger, C., 1963, Metabolic regulatory circuits and carcinogenesis, *Cancer Res.* **23**:1694.

Portelius, P., Saksela, E., and Saxen, E., 1960, A HeLa clonal line lacking alkaline phosphatase activity, *Exp. Cell Res.* **21**:616.

Potter, V. R., 1958, The biochemical approach to the cancer problem, *Fed. Proc.* **17**:691.

Quastler, H., and Sherman, F. G., 1959, Cell population kinetics in the intestinal epithelium of the mouse, *Exp. Cell Res.* **17**:420.

Reich, E., 1973, Tumor-associated fibrinolysis, *Fed. Proc.* **32**:2174.

Rennert, O. M., 1971, Transfer RNA's of embryonic tissues, *Cancer Res.* **31**:637.

Rule, A. H., and Goleski-Reilly, C., 1974, Phase-specific oncocolon antigens: A theoretical framework for "carcinoembryonic antigen" specificities, *Cancer Res.* **34**:2083.

Rusch, H. P., 1969, Some biochemical events in the growth cycles of *Physarum polycephalum, Fed. Proc.* **28**:1761.

Rustigian, R., Kelly, J. P. W., Ellis, D. A., Clark, L. A., Inglis, N. R., and Fishman, W. H., 1974, Regan type of alkaline phosphatase in a human heteroploid cell line, *Cancer Res.* **34**:1908.

Sasaki, M., and Fishman, W. H., 1973, Ultrastructural studies on Regan and non-Regan isoenzymes of alkaline phosphatase in human ovarian cancer cells, *Cancer Res.* **33**:3008.

Schapira, F., 1973, Isozymes and cancer, *Adv. Cancer Res.* **18**:77.

Schapira, F., Dreyfus, J. C., and Schapira, G., 1963, Anomaly of aldolase in primary liver cancer, *Nature (London)* **200**:995.

Schidlovsky, G., and Ahmed, M., 1973, C-type virus particles in placentas and fetal tissues of rhesus monkeys, *J. Natl. Cancer Inst.* **51**:225.

Schwalbe, E., 1907, *Die Morphologie und Missbildungen des Menschen und der Tiere,* II, Jena.

Shinkai, K., and Akedo, H., 1972, A multienzyme complex in serum of hepatic cancer, *Cancer Res.* **32**:2307.

Singer, R. M., and Fishman, W. H., 1974a, Characterization of two HeLa sublines: TCRC-1 produces Regan isoenzyme and TCRC-2 non-Regan isoenzyme, *J. Cell Biol.* **60**:777.

Singer, R. M., and Fishman, W. H., 1975, Specific isozyme profiles of alkaline phosphatase in prednisolone-treated human cell populations, in: *Isozymes; Developmental Biology* (C. L. Markert, ed.), Academic Press, New York, Volume 3, p. 753.

Singer, R. M., Lin, C. W., Sasaki, M., and Fishman, W. H., 1973, Evidence for a plasma membrane localization of alkaline phosphatase in HeLa cells, *J. Histochem. Cytochem.* **22**:286.

Sjogren, H. O., Hellstrom, I., and Klein, G., 1961, Transplantation of polyoma virus-induced tumors in mice, *Cancer Res.* **21**:329.

Spencer, T., 1970. Some factors controlling alkaline phosphatase isoenzymes in HeLa cells, *Biochem. J.* **116**:927.

Stolbach, L. L., Krant, M. J., and Fishman, W. H., 1969, Ectopic production of an alkaline phosphatase isoenzyme in patients with cancer, *New Engl. J. Med.* **281**:757.

Subak-Scharpe, J. H., 1969, The doublet pattern of the nucleic acid in relation to the origin of viruses, in: *Handbook of Molecular Cytology* (A. Lima-de-Faria, ed.), pp. 68–87, North-Holland, Amsterdam.

Tanaka, T., Harano, H., Sue, F., and Morimura, 1967, Crystallization, characterization and metabolic regulation of two types of pyruvate kinase isolated from rat tissues, *J. Biochem. (Tokyo)* **62**:71.

Taylor, A. T., Stafford, M. A., and Jones, O. W., 1972, Properties of thymidine kinases partially purified from fetal and adult tissues, *J. Biol. Chem.* **247**:1930.

Temin, H. M., 1963, The effects of actinomycin D on growth of Rous sarcoma virus *in vitro, Virology* **20**:577.

Temin, H. M., 1964, Homology between RNA from Rous sarcoma virus and DNA from Rous sarcoma virus-infected cells, *Natl. Acad. Sci. U.S.A.,* **52**:323.

Temin, H. M., and Mizutani, S., 1972, RNA-dependent DNA polymerase in virions of Rous sarcoma virus, *Nature (London)* **226**:1211.

Tiedemann, H., 1959, Neue Ergebnisse zur Frage nach der chemischen Natur de Induktionsstaffe beim Organisator-effekt Spemamns, *Naturwissenschafften* **46**:613.

TIEDEMANN, H., AND TIEDEMANN, H., The induction capacity of purified induction factors in combination, *Rev. Suisse Zool.* **71:**117.

TIMPERLEY, W. R., 1968, Alkaline phosphatase secreting tumor of the lung, *Lancet* **2:**356.

TJIO, J. H., CARBONE, P. P., WHANG, J., AND FREI, E., III, The Philadelphia chromosome and chronic myelogenous leukemia, *J. Natl. Cancer Inst.* **36:**567.

TOIVONEN, S., 1950, Stoffliche Induktoren, *Rev. Suisse Zool.* **57:**41.

TOIVONEN, S., SAXEN, L., AND VAINIO, T., 1961, Quantitative evidence for the two-gradient hypothesis for primary induction, *Experientia* **17:**86.

TSUIKI, S., SATO, K., MIYAGI, T., AND KIKUCHI, H., 1972, Isozymes of fructose 1,6-diphosphatase 6-diphosphatase glycogen synthetase and glutamine: Fructose 6-phosphate aminotransferase, in: *Isozymes and Enzyme Regulation in Cancer* (T. Ono and S. Weinhouse, eds.), pp. 153–165, Gann Monograph No. 13, University of Tokyo Press, Tokyo.

UNKELESS, J., DANØ, K., KELLERMAN, G. M., AND REICH, E., 1974, Fibrinolysis associated with oncogenic transformation, partial purification and characterization of the cell factor, a plasminogen activator, *J. Biol. Chem.* **249:**4295.

USATEGUI-GOMEZ, M., YEAGER, F. M., AND DE CASTRO, A. F., 1973, A sensitive immunochemical method for the determination of the Regan isoenzyme in serum, *Cancer Res.* **33:**1574.

VAITUKAITIS, J. L., BRAUNSTEIN, G. D., AND ROSS, G. T., 1972, A radioimmunoassay which specifically measures human chorionic gonadotrophin in the presence of human luteinizing hormone, *Am. J. Obstet. Gynecol.* **113:**751.

VARGA, J. M., DIPASQUALE, A., PAWELEK, J., MCGUIRE, J. S., AND LERNER, A. B., 1974, Regulation of melanocyte stimulating hormone action at the receptor level: Discontinuous binding of hormone to synchronized mouse melanoma cells during the cell cycle, *Proc. Natl. Acad. Sci. U.S.A.* **71:**1590.

VERNON, M. L., LANE, W. T., AND HUEBNER, R. J., 1973, Prevalence of type-C particles in visceral tissues of embryonic and newborn mice, *J. Natl. Cancer Inst.* **51:**1171.

VOLPE, P., 1969, Depression of ornithine-δ-transaminase synchronized with the life cycle of HeLa cells cultivated in suspension, *Biochem. Biophys. Res. Commun.* **34:**190.

WARBURG, O., 1930, *Metabolism of Tumors* (trans. by F. Dickens), Constable Press, London.

WARNOCK, M. L., AND REISMAN, R., 1969, Variant alkaline phosphatase in human hepatocellular cancers, *Clin. Chim. Acta* **24:**5.

WATTS, C., AND GOLDBERG, D. M., 1969, New observations on β-glucuronidase in human cervical cancer, *Eur. J. Cancer* **5:**465.

WEINHOUSE, S., 1972, Glycolysis, respiration and anomalous gene expression in experimental hepatomas: G. H. A. Clowes' Memorial Lecture, *Cancer Res.* **32:**2007.

WEINHOUSE, S., 1973, Metabolism and isozyme alterations in experimental hepatomas, *Fed. Proc.* **32:**2162.

WEINTRAUB, B. D., AND ROSEN, S. W., 1971, Ectopic production of human chorionic somatomammotropin by non-trophoblastic cancers, *J. Clin. Endocrinol. Metab.* **32:**94.

WITSCHI, E., 1952, Overripeness of the egg as a cause of twinning and teratogenesis: A review, *Cancer Res.* **12:**763.

WOLFF, E., AND GINGLINGER, A. C., 1935, Sur les doses de folliculine necessaires pour realiser des intersexues et sur le stade limite de l'intervention, *C. R. Soc. Biol.* **120 (129):**114.

YOUNG, R. C., AND DEVITA, V. T., 1970, Cell cycle characteristics of human solid tumors *in vivo*, *Cell Tissue Kinet.* **3:**285.

4

Ectopic Hormone Secretion by Tumors

WILLIAM D. ODELL AND ADA WOLFSEN

1. Introduction

In addition to symptoms produced directly by tumor presence in a specific anatomical location, cancers frequently produce *systemic* symptoms by means of production of a variety of humoral or hormonal substances. At times, these systemic symptoms may be the first clue to the presence of a cancer, preceding other clinical manifestations by weeks, months, or even years. Table 1 lists a variety of humoral substances or syndromes known to be associated with neoplasms. It is to be noted that these are the *clinically recognized* cancer-associated syndromes. Table 2 lists the hormones reported to be produced by nonendocrine neoplasms. Note that all of the hormones listed in Table 2 are polypeptide hormones or prostaglandins; the ectopic hormonal syndromes are not associated with steroid hormone or iodothyronine (thyroxine, triiodothyronine) production. While it is not certain why this is true, we hypothesize that localized chromosomal events (mutations, depression, introduction of new viral DNA, reverse transcription, or derangement of DNA transcription and translation) may result in aberrant peptide synthesis, but production of steroids or iodothyronines requires an orderly sequence of controlled enzyme steps involving a number of enzyme systems. Singular nuclear events would seem more likely to be associated with the process of neoplasia than the development of new controlled series of enzymatic reactions. Whether or not this is the explanation, it is a general observation that humoral syndromes are almost invariably caused by peptide substances. The

WILLIAM D. ODELL and ADA WOLFSEN • Department of Medicine, Harbor General Hospital Campus, UCLA School of Medicine, Torrance, California.

TABLE 1

Examples of Humoral Syndromes Associated with Neoplasms

1. Ectopic hormone production
2. Carcinoembryonic antigen
3. α-Fetal globulin (a fetal thyroxine-binding globulin)
4. Enzymes (alkaline phosphatase, thymidine kinase, ribonuclease, etc.)
5. Central nervous system degenerative conditions
6. Myopathies
7. Myasthenic syndromes
8. Dermatological diseases (i.e., dermatomyositis, acanthosis nigricans, pachydermia)
9. Digital clubbing and arthropathies
10. Hematological diseases (i.e., aplastic anemias, γ-globulin abnormalities, thrombophlebitis)
11. Cardiovascular syndromes (i.e., nonbacterial endocarditis)
12. Fever
13. Chemotactic-factor inactivator (CFI)

synthesis of prostaglandins (substances related to fatty acids) is not completely understood.

Each of the clinically recognized syndromes is associated with a spectrum of neoplasms. For example, about 60% of patients with the ectopic ACTH syndrome have carcinoma of the lung or thymus. Similarly, about 60% of patients with ectopic parathormone production have carcinoma of the kidney or lung. In each instance, however, a few patients have been reported with the ectopic ACTH syndrome or hypercalcemia associated with other types of carcinoma. Thus, although syndromes of ectopic ACTH or PTH production are typically associated with neoplasms, any carcinoma may elaborate ectopic ACTH or parathormone.

As we indicate by specific examples later, there is now evidence to suggest that in some instances peptides with structures very similar to those of native hormones, but possessing *no biological activity*, are produced by neoplasms. We believe, in fact, that the clinically recognized ectopic hormonal syndromes serve to call attention to only a small fraction of the neoplasms which synthesize aberrant peptides and that in many instances these peptides may possess no biological activity. We hypothesize that peptide elaboration by neoplasms may be extraordinarily common and may represent a universal concomitant of neoplasia. Identification

TABLE 2

Hormones Reported to Be Produced by Nonendocrine Neoplasms[a]

1. ACTH	11. Corticotropin-releasing hormone
2. α- and β-MSH	12. Prolactin
3. Gonadotropin	13. Growth hormone
4. Vasopressin	14. Kinins
5. Parathormone	15. Prostaglandins
6. Hypoglycemia-producing factor	16. Secretin
7. Erythropoietin	17. Glucagon
8. Gastrin	18. Chorionic somatomammotropin
9. Thyroid-stimulating factor	19. Insulin
10. Hypophosphatemia-producing factor	

[a] The order is approximately in relation to numbers of patients reported with these syndromes.

of additional tumor-associated peptides requires the development of specific sensitive radioimmunoassays; the incidence of detection is proportional to the sensitivity of the method employed.

2. Quantification of Hormones

2.1. Prohormones

The synthesis of a prohormone with decreased biological activity was first demonstrated for insulin. The hormone insulin is composed of two polypeptide chains connected by disulfide bridges between cysteine residues. For many years, it was debated whether the two chains were separately synthesized and assembled within the β-cell of the pancreas, or, alternatively, whether the two chains were synthesized as part of a larger single peptide chain which was then cleaved to form the two-chained peptide. In 1967, Steiner and Oyer, using insulinoma tissue and radioactive amino acid precursors, demonstrated that insulin is synthesized as a prohormone (proinsulin), a single-chained peptide containing 81–86 amino acids (depending on species) covalently linked by disulfide bonds to form a single molecule. Native, two-chained insulin is formed by enzymatic removal of the peptide connecting piece, a 33 amino acid segment (Fig. 1). This synthetic system

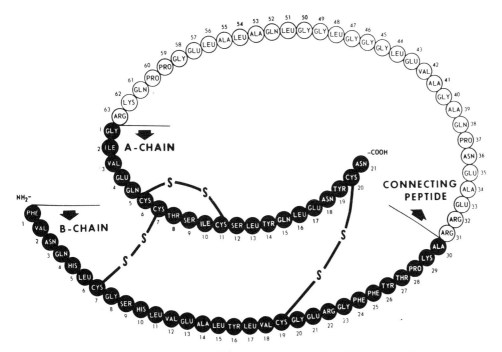

FIGURE 1. Structure of human proinsulin. This prohormone consists of 84 amino acids and possesses little biological activity. Enzymatic removal of the connecting peptide (α 31–63) results in the formation of the dipeptide insulin, which has full biological activity. Both proinsulin and insulin have full immunological potency in most insulin radioimmunoassays With permission of Ronald E. Chance, Ph.D., from Fig. 1, *Diabetes 21* (Suppl. 2): 461 (1972).

has been accepted as a general model for the synthesis of many *covalently* linked two-chained peptides. Pertinent to this discussion is the fact that proinsulin possesses markedly less biological activity than native insulin (the exact potency varies among bioassays) yet possesses full immunological potency as measured by most radioimmunoassays (Rubenstein and Steiner, 1971). By use of Sephadex columns, proinsulin can be separated from standard insulin (mol wt 6000) and can be enzymatically modified to produce insulin *in vitro* by incubation with trypsin (Steiner *et al.*, 1968).

Large forms of other hormones (possibly prohormones) have been described. These include ACTH (Gewirtz and Yalow, 1973), gastrin (Yalow and Berson, 1970), and parathormone (Habener *et al.*, 1972). The existence of such prohormones is not so easily understood as is that of proinsulin; polypeptides containing only a single polypeptide chain would appear to have no "need" to exist in a prohormone form. Nevertheless, it is clear that in some instances these large forms of hormones are elaborated in a larger quantity by neoplasms than in the conventional hypersecretory endocrine state. Such prohormones may thus serve as quantitative tumor markers. Moreover, they may react (as does large ACTH and proinsulin) in radioimmunoassays which depend on recognition of antigenic sites (which have an estimated mol wt of 600–900) but fail to react in radioreceptor assays or bioassays. Radioreceptor assays are based on the same principles as radioimmunoassays but utilize a target-tissue hormone receptor as the assay binding protein, instead of an antibody. Thus for ACTH the adrenal cortex membrane receptor for ACTH is used. The regions of the ACTH molecule needed for *binding* of hormone to receptor (amino acids 11–20) were distinguished from those necessary for hormone–receptor complex *to activate* the cell (amino acids 1–10) by the use of synthetic ACTH derivatives and fragments (Hofmann *et al.*, 1970). Evidence from controlled trypsinization suggests that small ACTH is covalently linked at its amino terminal to a basic amino acid of a larger peptide and thus the amino acid sequence necessary for activation of the target cell may be unavailable (Yalow and Berson, 1973). In addition, Schneider *et al.* (1973) have shown that "big ACTH" does not react *in vitro* in a dispersed adrenal cell assay system, but possesses full immunological activity when measured by radioimmunoassay. Theoretically a neoplasm might elaborate "big ACTH" and produce no recognizable clinical symptoms. Since in the study of Gewirtz and Yalow all of a small number of extracts of bronchogenic carcinomas contained "big ACTH", production of "big ACTH" may represent a universal concomitant of bronchogenic carcinoma. In addition to tumor-associated high molecular weight forms of ACTH, Orth *et al.* (1973) reported that tumors associated with the clinically recognized ectopic ACTH syndrome contain *N*-terminal and *C*-terminal ACTH fragments which possess no biological activity.

2.2. Glycopeptide Hormones

In the early years of 1963–1968, during which radioimmunoassays for the glycopeptide hormones, thyroid-stimulating hormone, luteinizing-stimulating hormone, follicle-stimulating hormone, and human chorionic gonadotropin

(TSH, LH, FSH, and hCG), were being developed, it became painfully apparent that there were immunological and hence structural similarities among all these hormones. Although some specific antisera against FSH were found, many antisera prepared against human FSH did not distinguish FSH from the other three glycopeptides. All antisera against human TSH also showed cross-reaction with LH and hCG. Subsequently, the structures of these hormones were elucidated and the reasons for this immunological similarity became clear. Biochemically these four hormones are composed of two peptide chains, an α- and a β-chain. The α-chain of all four hormones is similar or identical in structure; the β-chain of each is unique and confers biological specificity. Thus antisera prepared against one of the intact hormones which were partially or totally directed against the α-chain showed partial or complete reaction with the other three hormones; antisera directed against the β-chain showed specificity. Based on this fact, the use of isolated, purified β-chains resulted in very specific radioimmunoassays for hCG and TSH. The spatial structure of the β-chain in isolated form appears to be subtly different from that structure when the β-chain is combined with the α-chain. Because of this, the *affinity* of a β-chain antiserum is less for the intact hormone than for the isolated β-chain. Thus the β-chain radioimmunoassay is better for measuring β-chain than intact hormone (Binoux *et al.*, 1974). Recent structural biochemical work has shown that neither the immunoreactive α- nor β-chain alone possesses biological activity in *in vivo* or *in vitro* receptor assays. α-Chain and β-chain mixed *in vitro* will combine *without covalent bonding* to form intact, biologically active hormone—the nature of the biological activity is determined by the β-chain.*

It is not certain at present whether the two chains of these glycopeptides are synthesized and linked intracellularly or whether they are synthesized and secreted independently—combining during secretion from the cell or in the bloodstream to form the intact hormone. Data supporting the first hypothesis now exist. Studies from our laboratory have shown that the α-chain is secreted by the pituitary after stimulation with thyrotropin or luteinizing hormone releasing hormone (TRH and LRH): α-chains are not formed by degradation of intact TSH or LH (Edmonds *et al.*, 1974). Furthermore, Weintraub and Rosen (1973) described a patient with a pancreatic neoplasm that elaborated free β-chain of hCG. In a screen of 405 cancer sera from nontrophoblastic nongonadal neoplasms, hCG β-subunit was identified in 7% (Braunstein *et al.*, 1973). It is thus possible that free α- or β-chains are synthesized by a variety of neoplasms and such synthesis might not be recognized, since no biological activity exists. If this is true and quantitative differences between normals and cancer patients exist, such α- or β-peptides might also serve as tumor markers.

3. Ectopic Hormone Production

As discussed earlier, the cancer patient may present to the physician with clinical symptoms or laboratory findings arising from tumor elaboration of peptide

*For a review of this subject, see Pierce *et al.* (1971).

TABLE 3
Neoplasms Associated with Ectopic ACTH Production

Tumor type	Approximate percentage of cases
Carcinoma of lung	50
Thymic carcinoma	10
Pancreatic carcinoma (including islet cell and carcinoid)	10
Neoplasms from neural crest tissue (pheochromocytoma, neuroblastoma, paraganglioma, ganglioma)	5
Bronchial adenoma (including carcinoid)	2
Medullary carcinoma of the thyroid[a]	5
Miscellaneous[b]	each <2

[a] These interesting neoplasms also elaborate thyrocalcitonin and are associated frequently in the same patient with pheochromocytomas, hyperparathyroidism, Marfan's habitus, increased frequency of peptic ulcers, intestinal diverticulosis, and humoral-caused diarrhea. According to our definition, calcitonin elaboration by medullary carcinoma is not an example of *ectopic* hormone production.

[b] Carcinoma of ovary, prostrate, breast, thyroid, kidney, salivary glands, testes, stomach, colon, gallbladder, esophagus, appendix, etc.

hormones. We stress that these relatively infrequent presentations represent only the *clinically recognized* syndromes, and that elaboration of peptides related in structure to hormones but without biological activity may be very common. Nevertheless, recognition of the significance of the clinical syndromes is important to the practicing physician. Each of these is discussed briefly in the following sections.

3.1. Ectopic ACTH Production

The theoretical and biochemical information available on the syndrome of ectopic ACTH production was discussed at the beginning of this chapter. At present, the clinical or laboratory findings of the syndrome are associated with a relatively small number of neoplasms. Table 3 lists the approximate incidence of various neoplasms associated with the ectopic ACTH syndrome. About 70% of these patients have carcinoma of the lung, thymus, or pancreas. However, a variety of miscellaneous carcinomas have been described to cause this syndrome and any carcinoma should be considered as a potential source. In children, the distribution of types of neoplasms associated with this syndrome is different; most are neoplasms derived from the neural crest. The syndrome of hypercortisolism may appear coincidentally with the diagnosis of the neoplasm, after the neoplasm has been diagnosed, or at times up to 3 years *before* the neoplasm is apparent. In addition to all of the expected alterations usually related to Cushing's syndrome,*

---

* Cushing's syndrome has been defined as the clinical spectrum of excess cortisol secretion, Cushing's disease as bilateral adrenal hyperplasia associated with a hypothalamic-pituitary defect in control of ACTH secretion.

patients with ectopic ACTH production usually have laboratory evidence of hypokalemia and markedly increased excretion of 17-ketosteroids; these are not usually present in patients with Cushing's disease. In many patients, the duration of hypercortisolism is relatively short and the increase in cortisol secretion very great. Thus the metabolic abnormalities (hypokalemia, hypochloremic alkalosis, abnormal glucose tolerance) may be major clues; the physical appearance of Cushing's syndrome may not be apparent. Any patient with cancer and hypokalemia or abnormal glucose tolerance should be suspected of having the ectopic ACTH syndrome. Additional diagnostic assistance is available by suppression of ACTH (and cortisol secretion) with potent exogenous synthetic glucorticoids such as dexamethasone. Patients with Cushing's disease show such suppression in plasma ACTH (by radioimmunoassay) when 2 mg of dexamethasone is given every 6 h for 2–3 days; patients with ectopic ACTH or pituitary tumors elaborating ACTH usually do not. ACTH measurements assist also in distinguishing *adrenal* neoplasms elaborating cortisol (ACTH low) from ectopic ACTH syndrome or pituitary tumor (ACTH high). Routine measurements to distinguish "big ACTH" from normal ACTH are not currently available.

The dose–response relations between average ACTH and average cortisol concentrations (for normal subjects and patients with standard Cushing's disease) have been carefully established by Wolfsen and Odell (1975). Figure 2 depicts these relations and shows that in subjects with Cushing's disease significant ACTH suppression occurred when average plasma cortisol concentrations were as low as 1.2 μg/100 ml and that ACTH suppressed to zero at average cortisol concentrations of about 100 μg/100 ml. Measurement of average plasma ACTH and cortisol concentrations may help to distinguish ectopic ACTH-producing tumors and autonomous pituitary tumors from the standard Cushing's disease.*

An exception to the statement that dexamethasone will usually not suppress ACTH (and hence cortisol) secretion in the ectopic ACTH syndrome exists. Approximately 50% of patients with bronchial carcinoids show suppression. A possible explanation is available; Upton and Armatruda (1971) reported studies on two patients with carcinoma of the lung and two with pancreatic carcinoma. These neoplasms elaborated a peptide with ability to stimulate ACTH secretion by the pituitary (corticotropin-releasing hormone, CRH). Thus dexamethasone presumably inhibits the pituitary response to this ectopic CRH.

As was discussed earlier, the ectopic ACTH possessing biological potency is indistinguishable from standard pituitary ACTH. However, larger forms of ACTH, "big ACTH," and fragments of the ACTH peptide are also elaborated and possess no biological activity. Development of assay systems which can specifically and easily identify these peptides should make diagnosis of the ectopic ACTH syndrome easier.

---

*Separating standard Cushing's disease from pituitary tumors causing Cushing's syndrome may not be possible. Burke *et al.* (1973) reported that 64% of 33 patients with Cushing's disease had pituitary tumors present on needle biopsy; seven of these patients had normal sellar X-rays.

WILLIAM
D. ODELL
AND ADA
WOLFSEN

The α- and β-melanocyte-stimulating hormones (MSH) are structurally related to ACTH (Fig. 3). Phifer *et al.* (1970) have shown that in the *human* pituitary MSH and ACTH may be secreted by the same cell. This is different from the situation in the amphibian, where MSH is secreted by cells in a distinct intermediate pituitary lobe and ACTH is secreted by cells in the anterior lobe. In humans, ectopic MSH syndromes have been described, but to date such syndromes have always been associated with the ectopic ACTH syndrome. MSH assays have not usually been available and it is possible that this syndrome is commonly produced. Since increased MSH (even if in a biologically active form) produces few symptoms, such syndromes might not be clinically apparent. It is quite possible that large

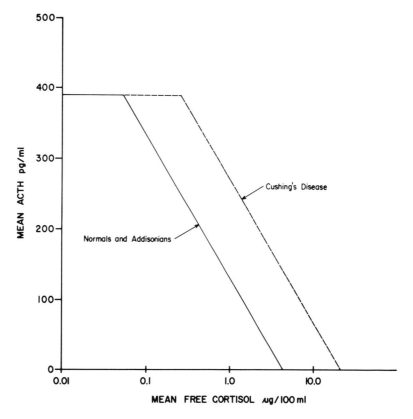

FIGURE 2. Dose–response curves for average free plasma cortisol and average ACTH between 6 and 10 A.M. in normal subjects and subjects with primary adrenal insufficiency as compared to patients with Cushing's disease. Cushing's disease may be defined as bilateral adrenal hyperplasia associated with an abnormality of hypothalamic-pituitary control. Note the following: (1) The two dose–response curves are parallel, but that for Cushing's disease is shifted to the right, indicating decreased feedback sensitivity. (2) Maximal ACTH secretion at unmeasurable cortisol concentration is similar for both groups of patients. (3) Patients with Cushing's disease remain very sensitive to cortisol suppression of ACTH, showing significant suppression of ACTH with plasma cortisol levels as low as 0.3 μg%. Patients with ectopic ACTH show even less feedback sensitivity and often fail to suppress with very high free cortisols. From data published by Wolfsen and Odell (1975).

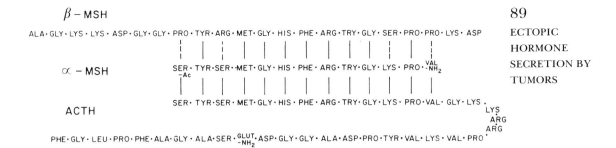

FIGURE 3. Structure of human ACTH, α-MSH, and human β-MSH. There are distinct species differences in amino acid sequence of ACTH and β-MSH; α-MSH appears to have a constant structure among all mammals and is not normally found in blood, but is present in pituitary extracts.

forms of either α- or β-MSH not possessing full biological activity may exist. Furthermore, α-MSH is not believed to be normally secreted by the human pituitary and the presence in blood may *per se* indicate the presence of a neoplasm.

3.3. Ectopic Gonadotropin Production

As was indicated earlier, the gonadotropins are glycopeptide hormones consisting of two peptide chains, α and β, neither of which possesses biological activity *per se*. The gonadotropin elaborated by neoplasms is similar or identical to human chorionic gonadotropin (hCG), the gonadotropin normally elaborated by the trophoblastic cells during gestation. Neoplasms derived from trophoblastic cells (choriocarcinoma, hydatid mole, etc.) elaborate such a hormone as a cellular property retained by the neoplasm and thus, strictly speaking, do not represent examples of ectopic production. Teratomas containing trophoblastic cells may also elaborate such a gonadotropin. In addition, as a true ectopic production, carcinomas of the lung, malignant melanomas, and possibly bladder tumors may elaborate a gonadotropin. Table 4 lists the known examples of ectopic gonadotropin production. We have recently shown (Edmonds *et al.*, 1974) that α-chains are secreted by the pituitary gland. Thus it is possible that neoplasms may elaborate α-chains possessing no biological activity but recognizable as tumor markers. Weintraub and Rosen (1973) recently described a patient with a pancreatic cancer that elaborated free β-chains of hCG.

Interestingly, pituitary glycopeptide production by neoplasms (as opposed to *chorionic* gonadotropin) appears to be very rare. Only one patient has been described for whom such a claim is made; Faiman *et al.* (1967) found

TABLE 4
Ectopic Production of Gonadotropin

Carcinoma of the lung
Teratomas (testes, ovary, pineal, mediastinum)
Miscellaneous (hepatoblastoma, malignant melanoma, bladder papilloma)

arterial–venous differences for both FSH and LH using specific radioimmunoassays. Pituitary thyrotropin has not been described to be produced by a nonpituitary neoplasm, although elaboration of chorionic thyrotropin by testicular teratocarcinomas also producing a gonadotropin has been described (Steigbigel *et al.*, 1964). Human chorionic thyrotropin (HCT) is also a glycopeptide hormone, but possesses less intrinsic potency (biological activity/mass of hormone) than pituitary TSH. It is immunologically more closely related to bovine TSH than to human. Since its biological potency is low and specific immunoassays do not exist, the frequency of its elaboration by neoplasms is uncertain.

3.4. Ectopic Vasopressin Production

Vasopressin is an eight amino acid* peptide predominantly elaborated in ectopic syndromes by carcinomas of the lung. When this biologically active peptide is produced, a syndrome of hyponatremia, persistently hyperosmotic urine, and difficulty with sodium conservation is produced. As we have reviewed separately (Odell, 1974), the peptide has been identified by bioassays and also shown to be structurally similar or identical to arginine vasopressin by radioimmunoassays. Bartter and Schwartz (1967) and Vorherr *et al.* (1968) reported a large series of patients in whom the tumor vasopressin reacted identically to arginine vasopressin in radioimmunoassays. Interestingly, a series of octapeptides exist in nature. These are shown in Table 5. It is not known whether neoplasms commonly elaborate these other peptides than arginine vasopressin, but Viszolyi and Perks (1969) have shown by bioassay and Skowsky and Fisher (1973) by radioimmunoassay that the fetal pituitary does elaborate *arginine vasotocin*. Since fetal peptides are being shown with increasing frequency to be elaborated by neoplasms (α-fetal protein, chorionic gonadotropin, chorionic thyrotropin, carcinoembryonic antigen, placental alkaline phosphatase, thymidine kinase, human chorionic somatomammotropin), it is intriguing to believe that vasotocin and some of the other peptides shown in Table 5 may be elaborated by neoplasms. It is not known, furthermore, whether these other peptides possess biological potency in man or whether "big forms" may exist as for ACTH, parathormone, insulin, etc.

3.5. Hypercalcemia and Cancer

Control of blood calcium concentrations involves a number of dynamic processes and several hormones. Disturbances of nonhormonal parameters may at times exceed the abilities of hormonal control mechanisms to maintain calcium constant and result in hypercalcemia. Thus profound immobilization such as is seen with bulbar poliomyelitis may cause hypercalcemia when bone mobilization exceeds body disposal mechanisms. Alternatively, excessive calcium ingestion in milk-alkali syndrome may also produce hypercalcemia. Such factors as decreased

---

* The two half-cysteine residues are considered as one amino acid (cystine).

TABLE 5
Amino Acid Sequences of Some Neurohypophyseal Hormones

Hormone	Residue position									Species
	1^a	2	3	4	5	6^a	7	8	9	
Glumitocin	Cys-	Tyr-	Ile-	Ser-	Asn-	Cys-	Pro-	<u>Gln</u>-	GlyNH$_2$	Cartilaginous fishes
Isotocin	Cys-	Tyr-	Ile-	Ser-	Asn-	Cys-	Pro-	<u>Ile</u>--	GlyNH$_2$	Bony fishes
Mesotocin	Cys-	Tyr-	Ile-	<u>Gln</u>-	Asn-	Cys-	Pro-	<u>Ile</u>-	GlyNH$_2$	Amphibians
Vasotocin	Cys-	Tyr-	Ile-	<u>Gln</u>-	Asn-	Cys-	Pro-	<u>Arg</u>-	GlyNH$_2$	Bony fishes, amphibians
Oxytocin	Cys-	Tyr-	Ile-	<u>Gln</u>-	Asn-	Cys-	Pro-	<u>Leu</u>-	GlyNH$_2$	Mammals
Vasopressin	Cys-	Tyr-	<u>Phe</u>-	<u>Gln</u>-	Asn-	Cys-	Pro-	<u>Arg</u>-	GlyNH$_2$	Mammals except pig
Vasopressin	Cys-	Tyr-	<u>Phe</u>-	<u>Gln</u>-	Asn-	Cys-	Pro-	<u>Lys</u>-	GlyNH$_2$	Pig

[a] A disulfide bridge links residues 1 and 6 in each case. The variations in amino acid residues among these hormones are indicated by underlining.

activity, decreased solute load, and increased calcium intake may affect the clinical recognition of a calcium-modifying peptide hormone elaborated by neoplasms. Thus a patient with ectopic parathormone elaboration (or a nonparathormone, "calcium-effecting" peptide) may not have hypercalcemia when physically active and ingesting high solute loads, but may manifest hypercalcemia if put to bed and/or deprived of salt and water. Hypercalcemia has been found in association with a large number of neoplasms; many of such neoplasms have metastasized. Most hypercalcemic patients have bony metastases, but a significant number do not. Table 6 lists the neoplasms described to produce this syndrome in the absence of bony metastases. This does not imply that tumors spreading to bone do not elaborate a hypercalcemia-producing peptide, but merely that the association or cause is less certain in those instances. The material elaborated by these neoplasms appears not to be identical in all patients. In many it is similar or identical to parathormone; in others it is not. Munson *et al.* (1965), using hemagglutination inhibition immunoassays, and Sherwood *et al.* (1967), using a more precise radioimmunoassay, identified a material indistinguishable from parathormone in tumor extracts from several patients. Buckle *et al.* (1970) thoroughly studied a

TABLE 6
Neoplasms Associated with Ectopic Parathyroid Hormone Production[a]

Tissue of origin	Approximate frequency (%)
Carcinoma of lung	35
Carcinoma of kidney	24
Carcinoma of ovary	<8
Miscellaneous[b]	each <3

[a] Reproduced from W. Odell, in: *Textbook of Endocrinology* (R. H. Williams, ed.), Saunders, Philadelphia (1974).
[b] Carcinoma of breast, uterus, pancreas, urinary bladder, colon, prostate, penis, esophagus, parotid gland, testis (a child), hepatoblastoma (a child), hemangiosarcoma.

patient with renal adenocarcinoma and hypercalcemia. Plasma and tumor extracts gave a dose–response curve identical to that for bovine parathormone (as did standard human parathormone). A sharp tumor A-V difference in parathormone existed, and after surgical removal of the tumor blood parathormone concentrations fell to normal. In contrast to this, Powell *et al.* (1973) have described several patients with cancer and hypercalcemia in whom no material capable of reacting in several radioimmunoassays, each directed to different portions of the peptide sequence of parathormone, could be found. Tumor extracts produced calcium resorption from bone *in vitro*. Presumably these neoplasms elaborated a peptide that could produce hypercalcemia but that was structurally different from parathormone.

Habener *et al.* (1972) described a large form of parathormone in extracts of parathyroid adenomas obtained from patients with hyperparathyroidism. These workers also showed that this was a true prohormone by incubating adenoma tissue *in vitro* with labeled amino acids. The specific activity of large parathormone was greater than that of standard parathormone. Whether such forms exist in patients with cancers is uncertain. The relative biological potency of such proparathormones is also unknown. It is conceivable that these large forms are biologically inert and might be excellent tumor markers.

3.6. Hypoglycemia and Cancer

Another interesting syndrome associated with selected nonpancreatic neoplasms is hypoglycemia. Approximately two-thirds of patients with this syndrome have a relatively rare neoplasm in the general family of mesenchymal tumors and typified by the fibrosarcoma. Such tumors are located in the peritoneal (40%), retoperitoneal (24%), and thoracic (36%) areas (Odell, 1974). All these mesenchymal neoplasms have been large, weighing 800–10,000 g, and many are benign. Table 7 lists the estimated frequency and types of neoplasms associated with hypoglycemia. The nature of the humoral agent producing hypoglycemia is uncertain. Although it has biological properties indistinguishable from those of

TABLE 7
Types of Neoplasms Causing Hypoglycemia[a]

Tumor types	Approximate percentage of cases
Mesenchymal[b]	64
Heptatic	21
Adrenal carcinomas	6
Miscellaneous (anaplastic carcinomas, adenocarcinomas, pseudomyxomas, cholangiomas)	9

[a] Reproduced from W. Odell, in: *Textbook of Endocrinology* (R. H. Williams, ed.), Saunders, Philadelphia (1974).
[b] Included in this category are fibrosarcomas, mesotheliomas, enurofibromas, neurofibrosarcomas, spindle cell sarcomas, rhabdomyosarcomas, and leiomyosarcomas.

insulin in *in vitro* bioassays, it does not react in radioimmunoassays for insulin. Boshell *et el.* (1964) reported neutralization of bioassay potency of material from one neoplasm by excess anti-insulin antibody, but no reports of insulin radioimmunoassay reaction exist. Field *et al.* (1963) studied extracts of four neoplasms associated with hypoglycemia in detail: two had no activity by either bioassay or insulin radioimmunoassay. Two extracts had bioassayable activity similar to that of insulin, but this material failed to react in the radioimmunoassay for insulin. This strong evidence that the hypoglycemia-producing factor is not identical to insulin. Recently, the peptide somatomedin (formerly called "sulfation factor"), an intermediary in growth hormone action, has been shown to have insulinlike biological properties and to compete with labeled insulin for insulin receptors *in vitro*. It is probably equivalent to what previously was termed "nonsuppressible insulinlike activity" in serum, which also competes with labeled insulin for the insulin receptor *in vitro*. Conceivably this or a similar material is the one elaborated by these neoplasms. Studies in progress will clarify these points.

3.7. Other Hormonal Syndromes

Several other peptides with hormonal properties are known to be elaborated by neoplasms. Erythremia—or erythrocytosis caused by production of erythropoietin—has been described in association with the several types of neoplasms listed in Table 8. Such neoplasms are not readily apparent in many instances and specific studies directed to discovering such neoplasms as renal carcinoma are indicated in patients with erythrocytosis. Since the kidney is the normal site of erythropoietin production, this syndrome as caused by renal carcinoma may not strictly speaking represent ectopic hormone production. As judged by bioassay techniques, and some chemical manipulation, this material is similar to native erythropoietin. Since erythropoietin has not been highly purified, specific radioimmunoassays do not yet exist, and subtle differences in

TABLE 8
Neoplasms Associated with Polycythemia[a]

Neoplasm	Approximate percentage of cases
Renal carcinomas	46
Cerebellar hemangioblastomas	21
Benign renal lesions[b]	16
Uterine fibromas	6
Adrenal cortical carcinoma or hyperplasia	3
Ovarian neoplasms	3
Hepatomas	3
Pheochromocytomas	1

[a] Reproduced from W. Odell, in: *Textbook of Endocrinology* (R. H. Williams, ed.), Saunders, Philadelphia (1974).
[b] Such as hydronephrosis, cysts, and adenomas.

molecular structure may not have been detected by the chemical or bioassay techniques used to date.

Secretion of gastrin, secretin, or kinins may be involved in a spectrum of cancer-related syndromes. The best known is the Zollinger–Ellison syndrome, associated with single or multiple non-β-cell adenomas of the pancreas, severe peptic ulcer disease, and, at times, severe diarrhea. The peptic ulcer disease is caused by gastrin elaboration (a peptide normally produced by the gastric antrum which stimulates acid secretion). The diarrhea may be caused by excess gastric fluid production or by kinin or prostaglandin production by the neoplasm.

Another interesting but rare syndrome associated with neoplasms is hypophosphatemia (with normal calcium). The hypophosphatemia leads to osteomalacia, severe generalized bony pain, and, at times, muscle spasms and profound weakness. Yoshikawa et al. (1964) obtained a hypophosphatemia-producing substance in urine from a patient with this syndrome. Salassa et al. (1970) found no detectable parathormone in the blood of a patient with this syndrome; after tumor removal, parathormone concentrations and serum calcium were normal.[*]

Ectopic growth hormone has been reported but rarely. Steiner et al. (1968) described a patient with bronchogenic carcinoma and osteoarthropathy and tumor production of growth hormone. Greenberg et al. (1972) reported increased growth hormone content in 18 bronchogenic and eight gastric carcinomas. Since increased growth hormone elaboration in adults produces few symptoms unless present for several years, such syndromes may be more common than the literature suggests. It is also possible that peptides related to growth hormone but having few or no biological properties may be elaborated.

Weintraub and Rosen (1971) described several neoplasms that elaborated chorionic somatomammotropin, a single-chained peptide related structurally to prolactin and growth hormone, yet possessing very weak biological potency, and this activity related to carbohydrate control. Patients with neoplasms elaborating this peptide would suffer little or no clinically recognizable symptoms except possibly mild alteration in carbohydrate tolerance.

4. Elaboration of Nonhormonal Peptides

As was discussed at the beginning of this chapter, these ectopic hormone syndromes may represent only a fraction of a more generalized phenomenon—peptide elaboration by neoplasms. Peptides normally produced by the fetus appear to be also commonly elaborated by neoplasms. Thus carcinoembryonic antigen and α-fetal globulin are commonly elaborated by a large variety of neoplasms. These peptides possess no known biological effect that would produce clinically recognized symptoms, yet their presence is useful for cancer detection or to follow response to treatment. Fisher and Lam (1974) have shown that α-fetal protein is similar or identical to fetuin, a thyroxine-binding

---

[*] For a review of this syndrome, see Stanbury (1972).

globulin present in fetal sera. Fetal enzymes are also elaborated by neoplasms; for example, thymidine kinase (Bresnick and Burleson, 1970; Stafford and Jones, 1972) and placental alkaline phosphatase (Fishman, 1973).

Review of Table 1 indicates the immense spectrum of cancer-related humoral syndromes. Many are at present poorly or not at all explained. One group of nine functionally related peptides, the complement system, interrelates to a variety of body functions. Figure 4 depicts schematically this cascade peptide system, which is known to influence the following functions:

1. The complement system is involved in antigen–antibody interaction.
2. Damage of red cell membrane is produced by two terminal complement proteins after it is altered or prepared by preceding complement components.
3. Inflammation may be caused by complement through histamine release from mast cells and platelets.
4. Leukocyte chemotactic activity is promoted by complement components.
5. Immune adherence of leukocytes is enhanced.
6. Mobilization of leukocytes from bone marrow is enhanced.
7. Complement factors promote blood coagulation by mechanisms not clearly defined. Complement is involved in normal coagulation (Götze and Müller-Erberhard, 1971).

In addition to the many actions of these peptides, some evidence suggests that each protein component is further controlled by inhibitor peptides which can thereby modify action.

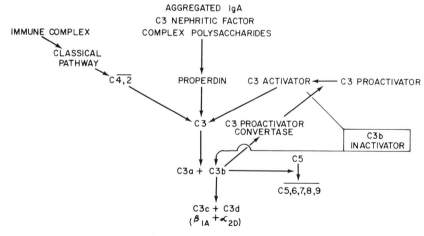

FIGURE 4. Schematic representation of the complement cascade. This peptide group is involved in many physiological reactions including red cell lysis, antigen–antibody interaction, inflammation via histamine release, leukocyte chemotactic activity, immune adherence of leukocytes, mobilization of leukocytes from bone marrow, and blood coagulation. Reproduced from drawing prepared by Dr. R. Glassock, Harbor Hospital Campus, UCLA School of Medicine.

Thus it appears possible that tumor elaboration of one or more of these complement peptides or the postulated inhibitor peptides might explain some of the poorly understood humoral syndromes associated with neoplasms, such as thrombophlebitis, fever, or chemotaxis inhibition. This exciting area holds promise of wide development and utilization in early recognition, localization, and effective treatment of neoplastic states in man.

5. References

BARTTER, F. C., AND SCHWARTZ, W. B., 1967, The syndrome of inappropriate secretion of antidiuretic hormone, *Am. J. Med.* **42:**790.

BINOUX, M., PIERCE, J. G., AND ODELL, W. D., 1974, Radioimmunoassay characterization of human thyrotropin and its subunits: Applications for measurement of human TSH, *J. Clin. Endocrinol. Metab.* **38:**674.

BOSHELL, B. R., KIRSCHENFELD, J. J., AND SOTERES, P. S., 1964, Extrapancreatic insulin-secreting tumor, *New Engl. J. Med.* **270:**338.

BRAUNSTEIN, G. D., VAITUKAITIS, J. L., CARBONE, P. P., AND ROSS, G. T., 1973, Ectopic production of human chorionic gonadotropin by neoplasms, *Ann. Intern. Med.* **78:**39–45.

BRESNICK, E., AND BURLESON, S. S., 1970, Rates of turnover of deoxythymidine kinase and its template RNA in Novikoff hepatoma and neonatal liver, *Cancer Res.* **30:**1060.

BUCKLE, R. M., McMILLAN, M., AND MALLINSON, C., 1970, Ectopic secretion of parathyroid hormone by a renal adenocarcinoma in a patient with hypercalcemia, *Br. Med. J.* **4:**724.

BURKE, C. W., DOYLE, F. H., JOPLIN, G. F., ARNOT, R. N., MACERLEAN, D. P., AND FRASER, T. R., 1973, Cushing's disease, treatment by pituitary implantation of radioactive gold or yttrium seeds, *Quart. J. Med.* **42:**693.

EDMONDS, M., MOLITCH, M., AND ODELL, W., 1974, Secretion of alpha subunits by the anterior pituitary (abst.), p. A68, Endocrine Society Meeting, June 12–14, 1974, Atlanta, Ga.

FAIMAN, C., COLWELL, J. A., RYAN, R. J., HERSHMAN, J. M., AND SHIELDS, T. W., 1967, Gonadotropin secretion from a bronchogenic carcinoma: Demonstration by radioimmunoassay, *New Engl. J. Med.* **277:**1395.

FIELD, J. B., KEEN, H., JOHNSON, P., AND HERRING, B., 1963, Insulinlike activity of nonpancreatic tumors associated with hypoglycemia, *J. Clin. Endocrinol. Metab.* **23:**1229.

FISHER, D. A., AND LAM, R. W., 1974, Thyroid hormone binding by bovine and ovine fetuin, *Endocrinology* **94:**49.

FISHMAN, W. H., 1973, *Advances in Enzyme Regulation*, Vol. II, Pergamon Press, Elmsford, N.Y.

GEWIRTZ, G., AND YALOW, R. S., 1973, Ectopic ACTH production: Big and little forms (abst.), p. A53, Endocrine Society Meeting, June 20–22, 1973, Chicago, Ill.

GÖTZE, O., AND MÜLLER-EBERHARD, H. J., 1971, The C_3 activator system: An alternate pathway of complement activation, *J. Exp. Med.* **134:**90.

GREENBERG, P. B., MARTIN, T. J., BECK, C., AND BURGER, H. G., 1972, Synthesis and release of human growth hormone from lung carcinoma in cell culture, *Lancet* **1:**350.

HABENER, J. F., KEMPER, B., POTTS, J. T., JR., AND RICH, A., 1972, Proparathyroid hormone: Biosynthesis by human parathyroid adenomas, *Science* **178:**630.

HOFMANN, K., WINEGENDER, W., AND FINN, F. M., 1970, Correlation of adrenocorticotropic activity of ACTH analogs with degree of binding to an adrenal corticol particulate preparation, *Proc. Natl. Acad. Sci. U.S.A.* **67:**829.

MUNSON, P. L., TASHJIAN, A. H., JR., AND LEVINE, L., 1965, Evidence for parathyroid hormone in nonparathyroid tumors associated with hypercalcemia, *Cancer Res.* **25:**1062.

ODELL, W. D., 1974, Humoral manifestations of nonendrocrine neoplasms—Ectopic hormone production, in: *Textbook of Endocrinology* (R. H. Williams, ed.), 5th ed., pp. 1105–1115, Saunders, Philadelphia.

ORTH, D. N., NICHOLSON, W. E., MITCHELL, W. M., ISLAND, D. P., AND LIDDLE, G. W., 1973, Biologic and immunologic characterization and physical separation of ACTH and ACTH fragments in the ectopic ACTH syndrome, *J. Clin. Invest.* **52:**1756.

PHIFER, R. F., SPICER, S. S., AND ORTH, D. N., 1970, Specific demonstration of the human hypophyseal cells which produce adrenocorticotropic hormone, *J. Clin. Endocrin.* **31**:347–61.

PIERCE, J. G., LIAO, T., HOWARD, S. M., SHOME, B., AND CORNELL, J. S., 1971, Studies on the structure of thyrotropin: Its relationship to luteinizing hormone, in: *Recent Progress in Hormone Research*, Vol. 27 (E. B. Astwood, ed.), pp. 165–212, Academic Press, New York.

POWELL, D., SINGER, F. R., MURRAY, T. M., MINKIN, C., AND POTTS, J. T., JR., 1973, Nonparathyroid humoral hypercalcemia in patients with neoplastic diseases, *New Engl. J. Med.* **289**:176.

RUBENSTEIN, A. H., AND STEINER, D. F., 1971, Proinsulin, *Ann. Rev. Med.* **22**:1.

SALASSA, R. M., JOWSEY, J., AND ARNAUD, C. D., 1970, Hypophosphatemic osteomalacia associated with "nonendocrine" tumors. *New England J. Med.*, **283**:65–70.

SCHNEIDER, B., GEWIRTZ, G., KRIEGER, D., AND YALOW, R. S., 1973, Big ACTH: Conversion to biologically active ACTH by trypsin (abst.), p. A52, Endocrine Society Meeting, June 20–22, 1973, Chicago, Ill.

SHERWOOD, L. M., O'RIORDAN, J. L., AURBACH, G. D., AND POTTS, J. T., JR., 1967, Production of parathyroid hormone by non-parathyroid tumors, *J. Clin. Endocrinol. Metab.* **27**:140.

SKOWSKY, W. R., AND FISHER, D. H., 1973, Immunoreactive arginine vasopressin (AVP) and arginine vasotocin (AVT) in the fetal pituitary of man and sheep, *Clin. Res.* **21**:205.

STAFFORD, M. A., AND JONES, O. W., 1972, The presence of "fetal" thymidine kinase in human tumors, *Biochim. Biophys. Acta* **277**:439.

STANBURY, S. W. (ed.), 1972, *Clinics in Endocrinology and Metabolism*, Vol. 1, p. 256, Saunders, Philadelphia.

STEIGBIGEL, N. H., OPPENHEIM, J. J., FISHMAN, L. M., AND CARBONE, P. P., 1964, Metastatic embryonal carcinoma of the testis associated with elevated plasma TSH-like activity and hyperthyroidism, *New Engl. J. Med.* **271**:345.

STEINER, D. F., AND OYER, P. E., 1967, The biosynthesis of insulin and a probable precursor of insulin by a human islet cell adenoma, *Proc. Natl. Acad. Sci. U.S.A.* **5**:473.

STEINER, D. F., HALLUND, O., RUBENSTEIN, A., SOOJA, C., AND BAYLISS, C., 1968, Isolation and properties of proinsulin, intermediate forms, and other minor components from crystalline bovine insulin, *Diabetes* **17**:725.

STEINER, H., DAHLBACK, O., AND WALDENSTROM, J., 1968, Ectopic growth-hormone production and osteoarthropathy in carcinoma of the bronchus, *Lancet* **1**:783.

UPTON, G. V., AND ARMATRUDA, T. T., JR., 1971, Evidence for the presence of tumor peptides with corticotropin-releasing-factor-like activity in the ectopic ACTH syndrome, *New Engl. J. Med.* **285**:419.

VISZOLYI, E., AND PERKS, A. M., 1969, New neurohypophysial principle in foetal mammals, *Nature (London)* **223**:1169.

VORHERR, H., MASSRY, S. G., UTIGER, R. D., AND KLEEMAN, C. R., 1968, Antidiuretic principle in malignant tumor extracts from patients with inappropriate ADH syndrome, *J. Clin. Endocrinol. Metab.* **28**:162.

WEINTRAUB, B. D., AND ROSEN, S. W., 1971, Ectopic production of human chorionic somatomammotropin by nontrophoblastic cancers, *J. Clin. Endocrinol. Metab.* **32**:94.

WEINTRAUB, B. D., AND ROSEN, S. W., 1973, Ectopic production of the isolated beta subunit of human chorionic gonadotropin, *J. Clin. Invest.* **52**:3135.

WOLFSEN, A. R., AND ODELL, W. D., 1975, The dose response relation between ACTH and cortisol in Cushing's disease, in press.

YALOW, R. S., AND BERSON, S. A., 1970, Size and charge distinctions between endogenous human plasma gastrin in peripheral blood and heptadecapeptide gastrins, *Gastroenterology* **58**:609.

YALOW, R. S., AND BERSON, S. A., 1973, Characteristics of "big ACTH" in human plasma and pituitary extracts, *J. Clin. Endocrinol. Metab.* **36**:415.

YOSHIKAWA, S., KAWABATA, M., HATSUYAMA, Y., HOSOKAWA, O., AND FUJITA, T., 1964, Atypical vitamin-D resistant osteomalacia, report of a case, in: *J. of Bone & Joint Surgery*, **46A**:998–1007.

5

Tumor Progression

Daniel Medina

1. Introduction: A Historical Perspective

The process of neoplastic development is generally conceded to be a multistage phenomenon. On exposure to an oncogen, a cell(s) undergoes' a series of qualitative and quantitative changes which ultimately are expressed as a neoplasm. In addition, neoplasms further undergo a series of qualitative changes which determine their biological behavior patterns. The concept that explains the qualitative changes which determine neoplasms' behavior has been termed "tumor progression" (Foulds, 1949*a,b*, 1954, 1964, 1969). In simple terms, the concept states that neoplasms develop and progress, from their earliest inception, by the acquisition of new properties which are expressed in their behavior patterns. As will be indicated later, the process of neoplastic progression starts at the initial interaction between a cell and oncogen. These qualitative and quantitative changes undergone by a normal cell population exposed to an oncogen can be conceived of as preneoplastic progression. Once a neoplasm has developed, the process of progression continues, and is facilitated by experimental manipulations such as serial passage of the neoplasm either *in vivo* or *in vitro*. These experimental manipulations provide the investigator with a means to analyze the process of progression and should by no means be considered an artifact. The occurrence of neoplastic progression is evident in the problem of metastases, where it is well documented that a malignant tumor that appears as a metastasis is a different entity than was present in the original palpable tumor or original neoplastic cell. The importance of selection pressures and host factors (hormones, mutational changes, immunological pressures) on the course of neoplastic pro-

DANIEL MEDINA ● Department of Cell Biology, Baylor College of Medicine, Houston, Texas

gression is a subject of practical and theoretical importance that will be considered here.

The phenomenon of progressive stages in the development of neoplasms is an old idea which was recognized at the turn of the century. Haaland (1911) recognized the existence of multiple stages and stressed the significance of progressive stages during the genesis of mammary cancer. The concept of multistage development of neoplasia gained general acceptance after the studies by Rous and coworkers (Rous and Beard, 1935; Rous and Kidd, 1941; McKenzie and Rous, 1941; Friedewald and Rous, 1950), Berenblum and Shubik (1947, 1949), and Greene (1940) on experimental skin and mammary tumorigenesis. They demonstrated that the neoplastic transformation was a multistage phenomenon rather than a single-stage event. The idea that tumors develop by acquisition of new characters from the initial altered cell to the established neoplasm can be viewed as a logical extension of the concept of multistage carcinogenesis. The idea of a cell population undergoing progressive changes was stressed early by Rous and coworkers (Rous and Beard, 1935; Rous and Kidd, 1941). In their study on the progression of Shope papillomas to carcinomas, they indicated that the progression occurred by "graded alterations." They demonstrated that papillomas progressed toward malignancy from their earliest inception and attained malignancy by a continuous series of alterations. Furthermore, neoplasms continued to evolve further morphological and behavioral changes even after the malignant characteristic was attained. Finally, they pointed out that malignant progression was generally focal and that it occurred as discrete qualitative changes.

Greene (1940) in his study on the evolution of the transplantability of mammary cancer in the rabbit demonstrated that the characteristics of cytological malignancy, invasiveness, and transplantability were not correlated with each other. Many noninvasive tumors demonstrated morphological changes in cells characteristic of malignancy. In his view, "invasiveness and metastasis represented progressive steps in a graded evolutionary process."

The concept of progression in neoplasms was definitively established and illustrated by the classical studies of Foulds (1949a,b, 1954, 1956a,b, 1958, 1964, 1965, 1969) on the evolution of hormonal independence in mammary tumors. He defined progression as the "acquisition of permanent, irreversible qualitative changes of one or more characteristics in a neoplasm" (Foulds, 1958). Foulds observed that tumor cell populations continued to evolve even after the acquisition of the neoplastic characteristic. The evolution of tumor patterns represented a series of stepwise changes which were unique and discrete. The analysis of these changes will be considered in the next section. It is perhaps pertinent to indicate that the concept of tumor progression is widely applicable to a tremendous variety of characteristics seen at both the cellular and the molecular level of neoplasms. Although the concept is sometimes narrowly interpreted, mainly in the consideration of hormonal dependence and the evolution of malignancy, other characteristics such as drug resistance, chromosome patterns, ascites conversion, transplantability, histoarchitecture, and enzymatic patterns have contributed much to the understanding of the·process and mechanism of neoplastic progression. While

the principles of neoplastic progression will be illustrated mainly from Foulds'
studies on the evolution of hormonal independency, it is the ultimate aim of this
chapter to discuss neoplastic progression in its broader sense as a process of
epigenetic and genetic development. Additionally, it will be emphasized that
progression, viewed as the acquisition of new characters, occurs at the earliest
stages, even before neoplasia becomes biologically or cytologically evident.
Progression in conjunction with the selection of cell populations altered genetically or epigenetically explains the evolution of neoplasms from the incipient stage
to the most anaplastic stage.

2. Concept of Tumor Progression

2.1. Evolution of Hormone Independence

2.1.1. Mammary Tumors

The study of spontaneous mammary tumors in different strains of inbred mice
has provided an ideal system for studying the evolution of tumor phenotypes. In
particular, Foulds (1949a,b 1956a,b) took advantage of the hormone-dependent
mammary tumors which arose in (C57BL × RIII)F$_1$ female mice and studied in
detail the acquisition of hormone independency in these tumors. Similar tumors
have subsequently been demonstrated to arise in other inbred mouse strains,
namely, RIII (Squartini, 1962), GR/A (Mühlbock, 1965; vanNie and Thung,
1965; vanNie and Dux, 1971), DD (Heston et al., 1964), and DDD (Matsuzawa et
al., 1974). Mammary tumors arising in the common American derived strains are
primarily hormone independent. This is true both for tumors induced by
mammary tumor virus (MTV) and for those induced by chemical carcinogens.

The hormone-dependent tumors are termed "plaques," which have been
described by Foulds (1949a,b, 1956a,b) as "symmetrical, organoid structures."
Histologically, plaques contain a core of fatty stroma and peripheral radiating
tubules. Under the stimulus of pregnancy and subsequent lactation, the tubules
undergo epithelial hyperplasia to give the appearance of an adenocarcinoma. At
weaning, the epithelium degenerates. Interestingly, experiments using the fat
pad transplantation technique of DeOme et al. (1959) have shown that plaques
transplanted into the mammary fat pads of young syngeneic virgin mice fill the fat
pad as ductal structures resembling the normal mammary gland of nonpregnant
mice (Aidells and Daniel, 1974). These tissues, serially transplanted for nine
generations, retained the ability to form hormone-dependent tumors in pregnant
mice and ducts in nonpregnant mice. It is within the alveolar hormone-dependent
tumors that foci of hormone-independent tumors arise focally or multifocally
(Foulds, 1949b, 1956b). Once the property of hormone independence is attained,
there is no reversion to the original phenotype; i.e., tumors do not produce
"normal" ducts in nonpregnant mice nor do they regress to hormone dependence. Progression of the characteristic for hormone independence thus is
irreversible.

In Foulds' original studies (1949a,b, 1954, 1956a,b), he noted that these mammary tumors were often multiple and that as many tumors were hormone independent as hormone dependent. By measuring the growth rates of tumors in pregnant mice and after parturition, he observed the various parameters associated with hormone-dependent and -nondependent tumors. Generally speaking, hormone dependency was not associated with size and age of the tumors, it persisted for many pregnancies, and the change from dependence to independence was generally abrupt but always irreversible. These studies and the conclusions derived from them established the concept of tumor progression firmly in the annals of tumor biology. It became quickly apparent that this concept was widely applicable.

2.1.2. Endocrine Tumors

Tumors arise in endocrine organs often as a result of a hormone imbalance (Furth, 1953; Furth et al., 1960). The hormonal imbalance may lead to a tumor in either the organ producing the hormone or the target organ, i.e., pituitary tumor (thyrotropic adenoma) in a host which has undergone thyroidectomy. Such tumors pass through at least two phases. In the initial phase, the continued growth of the adenoma depends on the abnormal hormone imbalance; i.e., in this phase, the thyrotropic adenoma is transplantable only when thyroxine is inhibited or absent. In the second phase, the thyrotropic tumor no longer requires the state of hormone imbalance for its continued growth; i.e., it has developed hormone independence. The time of onset of hormone independence may vary and be abrupt or casual. This progression from hormonal dependence to independence occurs in a variety of pituitary tumors, in ovarian tumors, in testicular tumors, and in chemical-carcinogen induced rat mammary tumors. In general, they follow the same patterns of growth as observed by Foulds in his study of spontaneous mammary tumors in (C57BL × RIII)F$_1$ hybrids. At this point, it is perhaps pertinent to indicate that hormonal independence is not equated with hormonal unresponsiveness. Hormone-independent tumors are still responsive to hormonal stimulation; however, they are no longer dependent on the original hormonal imbalance state for continued growth.

2.2. Principles of Tumor Progression

The concept of tumor progression was based on several principles outlined by Foulds which can be formulated as generalizations. The initial and most important generalization was that "progression is a permanent, irreversible change independent of other tumors." It was apparent to Foulds that the multiple tumors in the mammary gland attained hormonal independence separately and independently from each other. Thus only one or a few mammary tumors attained progressive development at any given time and each according to its own rate and pattern. This phenomenon is readily seen in other organs where tumors arise

multifocally. The conversion of papillomas to carcinomas in the skin of carcinogen-treated mice or rabbits occurs independently, and the conversion may be
either gradual or abrupt (Rous and Beard, 1935). Rous and Kidd (1941)
recognized and stressed that carcinoma arose as a result of a "stepwise change."
The change was not an exaggeration of previous papillomatosis, but a new event.
Other cancers where independent progression of tumors is thought to occur are
xeroderma pigmentosum (Foulds, 1958; Willis, 1967), familial intestinal polyps
(Foulds, 1958; Willis, 1967), liver cancer (Farber, 1968; Potter, 1969), and bladder
cancer (Schade, 1972; Koss *et al.*, 1974).

The second generalization states that the "individual characters of a tumor are
independently assortable." The morphological structure, biological behavior, and
biochemical characteristics of tumors are determined by many characters, each of
which may progress in an irreversible manner and independently. This independent variability of characters is seen in various experimental and human tumors.

The histoarchitecture of tumors is characterized by unique and unusual
examples of tissue patterns. Thus neoplasms of the mammary gland exhibit a
wide range of tissue configurations which include acinar, solid, papillary, cystic,
and metaplastic growths. The relative proportion of these can be used as a basis
for classification (Dunn, 1959). Progression of the histoarchitecture leads invariably to the most anaplastic tissue patterns. Similarly, Greene (1940) noted that
cytological changes characteristic of malignancy occurred 9–15 months before
invasiveness in the tumor, and that other tumors were locally invasive but not
metastatic. This dissociation of two characters is equally well established for
human tumors (Hamperl, 1957, 1967). Thus many human tumors undergo a
stage of being cytologically "malignant" but not invasive (Hamperl, 1967). The
interval between the two states is expressed in terms of years as in the case of
human cervical cancer. Although there is disagreement about the exact meaning
of the terminology "cytologically malignant" (Shabad, 1973; Scarpelli and Murad,
1973), it is evident that the observations of such different states can be interpreted
within the framework of the concept of tumor progression. Tumor progression
provides a means by which long latency periods between different developmental
states of altered cell populations become explainable. Chemical-carcinogen-
induced skin cancers of mice evolve changes in morphological pattern, growth
rate, and invasiveness independently of each other (Shubik *et al.*, 1953; Boutwell,
1964). This dissociation of characters has been analyzed in detail and provides
another example where characters of a neoplasm progress independently.

The analysis of the tumor phenotype at the molecular level documented that
tumors were biochemically distinct. The studies by Greenstein (1956) and others
(Weinhouse, 1960; Potter, 1969; Potter and Watanabe, 1968; Daoust and
Calamai, 1971) of the enzyme levels of normal and neoplastic cells demonstrated
that neoplastic tissue possessed enzymatic patterns which were unique—different
from those of normal tissues and different for tumors of the same tissue. In liver,
for which a great deal of information on enzyme patterns exists, it is clear that
individual tumors have characteristic enzyme patterns (Potter, 1969). One
mechanism, although by no means the only one, for the evolution of such tumor

phenotypes is the selection of cell populations which have acquired a given set of properties. The combinations resulting from progression of independent chartacters result in the wide variation seen in tumors.

The third generalization is that "tumor progression is potentially unlimited." The limits of tumor progression are frequently determined by the age and species of the hosts. In rabbits, chemical-carcinogen induced skin carcinomas rarely progress from papillomas, although papillomas induced by Shope papilloma virus progress frequently to carcinomas. In mice, skin carcinomas develop earlier and in greater frequency than in rabbits (Foulds, 1958). The method of serial transplantation of tumors clearly demonstrated that the extent of variability and the establishment of such variability are potentially unlimited. Alterations continue to arise spontaneously or to be induced in primary and transplanted tumors. Progression in hormone-induced tumors, mammary tumors of rodents, and chemical- or virus-induced papillomas is most clearly demonstrated by transplantation methods *in vivo* and *in vitro*.

The pathways progressed by tumors may be direct and indirect. In carcinogen-induced rat mammary tumors or papillomas, the progression to hormone independence and carcinoma, respectively, may be through observable stepwise changes or by indirect pathways which are traversed so rapidly as to be unnoticeable. In the neoplastic progression from mammary hyperplastic alveolar nodules (HAN) to adenocarcinomas in chemical-carcinogen-treated mice and rats, HAN are rarely seen, although carcinomas are frequent (Sinha and Dao 1971; Medina, 1974*a,b*). However, the potential for neoplastic development may be so great in carcinogen-induced HAN that the pathway of the nodule phenotype to adenocarcinoma is traversed very rapidly; thus nodules are rare under these conditions (Medina, 1974*a,b*).

A fourth generalization for which there is little appreciation is that "progression is independent of growth" (Foulds, 1954, 1958). This was originally based on the observation that regressed mammary tumors reappeared as hormone-independent tumors without the stimulus of pregnancy. A similar situation exists in initiation–promotion sequence for carcinogen-induced skin cancers. In both cases, progression occurs in a cell population not under the influence of the initial inciting stimulus. However, the cellular kinetics in neither of these two cases is well established; thus one is not sure of the actual mitotic activity of these altered cells. In light of subsequent experimentation, it is perhaps more appropriate to consider that progression can occur in the absence of the original inciting stimulus, while still remaining responsive to the original stimulus. This is surely true for carcinogen-induced mammary tumors, spontaneous hormone-dependent mammary tumors, and hormone-dependent endocrine tumors. In all of these cases, progression is probably enhanced under the influence of the inciting stimulus. The stronger and longer the stimulus, the greater the capacity for progression.

The criteria used to study the property of tumor progression are multiple characters, although they behave and are studied as unit characteristics. The original descriptions of progression to hormone independence and progression

of skin papillomas to carcinomas considered these characteristics as units.
However, it is clear that the response of a tumor to hormones involves uptake, translocation, and fixation (O'Malley and Means, 1974). Progression can take place at any of these levels, with the end result being the same, i.e., altered growth pattern, which is observed as a unit phenomenon. This becomes important in considering practical aspects of hormone therapy, chemotherapy, and immunotherapy since the permutations and combinations giving rise to variability in neoplasms assume immense proportions.

It should be clear that neoplastic progression signifies an empirically observed phenomenon and implies nothing about mechanisms, mutation, or differentiation. Progression merely signifies the acquisition of new characters by neoplastic cell populations and serves as a useful concept to understand the behavior of tumors and the wide variety of characteristics seen in neoplasms of the same organ.

3. Progression in Preneoplastic States

3.1. Mammary Hyperplastic Alveolar Nodules

The concept of progression can be applied advantageously to preneoplastic states to explain the numerous variants occurring in some of these populations. Although preneoplastic states exist in many tissues (i.e., cervix, bladder, intestine, liver, skin, mammary gland, endocrines), they have been studied to advantage only in the liver and the mammary gland. However, the ability to transplant normal and preneoplastic mammary tissue into isotopic sites has permitted extensive analysis of the nature of the nodule variants that arise within the mammary gland. The studies of DeOme and coworkers (DeOme *et al.*, 1959; DeOme, 1965), Ingraham (1966), and Slemmer (1972, 1974) have given rise to the following concepts concerning mammary nodule variation and progression of these variants.

The mammary nodule most frequently encountered is the hyperplastic alveolar nodule (HAN). The working scheme developed by DeOme and coworkers (DeOme, 1967; Medina and DeOme, 1968) suggests that nodules, at their earliest inception, represent a deviation from normal mammary tissue. The etiological factors and the mechanisms giving rise to nodule cell variants are not well understood, although it is clear that mammary tumor viruses and/or the hormonal milieu modulated by the appropriate genetic inheritance are primarily responsible for the majority of the nodules arising in most mouse strains (DeOme, 1967; Medina, 1973a). HAN do not represent areas of "latent tumor cells," "incipient" neoplasia, or regional neoplasia (Foulds, 1964, 1965), but represent cell populations different from both normal and neoplastic cells (DeOme, 1965). The HAN are characterized by a set of criteria which distinguish them from normal and neoplastic tissues. Table 1 lists the criteria which have been accumulated so far. It is clear that nodules represent cell populations which deviate from

TABLE 1

Characteristics of Normal, HAN, and Neoplastic Mammary Tissues

Criteria	Normal	HAN	Neoplastic
Morphological and physiological			
Myoepithelium	+	+	−
Apical alkaline phosphatase	−	−	+
Virus particles (A and B)	+	++	+++
^{32}P uptake	+	+	++
Polyploid DNA	−	−	++
Nuclear magnetic resonance[a]	Low	Intermediate	High
Transplantation			
Survival	+	+	+
Growth inhibition by cortisol	N.D.	−	+
Transformation	→	→	→
Progressive growth	−	−	+
Serial transplantation	−	+	+
Fat pad dependent	+	+	−
Subject to local growth regulation	+	+	−
Hormone dependency			
Ovariectomy: growth	+	+/−	+
alveolarity	−	+/−	+
Hypophysectomy: growth	−	−	+
alveolarity	−	−	+

[a] Value for relaxation time of water protons.

normal in many characteristics: hormonal responsiveness, responsiveness to growth regulatory factors, tumor potential, secretory status, growth rate, immunogenicity, etc. Extensive experiments in which the morphological and developmental characteristics of a series of nodule lines were analyzed over numerous serial transplant generations have established that these characteristics are stable, inherent, independently assortable properties of each nodule line (Blair *et al.*, 1962; Medina, 1973a).

If nodules represent an alteration from normal mammary gland at its very earliest inception, the observation that nodule outgrowth lines established from the transplantation of primary HAN into the fat pads of syngeneic mice subsequently differ in their morphological and behavioral characteristics suggests that variation from normal can be extended further and occurs frequently. A particular nodule outgrowth line with a low tumor potential progresses to neoplasia infrequently, yet may still deviate significantly from normal with respect to hormonal dependencies, morphological differentiation, and other criteria.

The variety of characteristics seen in mammary nodule tissue may occur independently. The development of hormone independence need not correlate with the development of neoplasia. In this respect, DeOme (1965) speaks of "essential" and "non-essential" characteristics. Some variants are obviously essential for the neoplastic transformation to occur in nodule lines (i.e., capability to override local growth regulatory factors, capability to produce neoplasms), and some are obviously not essential (i.e., secretory status, specialized protein products expressed as antigens, growth rate); however, all are expressed as stable, inherent properties. In this model, then, nodules are represented as a cell population comprised of cells with essential and nonessential variants, any of which are capable of independent progression. The critical question remains as to which variants are truly essential for the neoplastic population. Thus the behavioral and morphological characteristics of a nodule cell population will be determined by the proportion of cells showing any given variant.

It can be hypothesized that a similar situation exists in chemical-carcinogen-induced liver nodules, where subpopulations can be demonstrated for particular phenotypic characteristics (Becker and Klein, 1971; Daoust and Calamai, 1971; Rabes et al., 1972; Bruni, 1973). The carcinogen-induced liver nodules appear as hyperbasophilic foci which exhibit alterations in cell cycle, mitotic activity, dedifferentiation, and histochemical changes (Daoust and Calamai, 1971). These foci are thought to represent transitional populations between normal and neoplastic liver. Subpopulations of hepatocytes occur with chemical-carcinogen-induced liver nodules which are mitotically responsive but resistant to L-asparaginase-induced mitotic inhibition (Becker and Klein, 1971). These L-asparaginase-resistant hepatocytes are localized randomly in occasional nodules, are diploid, and persist throughout the evolution of the hepatic neoplasm (Becker and Klein, 1971). Additional studies by Rabes et al. (1972) using enzyme histochemical techniques demonstrated that carcinogen-induced liver nodules are not a homogeneous preneoplastic population but rather subpopulations in various stages of development. These areas of altered cells can be demonstrated by 30 days after carcinogen feeding. While these initial changes are seen in many cells, further alterations are necessary before the appearance of neoplasms. Finally, Bruni (1973) demonstrated that some cells in carcinogen-treated liver are morphologically distinguishable on the basis of the lack of development of smooth endoplasmic reticulum. These studies taken together suggest the great heterogeneity of cells during the early stages of chemical carcinogenesis and provide the framework for neoplastic progression.

Variant cells may exist in large numbers in a normal-appearing mammary gland, but their presence not be revealed as recognizable morphological structures. In such cases, a biochemical change may have occurred which has segregated a variant cell from normal cells in the population (i.e., increased ability to proliferate); however, the essential variant for expression as nodules has not occurred (i.e., the development of hormonal unresponsiveness resulting in the ability to differentiate into alveoli in the absence of mammotropin). That such variants do exist in a normal population is supported by several inferences and recent direct experimental observations. It has been extensively documented in both mice and rats that HAN precede and give rise to mammary neoplasms (DeOme et al., 1959; Beuving, 1968; Medina, 1973a). However, in certain instances, one can observe the development of mammary tumors with high frequency in the absence of HAN or with few HAN (Sinha and Dao, 1971; Medina, 1974a,b). These events generally occur in chemical-carcinogen-treated mice and rats. One can hypothesize that the progression from normal tissue to nodule to neoplasm is extremely rapid so that the probability of observing a high frequency of nodules is minimal. Nodules that do occur would have high tumor potentials. Alternatively, it is possible that tumors arise directly from normal tissues. Several observations support the former prediction. Nodule lines that have been derived from nodules occurring in carcinogen-treated mice do have very high tumor potentials (Medina, unpublished). Even more important, DeOme (personal communication) has demonstrated that nodule cells are present in normal-appearing mammary gland long before they are observed as primary HAN. Thus whereas HAN are initially seen as discrete foci in 10- to 12-month-old virgin BALB(cfC3H mice, they can be demonstrated to exist as unexpressed nodule variants in the mammary glands of 3-month-old mice by transplantation of cells collected from an enzyme-dissociated mammary gland preparation.

Progression at the preneoplastic level can be explained by the emergence of a few essential variants followed by increasing divergence of the previous population. The acquisition of the critical properties which allow the cells to be expressed first as a nodule and then as a neoplasm may occur independently from the acquisition of other nonessential variants at any time in the life span of the nodule cell population. The neoplastic population represents the selection of cells within a nodule cell population possessing the essential variant characteristics. The critical essential variant characteristics are not defined, although several have been hypothesized. DeOme (Faulkin and DeOme, 1960; DeOme, 1965) considers the independence from local growth factors elaborated by normal ducts (and/or fat pad stroma) to be a critical variant. Slemmer (1974) believes the independence from myoepithelial cell control to be critical for the emergence of malignant neoplasms. The important point is that both the nodule cell and neoplastic cell populations are comprised of essential and nonessential variants. The concept of progression then can be extended down to the level of the original deviation from normal, which occurs long before neoplasms arise. The dual events of progression (acquisition of new characters at the cellular level) and selection act throughout the life span of cell populations to forge the emergence of preneoplastic and neoplastic populations, and, as stated in the earlier sections, these forces are infinitely at play.

3.2. Factors Influencing Progression at the Preneoplastic Level

In the life span of a cell population, the acquisition of new, inheritable characteristics may be influenced by various environmental and host factors. It is not clear whether the mechanisms involved are direct or indirect since the role of host factors (viruses, hormones) on tumor progression has not been investigated *per se*. That is not to say that little is known about whether hormones, viruses, and drugs inhibit or enhance tumorigenesis, since the literature on this subject is extensive. But the relationship of these agents in the context of tumor progression is unclear.

There is some information which suggests that chemical carcinogens and perhaps viruses may enhance the emergence of neoplastic cell variants in the mammary nodule system. It has been amply documented that the same agents which give rise to nodules also enhance the nodule-to-tumor transformation. Thus mammary tumor viruses (Medina and DeOme, 1968), chemical carcinogens (Medina and DeOme, 1970a), and hormonal stimulation (Medina and DeOme, 1970b) all enhance tumorigenesis. If one considers a preneoplastic state to exist in skin, then many agents are known which enhance or promote tumorigenesis (Boutwell, 1964; Major, 1970; Hennings and Boutwell, 1970; Slaga and Scribner, 1973; Raick, 1974). The mechanism behind such skin promoting agents remains unknown.

A critical achievement with respect to the role of oncogenic agents modifying the process of tumor progression would be to demonstrate the emergence of cell variants which have an increased responsiveness or susceptibility to otherwise innocuous stimuli. Thus the acquisition, after carcinogen treatment, of the ability to produce neoplastic cell variants in response to normal stimuli would be a clear demonstration that tumor progression may be modulated by environmental factors. One such example occurs in the mouse mammary nodule system. In this case, treatment with 3-methylcholanthrene leads to the appearance of cell variants which produce mammary tumors in response to a hormonal milieu that would be otherwise nontumorigenic (Medina, 1972). Such nodule outgrowth lines treated with 3-methylcholanthrene produce tumors in response to prolonged hormonal stimulation (Medina, 1972) and the undefined hormonal alterations of a host treated neonatally with 17β-estradiol (Medina, unpublished). The untreated tissue does not respond to these hormonal environments with enhanced tumorigenesis and the carcinogen-treated tissue does not produce tumors in the untreated mouse. Similarly, the tumors that arise are not hormone dependent (Medina, 1973b). The mechanisms underlying the phenomenon are unclear; thus it is not known whether the carcinogen is selecting preexisting hormone-sensitive cell variants or inducing the property within the cell. The former alternative appears unlikely since the cell variants can be demonstrated 1 day after carcinogen treatment and do not increase with time (Medina, 1972).

Preneoplastic progression at the cellular level during the evolution of histogenetic unique mammary tumors was documented in an elegant study by Slemmer (1974). Using the fat pad transplantation method of DeOme et al. (1959), and cell suspensions of normal and neoplastic cells with different histocompatibility markers, Slemmer (1974) examined the cellular compositions of mammary tumors of different histoarchitecture. Slemmer (1974) provided evidence that normal mammary glands are composed of at least three cell populations, ductal epithelial, alveolar epithelial, and myoepithelial. It was postulated that various oncogenic agents caused the transformation of the different cell types, each of which produced a unique class of preneoplastic lesion which progressed sequentially to a malignant tumor characteristic of one of the three cell types. Although there is little direct evidence that each cell type gives rise to a morphologically characteristic tumor, it was evident that the progression of neoplasms from benign to malignant resulted from the acquisition of the property to survive and proliferate independently from associated normal myoepithelial or normal ductal cells (Slemmer, 1974). The experiments demonstrated that normal cell components were progressively lost as hyperplastic alveolar nodules progressed to adenomas and subsequently malignant tumors. These studies documented in an elegant fashion the phenomenon of neoplastic progression at the cytological level.

A second case of host-related modification of tumor progression is the problem of isoantigenic variation, which is discussed further in this chapter. The general problem of inhibition and enhancement of tumor growth lies outside the context of the general discussion of tumor progression and is discussed elsewhere in these volumes.

4. Other Examples of Tumor Progression

The phenomenon of tumor progression has been studied in other systems which have yielded additional information on the process and the mechanisms underlying the process. The more important of these studies have been on ascites conversion, drug resistance, evolution of chromosome patterns, and isoantigenic variation.

4.1. Ascites Conversion

An ascites tumor is defined as a neoplastic population able to grow in free suspension within the peritoneal fluid of the peritoneal body cavity. The ascites tumor can grow as either single cells or small aggregates in the peritoneal fluid in the absence of capillaries or stroma. Probably any type of tumor is capable of growing in the ascites form. Leukemias, lymphomas, sarcomas (Goldie *et al.*, 1953), mammary adenocarcinomas, hepatomas, and a variety of other solid tissues (G. Klein and E. Klein, 1956) have been grown in the ascites form. Ascites tumors arise from solid tumors which have been finely minced and injected intraperitoneally. The conversion to ascites form is usually a long process and the result of serial passage of peritoneal exudate. G. Klein and E. Klein (1955, 1956) have studied the ascites conversion in detail as an excellent example of tumor progression. They found that the conversion from solid tumor to ascites form occurred in one of three patterns. Tumors were either immediately convertible, gradually convertible, or unconvertible. The majority of the tumors (75%) fell into the last category. However, there was no general correlation between convertibility and morphogenetic origin, although spontaneous primary solid mammary adenocarcinomas were inconvertible as a whole. The process to conversion was facilitated by rapid growth rate, anaplasia, and ability to survive in a liquid exudate (G. Klein and E. Klein, 1955, 1956). The inability to convert was correlated with failure to survive in the fluid.

The conversion to ascites form is stable and irreversible. Tumors which were converted to ascites and then serially transplanted subcutaneously as solid tumors retained the ability to form ascites tumors immediately on injection of the cells into the peritoneal cavity regardless of the length of time it took for the original ascites transformation. This was true for both carcinomas and sarcomas. The cellular changes which were required for progressive growth in suspension were independent from those that facilitated survival in suspension. The conclusion drawn by the Kleins (E. Klein and G. Klein, 1956) was that the conversion from solid tumors to ascites tumor was the result of a sequential progression of events. The cellular and molecular mechanisms responsible are discussed in Section 5.

4.2. Drug Resistance

The development of resistance to the cytotoxic effects of drugs provides another system which parallels the process of tumor progression outlined in the evolution of hormonal autonomy and ascites conversion. Early workers in the field of cancer chemotherapy noticed the development of resistance on the part of tumors to a variety of drugs, including folic acid antagonist (Burchenal *et al.*, 1950), 8-azaguanine (Law, 1951), and 6-mercaptopurine (Law, 1953). The variant cell populations arose as a consequence of continued treatment of the tumor over a period of several transplant generations. This phenomenon, termed "drug resistance," varied extensively even among histogenetically similar neoplasms responding to a single drug. The response of cells varied from complete resistance to varying degrees of sensitivity (G. Klein, 1963). Resistance developed either with prolonged passage in the presence of the drug (Potter, 1958) or immediately (G. Klein, 1963; Law, 1958). Resistance developed at different functional loci within a given tumor line (Potter, 1958).

The acquisition of drug resistance is a stable, primarily irreversible event which is maintained in the absence of the original drug. The random appearance and clonal growth of variant populations suggest that the phenomenon is broadly based and may be the result of a general preexisting refractoriness in the population (G. Klein, 1963).

The molecular basis for the development of resistance is manifold and includes the decreased activity or deletion of metabolic enzymes in nucleotide synthetic pathways (Handschumacher and Welch, 1960), increase in enzyme activities (Fischer, 1961), appearance of genetically altered enzymes (Heidelberger, 1961), and changes in cell permeability (Fischer, 1962). Although the mechanism underlying these changes has been presumed to be genetic, there is some evidence that epigenetic mechanisms (G. Klein, 1963; Harris, 1973, 1974) may play an important role in the appearance of cell variants in tumor populations.

4.3. Chromosome Patterns

Since Boveri's (1912) postulation that alterations in chromosome number were causally significant in the genesis of neoplasms, the evolution of aneuploid chromosomal patterns in neoplasms and *in vitro* permanent cell lines has been a central theme in tumor biology. Additionally, the demonstration that chromosomal alterations continue throughout the evolution of a neoplasm illustrates another pattern in tumor progression.

Neoplasms are commonly diploid (Bayreuther, 1960; Koller, 1972), hypodiploid (Koller, 1972), or hypotetraploid (Koller, 1972). On serial transplantation, the karyotype of tumors often shifts to form aneuploid patterns (Hsu, 1961; Hauschka, 1961). The development of a tumor with a characteristic aneuploid number is dependent on at least two events: (1) development of polyploidy where both low-ploid and high-ploid cells exist in balance within the tumor cell population and (2) selection of variants with a modal chromosome number (Makino, 1956, 1957; Hsu, 1961). The clonal evolution of subpopulations comprising various karyotypes resulted in the hypothesis of stem lines (Makino, 1956, 1957; Hauschka, 1961). Essentially the stem line concept states that neoplasms are represented by a population of stem cells from which all other cells are derived. The stem cell in the neoplasm is the modal cell karyotype which gives rise to the bulk of the population through mitosis. Any cell population of a neoplasm may have several stem cells (Makino, 1956, 1957; Hauschka, 1961). The evolution of karyotype patterns is continuous, with no implication of an endpoint (Hsu, 1961).

Although the mechanism of karyotype variability is not understood in molecular or genetic terms, most authorities agree that karyotype variability is not causal in the genesis of neoplasm (Koller, 1972). The extent of karyotype variability and instability has caused one noted authority to sum up the state of the significance of karyotype instability in neoplasms as follows: "variations in chromosome numbers occur in tumors not because they matter more, but because they matter less, than elsewhere" (Darlington, 1959).

One of the more plausible suggestions regarding the significance of karyotype variability was the suggestion by Makino (1956) that progeny of stem-like cells are "better adapted" toward autonomous growth. This hypothesis is probably oversimplified. Environmental conditions influence markedly the stem line of neoplasms. Thus stem lines vary with the site of transplantation and the form of growth. For example, the stem line of Yoshida sarcoma (CB subline) is 4 times greater if the neoplasm is grown as a solid tumor than if grown as an ascites tumor intraperitoneally. However, once the solid tumor is reconverted into an ascites form again, the stem line adapts toward growth in the particular environment (Koller, 1960, 1972).

Additionally, it is clear that cell populations of neoplasms contain variants of various kinds (drug resistance, antigenicity, hormone dependency) which may or may not be correlated with the particular chromosome constitution of the neoplasm (Koller, 1972). The variation of karyotype provides cell populations which are adapted to specific functions and can be selected to replace parental cells under appropriate pressures. Thus karyotype variability behaves as a unit character independent of other characteristics associated with the neoplastic state and subject to the same laws of neoplastic progression, as illustrated in the discussion on the evolution of hormonal independence. The importance of

karyotype variability in preneoplastic progression has not been investigated
extensively, although the use of newer chromosomal staining techniques might
prove useful in identifying critical and subtle chromosomal changes in the initial
stages of progression (Rowley, 1974).

113

TUMOR
PROGRESSION

4.4. Tumor Transplantability (Isoantigenic Variation)

The transplantability of tumors is governed by protein determinants on the cell
membrane called histocompatibility proteins. The most extensively studied and
strongest histocompatibility locus in the mouse is the multiallelic *H-2* locus. The
degree and length of a successful tumor transplant are generally proportional to
the exactness of the identity between the donor and recipient. There are many
exceptions to the rule, the most notable being the universal tumors (i.e., Jenson
sarcomas; Krebs, Ehrlich ascites; Brown–Pierce rabbit carcinoma), which have
acquired a nonspecific host range. These "universal" tumors generally have lost
their *H-2* alleles and are aneuploid.

Tumors which acquire the ability to grow in histoincompatible hosts exhibit a
deletion of isoantigens which may or may not be correlated with aneuploidy. The
reduction in isoantigens is one of degree since these tumors may be antigenic
under other specific circumstances. The phenomenon of isoantigenic variation
has been noted in a variety of tumors, and has been studied most extensively by
Klein and coworkers (E. Klein, 1961; G. Klein, 1963; E. Klein *et al.*, 1960; Weiner
et al., 1974; Cikes *et al.*, 1973). The changes which occur are always loss changes;
thus they proceed in the direction of decreased specificity (G. Klein, 1963). The
events are stable, random, and persistent throughout successive generations.
Different tumors vary with regard to the occurrence and frequency of a particular
variant, and, conversely, different isoantigenic variants can be obtained from the
same tumor (G. Klein, 1963). Isoantigenic variants can occur immediately or after
many serial transplants.

The formation of isoantigenic variants in tumors arising in hybrid mice
provides the basic information on the process of variant formation (G. Klein,
1963). Tumors which arise in hybrid mice can be transplanted into the parental
strains. Under these conditions, the parental strain, especially if immunized,
should reject the hybrid tumors on the basis of the heterozygous *H-2* allele. If a
tumor grows in a given parent, this suggests a loss of one *H-2* allele. Several
different types of growth can be demonstrated. The first two, nonspecific growth
and false positives, are quickly recognized since they occur only in nonimmunized
parental strains. However, tumors exhibiting isoantigenic variants grow in one
parent and not the other. The antigenic loss is stable and specific even after
growth of the tumors in hybrids for several generations. All variants are generally
of the "loss" type and antigenic conversion is rarely if ever induced (G. Klein,
1963). The isoantigenic variant is not lost further; thus it is probably essential for
growth. In the Kleins' studies (G. Klein, 1963), further progression to a "universal" tumor similar to Krebs ascites was not demonstrated, although the possibility

was not investigated thoroughly. The acquisition of isoantigenic variants was hypothesized to be due to the selection of preexisting cell variants with the tumor cell population.

5. Mechanisms of Tumor Progression

The study of ascites conversion, drug resistance, and isoantigenic variation has provided the main insight into the mechanisms underlying tumor progression. These studies have been done primarily by Klein and his coworkers (G. Klein, 1963), although the recent work by Harris (1971, 1973, 1974) and the earlier work by DeOme and coworkers (DeOme, 1965; Blair *et al.*, 1962) have contributed much to the overall concept.

The initial experiments by G. Klein and E. Klein (1956) demonstrated that selection of a small population of variants, rather than physiological adaptation, was responsible for the changes in behavior demonstrated by tumors undergoing progression. Thus the Kleins demonstrated that a critical number of cells were necessary for a tumor to undergo ascites conversion and the percentage of cell variants was directly proportional to the time required for ascites conversion. A tumor population with 5% variants was immediately convertible; a population with 1% was convertible after two transfer generations, and populations with 0.1% were convertible after four transfer generations. Their conclusion was that the ascites conversion represented a minority proportion of the population giving rise to a majority under selective pressure. One estimate of the frequency of ascites variants in solid tumors was 2.4×10^{-6}. These variants preexisted but needed the selective pressure of a fluid environment to become dominant.

Not all phenomena need be explained on a variation-selection hypothesis. The Barrett–Deringer effect (Barrett *et al.*, 1953; E. Klein and G. Klein, 1956) is a classic example of host-induced adaptation. In this type of effect, tumor cells passaged once through a hybrid grow better in the backcross resistant hosts than tumors not so passaged. The stable change in the tumor cell populations is induced at the cellular level, is permanent, and is not enhanced with repeated passage through hybrids. Small inocula have the same effect as large inocula and cellular contact between tumor and F_1 host is not necessary (G. Klein, 1963). In addition, a shift in *H-2* alleles is not seen. In this phenomenon, the increase in transplantability is induced in tumors by factors within the hybrid host and is probably related to changes in weak histocompatibility genes.

These studies do not allow a conclusion on the merits of epigenetic vs. genetic mechanisms. The continuing work by Klein and coworkers on the evolution of isoantigenic variants has demonstrated that both crossing over (E. Klein, 1961) and, in special cases, chromosome loss (Weiner *et al.*, 1974) are responsible for isoantigenic variation. In an early series of experiments, the loss of *H-2* alleles in a hybrid tumor was correlated with growth of the tumor in the parental strain. Variant tumors lacked either *H-2^k*, or *H-2^d* and *H-2^k*, but never *H-2^d* alone. Selection against D yielded cell variants without D and K. This occurred when the determinants were in the *cis* position (G. Klein, 1963). This process was consistent with a somatic crossing-over mechanism. Recent experiments demonstrated that the loss of one parental *H-2* allele was associated with loss of both chromosomes bearing the locus (Weiner *et al.*, 1974). The phenomenon is different from the modulation of antigenic expression that occurs with the thymic-leukemia antigen (TL) studied by Boyse *et al.* (1967) and probably different from the phenomenon reported by Cikes *et al.* (1973) where the progressive loss of *H-2* alleles from tumor lines maintained *in vitro* was reversed after a single *in vivo* passage. These last two studies revealed a modulation of antigenic expression (i.e., a quantitative difference), whereas the loss of *H-2* allele was qualitative and permanent.

The experiments by Harris (1971, 1973, 1974) have demonstrated that epigenetic mechanisms must seriously be considered as another basis for tumor progression. Fluctuation tests showed that stable drug-resistant variants can occur spontaneously, and randomly (Harris, 1973). The mechanistic basis for these changes may be genetic (Albrecht *et al.*, 1972; Lee *et al.*, 1973) or epigenetic (Harris, 1971, 1973, 1974). Evidence supporting the latter mechanism arises from the high rate of ascites variants, which is inconsistent with known levels of somatic cell mutation (E. Klein, 1961; Harris, 1974). In addition, Harris (1971) demonstrated that the mutation rates for 8-azaguanine resistance did not change in diploid, tetraploid, and octaploid lines; thus the lack of an effect of ploidy supports the concept that variations arise in somatic cells by changes in phenotypic expression (Harris, 1971). The recent demonstration that the expression of either spontaneous or nitrosoguanidine-induced cell variants exhibiting resistance to vinblastine sulfate (dominant characteristic) and cytosine arabinoside (recessive characteristic) was independent of the dominant or recessive characteristic of the marker supports the concept that resistance to these markers may "arise by nonchromosomal changes" (Harris, 1974). Thus cellular variation may arise "by random shifts to new and stable patterns of gene expression" as well as by changes of genetic information in cytoplasmic and nuclear determinants (Harris, 1974).

6. Conclusions

It is evident that tumor cell populations rarely can be viewed as homogeneous. The studies performed over the past 20 years on the evolution of hormone independence, karyotype variation, ascites conversion, drug resistance, isoantigenic variation, and a number of other morphological and behavioral patterns have demonstrated that tumors are a heterogeneous population in which a broad range of variation permits the continuous operation of selective forces. This variation provides a pool which confers advantageous conditions in a selective environment. All characters in a tumor are subject to variation and progression, a process which proceeds generally in the direction of progressive freedom from all growth regulation mechanisms of the body.

Foulds' original description of the term "progression" excluded any suggestion as to the exact mechanisms underlying the process. In view of recent findings that both epigenetic and genetic mechanisms may play a crucial role in the "acquisi-tion" of new characters, Foulds was justified in his vagueness. Progression is useful in understanding the behavior of a tumor from its earliest inception through its final demise. In addition, the concept of progression can be usefully applied to the earliest inception of alterations, i.e., at the preneoplastic cell level. At all levels of organization, it is clear that cell populations are a complex of cell variants, which allows preneoplastic or neoplastic cells to grow in adverse and changing environments.

The final challenge in understanding tumor progression lies in unraveling the mechanisms producing the continued variation seen in tumor cell populations. Understanding of the roles played by genetic and epigenetic mechanisms will provide basic information pertinent to the ultimate neoplastic alteration. For these studies, the phenomena of both isoantigenic variation (G. Klein, 1963) and drug resistance (Harris, 1974) should provide critical information concerning the relative roles of genetic and epigenetic mechanisms in tumor progression.

7. References

AIDELLS, B. D., AND DANIEL, C. W., 1974, Hormone dependent mammary tumors in strain GR/A mice. I. Alteration between ductal and tumorous phases of growth during serial transplantation, *J. Natl. Cancer Inst.* **52:**1855.

ALBRECHT, A. M., BIEDLER, J. L., AND HUTCHISON, D. J., 1972, Two different species of dihydrolate reductase in mammalian cells differentially resistant to amethopterin and methasquin, *Cancer Res.* **32:**1539.

BARRETT, M. K., DERINGER, M. K., AND HANSEN. W. H., 1953. Induced adaptation in a tumor: Specificity of the change, *J. Natl. Cancer Inst.* **14:**381.

BAYREUTHER, K., 1960, Chromosomes in the primary neoplastic growth, *Nature (London)* **186:**6.

BECKER, F. F., AND KLEIN, K. M., 1971, The effect of L-asparaginase on mitotic activity during N-2-fluorenylacetamide hepatocarcinogenesis: Subpopulations of nodular cells, *Cancer Res.* **31:**169.

BERENBLUM, I., AND SHUBIK, P., 1947, The role of croton oil applications, associated with a single painting of a carcinogen, in tumor induction of the mouse's skin, *Br. J. Cancer* **1:**379.

BERENBLUM, I., AND SHUBIK, P., 1949, The persistence of latent tumor cells induced in the mouse's skin by a single application of 9:10-dimethyl-1:2-bezanthracene, *Br. J. Cancer* **3:**384.

BEUVING, L. J., 1968, Mammary tumor formation within outgrowths of transplanted hyperplastic nodules from carcinogen-treated rats, *J. Natl. Cancer Inst.* **40:**1287.

BLAIR, P. B., DeOME, K. B., AND NANDI, S., 1962, The characteristics of the preneoplastic state in mouse mammary carcinogenesis, in: *Biological Interactions in Normal and Neoplastic Growth* (M. J. Brennan and W. L. Simpson, eds.), pp. 371–389, Little, Brown, Boston.

BOUTWELL, R. K., 1964, Some biological aspects of skin carcinogenesis, *Prog. Exp. Tumor Res.* **4:**207.

BOVERI, T., 1912, Beitrag zum Studium des Chromatin in den Epithelzellen der Carcinome, *Beitr. Pathol. Anat.* **14:**249.

BOYSE, E. A., STOCKERT, E., AND OLD, L. J., 1967, Modification of the antigenic structure of the cell membrane by thymus-leukemia (TL) antibody, *Proc. Natl. Acad. Sci. U.S.A.* **58:**954.

BRUNI, C., 1973, Distinctive cells similar to fetal hepatocytes associated with liver carcinogenesis by diethylnitrosamine: Electron microscopic study, *J. Natl. Cancer Inst.* **50:**1513.

BURCHENAL, J. H., ROBINSON, E., JOHNSTON, S. F., AND KUSHIDA, M. N., 1950, The induction of resistance to 4-amino-N^{10}-methyl-pteroylglutamic acid in a strain of transmitted mouse leukemia, *Science* **111:**116.

CIKES, M., FRIBERG, S., JR., AND KLEIN, G., 1973, Progressive loss of H-2 antigens with concomitant increase of cell-surface antigens determined by Maloney leukemia virus in cultured murine lymphomas, *J. Natl. Cancer Inst.* **50:**347.

DAOUST, R., AND CALAMAI, R., 1971, Hyperbasophilic foci as sites of neoplastic transformation in hepatic parenchyma, *Cancer Res.* **31**:1290.

DARLINGTON, C. D., 1959, Plasmagene theory and cancer genesis, in: *Genetics and Cancer*, pp. 9–24, University of Texas Press, Austin.

DEOME, K. B., 1965, Multiple factors in mouse mammary tumorigenesis, *Cancer Res.* **25**:1348.

DEOME, K. B., 1967, The mouse mammary tumor system, in: *Proceedings of the Fifth Berkeley Symposium on Mathematical Statistics and Probability* (J. Neyman, ed.), pp. 649–655, University of California Press, Berkeley.

DEOME, K. B., FAULKIN, L. J., JR., BERN, H. A., AND BLAIR, P. B., 1959, Development of mammary tumors from hyperplastic alveolar nodules transplanted into gland-free mammary fat pads of female C3H mice, *Cancer Res.* **19**:515.

DUNN, T. B., 1959, Morphology of mammary tumors in mice, in: *Physiopathology of Cancer* (F. Homberger, ed.), pp. 38–84, Hoeber-Harper, New York.

FARBER, E., 1968, On the concept of minimum deviation in the study of the biochemistry of cancer, *Cancer Res.* **28**:1210.

FAULKIN, L. J., JR., AND DEOME, K. B., 1960, Regulation of growth and spacing of gland elements in the mammary fat pad of the C3H mouse, *J. Natl. Cancer Inst.* **24**:953.

FISCHER, G. A., 1961, Increased levels of folic acid reductase as a mechanism of resistance to amethopterin in leukemic cells, *Biochem. Pharmacol.* **7**:75.

FISCHER, G. A., 1962, Defective transport of amethopterin as a mechanism of resistance to the antimetabolite in L-5178Y leukemic cells, *Biochem. Pharmacol.* **11**:1233.

FOULDS, L., 1949a, Mammary tumors in hybrid mice: Hormone responses of transplanted tumors, *Br. J. Cancer* **3**:240.

FOULDS, L., 1949b, Mammary tumors in hybrid mice: Growth and progression of spontaneous tumors, *Br. J. Cancer* **3**:345.

FOULDS, L., 1954, Tumor progression: A review, *Cancer Res.* **14**:327.

FOULDS, L., 1956a, The histological analysis of mammary tumors of mice. I. Scope of investigations and general principles of analysis, *J. Natl. Cancer Inst.* **17**:701.

FOULDS, L., 1956b, The histological analysis of mammary tumors of mice. II. The histology of responsiveness and progression: The origins of tumors, *J. Natl. Cancer Inst.* **17**:713.

FOULDS, L., 1958, The natural history of cancer, *J. Chron. Dis.* **8**:2.

FOULDS, L., 1964, Tumor progression and neoplastic development, in: *Cellular Control Mechanisms and Cancer* (P. Emmelot and O. Mühlbock, eds.), pp. 242–258, Elsevier, Amsterdam.

FOULDS, L., 1965, Multiple etiological factors in neoplastic development, *Cancer Res.* **25**:1339.

FOULDS, L., 1969, *Neoplastic Development*, Academic Press, New York.

FRIEDEWALD, W. F., AND ROUS, P., 1950, The pathogenesis of deferred cancer: A study of the aftereffects of methylcholanthrene upon rabbit skin, *J. Exp. Med.* **91**:459.

FURTH, J., 1953, Conditional and autonomous neoplasms, *Cancer Res.* **13**:477.

FURTH, J., KIM, U., AND CLIFTON, K. H., 1960, On evolution of the neoplastic state: progression from dependence to autonomy, *Natl. Cancer Inst. Monogr.* **2**:149.

GOLDIE, H., BUTLER, C. H., ANDERSON, M. M., MAXWELL, M. C., AND HAHN, P. F., 1953, Growth characteristics of free C1498 (granulocytic leukemia) tumor cells in the peritoneal fluid and the blood of C57 mice, *Cancer Res.* **13**:125.

GREENE, H. S. N., 1940, Familial mammary tumors in the rabbit. IV. The evolution of autonomy in the course of tumor development as indicated by transplantation experiments, *J. Exp. Med.* **71**:305.

GREENSTEIN, J. P., 1956, Some biological characteristics of morphologically separable cancers, *Cancer Res.* **16**:641.

HAALAND, M., 1911, Spontaneous tumors in mice, *Sci. Rep. Imperial Cancer Res. Fund* **4**:1.

HAMPERL, H., 1957, Ueber die Entwicklung von Tumoren. *Wien. Klin. Wochenschr.* **69**:201.

HAMPERL, H., 1967, Early invasive growth as seen in uterine cancer *in situ* and the role of the basal membrane, in: *Mechanisms of Invasion in Cancer* (P. Denoix, ed.), pp. 17–25, Springer, Berlin.

HANDSCHUMACHER, R. E., AND WELCH, A. D., 1960, Agents which influence nucleic acid metabolisms, in: *The Nucleic Acids*, Vol. 3 (E. Chargaff and J. N. Davidson, eds.), pp. 453–526, Academic Press, New York.

HARRIS, M., 1971, Polyploid series of mammalian cells, *Exp. Cell Res.* **66**:329.

HARRIS, M., 1973, Phenotypic expression of drug resistance in hybrid cells, *J. Natl. Cancer Inst.* **50**:423.

HARRIS, M., 1974, Comparative frequency of dominant and recessive markers for drug resistance in Chinese hamster cells, *J. Natl. Cancer Inst.* **52**:1811.

HAUSCHKA, T. S., 1961, The chromosome in ontogeny and oncogeny, *Cancer Res.* **21:**957.

HEIDELBERGER, C., 1961, Nucleic acid synthesis and mechanism of action of fluoropyrimidines, in: *Biological Approaches to Cancer Chemotherapy* (R. J. C. Harris, ed.), pp. 47–58, Academic Press, New York.

HENNINGS, H., AND BOUTWELL, R. K., 1970, Studies on the mechanism of skin tumor formation, *Cancer Res.* **30:**312.

HESTON, W. E., VLAHAKIS, G., AND TOUBURA, Y., 1964, Strain DD, a new high mammary tumor strain and comparison of DD with strain C3H, *J. Natl. Cancer Inst.* **32:**237.

HSU, T. C., 1961, Chromosome evolution in cell populations, *Int. Rev. Cytol.* **12:**69.

INGRAHAM, R. L., 1966, Analysis of variation in preneoplastic tissues from the mouse mammary gland by means of organ-culture techniques, Ph.D. thesis in zoology, University of California, Berkeley.

KLEIN, E., 1961, Studies on the mechanism of isoantigenic variant formation in heterozygous mouse tumors. I. Behavior of H-2 antigens D and K: Quantitative absorption tests on mouse sarcomas, *J. Natl. Cancer Inst.* **27:**1069.

KLEIN, E., AND KLEIN, G., 1956, Mechanism of induced change in transplantation specificity of a mouse tumor passed through hybrid hosts, *Transpl. Bull.* **3:**136.

KLEIN, E., KLEIN, G., AND HELLSTROM, K. E., 1960, Further studies on isoantigenic variation in mouse carcinomas and sarcomas, *J. Natl. Cancer Inst.* **25:**271.

KLEIN, G., 1963, Genetics of somatic cells, in: *Methodology in Mammalian Genetics* (W. J. Burdette, ed.), pp. 407–468, Holden-Day, San Francisco.

KLEIN, G., AND KLEIN, E., 1955, Variation in cell population of transplanted tumors as indicated by studies on the ascites transformation, *Exp. Cell Res. Suppl.* **3:**218.

KLEIN, G., AND KLEIN, E., 1956, Conversion of solid neoplasms into ascites tumors, *Ann. N.Y. Acad. Sci.* **63:**640.

KOLLER, P. C., 1960, Chromosome behavior in tumors: Readjustments to Boveri's theory, in: *Cell Physiology of Neoplasia*, pp. 9–48, University of Texas Press, Austin.

KOLLER, P. C., 1972, The role of chromosomes in cancer biology, *Recent Results Cancer Res.* **38:**14.

KOSS, L. G., ESPERANZA, M. T., AND ROBBINS, M. A., 1974, Mapping cancerous and precancerous bladder changes, *J. Am. Med. Assoc.* **227:**281.

LAW, L. W., 1951, Resistance in leukemic cells to a guanine analog, 8-azaguanine, *Proc. Soc. Exp. Biol. Med.* **78:**499.

LAW, L. W., 1953, Resistance in leukemic cells to an adenine antagonist, 6-mercaptopurine, *Proc. Soc. Exp. Biol. Med.* **84:**409.

LAW, L. W., 1958, Some aspects of drug resistance in neoplasms, *Ann. N.Y. Acad. Sci.* **71:**976.

LEE, R. W., GILLHAM, N. W., VAN WINKLE, K. P., AND BOYNTON, J. E., 1973, Preferential recovery of uniparental streptomycin resistant mutants from diploid *Chlamydomonas reinhardti*, *Mol. Gen. Genet.* **121:**109.

MAJOR, I. R., 1970, Correlation of initial changes in the mouse epidermal cell population with two-stage carcinogenesis: A quantitative study, *Br. J. Cancer* **24:**149.

MAKINO, S., 1956, Further evidence favoring the concept of the stem cell in ascites tumors of rats, *Ann. N.Y. Acad. Sci.* **63:**818.

MAKINO, S., 1957, The chromosome cytology of the ascites tumors of rats, with special reference to the concept of the stemline cell, *Int. Rev. Cytol.* **6:**25.

MATSUZAWA, A., YAMAMOTO, T., AND SUZUKI, K., 1974, Pregnancy dependence of mammary tumors in strain DDD mice, *J. Natl. Cancer Inst.* **52:**449.

McKENZIE, I., AND ROUS, P., 1941, The experimental disclosure of latest neoplastic changes in tarred skin, *J. Exp. Med.* **73:**391.

MEDINA, D., 1972, Serial transplantation of methylcholanthrene-treated nodule outgrowth lines, *J. Natl. Cancer Inst.* **48:**1363.

MEDINA, D., 1973*a*, Preneoplastic lesions in mouse mammary tumorigenesis, *Methods Cancer Res.* **7:**3.

MEDINA, D., 1973*b*, Serial transplantation of carcinogen-treated mammary nodule outgrowths. III. Dissociation of carcinogen-induced cell variants by dose and chemical structure of carcinogen, *J. Natl. Cancer Inst.* **50:**1555.

MEDINA, D., 1974*a*, Mammary tumorigenesis in chemical carcinogen-treated mice. I. Incidence in Balb/c and C57BL mice, *J. Natl. Cancer Inst.* **53:**213.

MEDINA, D., 1974*b*, Mammary tumorigenesis in chemical carcinogen-treated mice. II. Dependence on hormone stimulation for tumorigenesis, *J. Natl. Cancer Inst.* **53:**223.

MEDINA, D., AND DeOME, K. B., 1968, Influence of mammary tumor virus on the tumor-producing capabilities of nodule outgrowths free of mammary tumor virus, *J. Natl. Cancer Inst.* **40:**1303.

MEDINA, D., AND DEOME, K. B., 1970a, Carcinogen-induced mammary tumors from preneoplastic nodule outgrowths in Balb/c mice, *Cancer Res.* **30**:1055.

MEDINA, D., AND DEOME, K. B., 1970b, Effects of various oncogenic agents on the tumor-producing capabilities of the D series of Balb/c mammary nodule outgrowth lines, *J. Natl. Cancer Inst.* **45**:353.

MÜHLBOCK, O., 1965, Note on a new inbred mouse-strain GR/A, *Eur. J. Cancer* **1**:123.

O'MALLEY, B. W., AND MEANS, A. R., 1974, Female steroid hormones and target cell nuclei, *Science* **183**:610.

POTTER, M., 1958, Variation in resistance patterns in different neoplasms, *Ann. N.Y. Acad. Sci.* **76**:630.

POTTER, V. R., 1969, Recent trends in cancer biochemistry: The importance of studies on fetal tissue, *Can. Cancer Conf.* **8**:9.

POTTER, V. R., AND WATANABE, M., 1968, Some biochemical essentials of malignancy: The challenge of diversity, in: *Proceedings of the International Conference on Leukemia-Lymphoma* (C. J. D. Zarafonetis, ed.), pp. 33–46, Lea and Febiger, Philadelphia.

RABES, H. M., SCHOLZE, P., AND JANTSCH, B., 1972, Growth kinetics of diethylnitrosamine-induced, enzyme deficient "preneoplastic" liver cell populations *in vivo* and *in vitro, Cancer Res.* **32**:2577.

RAICK, A. N., 1974, Cell proliferation and promoting action in skin tumorigenesis, *Cancer Res.* **34**:920.

ROUS, P., AND BEARD, J. W., 1935, The progression to carcinoma of virus-induced papillomas (Shope), *J. Exp. Med.* **62**:523.

ROUS, P., AND KIDD, J. G., 1941, Conditional neoplasms and subthreshold neoplastic states: A study of the tar tumors of rabbits, *J. Exp. Med.* **73**:365.

ROWLEY, J. D., 1974, Do human tumors show a chromosome pattern specific for each etiologic agent? *J. Natl. Cancer Inst.* **52**:315.

SCARPELLI, D. G., AND MURAD, T. M., 1973, Recent contributions to our knowledge about the pathology of breast cancer, *Recent Results Cancer Res.* **42**:42.

SCHADE, R. O. K., 1972, Some observations on the pathology and natural history of urothelial neoplasms, *Beitr. Pathol.* **145**:325.

SHABAD, L. M., 1973, Precancerous morphologic lesions, *J. Natl. Cancer Inst.* **50**:1421.

SHUBIK, P., BASERGA, R., AND RITCHIE, A. C., 1953, The life and progression of induced skin tumors in mice, *Br. J. Cancer* **7**:342.

SINHA, D., AND DAO, T., 1971, A direct mechanism of mammary carcinogenesis, *Proc. Am. Assoc. Cancer Res.* **62**:370.

SLAGA, T. J., AND SCRIBNER, J. D., 1973, Inhibition of tumor initiation and promotion by anti-inflammatory agents, *J. Natl. Cancer Inst.* **51**:1723.

SLEMMER, G., 1972, Host response to premalignant mammary tissues, *Natl. Cancer Inst. Mongr.* **35**:57.

SLEMMER, G., 1974, Interactions of separate types of cells during normal and neoplastic mammary gland growth, *J. Investigative Dermatology* **63**:27–47, 1974.

SQUARTINI, F., 1962, Responsiveness and progression of mammary tumors of high cancer strain mice, *J. Natl. Cancer Inst.* **28**:911.

VANNIE, R., AND DUX, A., 1971, Biological and morphological characteristics of mammary tumors in GR mice, *J. Natl. Cancer Inst.* **46**:885.

VANNIE, R., AND THUNG, P. J., 1965, Responsiveness of mouse mammary tumors to pregnancy, *Eur. J. Cancer* **1**:41.

WEINER, F., DALIANIS, T., KLEIN, G., AND HARRIS, H., 1974, Cytogenetic studies on the mechanism of formation of isoantigenic variants in somatic cell hybrids. I. Banding analysis of isoantigenic variant sublines derived from the fusion of TA3Ha carcinoma with MSWBS sarcoma cells, *J. Natl. Cancer Inst.* **52**:1779.

WEINHOUSE, S., 1960, Enzyme activities and tumor progression, in: *Amino Acids, Proteins, and Cancer Biochemistry* (J. T. Edsall, ed.), pp. 109–119, Academic Press, New York.

WILLIS, R. A., 1967, *The Pathology of Tumors*, Butterworths, London.

6

Metabolic Controls and Neoplasia

HENRY C. PITOT

1. The Regulation of Genetic Expression in Eukaryotes

Since the advent of major advances in our fundamental understanding of the interrelationships of DNA, RNA, and protein within all living cells, one of the most pressing problems in biology has been to understand the mechanisms involved in the cellular regulation of expression of the information coded in DNA as the ultimate phenotype of enzymes and complex cellular structures seen in multicellular organisms.

Because of the simplicity of prokaryotic organisms, the earliest studies directed toward an understanding of these complex processes were fruitfully carried out in such systems. On the basis of both genetic and biochemical evidence, Jacob and Monod (1961) promulgated their now famous "operon" hypothesis. This hypothesis, which concerns both positive and negative regulation of genetic transcription on the DNA molecule itself, has now been substantiated in a number of prokaryotic systems. The manipulability of the genetics of the system as well as the success in the technology needed to substantiate chemically the concepts formulated genetically has allowed this field to advance quite rapidly. In fact, some molecular biologists now consider most of the problems in the area of regulation solved for prokaryotes and feel that further information will merely substantiate these mechanisms in other systems rather than provide surprising new basic concepts. Whether such considerations resulting from studies in bacteria prove to be fact or fallacy, it is strikingly clear that major new conceptual

HENRY C. PITOT ● Departments of Oncology and Pathology, McArdle Laboratory for Cancer Research, University of Wisconsin, Madison, Wisconsin

advances will be required before we can even begin to understand the genetics and, in all likelihood, the basic mechanisms of the regulation of genetic expression in eukaryotic cells, with their extremely complex polyploid genomes and intracellular structures, as well as we presently do those of prokaryotes.

In the prokaryote system, the entire sequence of genetic expression from the transcription of DNA by RNA polymerase to the final production of protein occurs in a physically linked sequence of events. As RNA polymerase is transcribed by DNA, ribosomes initiate protein synthesis on the growing strand of RNA prior to its release from the transcribing system. In the eukaryote, the system is considerably different. One of the major reasons is that the structural relationships in the eukaryotic cell with its delimiting nuclear membrane separating the transcribing units from the translating units are quite distinct from those of the prokaryotes. Figure 1 is a schematic diagram of the flow of genetic information from DNA to enzyme protein in eukaryotes. Numerous studies have now demonstrated the presence of repetitive sequences in the genome in mammalian DNA as well as in that of many other eukaryotic organisms (Saunders *et al.*, 1972; Hough and Davidson, 1972). Some of the repetitive sequences are present in thousands of copies. These sequences do not code for specific proteins and their function is not clearly understood, although many argue that they play a principal role in the regulation of transcription in the nucleus. As can be seen from Fig. 1, RNA polymerase in the presence of the four nucleoside triphosphates transcribes one of the DNA strands into a comparable copy of RNA. The repetitive region and the unique region are transcribed and form a single molecule to which is subsequently added a stretch of polyadenylate by a mechanism not involving direct genetic transcription (Adesnik *et al.*, 1972; Penman *et al.*, 1970). Obviously, Fig. 1 does not indicate the complex structural relationships of DNA with proteins

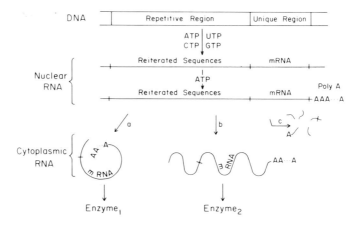

FIGURE 1. Basic aspects of the expression of genetic information in mammalian cells. The diagram demonstrates the process of transcription of both the repetitive and unique regions of a segment of the chromosome, with the subsequent addition of adenylate residues within the nucleus. Cytoplasmic RNA is demonstrated as a cochlear configuration representing the stable messenger RNA template (pathway a), as an elongated molecule representing the short-lived messenger RNA template (pathway b), and as fragments resulting from degradation either within the nucleus or in the cytoplasm as nonfunctional messages (pathway c). See text for further discussion.

and other molecules forming the chromatin structure. Such protein–DNA interactions appear to modify the expression of large segments of the genome in various cell types (Bonner *et al.*, 1968).

After the formation of the polyadenylated messenger RNA, this material is further processed by cleavage of many of the reiterated sequences from the 5'-end of the unique messenger RNA sequence with its 3'-polyadenylated tail. It is not clear whether some messages are also cleaved at this point and never become available for translation although they are transcribed. Those messenger RNAs destined for translation within the cytoplasm of the cell then pass through the nuclear pores in association with proteins, the entire unit being termed the "informasome" by Spirin (1969).

In the cytoplasm of the cell, messenger RNA–protein complexes associate with ribosomes to form polysomes. In all mammalian cells, these can be physically divided into membrane-bound polysomes and those that are not membrane associated. Functionally speaking, it is not possible at the present time to ascribe the synthesis of specific classes of proteins to the free or bound polysomes (Shires *et al.*, 1974). Despite the more recent studies demonstrating direct effects of actinomycin D on the stability of cellular messenger RNA both *in vivo* and *in vitro* (Endo *et al.*, 1971; Singer and Penman, 1972), the earlier studies of Wilson and Hoagland demonstrating a rapidly turning-over messenger RNA population as well as a longer-lived population in liver have now been substantiated without the use of inhibitors in two distinct systems (Schultz, 1974; Edström and Tanguay, 1974). While the relationship between the free and bound polysomes and the short-lived and long-lived messenger RNA population has not been totally elucidated, at least two studies utilizing actinomycin D have demonstrated the rapid decay of free polysomes and the relative stability of membrane-bound polysomes (Sarma *et al.*, 1969; Hill and Saunders, 1971).

These two pathways of short- and long-lived messenger RNA molecules are seen in Fig. 1 as pathways (b) and (a), respectively. While the lifetime of messenger RNAs in eukaryotic systems appears to be generally longer than that of rapidly dividing prokaryotes, the short-lived class of messenger RNAs are comparable to the messenger RNA molecules seen in prokaryotes. Pathway (a), the long-lived or stable messenger RNA, may be relatively unique to the eukaryotic system. These molecules may be stabilized within the cytoplasm of the cell and maintain their translating functions for periods of time extending to days, week, or months. As indicated earlier, the third pathway, (c), represents the possibility that messenger RNA molecules may be transcribed but never translated, being broken down either in the nucleus or in the cytoplasm of the cell.

While the scheme in Fig. 1 is obviously oversimplified, even at our present state of knowledge, it points out the numerous sites available for the regulation of genetic expression in eukaryotic systems. The regulation at the level of RNA polymerase by various hormones has now been described in several systems (Tata *et al.*, 1963; O'Malley, 1971). While as yet no specific controlling mechanism has been shown at other sites within the nucleus itself, it is quite likely that regulation may occur during polyadenylation or the interaction of the newly formed messenger RNA with protein to form the informasome complex (Spirin, 1969).

A site of regulation which several investigators have argued must exist is that for the transport of the messenger RNA–ribonucleoprotein complex into the cytoplasm. Presumably such regulation would occur at the level of the nuclear membrane. The complexing of the newly formed message with ribosomes, tRNA, and initiation factors offers an obvious site for regulation at the translational level of genetic expression. Chain elongation of the protein during synthesis is another possible site of control, as is the release of protein from the functioning polysome complex. While the folding of a protein may occur spontaneously, as do all biologically important reactions, enzymes are available which catalyze the rapid formation of the three-dimensional structure (Givol *et al.*, 1965). Such enzymes have been implicated in the binding of polysomes to the surface of the endoplasmic reticulum (Williams and Rabin, 1969).

Since, in the mammalian organism at least, all proteins are in a dynamic state of synthesis and degradation, the regulation of this latter process offers a very important site for the control of genetic expression at a posttranslational level. Finally, the regulation of the activity of the enzyme itself by specific allosteric effectors or by ionic, pH, or physical and chemical means is a factor, as with all biological catalysts.

Thus it is clear that the process of genetic expression in eukaryotes is extremely complex and that our knowledge of such mechanisms is relatively embryonic. On the other hand, it is possible to point out sites for the potential regulation of genetic expression and then to examine experimentally situations of metabolic control in specific systems such as will be considered in the remainder of this review.

2. Mechanisms for the Regulation of Genetic Expression in Normal and Neoplastic Eukaryotic Cells

2.1. Regulation of DNA Synthesis

While in our introductory considerations we did not consider separately the problem of DNA synthesis, cell replication, and its control, nevertheless this complex phenomenon is one of the principal problems facing us in our understanding of neoplasia. Although the rate of cell replication is not uniformly more rapid in neoplasms than in their cell of origin (e.g., carcinoma of the small intestine, chronic leukemia), still in virtually all instances neoplasms would operationally not exist unless they had the advantage of cell replication over their cell of origin and most other normal cells within the host. In fact, many investigators feel that the solution to the problem of the regulation of cell replication and DNA synthesis will carry with it the solution to the problem of cancer.

As with other mechanisms of regulation, studies in the prokaryote have far outdistanced those in mammalian cells either *in vitro* or *in vivo*. The model system for studying the control of DNA synthesis *in vivo* has been the regenerating liver (see review by Becker, 1974). On the other hand, the most popular studies of late have been on the regulation of DNA synthesis in cell culture.

While the subject of cell replication is covered extensively in another chapter, it is important to mention a few of the highlights of our knowledge of the regulation of DNA synthesis in eukaryotes. The description of the replicating unit of DNA in prokaryotes, termed the "replicon" (Jacob and Brenner, 1963), has led investigators to look for similar units in mammalian cells. It is quite certain that such units exist since the rate of DNA synthesis varies in different parts of the chromosome and at different times during the synthesis period (Painter and Schaefer, 1969). Although replicons in the DNA of mammalian cells are not as clearly defined as those of prokaryotes (Okada, 1968), Taylor (1973) has described evidence for the isolation of replicating segments in mammalian chromosomes.

More recently, studies in prokaryotic systems have indicated that the initiation of DNA synthesis may involve the synthesis of a short segment of RNA linked covalently to DNA (Sugino and Okazaki, 1973). That such a phenomenon may occur in prokaryotic cells has recently been claimed by Fox et al. (1973) and by Eliasson et al. (1974) for the case of polyoma virus synthesis. The fact that small molecules are capable of stimulating the environmental regulation of DNA synthesis has been known for some time. Isoproterenol administration results in marked cellular proliferation of the cells of the salivary gland (Barka, 1965; Whitlock et al., 1968). In addition, the administration of folic acid stimulates a dramatic mitotic response in the kidney (Byrnes et al., 1972). Becker (1969) has reviewed the control of cell division in normal mammalian tissue.

In prokaryotes, DNA synthesis is initiated at a site on the chromosome which is an association with the cell membrane. These studies have stimulated numerous investigations in eukaryotic systems designed to determine whether or not DNA synthesis is initiated or even occurs in association with the nuclear membrane. Thus far, the results have been somewhat conflicting (Wise and Prescott, 1973; Yamada and Hanaoka, 1973), although a number of publications have demonstrated nuclear-membrane-associated DNA (Hall et al., 1971; Infante et al., 1973; Franke et al., 1973).

Although few investigations designed to study the regulation of DNA synthesis in neoplasms have been carried out, one experimental system—study of the effect of partial hepatectomy on hepatoma cell proliferation—has been used. An early investigation by Trotter (1961) demonstrated that the mitotic indices of all hepatomas studied were the same in partially hepatectomized and sham-operated animals. These studies were extended by Maini and Stich (1962), who also demonstrated that this operative procedure did not stimulate mitotic activity in animals undergoing chemical hepatocarcinogenesis. On the other hand, a more recent study by Lee (1971) did demonstrate that two transplanted hepatomas in hepatectomized animals had a transient increase in their DNA synthesis as measured by the incorporation of [^{3}H]thymidine as well as an apparent increase in growth rate. Another example of humoral substances regulating DNA synthesis may be seen in the case of chalones, considered more completely in Chapter 11.

Laurence and Elgjo (1971) could not demonstrate any effect of the epidermal chalone on mitotic activity of a transplantable hamster squamous cell carcinoma in culture, although the neoplasm appeared to produce the substance. On the other hand, Bullough and Deol (1971) were able to demonstrate an inhibitory effect of the epidermal chalone on mitosis of mouse squamous cell carcinoma.

While the studies cited above are all suggestive of new directions for experimentation, to this reviewer's knowledge none has been adequately applied to a detailed investigation of the regulation of DNA synthesis in neoplastic cells. Thus the future holds much promise in this area not only for our understanding of the normal control of growth but also for the potential to control neoplastic and other disease states.

2.2. Transcriptional Regulation in Normal and Neoplastic Cells

In this section, we will consider the regulation of DNA-directed synthesis of RNA which occurs in the nucleus of eukaryotic cells. Other nuclear functions such as polyadenylation, nucleic acid maturation, and the phenomenon of transport of ribosomal and messenger RNA into the cytoplasm will not be specifically considered since knowledge of their regulation is very sparse.

2.2.1. Histones and Other Nuclear Proteins in the Regulation of Genetic Expression

In view of the fact that Chapter 15 will cover the subject of nucleoproteins in detail, only a few points will be considered here as they bear on the regulation process itself.

In general, one may divide nuclear proteins into the basic histones and the other proteins, the so-called nonhistone chromosomal proteins. If one assumes that histones themselves act primarily in the quantitative restriction of DNA, which is determined by differentiation and probably maintained during all subsequent cell divisions of any differentiated phenotype, then one would expect a close relationship between histone and DNA synthesis. Such has been described, as reviewed by McClure and Hnilica (1972). On the other hand, there is no such relationship between the synthesis of nonhistone chromosomal proteins and specific differentiated tissues. These latter protein components appear to be synthesized differentially during periods of the cell cycle, thus suggesting a role in the control of cell proliferation (Stein et al., 1974). Also, the population of these proteins differs in different tissues (Wu et al., 1973). On the other hand, Pederson (1974) has proposed that such alterations in the nonhistone chromosomal proteins may be the result rather than the cause of genetic activation.

Clearly the essential point is the actual and potential relationship of these proteins to the chromatin structure in normal and neoplastic tissues and thus possibly to both the regulation of genetic expression and the control of cell division. Early studies by Sporn and Dingman (1966) suggested that there were no differences in the histone content of protein between normal and tumor tissues. Furthermore, Laurence and Butler (1965) demonstrated no differences in the

turnover of histones in the normal and neoplastic tissues that they studied. A
study by Arnold *et al.* (1973) suggested differences in the chromatin of a relatively rapidly proliferating hepatocellular carcinoma compared to liver, whereas a slowly growing, very highly differentiated hepatic carcinoma exhibited no significant differences in its chromatin.

In general, it may be said that no characteristic or completely understood differences can be seen in nuclear proteins of normal vs. neoplastic tissues. On the other hand, not enough studies have been carried out to make it possible to distinguish absolute significant differences between these protein populations when a neoplasm is carefully compared with its cell of origin, both cells having the same karyotype.

2.2.2. Hormones, Hormone Receptor Proteins, and Transcriptional Regulation

In the multicellular organism, the unity and concert of the whole are maintained by a combination of cell-to-cell interaction mediated through direct contact and the presence of controlling factors known in general as hormones. Certain cell populations within the organism differentiate into cells whose principal function is the production of one or a set of such internal mediators. The cells that respond to these mediators have acquired this characteristic during development, also. The mechanisms within the cell allowing for such interaction depend on specific molecular structures on the surface or within the cell itself which react with selected hormones with a high degree of specificity (Lefkowitz, 1973). Such hormone–receptor interactions result in an alteration in the phenotype of the cell, usually reflected in changes in the levels of enzymes therein (Pitot and Yatvin, 1973).

a. Receptors and Receptor Proteins. In general, one may subdivide the field of hormonal receptors into two general areas. Those receptors that are present on the plasma membrane in general are concerned with polypeptide hormone–cell relationships. Such a mechanism is eminently reasonable since, with the exception of the process of pinocytosis, polypeptide hormones usually do not survive entrance into the cell without being degraded. One of the principal examples of this mechanism is the interaction of mammalian cells with insulin, as has been reviewed by Cuatrecasas (1973).

Hormones may also interact with cells by direct combination with cytoplasmic proteins. The principal studies on this phenomenon were carried out initially by Jensen *et al.* (1971). In this instance, the steroid hormones are the principal examples of such hormone–receptor interaction. The complexity of this interaction has been described by several laboratories (Jensen and DeSombre, 1973; Stancel *et al.*, 1973; Yamamoto and Alberts, 1972). That estrogen–receptor complex probably does stimulate phenotypic changes within end organs was first studied from a detailed biochemical standpoint by Mueller and his associates in the rat uterus (Mueller, 1965). Since that time, extensive studies on the mechanism of action of this hormone in the immature rat uterus (Hamilton, 1968; Means and O'Malley, 1972) have demonstrated very rapid and numerous effects.

The actual mechanism whereby these hormone–receptor complexes exert their effects is not totally understood. In the case of the polypeptide hormones, it would appear that the receptor complex affects adenyl and/or guanyl cyclase, resulting in an alteration in the concentration of cyclic nucleotides within the cell. This "second hormone" then functions within the intracellular environment to regulate the expression of genetic information (Pitot and Yatvin, 1973). On the other hand, the steroid–receptor protein complex undergoes some conformational or molecular weight changes and enters the nucleus. It is presumed that this complex then somehow interacts with the transcription mechanism to enhance (Dingman *et al.*, 1969) or repress (Van der Meulen *et al.*, 1972) the synthesis of RNA. In order to function in this way, estrogen receptors should bind to chromatin to regulate transcription. Such a phenomenon has been demonstrated for the mammalian uterus and the chick oviduct (McGuire *et al.*, 1972; Palmiter *et al.*, 1973).

The system in which the transcriptional regulation of genetic expression by hormones has been best documented is that of the estrogenic induction of ovalbumin in the chick oviduct. By quantitatively measuring the amount of ovalbumin messenger RNA produced in this system after stimulation by estrogen, Schimke and his associates (Rhoads *et al.*, 1973) have demonstrated the direct effect of estrogens on transcription of this specific gene. This was further substantiated by Palmiter (1973) as well as by O'Malley and his associates (Harris *et al.*, 1973), the latter workers demonstrating that while ovalbumin comprises 65% of the total oviduct protein after estrogen administration only one copy of the ovalbumin gene exists for each haploid component of the genome. Thus in this model system it is very clear that the estrogen, and in all probability the estrogen–receptor protein complex, modulates transcription of the ovalbumin gene. With this as a model, it is not unreasonable to argue that steroid hormones produce similar effects in other tissues of the mammalian organism.

b. The Regulation of Transcription by Hormones. In view of the most recent investigations cited above (McGuire *et al.*, 1972; Palmiter *et al.*, 1973) demonstrating the direct effect of steroid hormones on the transcriptional apparatus resulting in the production of a specific messenger RNA, many earlier investigations demonstrating the effect of inhibitors of RNA synthesis such as actinomycin D can now be considered in terms of transcriptional regulation.

As has been discussed in an earlier review (Pitot and Yatvin, 1973), inhibition of RNA synthesis affects the action of a number of hormones *in vivo*. In particular, the effects of both the steroid hormones (O'Malley, 1971; Karlson and Sekeris, 1966) and the thyroid hormones (Tata, 1969) have been shown to be accompanied by increases in RNA synthesis. A number of the functional effects of these hormones are blocked by the administration of actinomycin D *in vivo*. In addition, several of the polypeptide hormones such as insulin (Wool and Munro, 1963), growth hormone (Dawson *et al.*, 1966), and parathormone (Rasmussen *et al.*, 1964) have been shown to induce actinomycin-sensitive processes. On the other hand, the manner of action of the polypeptide hormones, all of which appears to be through cyclic nucleotides (Pitot and Yatvin, 1973), might suggest indirect effects on transcription by these hormones. Significantly, Garren and his associates (Davis and Garren, 1968) have demonstrated that the primary effect of ACTH appears to be related to translation.

Because so much material is available on the hormonal regulation of genetic expression (Tata, 1969; O'Malley, 1971; Pitot and Yatvin, 1973), we will not attempt to repeat it here. Rather, the abnormalities of hormonal control that have been seen in a number of neoplasms will be discussed further. One of the early demonstrations of the lack of transcriptional control by cortisone was the absence of cortisone induction of tryptophan pyrrolase in the Morris 5123 hepatoma (Pitot and Morris, 1961). In later studies from this same laboratory, Cho *et al.* (1964) demonstrated that while most highly differentiated hepatocellular carcinomas did not exhibit the cortisone induction of tryptophan pyrrolase at least two such neoplasms did exhibit substrate induction in the intact host but not in the adrenalectomized animal. Administration of low doses of cortisone to the tumor-bearing adrenalectomized animal restored this low level of substrate induction. Studies by Dyer *et al.* (1964) also demonstrated hormonal induction of this enzyme in several highly differentiated hepatocellular carcinomas. These authors, however, did not study the adrenalectomized host. Furthermore, the induction of tryptophan pyrrolase by cortisol was markedly inhibited during the administration of a number of hepatocarcinogens (Kizer *et al.*, 1969).

The enzyme tryosine aminotransferase was found to be present at a very high concentration in a number of highly differentiated hepatocellular carcinomas, but on adrenalectomy the level decreased to that found in normal and host liver (Pitot, 1963). However, some neoplasms possessed normal or lower than normal levels of this enzyme. In all tumors thus far studied—either in the adrenalectomized host or in the normal host—where tyrosine aminotransferase activities are low, cortisone administration does induce the enzyme. The concentration of another enzyme of gluconeogenesis, serine dehydratase, was found to be very high in several hepatomas, a level which adrenalectomy lowered precipitously (Bottomley *et al.*, 1963). Administration of cortisone to the adrenalectomized host did stimulate the level of the enzyme in the hepatoma.

A number of investigations have been directed toward the induction of tyrosine aminotransferase in hepatoma cells in cell culture. The induction of this enzyme by cortisone in cell cultures of the Reuber H-35 hepatoma was first demonstrated by Pitot *et al.* (1963). Subsequent to that investigation, numerous studies by several authors (Thompson *et al.*, 1966; Lee *et al.*, 1970; Sellers and Granner, 1974) have utilized this finding in attempts to study the actual mechanism of the hormal induction of this enzyme in cell culture.

An interesting effect of transcriptional control was reported by Wu and Morris (1970), who demonstrated that cortisol administration to animals bearing highly differentiated hepatomas could induce glutamine synthetase to quite high levels in several of these neoplasms while having virtually no effect on the level of the enzyme in host liver. In addition, thyroxine administration induced the level of glutamine aminotransferase in two Morris hepatomas while not affecting the level of this enzyme in the liver. Work from the same laboratory also demonstrated that administration of cortisol induced arginase activity more efficiently in the hepatomas than in host liver while elevating arginosuccinate synthetase activity in one hepatoma but not in host liver (Wu *et al.*, 1971).

Another example of the defectiveness of the regulation of enzyme synthesis by thyroid hormone is seen with hepatic glycerophosphate dehydrogenase, a mitochondrial enzyme. Karsten *et al.* (1971) demonstrated that while the administration of T_3 induced this enzyme in livers of normal animals and those fed diethylnitrosamine, transplantable hepatomas produced by this regimen showed no induction of the enzyme after T_3 administration.

In a number of rather extensive studies, Hilf *et al.* (1967) have demonstrated some aspects of the regulation of several enzymes in a highly differentiated rat mammary adenocarcinoma by estrogen administration. While few changes occur in the mammary gland, the neoplasm responds dramatically to several enzymes including glucose-6-phosphate dehydrogenase. This response in the hepatoma appears to be sensitive to extremely high doses of actinomycin. The results of such experiments are probably related to the removal of the principal steroid-hormone-producing organ affecting these neoplasms (Banerjee, 1969) and neoplasms of the ovary itself (Bruzzone, 1970).

The regulation of enzyme synthesis by polypeptide hormones also appears to be defective in several neoplasms. Insulin regulation of pyruvate kinase was absent in several highly differentiated hepatocellular carcinomas (Campadelli-Fiume *et al.*, 1970; Criss and Morris, 1973*b*), although the enzyme was "hyperresponsive" to hydrocortisone in the hepatomas studied. Studies by Sharma and Brush (1974) had indicated that the effect of ACTH on the synthesis of corticosterone in isolated adrenocortical carcinoma cells compared to normal adrenal cells is significantly abnormal.

Thus it would appear even from this incomplete survey of transcriptional mechanisms regulating enzyme levels in neoplasia that most if not all such mechanisms are absent in tumors or are abnormal compared to their cell of origin. What perhaps may not be so evident is the extreme heterogeneity that is seen with these defective regulatory mechanisms. As we look at other mechanisms of environmental regulation, it will become apparent that the defective control characteristic of the biology of all neoplasms may be demonstrated just as ubiquitously at the biochemical level.

2.2.3. *Cyclic Nucleotides and Metabolic Regulation*

While the exact site of action of cyclic nucleotides in regulating enzyme synthesis in the eukaryotic cell is unknown, the prokaryotic model (Pastan and Perlman, 1970) demostrating the transcriptional effect of these small molecules allows us to consider them here. However, the reader should realize that the exact site(s) of action of cyclic nucleotides in regulating genetic expression is not understood at the present time in eukaryotic systems. On the other hand, the demonstration of changes in levels of cyclic AMP with the growth rate of eukaryotic cells *in vitro* (Otten *et al.*, 1972) and the stimulation of histone phosphorylation by this nucleotide *in vitro* (Langan, 1968) are certainly suggestive of effects of this small molecule in regulating DNA synthesis itself. In addition, Jost and Sahib (1971) have demonstrated an effect of dibutyryl cyclic AMP on RNA synthesis in rat liver nuclei.

There has been considerable experimental work directed toward the possible role of cyclic nucleotides in the neoplastic transformation in cell culture (Chandra and Gerick, 1972; Sheppard, 1972; Anderson *et al.*, 1973).

It is well known that many cells transformed *in vitro* lose their density-dependent inhibition of cell replication (contact inhibition of growth) and gain the character of agglutinability by plant lectins (Rapin and Burgin, 1974). Addition of dibutyryl cyclic AMP to neoplastic cells in culture restored contact inhibition of growth (Teel and Hall, 1973). Willingham and Pastan (1974) have demonstrated that levels of cyclic AMP in both normal and neoplastic cells *in vitro* correlate with the degree of agglutinability by concanavalin A. Thus in the *in vitro* situation changes in cyclic nucleotides appear to be correlated with membrane changes, which have been implicated in the primary neoplastic transformation event.

A comparable experimental effort has not been directed toward neoplasms growing *in vivo* other than hepatomas. Adenyl cyclase activity is present in highly differentiated hepatocellular carcinomas (Brown *et al.*, 1970). Northup *et al.* (1972) have described the presence of guanyl cyclase activity as well in several such neoplasms. At the effector end of the cyclic nucleotide metabolic pathway, Criss and Morris (1973*a*) have demonstrated the presence of cyclic-AMP-activated protein kinase in two highly differentiated hepatocellular carcinomas and one somewhat more anaplastic hepatoma. These investigators found that more highly differentiated neoplasms possessed a higher level of cyclic nucleotide activable protein kinase than did the less well-differentiated tumors, although all neoplasms studied appeared to have a similar pattern of activity of this enzyme as demonstrated by isoelectric focusing.

Changes in the regulation of liver adenyl cyclase during carcinogenesis (Christofferson *et al.*, 1972) as exemplified by an increased sensitivity of the enzyme to catecholamines are indicative that such alterations should occur in the final carcinomas. Christofferson *et al.* (1972) demonstrated that, in addition to the increased response of adenyl cyclase induced by feeding 2-acetylaminofluorene, the fully developed hepatocellular carcinomas exhibited a high basal adenyl cyclase activity but a very small response to either epinephrine or glucagon, the normal hormonal effectors of hepatic adenyl cyclase. Allen *et al.* (1971) surveyed a series of hepatomas extending from highly differentiated to poorly differentiated lesions and showed that in the most highly differentiated and slowly growing hepatomas the response of adenyl cyclase to glucagon was in the same range as that seen in liver. However, as the degree of differentiation of the neoplasm decreased, the response of adenyl cyclase to glucagon also decreased, although the activity of the enzyme did not follow this change. Somewhat similar results were reported by Emmelot and Bos (1971). In their continuing studies on plasma membranes of liver and hepatomas in a highly differentiated mouse hepatocellular carcinoma, the response of the adenyl cyclase activity in isolated plasma membranes of liver and hepatoma to glucagon and epinephrine was quite comparable to that seen in host liver. However, in the plasma membranes from an anaplastic hepatic neoplasm in the rat almost no response to epinephrine was elicited while that to glucagon was markedly reduced. More recent studies by Klein *et al.* (1974) did not support these earlier conclusions; these authors were able to demonstrate that while maximal increases in enzyme activity in response to glucagon were clearly lower in hepatocellular carcinomas the half-maximal enzyme activation occurred at identical concentrations in both liver and hepatoma.

Furthermore, the binding of [^{125}I]glucagon to washed membrane particles was in the same range in the hepatomas studied as that seen with normal liver. These authors have concluded that either defects in hormonal activation of adenyl cyclase reported earlier do not exist in the two hepatomas studied by them or the defects are beyond the adenyl cyclase enzyme system in hepatomas. In primary hepatocellular carcinomas induced by ethionine as well as in the earlier premalignant lesion, the hyperplastic nodule, Chayoth *et al.* (1973) demonstrated that prostaglandin stimulated cyclic AMP levels to normal and greater than normal levels in the nodules and hepatomas, respectively. Glucagon increased cyclic AMP levels in a similar fashion in all three tissues, although its stimulation of adenyl cyclase activity in the hepatoma was below normal. These studies are therefore in support of those of Klein *et al.* and suggest that the cyclic nucleotide metabolic picture in hepatocellular carcinomas is quite variable.

In neoplasms of tissues other than the liver, Brown *et al.* (1970) demonstrated a significantly higher level of adenyl cyclase in mammary tumor tissue of the rat as compared to normal or even lactating breast. Furthermore, epinephrine appeared to stimulate the activity of the enzyme in the neoplasm but not in the abnormal tissue. On the other hand, in a transplantable thyroid tumor of the rat the adenyl cyclase activity of normal thyroid but not of the tumor tissue was significantly stimulated by TSH (Macchia *et al.*, 1972). In a series of human endocrine tumors, Schorr *et al.* (1972) showed a varied response of adenyl cyclase to the various tropic hormones of the pituitary. Therefore, unlike the apparent significant role of cyclic AMP levels in *in vitro* transformation, the responses of adenyl cyclase and the levels of cyclic nucleotides in neoplasms *in vivo* do not appear to conform to any specific regulatory pattern.

2.2.4. Regulation of "Drug-Metabolizing" Enzymes

The so-called drug-metabolizing enzymes found in all tissues of higher vertebrates have been studied in many laboratories (Hucker, 1973; Conney, 1969). The level of genetic expression at which the synthesis of these enzymes is controlled appears to be somewhat complex, but there is substantial evidence suggesting transcriptional regulation. The stimulatory effect of 3-methylcholanthrene on benzpyrene hydroxylase was demonstrably inhibited by actinomycin D in studies performed more than a decade ago by Gelboin and Blackburn (1964). More recently, Jacob *et al.* (1974) have demonstrated that the phenobarbital induction of cytochrome P_{450} and *N*-demethylase activity also requires the *de novo* synthesis of RNA, probably messenger RNA as judged by its inhibition by α-amanitin. On the other hand, it is not clear whether phenobarbitol actually induces the formation of new ribosomal precursor RNA or enhances maturation of the precursor (Smith *et al.*, 1974). Phenobarbital does appear to enhance the synthesis of chromosomal proteins (Blankenship and Kuehl, 1973) as well as the phosphorylation of acidic nuclear proteins in rat liver (Blankenship and Bresnick, 1974). Both of these effects may, however, be related to a relatively nonspecific stimulation of growth of the liver. In the cytoplasm, phenobarbital administration appears to cause both an increased rate of synthesis and a decreased rate of breakdown of microsomal protein (Shuster and Jick, 1966).

While these multiple investigations do not prove a primary transcriptional control of the synthesis of these enzymes, they are certainly compatible with such a conclusion. With this reservation, one can still compare the regulation of the synthesis of this group of enzymes in both normal and neoplastic tissues. In an earlier study of primary tumors induced by 3'-methyl-4-dimethylaminoazo-benzene as well as the transplanted Novikoff and Morris 5123 hepatomas, it was shown that all tumors were either completely incapable of or of markedly defective ability to metabolize a wide assortment of drugs including acetanilide, chlorpromazine, codeine, hexobarbital, neoprontosil, and *p*-nitrobenzoic acid (Rogers *et al.*, 1967). Hydroxylation, oxidation, reduction of aromatic nitro groups, reductive cleavage of azo linkages, and dealkylation were all subsequently shown to be reduced in five different Morris hepatomas of different growth (Hart *et al.*, 1965). All values were less than 50% of the control rates except for aniline hydroxylation, which was twice as high as the host liver value for the Morris 7800 hepatoma. Phenobarbital caused the induction of at least one of these drug-metabolizing pathways in every one of the Morris hepatomas. The generally low levels of drug metabolism in the hepatomas in this study could not be attributed to poor perfusion of the tumor due to decreased blood supply, since the concentrations of phenobarbital in liver, tumors, and blood were similar. In an even earlier study, the inducibility of azo dye *N*-demethylation by 3-methylcholanthrene had been demonstrated in the Morris hepatoma 5123 to occur to the same high levels as in the host liver (Conney and Burns, 1963). The methylcholanthrene induction of another mixed-function oxidase, benzpyrene hydroxylase, was also demonstrated in a group of Morris hepatomas (Watanabe *et al.*, 1970). Basal activity of this enzyme was negligible in the five different Morris hepatomas studied by the enzyme but could be induced from 13- to 122-fold. There appeared to be no correlation between growth rate and inducibility of this drug metabolic pathway. As noted earlier with phenobarbital induction (Hart *et al.*, 1965), the highest induced level with methylcholanthrene was not dissimilar in hepatoma and rat liver. Basal levels for polycyclic hydrocarbon hydroxylases have also been reported to be very low in two subsequent studies. Benzpyrene hydroxylase in the Morris 7777 hepatoma was reported to be 25% of normal liver enzyme levels (Brown *et al.*, 1971) and aryl hydrocarbon hydroxylase was undetectable in this same tumor (Miyake *et al.*, 1974). Aniline hydroxylase was studied in four different Morris hepatomas (Sugimura *et al.*, 1966). The activity was less than one-seventh that of the normal liver in the most deviated Morris 7316A hepatoma and up to 50% of normal in the better-differentiated 7793 hepatoma.

In recent studies, technical improvements for measurement of the cytochrome components have made possible quantitation of the different forms of the carrier cytochromes (Miyake *et al.*, 1974). It was found that while cytochrome P_{450} existed in three spectrally different forms in normal microsomes only two of these forms were present in the Morris hepatoma 5123C and only one in the more rapidly growing 7777 hepatoma. The induction of components of the mixed-function oxidases was also studied in detail in the 7777 hepatoma; whereas phenobarbital could not induce cytochrome P_{450}, methylcholanthrene did cause as great an increase in the P_{448} cytochrome in the neoplasm as it did in the host liver. Although methylcholanthrene did not induce and in fact lowered NADPH cytochrome reductase in host and tumor microsomes, there were still relatively large amounts of this enzyme in both types of tissue.

No distinct pattern correlating the degree of differentiation of hepatomas with their ability to metabolize drugs has emerged from any of these studies. In several (Watanabe *et al.*, 1970; Sugimura *et al.*, 1966), embryonal liver was shown to contain concentrations of cytochromes, flavoprotein enzymes, and overall drug hydroxylation enzymes that were even lower than those in minimal-deviation hepatomas. Furthermore, benzpyrene hydroxylase could not be induced *in utero* (Watanabe *et al.*, 1970). Regenerating liver closely resembles adult normal liver with regard to drug hydroxylation and related enzymes and the cytochromes (Sugimura *et al.*, 1966).

2.3. Translational Regulation of Genetic Expression

With respect to the fate of messenger RNA synthesized in eukaryotic systems, pathway (a) of Fig. 1 implies the phenomenon of translational regulation. As long as a messenger RNA may exist stably within the cytoplasm of a cell, the possibility of altering the rate of translation always exists. In this section, we will concern ourselves with examples of such regulation of protein synthesis, some of which occur in conjunction with initial transcriptional effects.

2.3.1. Stabilization of Messenger RNA

It is now reasonably well accepted that messenger RNA molecules in mammalian systems and probably in most other eukaryotes and even a few prokaryotes may exist for finite periods of time as stable translatable units.

Until recently, most studies concerned with the determination of messenger RNA stability were carried out by means of inhibitors of RNA synthesis, especially actinomycin D. Studies from our laboratory almost a decade ago utilized the inhibitory effects of this antibiotic to measure the messenger RNA template lifetimes of several hepatic enzymes in both normal and neoplastic liver (Pitot *et al.*, 1965). Earlier, Greengard and Acs (1962) demonstrated that synthesis of the hepatic enzyme, tryptophan pyrrolase, which had been stimulated by administration of its substrate *in vivo* occurred even in the presence of this inhibitor. One of the more interesting and definitive demonstrations of stable messenger RNA template in the cytoplasm of the liver cell was carried out by Stewart and Farber (1967). In this experiment, polysome breakdown in liver was stimulated by the administration of ethionine. After complete degradation of the polysome patterns to monosomes, relief of the ethionine block by administration of methionine and adenine *in vivo* restored the polysome pattern even when actinomycin D was administered concomitantly. A number of examples of messenger RNA template stability in other mammalian systems have since appeared. The hemoglobin mRNA in the reticulocyte is probably among those whose translation has been most thoroughly studied. Secretory proteins have been shown to be synthesized on stable templates in several instances (Seed and Goldberg, 1963; Wilson *et al.*, 1967). In addition, the stability of messenger RNA during early development of both plants and animals has been well documented (Tasca and Hillman, 1970; Terman, 1970; Dure and Waters, 1965). Alterations in template stability occurring during normal development of mammalian and other systems have also been reported by many authors (Kafatos, 1972; Rutter *et al.*, 1968; Shires *et al.*, 1974).

In view of the considerable amount of information on messenger RNA template stabilization in eukaryotes, it is reasonable to investigate template stability in neoplastic tissues. As has been pointed out in several papers by this reviewer (Pitot, 1964, 1969, 1971), in the liver–hepatoma system all messenger RNA templates thus far studied through the use of inhibitors appear to have different lifetimes in neoplasms than do the templates for the same enzymes in liver. Although only two neoplasms were studied, the patterns of messenger RNA template stabilities differed between these two tumors themselves. In addition to the liver system, Hilf *et al.* (1965) demonstrated distinct differences in the actinomycin sensitivity of the response of enzyme levels to estrogen in normal and neoplastic rat mammary glands.

All of these studies at the cellular level have not been concerned with the actual mechanism of template RNA stabilization in the cytoplasm of eukaryotic cells. At present, the exact mechanism for this stabilization is unknown, although this reviewer and his associates have presented a theoretical model for the stable messenger RNA template (Shires *et al.*, 1974). This model has been termed the "membron." Basically, the hypothesis is that the stabilization of messenger RNA templates occurs within differentiated mammalian cells through an association of the messenger RNA molecule with the membranes of the endoplasmic reticulum and possibly other intracellular membranes. The experimental data in support of this model have been previously reviewed (Pitot, 1969; Shires *et al.*, 1974) and thus will not be considered here. However, one of the principal predictions of the model is that messenger RNA will be found to be directly associated with the surface of membranes of the endoplasmic reticulum, a point not in accord with models described by other investigators (Sabatini *et al.*, 1966; Sabatini and Blobel, 1970). Recent unpublished experiments from this laboratory which are in line with those briefly described from the laboratory of Sabatini (Lande *et al.*, 1974) demonstrate a direct association of polyadenylated RNA with membranes of the endoplasmic reticulum. Thus these data are in further support of the original model of template stabilization by membrane association. However, it is clear that much more work must be carried out before the mechanism of template stabilization in normal cells and its apparent variation in neoplastic cells will be understood completely.

2.3.2. Small Molecule Regulation of Translation

In prokaryotic systems, substrate and product regulation of enzyme synthesis usually occurs at the transcriptional level. As we have already seen, hormones, especially steroid hormones, regulate the rate of transcription in many eukaryotic systems. However, it is apparent that small molecules may also regulate the rate of translation in eukaryotic systems. Studies from this laboratory demonstrated that the administration of glucose *in vivo* completely suppressed the synthesis of the hepatic enzyme serine dehydratase during periods when the synthesis was totally independent of transcription (Jost *et al.*, 1968). While the mechanism of this regulation is still not understood, certain factors have been determined. No single hormonal ablation or replacement is capable of substituting for the effect of glucose (Soling *et al.*, 1969). Furthermore, unlike prokaryotic systems there does not appear to be a significant effect of glucose administration on the transient high levels of hepatic cyclic AMP resulting from induction of the enzyme by glucagon (Sudilovsky *et al.*, 1971). It is also not clear whether glucose may affect the transcription of specific messenger RNAs, although it does not appear to affect the ATP concentration present in liver (Peraino and Pitot, 1964). Furthermore, the glucose effect is by no means unique to the enzyme serine dehydratase, but has now been described in several other enzyme systems (Jervell *et al.*, 1965; Venkatesan *et al.*, 1970; Bonkowsky *et al.*, 1973; Treadow and Khairallah, 1972; Tilghman *et al.*, 1974).

Lack of the glucose effect in neoplasms has been reported for several hepatocellular carcinomas (Jost and Pitot, 1970). In these studies, the absence of a glucose effect was not the result of failure of the substrate to enter the neoplastic cell. The synthesis of serine dehydratase comprised 4–5% of the total soluble cellular protein synthesis in the Morris hepatoma 5123, and this high rate of synthesis was not affected by the administration of glucose. On the other hand, an effect of glucose on the synthesis of tyrosine aminotransferase in hepatoma cells growing in culture has been reported (Mendelson *et al.*, 1971). Thus it would appear that *in vivo* the induction of serine dehydratase is not sensitive to glucose while possibly that of tyrosine aminotransferase is. Again, the defective regulatory mechanisms which we have already seen to occur at the transcriptional level also are present at the translational level in those neoplasms studied and the defects appear to be quite variable and heterogeneous.

In addition to glucose as a regulator of translation in mammalian systems, Cho-Chung and Pitot (1968) were able to demonstrate that tryptophan could

double the rate of tryptopan pyrrolase synthesis in liver in the absence of RNA
synthesis while nicotinamide suppressed the synthesis of the enzyme. As yet, these
studies have not been applied to specific neoplastic situations, although the lack of
effect of tryptophan in inducing the synthesis of tryptophan pyrrolase in most
neoplasms is now well known (Cho-Chung and Pitot, 1968).

2.3.3. Isozymes as Manifestations of Translational Regulation

The demonstration of various multiple molecular forms of enzymes in both
normal and neoplastic tissues has recently assumed considerable importance not
only because of the potential diagnostic usefulness of such studies but also because
of the relationship of differential isozyme formation to the altered regulation of
gene expression characteristic of neoplasms. Since the former subject is covered
elsewhere in this book, we will attempt to restrict the discussion here to the role of
multiple molecular forms of enzymes in the regulation of genetic expression.

There are a number of reviews on isozymes in neoplastic cells (Weinhouse and
Ono, 1972; Weinhouse, 1973; Schapira, 1970).

In all hepatomas thus far studied, the regulable isozyme, glucokinase, is almost
always missing or exhibits very low activity (Sato et al., 1969). It is not clear as yet
whether the distinction between glucokinase and hexokinase is the result of
transcription or translation. Recent studies from this laboratory have demonstrated multiple molecular forms of two hepatic enzymes, each of these forms
being regulated by different hormones. Specifically, serine dehydratase occurs in
two forms, the synthesis of one being regulated by cortisone and that of the other
by glucagon (Inoue et al., 1971). Tyrosine aminotransferase occurs in four
physically separable forms, one of which appears to be constitutive and is in fact
probably a different enzyme; the synthesis of one of the other three forms is
regulated by insulin while that of the other two is regulated by steroids and cyclic
nucleotides (Iwasaki et al., 1973). Although the exact regulation of all three forms
of tyrosine aminotransferase is not as clear as in the case of serine dehydratase, the
synthesis of form IV is regulated by insulin and apparently at the translational
level (Iwasaki et al., 1973).

When these multiple forms are determined in several hepatomas, the two forms
of serine dehydratase are found to be present in the tumors but in reciprocal
amounts to that in the liver; the synthesis of these forms is unchanged by hormone
administration or endocrine ablation (Inoue and Pitot, 1970). In several Morris
hepatomas, the insulin-regulated form of tyrosine aminotransferase is absent
(Pitot et al., 1972).

The exact chemical differences of these several forms are not known, but
preliminary investigations in our laboratory have indicated that the differences
may be the result of the oxidation–reduction states of sulfhydryl–disulfide
components of the multiple molecular forms. Evidence for this is seen from the
fact that form I of serine dehydratase, the cortisone-regulated form, may be
converted to the glucagon-regulated form in the test tube by very high concentrations of mercaptoethanol. In addition, Dr. J. Rodriguez has demonstrated that the

multiple forms of tyrosine aminotransferase differ in their sulfhydryl content—form II, that regulated by cortisone, having two or three more free sulfhydryl groups than form IV. Exactly how these factors are involved in the regulation of the synthesis of these forms at the translational level is not clear, although it is interesting to speculate that the disulfide-interchange enzyme described by Anfinsen (1962) and others (Ansorge *et al.*, 1973) may be the regulating feature in the final synthesis of these enzymes, as has been suggested by Rabin and his associates in the steroid regulation of polysome–membrane interaction (Williams and Rabin, 1969).

2.3.4. Regulation of the Rate of Enzyme Degradation, a Translational or Posttranslational Event in the Regulation of Genetic Expression

The importance of the regulation of enzyme degradation in controlling the levels of enzymes seen in eukaryotic cells was pointed out very distinctly by Schimke *et al.* (1965), who demonstrated the stabilization *in vivo* of tryptophan pyrrolase by its substrate, tryptophan. Since this, other examples of this relatively unique role of tryptophan in stabilizing several gluconeogenic enzymes have been reported (Cihak *et al.*, 1973*a*; Ballard and Hopgood, 1973). That other intracellular compounds such as glucose and pyridoxine may regulate the rate of enzyme degradation has also been demonstrated for the enzyme serine dehydratase (Khairallah and Pitot, 1968). A volume covering many of the aspects of enzyme degradation has been published (Rechcigl, 1971*a*).

The exact mechanisn of the dynamic degradation of proteins in higher eukaryotic organisms is at present unknown. Katunuma *et al.* (1972) have demonstrated the existence of enzymes relatively specific for the degradation of other enzymes within the liver. The lysosome has also been implicated in dynamic protein degradation, as have ATP and the need for an energy system (Hayashi *et al.*, 1973; Haider and Segal, 1972).

In addition to these studies, Schimke and his associates (Arias *et al.*, 1969; Dice *et al.*, 1973) have proposed that one of the major factors in protein degradation is the relationship of the size of the protein to the rate of its degradation. Larger proteins are degraded more rapidly than smaller ones. However, it is clear that both this theory and the importance of lysosomes in protein degradation cannot account for the specific degradation of individual proteins and the environmental regulation of this degradation.

Studies on the regulation of turnover of specific proteins in neoplastic cells have not been very extensive. Rechcigl (1971*b*) reviewed the studies on the turnover of catalase in neoplastic tissues of the rat. These experiments demonstrated significant differences between the turnover of the enzyme in normal and in neoplastic tissues. The degradation of protein alkylated by the carcinogen *N*-methyl-*N*-nitrosourea *in vivo* is much slower in hepatomas than in liver (Lerman *et al.*, 1974). While in our laboratory it was demonstrated that 5-azacytidine inhibits the degradation of the enzyme tyrosine aminotransferase in liver (Cihak *et al.*, 1973*b*), Levitan *et al.* (1971) demonstrated that the cortisone-mediated induction of this

enzyme does not show enhancement of the level of the enzyme, probably
reflecting a decrease in degradation in the tumor as is seen in the liver. Moyer and
Pitot (1973) have demonstrated that the turnover of electrophoretically separable classes of proteins in membranes of the endoplasmic reticulum in two Morris
hepatomas occurred with a different pattern with respect both to each other and
to that seen in normal liver. Furthermore, the patterns of degradation did not
appear to follow the molecular weight of the protein classes as had been seen
earlier in the case of liver (Arias *et al.*, 1969). Dunaway *et al.* (1974) have
demonstrated that while the synthesis of the major phosphofructokinase isozyme
is two- or threefold greater in a hepatoma than in normal liver the rate of
degradation of the isozyme is identical in normal and neoplastic tissue. Unfortunately, there have been too few studies to permit any generalization about the
regulation of enzyme turnover in normal and neoplastic tissues. However, the
studies thus far undertaken clearly indicate significant differences in the dynamic
degradation of enzymes in normal cells as compared to their neoplastic counterparts.

2.4. Multifactorial Regulation of Genetic Expression in Eukaryotes

For the multicellular organism, it is doubtful whether it is possible to do
experiments using simple environmental factors and conclude that the effects
seen are directly the result of the administration or the presence of the environmental component. The hormonal alterations occurring on perturbation of the
internal environment by a single insult are known to be numerous. Thus studies in
cell culture are to be preferred when one is attempting to determine the specific
mechanism of the effect of a single environmental agent on one cell type. On the
other hand, the demonstration of alterations resulting from perturbations of the
environment *in vivo* is extremely important for determining the changes which
occur in the actual situation as it exists. In studies on the regulation of genetic
expression in eukaryotes, especially mammals, a number of complex methods for
altering genetic expression of several tissues, predominantly liver and endocrine
organs, have been devised.

The principal environmental change that has been utilized in such experiments
is alteration in the diet. While the influence of the diet both on tumor incidence
and on the relationship of the neoplasm and the host in which it grows is well
known (Ross and Bras, 1965; Costa, 1963), the direct effect of alteration in the diet
on changes in enzyme levels and metabolism in neoplasms has also been the
subject of a number of experiments. Early investigations in this laboratory
demonstrated that the level of serine dehydratase in the Morris hepatoma 5123
was extremely high and could not be altered by a number of dietary conditions
(Pitot *et al.*, 1961). Later studies by Bottomley *et al.* (1963) demonstrated a similar
phenomenon for another highly differentiated hepatocellular carcinoma but also
the fact that most hepatomas had low or nonexistent levels of this enzyme.
Furthermore, adrenalectomy of the tumor-bearing host reduced the high levels

of serine dehydratase, although this change was still not subject to dietary manipulation. In a more recent study, Tryfiates *et al.* (1974) extended these earlier studies and demonstrated that in animals deficient in vitamin B_6 no cortisone induction of tyrosine aminotransferase occurred in the hepatoma, although it was present in the tumor of a nondeficient animal as well as in the host liver under both dietary conditions. Under none of these conditions was serine dehydratase inducible in the hepatoma. Studies by Ono *et al.* (1963) demonstrated that the feeding of a high-protein diet did result in a slight but significant increase in the level of glucose-6-phosphate dehydrogenase in the Morris hepatoma 5123 but the usual fasting–feeding regimen had no effect on the enzyme in the hepatoma. Kopelovich and Sabine (1970) reported that this enzyme as well as several others involved in carbohydrate and lipid metabolism responded in one mouse hepatoma to the feeding of diets of various fat contents in a manner similar to that seen in both normal and host liver. Specifically, on feeding a fat-free diet the level of glucose-6-phosphate dehydrogenase increased almost threefold over that in the tumor in starved animals, as did both the malic enzyme and the citrate cleavage enzyme. On the other hand, pyruvate kinase was unresponsive to dietary carbohydrate in several highly differentiated hepatocellular carcinomas (Campadelli-Fiume *et al.*, 1970; Criss and Morris, 1973*b*). In a somewhat more complicated series of experiments involving a specific starving and feeding regimen accomplished in an oscillatory manner, Potter *et al.* (1966) demonstrated that the enzymes, tyrosine aminotransferase, serine dehydratase, and ornithine aminotransferase in the highly differentiated Morris 7793 hepatoma varied in their activity with the time of day. However, these variations were quite different from the same variations seen in normal liver and thus further reflected aspects of abnormal environmental regulation in this highly differentiated neoplasm.

One of the more interesting areas of multifactorial regulation in hepatomas has been the defect in the regulation of cholesterol synthesis described in both primary and transplanted hepatomas in several species. Normally, feeding of a high-cholesterol diet causes a prompt decrease in the synthesis of [^{14}C]cholesterol from [^{14}C]acetate in liver slices from control and tumor-bearing rats (Taylor and Gould, 1950; Gould, 1951). However, in all rat, mouse, human, and trout hepatomas studied to date (Siperstein and Fagan, 1964; Siperstein *et al.*, 1966; Siperstein and Luby, 1969) a total loss of this "feedback" control of cholesterol synthesis has been described. It was shown that the defective regulation of cholesterol synthesis was paralleled by the unresponsiveness of microsomal HMG-CoA reductase, the rate-controlling enzyme for cholesterol synthesis (Butcher *et al.*, 1960), in Morris hepatomas of different growth rates (Goldfarb and Pitot, 1971; Siperstein *et al.*, 1971). However, as expected, the enzyme activity in the host liver did increase rapidly with cholesterol feeding. In addition, cholestyramine feeding, which increases cholesterol synthesis and microsomal HMG-CoA reductase activity, presumably by increasing the fecal excretion of bile acids, resulted in an increase of HMG-CoA reductase activity in host liver but had no effect on the hepatoma enzyme (Goldfarb and Pitot, 1971). However, a diurnal cycling of the enzyme, seen in the livers of control and tumor-bearing rats, was evident in two of the more rapidly growing tumors—the 5123C and 7800—but not in the very slow-growing 9618A hepatoma (Goldfarb and Pitot, 1971). Since recent evidence suggests that the normal diurnal rhythm of the enzyme is hormonally mediated, possibly by insulin (Lakshmanan *et al.*, 1973), these studies suggest that a hormonal- but not a cholesterol-mediated control of HMG-CoA reductase is still somewhat intact in the Morris hepatomas. It should be noted that although cholesterogenesis and HMG-CoA reductase activity varied greatly in these different hepatomas, in general both are increased in the better-differentiated hepatomas compared to the more poorly differentiated ones (Siperstein *et al.*, 1966; Bucher *et al.*, 1960).

Several studies have suggested that the deranged feedback control may not be at the level of the enzyme but rather in the tumor's ability to accumulate the feedback regulator. The K_m and heat stability of HMG-CoA reductase of a mouse hepatoma were similar to those of normal mouse liver (Kandutsch and Hancock, 1971) and more importantly a clear-cut and striking decrease in the uptake and accumulation of dietary cholesterol in three Morris hepatomas has been reported (Harry *et al.*, 1971). In addition, several recent studies suggest that defective feedback control of HMG-CoA reductase noted *in vivo* could be secondary to the decreased and nonphysiological blood supply of the transplantable hepatomas. Cultured HTC cells derived from the Morris hepatoma 7288C do seem to maintain the feedback control of the cholesterol pathway since they show a threefold greater activity of HMG-CoA reductase when exposed to lipoprotein-poor serum that is depleted of cholesterol than when cultured in intact rat serum (Watson, 1973). Second, the best-differentiated primary hepatomas induced by acetylaminofluorene are as efficient as nontumorous liver in taking up dietary cholesterol from sera (Horton *et al.*, 1973). Therefore, considerably more study of the "feedback" regulation of HMG-CoA reductase in primary well-differentiated hepatomas is necessary before it can be concluded that the feedback control is due to an intrinsic defect of biochemical control in all hepatomas.

Several of the partial reactions of bile acid synthesis have recently been demonstrated in the Morris 5123C and 9618A hepatomas (Mott *et al.*, 1974). As much of the rate-controlling enzyme for bile acid synthesis, microsomal cholesterol-7α-hydroxylase, was found in the very-well-differentiated 9618A hepatoma as in host liver, while the less-differentiated 5123C tumor contained only about one-third as much of the enzyme. In view of the close synchrony of cholesterol and bile acid synthesis in normal liver under a variety of physiological conditions (Wilson, 1972), a similar ratio of the two rate-controlling enzymes, HMG-CoA reductase/cholesterol-7α-hydroxylase, in the 9618A and 5123C hepatomas suggests a similar synchronous control of cholesterol and bile acid synthesis in these tumors.

Following starving and refeeding of a fat-free diet, the liver normally responds by a great increase in fatty acid synthesis (Allman *et al.*, 1965). This response persists in host livers but has been found entirely lacking in many different transplantable mouse hepatomas (Sabine *et al.*, 1966, 1967) and Morris rat hepatomas (Sabine *et al.*, 1968; Zuckerman *et al.*, 1970; Elwood and Morris, 1968) over a wide spectrum of growth rates. There appears to be no correlation of growth rate with the degree of fatty acid synthesis (Sabine *et al.*, 1968). A detailed study of the regulation of acetyl coenzyme A carboxylase, the rate-controlling enzyme for fatty acid synthesis, and of fatty acid synthetase in the rapidly growing Morris hepatoma 7777 and véry slowly growing 9618A (Majerus *et al.*, 1968) showed that both enzymes increased by 12- to 29-fold in the host livers 48 h after refeeding but that there was no increase in the levels of these enzymes in the hepatomas. Kinetic studies of the purified acetyl CoA carboxylase from the 7777 hepatoma by these same workers showed that the tumor enzyme is essentially similar in behavior to the rat enzyme with regard to its affinity for acetyl coenzyme A and ATP, aggregation and activation by citrate, inhibition by malonyl CoA, biotin content, pH optima, and heat inactivation. The mechanism of this defective control in hepatomas is not known. It does not appear to be related to an absent portal blood flow in hepatomas, since median lobe autografts devoid of portal blood flow in rats that are starved and then refed still show a 6.5-fold increase in ^{14}C incorporation from [^{14}C]acetate into fatty acids and an 18-fold increase in fatty acid synthetase. These levels are comparable to those in the portions of the liver with intact blood supply (Bartley and Abraham, 1972). Lee *et al.* (1973) demonstrated that stearyl CoA desaturase activity increased significantly in liver and a transplantable sarcoma in rats fed a fat-free diet. However, no change occurred in the level of alkylacylglycerophosphorylethanolamine desaturase in the tumors of these animals.

While these studies further demonstrate the extensive defectiveness of environmental regulation not only in hepatocellular carcinomas but also in other neoplasms, we are still left with the dilemma that there is no common thread other than the fact of the extreme heterogeneity of the defective mechanisms of environmental control seen in neoplasms in general.

3. Conclusions

At the beginning of this brief survey, we indicated the general steps in the expression of genetic information in eukaryotes. In the remainder of our discussion, specific factors involved in the regulation of genetic expression at various levels were pointed out. By way of a concluding summary, Fig. 2 therefore portrays an expanded version of the steps in the regulation of genetic expression, pointing out potential and known sites of regulation, a number of which we have already alluded to.

Beginning with the regulation of DNA synthesis, a principal site (1) for the regulation of DNA synthesis is the actual enzyme mechanism performing this function. In Fig. 2, this entity is termed a "replisome," after Bleecken (1971). While such an entity may be analogous to the "replicon" of Jacob and Brenner (1963), the figure does not include the possible role of the nuclear membrane in the regulation of DNA synthesis (Franke *et al.*, 1973), although the involvement of

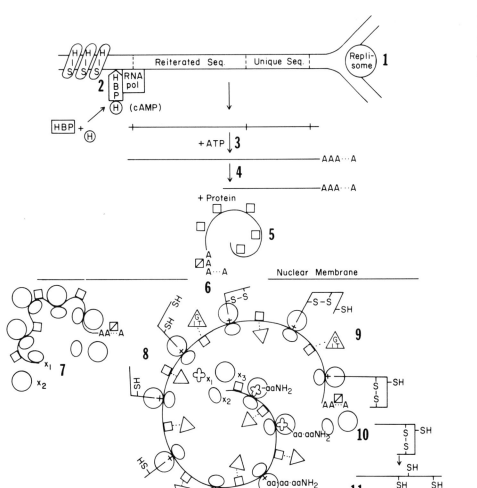

FIGURE 2. Components of genetic expression in mammalian cells. A segment of the DNA is demonstrated as in Fig. 1, but also a component of its replication may be seen (1) and on the left a portion of the DNA covered by histones (HIS). RNA polymerase is represented by a box (RNA pol) and the action of a hormone receptor (HBP) is shown together with the hormone (H within circle) and the possible effect of cyclic AMP (cAMP) (2). Transcription leads to the messenger RNA molecule, which in the presence of ATP is adenylated (3) and subsequently matured by cleavage of some of the reiterated sequences (4). This molecule is then associated with protein (boxes) (5) and transported out of the nucleus through the nuclear pore (6). The free polysome (7) is represented in a similar manner to that seen in Fig. 1 and is felt to be the more short-lived functional translating unit (see text). The bound polysome (8) is demonstrated in a much more complicated manner, with the initiation factors (X_1, X_2, X_3) initiating translation within the cochlear configuration. Transfer RNA is represented initially as a four-leaf clover and later as a small cross. The growing protein chain with its S—S and S—H components can be seen. The proteins associated with the message (boxes) are indicated to associate with triangles representing attachment points on the membrane (see text). In two of these instances, the triangle is shown to be the enzyme responsible for disulfide interchanges (GIT; see text for further details) (9). Chain termination (10) is demonstrated and the finished protein may then be degraded by reduction of its S—S bonds and subsequent proteolysis (11). See text for further discussion.

a short segment of RNA synthesis during the initiation of DNA synthesis is represented.

The restriction function of histones of DNA as well as the specific regulation of transcription by RNA polymerase (2) is noted schematically on the diagram. Since the exact function of cyclic AMP in the regulation of transcription is not known for eukaryotes, this molecule is noted in parentheses in the figure. The hormone-binding proteins (HBP) and the alteration of their conformation as well as their presumed interaction with the transcriptional mechanism are also denoted. The subsequent steps of adenylation (3), maturation with elimination of most of the repetitive sequences (4), and association of the mature messenger RNA with protein (5) are noted, although relatively little information about the regulation of these specific steps is presently known. On the other hand, studies of Webb and his associates (Schumm *et al.*, 1973; Schumm and Webb, 1974) have demonstrated that the release of messenger RNA from isolated nuclei is controlled by cytoplasmic proteins and is possibly related to polyadenylation. The proteins regulating the release of messenger RNA appear to be different in normal and neoplastic liver.

The lower portion of Fig. 2 is related to the translational regulation of genetic expression. The various steps of protein synthesis demonstrated include initiation (7), elongation (8), tertiary structural catalysis by glutathione-insulin transhydrogenase (GIT), as was suggested earlier in this review (9), and the phenomenon of chain termination and release from the enzyme-forming unit (10). While no specific examples of translational regulation at the point of the initiation of protein synthesis (7) or the elongation of polypeptide chains (8) were given, the glucose effect (Jost *et al.*, 1968) or the effect of tryptophan in regulating tryptophan pyrrolase synthesis (Cho-Chung and Pitot, 1968) possibly occur at one of these steps. Earlier studies in this laboratory suggested that cyclic AMP could effect the release of polysome-bound proteins *in vitro* (Khairallah and Pitot, 1967). More recently, Chong-Cheng and Oliver (1972) demonstrated that cyclic AMP together with a cytoplasmic factor could effect the release of tryosine aminotransferase from bound polysomes *in vitro*. It appears that the initiation factors involved in protein synthesis and denoted in Fig. 2 as X_1, X_2, and X_3 are similar in normal and neoplastic tissues (Murty *et al.*, 1974). Differences in the translational regulation of the synthesis of catalase in cell-free systems from liver and hepatoma have been described by Uenoyama and Ono (1973). In this study, it was not clear whether the regulating proteins act at chain initiation, termination, or elongation. Thus while understanding of the exact mechanism of the regulation of translation is still in its infancy, potential sites of regulation have been delineated.

Figure 2 distinguishes between the free polysome, on the lower left portion, and that bound to the endoplasmic reticulum, detailed on the right. The stabilization of the latter by an interaction of the informasome protein (small boxes) with some structure on the membrane (triangles), possibly GIT (Williams and Rabin, 1969), can also be seen in Fig. 2. Finally, the possible regulation of the degradation of proteins (11) may be seen as occurring in two steps, the initial one that of a disulfide interchange, as has been suggested to occur in the case of insulin (Varandani *et al.*, 1972).

Figure 2 as well as Fig.1 does not take into account the possibility of allosteric regulation of enzyme activity, which is clearly an important factor in the regulation of genetic expression. Besides the problem of insufficient space for such consideration, another significant reason is the fact that allosteric and feedback inhibitions of enzymes in neoplastic tissues are generally identical to those seen in their normal counterparts (Bresnick and Karjala, 1964; Gordon *et al.*, 1968). On the other hand, as should be apparent from this review, not only is the regulation of genetic expression involving the synthesis and degradation of proteins and nucleic acid generally abnormal in neoplasms compared to their cell or origin, but also the abnormalities noted form a pattern which appears to be unique to each neoplasm. While theoretical explanations for this biochemical diversity in both phenotype and regulatory mechanisms in neoplasia have been presented (Pitot *et al.*, 1974), the fact still remains that the most significant biological and biochemical distinctions defining the neoplastic phenomenon are the abnormalities seen in the regulation of genetic expression.

4. References

ADESNIK, M., SALDITT, M., THOMAS, W., AND DARNELL, J. E., 1972, Evidence that all messenger RNA molecules (except histone messenger RNA) contain poly(A) sequences and that the poly(A) has a nuclear function, *J. Mol. Biol.* **71**:21.

ALLEN, D. O., MUNSHOWER, J., MORRIS, H. P., AND WEBER, G., 1971, Regulation of adenyl cyclase in hepatomas of different growth rates, *Cancer Res.* **31**:557.

ALLMAN, D. W., HIBBARD, D. D., AND GIBSON, D. M., 1965, Fatty acid synthesis during fat free refeeding of starved rats, *J. Lipid Res.* **6**:63.

ANDERSON, W. B., JOHNSON, G. S., AND PASTAN, I., 1973, Transformation of chick embryo fibroblasts by wild-type and temperature-sensitive Rous sarcoma virus alters adenylate cyclase activity, *Proc. Natl. Acad. Sci. U.S.A.* **70**:1055.

ANFINSEN, C. B., 1962, Some observations on the basic principles of design in protein molecules, *Comp. Biochem. Physiol.* **4**:229.

ANSORGE, S., BOHLEY, P., KIRSCHKE, H., LANGNER, J., MARQUARDT, I., WIDERANDERS, B., AND HANSON, H., 1973, The identity of the insulin degrading thiol-protein disulfide oxidoreductase (glutathione-insulin transhydrogenase) with the sulfhydryl-disulfide interchange enzyme, *FEBS Letters* **37**:238.

ARIAS, I. M., DOYLE, D., AND SCHIMKE, R. T., 1969, Studies on the synthesis and degradation of proteins of the endoplasmic reticulum of rat liver, *J. Biol. Chem.* **244**:3303.

ARNOLD, E. A., BUKSAS, M. M., AND YOUNG, K. E., 1973, A comparative study of some properties of chromatin from two "minimal deviation" hepatomas, *Cancer Res.* **33**:1169.

BALLARD, F. J., AND HOPGOOD, M. F., 1973, Phosphopyruvate carboxylase induction by L-tryptophan, *Biochem. J.* **136**:259.

BANERJEE, M. R., 1969, Hormonal control of DNA synthesis: Altered responsiveness of hyperplastic alveolar nodules of mouse mammary gland, *J. Natl. Cancer Inst.* **42**:227.

BARKA, T., 1965, Stimulation of DNA synthesis by isoproterenol in the salivary gland, *Exp. Cell Res.* **39**:335.

BARTLEY, H. C., AND ABRAHAM, S., 1972, Dietary regulation of fatty acid synthesis in rat liver and hepatic autotransplants, *Biochim. Biophys. Acta* **260**:169.

BECKER, F. F., 1969, Cell division of normal mammalian tissues, *Ann. Rev. Med.* **20**:243.

BECKER, F. F., 1974, Regeneration, in: *The Liver: Normal and Abnormal Functions* (F. Becker, ed.), pp. 69–83, Dekker, New York.

BLANKENSHIP, J., AND BRESNICK, E., 1974, Effects of phenobarbital on the phosphorylation of acidic nuclear proteins of rat liver, *Biochim. Biophys. Acta* **340**:218.

BLANKENSHIP, J., AND KUEHL, L., 1973, Effects of phenobarbital and 3-methylcholanthrene on amino acid incorporation into rat liver chromosomal proteins, *Mol. Pharmacol.* **6**:247.

BLEECKEN, S., 1971, "Replisome"-controlled initiation of DNA replication, *J. Theor. Biol.* **32**:81.

BONKOWSKY, H. L., COLLINS, A., DOHERTY, J. M., AND TSCHUDY, D. P., 1973, The glucose effect in rat liver: Studies of δ-aminolevulinate synthase and tyrosine aminotransferase, *Biochim. Biophys. Acta* **320**:561.

BONNER, J., DAHMUS, M. E., FAMBROUGH, D., HUANG, R. C., MARUSHIGE, K., AND TUAN, D. Y. H., 1968, The biology of isolated chromatin, *Science* **159**:47.

BOTTOMLEY, R. H., PITOT, H. C., AND MORRIS, H. P., 1963, Metabolic adaptation in rat hepatomas. IV. Regulation of threonine and serine dehydratase, *Cancer Res.* **23**:392.

BRESNICK, E., AND KARJALA, R. J., 1964, End-product inhibition of thymidine kinase activity in normal and leukemic human leukocytes, *Cancer Res.* **24**:841.

BRICKER, L. A., MARRACCINI, J. V., ROSENBLATT, S., KOXLOVSKIS, P. L., AND MORRIS, H. P., 1974, Effects of dietary cholesterol on bile acid synthesis in liver and hepatomas, *Cancer Res.* **34**:449.

BROWN, H. D., CHATTOPADHYAY, S. K., MORRIS, H. P., AND PENNINGTON, S. N., 1970, Adenyl cyclase activity in Morris hepatomas 7777, 7794A and 9718A, *Cancer Res.* **30**:123.

BROWN, H. D., CHATTOPADHYAY, S. K., PENNINGTON, S. N., SPRATT, H. S., AND MORRIS, H. P., 1971, Mixed function oxidation in tumors, *Br. J. Cancer* **25**:135.

BRUZZONE, S., 1971, Differential response of ribonucleic acid polymerase in preneoplastic and neoplastic ovaries of mice following oestradiol treatment, *Br. J. Cancer* **25**:158.

BUCHER, N. L. R., OVERATH, P., AND LYNEN, F., 1960, β-Hydroxy-β-methylglutaryl coenzyme A reductase, cleavage and condensing enzymes in relation to cholesterol formation in rat liver, *Biochim. Biophys. Acta* **40**:491.

BULLOUGH, W. S., AND DEOL, J. U. R., 1971, Chalone-induced mitotic inhibition in the Hewitt keratinising epidermal carcinoma of the mouse, *Eur. J. Cancer* **7**:425.

BYRNES, K. A., GHIDONI, J. J., AND MAYFIELD, E. D., 1972, Response of the rat kidney of folic acid administration. I. Biochemical studies, *Lab. Invest.* **26**:184.

CAMPADELLI-FIUME, G., DELLA CORTE, E., AND STIRPE, F., 1970, Pyruvate kinase of Morris hepatoma 5123: Insensitivity to dietary changes, *Biochem. J.* **118**:195.

CHANDRA, P., AND GERICK, D., 1972, Regulation des Tumor Wachstums durch Adenosin-3',5'-monophosphat, *Naturwissenschaften* **59**:205.

CHATTOPADHYAY, S. K., BROWN, H. D., AND MORRIS, H. P., 1972, Further studies of electron transport components in a series of Morris hepatoma-bearing rats, *Br. J. Cancer* **26**:3.

CHAYOTH, R., EPSTEIN, S. M., AND FIELD, J. B., 1973, Glucagon and prostaglandin E$_1$ stimulation of cyclic adenosine 3',5'-monophosphate levels and adenylate cyclase activity in benign hyperplastic nodules and malignant hepatomas of ethionine-treated rats, *Cancer Res.* **33**:1970.

CHO, Y. S., PITOT, H. C., AND MORRIS, H. P., 1964, Metabolic adaptations in rat hepatomas. VI. Substrate–hormone relationships in tryptophan pyrrolase induction, *Cancer Res.* **24**:52.

CHO-CHUNG, Y. S., AND PITOT, H. C., 1968, Regulator effects of nicotinamide on tryptophan pyrrolase synthesis in rat liver *in vivo*, *Eur. J. Biochem.* **3**:401.

CHONG-CHENG, C., AND OLIVER, I. T., 1972, A translational control mechanism in mammalian protein synthesis modulated by cyclic adenosine monophosphate: Translational control of tyrosine aminotransferase synthesis in neonatal rat liver, *Biochemistry* **11**:2547.

CHRISTOFFERSEN, T., MOORLAND, J., OSNES, J. B., AND ELGJO, K., 1972, Hepatic adenyl cyclase: Alterations in hormone response treatment with a chemical carcinogen, *Biochim. Biophys. Acta* **279**:383.

CIHAK, A., LAMER, C., AND PITOT, H. C., 1973a, L-Tryptophan inhibition of tyrosine aminotransferase degradation in rat liver *in vivo*, *Arch. Biochem. Biophys.* **156**:188.

CIHAK, A., LAMAR, C., AND PITOT, H. C., 1973b, Studies on the mechanism of the stimulation of tyrosine aminotransferase activity *in vivo* by pyrimidine analogues: The role of enzyme synthesis and degradation, *Arch. Biochem. Biophys.* **1956**:176.

CONNEY, A. H., 1969, Drug metabolism and therapeutics, *New Engl. J. Med.* **280**:653.

CONNEY, A. H., AND BURNS, J. J., 1963, Induced synthesis of oxidative enzymes in liver microsomes by polycyclic hydrocarbons and drugs, in: *Advances in Enzyme Regulation*, Vol. 1 (G. Weber, ed.), pp. 189–214, Pergamon Press, Oxford.

COSTA, G., 1963, Cachexia, the metabolic component of neoplastic diseases, *Prog. Exp. Tumor Res.* **3**:321.

CRISS, W. E., AND MORRIS, H. P., 1973a, Protein kinase activity in Morris hepatomas, *Biochem. Biophys. Res. Commun.* **54**:380.

CRISS, W. E., AND MORRIS, H. P., 1973b, Influence of hormones on the growth of hepatomas and induction of adenylate and pyruvate kinases, *Cancer Res.* **33**:1023.

CUATRECASAS, P., 1974, Insulin receptor of liver and fat cell membranes, *Fed. Proc.* **32**:1838.

DAVIS, W. W., AND GARREN, L. D., 1968, On the mechanism of action of adrenocorticotropic hormone—The inhibition site of cycloheximide in the pathway of steroid biosynthesis, *J. Biol. Chem.* **243**:5153.

DAWSON, K. G., PATEY, P., RUBINSTEIN, D., AND BECK, J. C., 1966, Growth hormone and protein synthesis, *Mol. Pharmacol.* **2**:269.

DICE, J. F., DEHLINGER, P. J., AND SCHIMKE, R. T., 1973, Studies on the correlation between size and relative degradation rate of soluble proteins, *J. Biol. Chem.* **248**:4220.

DINGMAN, C. W., RONOW, A., BUNTING, S. L., PEACOCK, A. C., AND O'MALLEY, B. W., 1969, Changes in chick oviduct ribonucleic acid following hormonal stimulation, *Biochemistry* **8**:489.

DUNAWAY, G. A., TRAHAN, L. J., MORRIS, H. P., AND WEBER, G., 1974, Synthesis and degradation of the major hepatic phosphofructokinase isozyme in rat liver and hepatoma 3924-A, *Biochem. Res. Commun.* **59**:508.

DURE, L., AND WATERS, L., 1965, Long-lived messenger RNA: Evidence from cotton seed germination, *Science* **147**:410.

DYER, H. M., GULLINO, P. M., AND MORRIS, H. P., 1964, Tryptophan pyrrolase activity in transplanted "minimal deviation" type hepatomas, *Cancer Res.* **24**:97.

EDSTRÖM, J. E., AND TANGUAY, R., 1974, Cytoplasmic ribonucleic acids with messenger characteristics in salivary gland cells of *Chironomus tentans*, *J. Mol. Biol.* **84**:569.

ELIASSON, R., MARTIN, R., AND REICHARD, P., 1974, Characterization of RNA initiating the discontinuous synthesis of polyoma DNA, *Biochem. Biophys. Res. Commun.* **59**:307.

ELWOOD, H. C., AND MORRIS, H. P., 1968, Lack of adaptation in lipogenesis by hepatoma 9121, *J. Lipid Res.* **9**:337.

EMMELOT, P., AND BOS, C. J., 1971, Studies on plasma membranes. VI. Adenyl cyclase in plasma membranes isolated from rat and mouse livers and hepatomas and its hormone sensitivity, *Biochim. Biophys. Acta* **249**:285.

ENDO, Y., TOMINAGA, H., AND NATORI, Y., 1971, Effect of actinomycin D on turnover rates of messenger ribonucleic acid in rat liver, *Biochim. Biophys. Acta* **240**:215.

FOX, R. M., MENDELSOHN, J., BARBOSA, E., AND GOULIAN, M., 1973, RNA in nascent DNA from cultured human lymphocytes, *Nature New Biol.* **245**:234.

FRANKE, W. W., DEUMLING, B., ZENTGRAF, H., FALK, H., AND RAE, P. M. N., 1973, Nuclear membranes from mammalian liver. IV. Characterization of membrane-attached DNA, *Exp. Cell Res.* **81**:365.

GELBOIN, H. V., AND BLACKBURN, N. R., 1964, The stimulatory effect of 3-methylcholanthrene on benzpyrene hydroxlase activity in several rat tissues: Inhibition by actinomycin D and puromycin, *Cancer Res.* **24**:356.

GESSNER, T., 1974, Studies on glucuronidation and sulfation in tumor bearing rats, *Biochem. Pharmacol.* **23**:1809.

GIBOL, D., DELORENZO, F., GOLDBERG, R. F., AND ANFINSEN, C. B., 1965, Disulfide interchange and the three-dimensional structure of proteins, *Proc. Natl. Acad. Sci. U.S.A.* **53**:676.

GOLDFARB, S., AND PITOT, H. C., 1971, The regulation of β-hydroxy-β-methylglutaryl coenzyme A reductase in Morris hepatomas 5123C, 7800 and 9618A, *Cancer Res.* **31**:1879.

GORDON, H. L., BARDOS, T. J., CHMIELEWICZ, F., AND AMBRUS, J. L., 1968, Comparative study of the thymidine kinase and thymidylate kinase activities and of the feedback inhibition of thymidine kinase in normal and neoplastic human tissues, *Cancer Res.* **28**:2068.

GOULD, R. G., 1951, Lipid metabolism and atherosclerosis, *Am. J. Med.* **11**:209.

GREENGARD, O., AND ACS, G., 1962, The effect of actinomycin on the substrate and hormonal induction of liver enzymes, *Biochim. Biophys. Acta* **61**:652.

HAIDER, M., AND SEGAL, H. L., 1972, Some characteristics of the alanine aminotransferase- and arginase-inactivating system of lysosomes, *Arch. Biochem. Biophys.* **148**:228.

HALL, M. R., MEINKE, W., GOLDSTEIN, D. A., AND LERNER, R. A., 1971, Synthesis of cytoplasmic membrane-associated DNA in lymphocyte nucleus, *Nature New Biol.* **234**:227.

HAMILTON, T. H., 1968, Control by estrogen of genetic transcription and translation, *Science* **161**:649.

HARRIS, S. E., MEANS, A. R., MITCHELL, W. M., AND O'MALLEY, B. W., 1973, Synthesis of (^{3}H) DNA complementary to ovalbumin messenger RNA: Evidence for limited copies of the ovalbumin gene in chick oviduct, *Proc. Natl. Acad. Sci. U.S.A.* **70**:3776.

HARRY, D. S., MORRIS, H. P., AND MCINTYRE, N., 1971, Cholesterol biosynthesis in transplantable hepatomas: Evidence for impairment of uptake and storage of dietary cholesterol, *J. Lipid Res.* **12**:313.

HART, L. G., ADAMSON, R. H., MORRIS, H. P., AND FOUTS, J. R., 1965, The stimulation of drug metabolism in various rat hepatomas, *J. Pharmacol. Exp. Ther.* **149:**7.

HAYASHI, M., HIROI, Y., AND NATORI, Y., 1973, Effect of ATP on protein degradation in rat liver lysosomes, *Nature New Biol.* **242:**163.

HILF, R., MICHEL, I., SILVERSTEIN, G., AND BELL, C., 1965, Effect of actinomycin D on estrogen-induced changes in enzymes and nucleic acids of R3230AC mammary tumors, uteri, and mammary glands, *Cancer Res.* **25:**1854.

HILF, R., MICHEL, I., AND BILL, C., 1967, Biochemical and morphological responses of normal and neoplastic mammary tissues to hormonal treatment, *Recent Prog. Horm. Res.* **23:**229.

HILL, R. B., AND SAUNDERS, E. H., 1971, Cellular adaptation in rat liver. I. Decay of free and membrane-bound polysomes, *Lab. Invest.* **24:**321.

HORTON, B. H., MOTT, G. E., PITOT, H. C., AND GOLDFARB, S., 1973, Rapid uptake of dietary cholesterol by hyperplastic liver nodules and primary hepatomas, *Cancer Res.* **33:**460.

HOUGH, B. R., AND DAVIDSON, E. H., 1972, Studies on the repetitive sequence transcripts of *Xenopus* oocytes, *J. Mol. Biol.* **70:**491.

HUCKER, H. B., 1973, Intermediates in drug metabolism reactions, *Drug Metab. Rev.* **2:**33.

INFANTE, A. A., NAUTA, R., GILBERT, S., HOBART, P., AND FIRSCHEIN, W., 1973, DNA synthesis in developing sea urchins: Role of a DNA–nuclear membrane complex, *Nature New Biol.* **242:**5.

INOUE, H., AND PITOT, H. C., 1970, Regulation of the synthesis of serine dehydratase isozymes, in: *Advances in Enzyme Regulation*, Vol. 8 (G. Weber, ed.), pp. 289–296, Pergamon Press, New York.

INOUE, H., KASPER, C., AND PITOT, H. C., 1971, Studies on the induction and repression of enzymes in rat liver. VI. Some properties and the metabolic regulation of two isozymic forms of serine dehydratase, *J. Biol. Chem.* **246:**2626.

IWASAKI, Y., LAMAR, C., DANENBERG, K., AND PITOT, H. C., 1973, Studies on the induction and repression of enzymes in rat liver. VII. Characterization and metabolic regulation of multiple forms of tyrosine amino transferase, *Eur. J. Biochem.* **34:**347.

JACOB, F., AND BRENNER, F., 1963, Sur la regulation de la synthese du DNA chez les bacteries: l'Hypothese du replicon, *C. R. Acad. Sci.* **256:**298.

JACOB, F., AND MONOD, J., 1961, Genetic regulatory mechanisms in the synthesis of proteins, *J. Mol. Biol.* **3:**318.

JACOB, S. T., SCHARS, M. B., AND VESSEL, E. S., 1974, Role of RNA in induction of hepatic microsomal mixed function oxidases, *Proc. Natl. Acad. Sci. U.S.A.* **71:**704.

JENSEN, E. V., AND DESOMBRE, E. R., 1973, Estrogen–receptor interaction, *Science* **182:**126.

JENSEN, E. V., NUMATA, M., BRECHER, P. I., AND DESOMBRE, E. R., 1971, Hormone–receptor interaction as a guide to biochemical mechanism, in: *The Biochemistry of Steroid Hormone Action*, Biochemistry Society Symposium 32 (R. M. S. Smellie, ed.), pp. 133–159, Academic Press, London.

JERVELL, K. F., CHRISTOFFERSEN, T., AND MOORLAND, J., 1965, Studies on the 3-methylcholanthrene induction and carbohydrate repression of rat liver dimethylaminoazobenzene reductase, *Arch. Biochem. Biophys.* **111:**15.

JOST, J.-P., AND PITOT, H. C., 1970, Metabolic adaptations in rat hepatomas: Altered regulation of serine dehydratase synthesis by glucose and amino acid in hepatocellular carcinomas, *Cancer Res.* **30:**387.

JOST, J.-P., AND SAHIB, M. K., 1971, Role of cyclic adenosine 3',5' monophosphate in the induction of hepatic enzyme. II. Effect of $N^6,O^{2'}$-dibutyryl cyclic adenosine 3',5' monophosphate on the kinetics of ribonucleic acid synthesis in purified rat liver nuclei, *J. Biol. Chem.* **246:**1623.

JOST, J.-P., KHAIRALLAH, E. A., AND PITOT, H. C., 1968, Studies on the induction and repression of enzymes in rat liver. V. Regulation of the rate of synthesis and degradation of serine dehydratase by dietary amino acids and glucose, *J. Biol. Chem.* **243:**3057.

KAFATOS, F. C., 1972, mRNA stability and cellular differentiation, *Karolinska Symp. Res. Methods Reprod. Endocrinol.* **5:**319.

KANDUTSCH, A. A., AND HANCOCK, R. L., 1971, Regulation of the rate of sterol synthesis and the level of β-hydroxy-β-methylglutaryl coenzyme A reductase activity in mouse liver and hepatomas, *Cancer Res.* **31:**1396.

KARLSON, P., AND SEKERIS, C. E., 1966, Biochemical mechanisms of hormone action, *Acta Endocrinol.* **53:**505.

KARSTEN, U., SYDOW, G., WOLLENBERGER, A., AND GRAFFI, A., 1971, Rat liver glycerol phosphate dehydrogenase: Activity changes and induction by thyroid hormone of the mitochondrial enzyme in hepatomas and in precancerous and growing liver, *Acta Biol. Med. Germ.* **26:**1131.

KATUNUMA, N., KOMINAMI, E., KOMINAMI, W., AND KITO, K., 1972, Mode of action of specific inactivating enzymes for pyridoxal and NAD-dependent enzymes and their biological significance, in: *Advances in Enzyme Regulation*, Vol. 10 (G. Weber, ed.), pp. 289–308, Pergamon Press, New York.

KHAIRALLAH, E. A., AND PITOT, H. C., 1967, 3',5'-Cyclic AMP and the release of polysome-bound proteins *in vitro*, *Biochem. Biophys. Res. Commun.* **29**:269.

KHAIRALLAH, E. A., AND PITOT, H. C., 1968, Studies on the turnover of serine dehydratase: Amino acid induction, glucose repression and pyridoxine stabilization, in: *Symposium on Pyridoxal Enzymes* (K. Yamada, N. Katunuma, and H. Wada, eds.), pp. 159–164, Maruzen, Tokyo.

KIZER, D. E., COX, B., HOWELL, B. A., AND SHIRLEY, B. C., 1969, Effect of hepatocarcinogens on hepatocyte DNA synthesis and cortisone induction of tryptophan oxygenase, *Cancer Res.* **29**:2039.

KLEIN, I., LEVY, G. S., BRICKER, L. E., AND MORRIS, H. P., 1974, Glucagon and epinephrine activation of adenylate cyclase and glucagon binding in Morris hepatomas, *Endocrinology* **94**:279.

KOPELOVICH, L., AND SABINE, J. R., 1970, Control of lipid metabolism in hepatomas: Effects of fasting and dietary fat on the activities of several glycolytic and Krebs' cycle enzymes in mouse liver and hepatoma BW7756, *Biochim. Biophys. Acta* **202**:268.

LAKSHMANAN, M. R., NEPOKROEFF, C. M., NESS, G. C., DUGAN, R. E. AND PORTER, J. W., 1973, Stimulation by insulin of rat liver β-hydroxy-β-methylglutaryl coenzyme A reductase and cholesterol synthesizing activities, *Biochem. Biophys. Res. Commun.* **50**:704.

LANDE, M., SUMIDA, M., TASHIRO, Y., ADESNIK, M., AND SABATINI, D., 1974, Direct association of mRNA with microsomal membranes in human diploid fibroblasts, *J. Cell Biol.* **63**:183a.

LANGAN, T. A., 1968, Histone phosphorylation: Stimulation by adenosine 3',5-monophosphate, *Science* **162**:579.

LAURENCE, D. J. R., AND BUTLER, J. A. V., 1965, Metabolism of histones in malignant tissues and liver of the rat and mouse, *Biochem. J.* **96**:53.

LAURENCE, E. B., AND ELGJO, K., 1971, Epidermal chalone and cell proliferation in a transplantable squamous cell carcinoma in hamsters, *Virchows Arch. B: Zellpathol.* **7**:8.

LEE, J. C. K., 1971, Effects of partial hepatectomy in rats on two transplantable hepatomas, *Am. J. Pathol.* **65**:347.

LEE, K. L., REEL, J. R., AND KENNEY, F. T., 1970, Regulation of tyrosine α-ketoglutarate transaminase in rat liver. IX. Studies of the mechanisms of hormonal inductions in cultured hepatoma cells, *J. Biol. Chem.* **245**:5806.

LEE, T.-C., WYKLE, R. L., BLANK, M. L., AND SNYDER, F., 1973, Dietary control of stearyl CoA and alkylacylglycerophosphorylethanolamine desaturases in tumor, *Biochem. Biophys. Res. Commun.* **55**:574.

LEFKOWITZ, R. J., 1973, Isolated hormone receptors—Physiologic and clinical implications, *New Engl. J. Med.* **288**:1061.

LERMAN, M. I., ABAKUMOVA, O. Y., KUCENCO, N. J., GORBACHEVA, L. V., KUKUSHKINA, G. V., AND SEREBRYANYI, A. M., 1974, Different degradation rates of alkylated RNA protein and lipids in normal and tumor cells, *Cancer Res.* **34**:1536.

LEVITAN, I. V., MORRIS, H. P., AND WEBB, T. E., 1971, Tyrosine transaminase induction: Differential effect of 5-azacytidine on liver and hepatoma 5123D, *Biochim. Biophys. Acta* **240**:287.

LUEDERS, K. K., DYER, H. M., THOMPSON, E. B., AND KUFF, E. L., 1970, Glucuronyltransferase activity in transplantable hepatomas, *Cancer Res.* **30**:274.

MACCHIA, V., MELDOLISI, M. F., AND CHIARIELLO, M., 1972, Adenyl-cyclase in a transplantable thyroid tumor: loss of ability to respond to TSH, *Endocrinology* **90**:1483.

MAINI, M. N., AND STICH, H. F., 1962, Chromosomes of tumor cells. III. Unresponsiveness of precancerous hepatic tissues and hepatomas to a mitotic stimulus, *J. Natl. Cancer Inst.* **28**:753.

MAJERUS, P. W., JACOBS, R., AND SMITH, M. B., 1968, The regulation of fatty acid biosynthesis in rat hepatomas, *J. Biol. Chem.* **243**:3588.

MCCLURE, M. E., AND HNILICA, L. S., 1972, Nuclear proteins in genetic restriction. III. The cell cycle, sub-cell, *Biochemistry* **1**:311.

MCGUIRE, W. L., HUFF, K., AND CHAMNESS, G. C., 1972, Temperature-dependent binding of estrogen receptor to chromatin, *Biochemistry* **11**:4562.

MEANS, A. R., AND O'MALLEY, B. W., 1972, Mechanism of estrogen action: Early transcriptional and translational events, *Metabolism* **21**:357.

MENDELSON, D., GROSSMAN, A., AND BOCTOR, A., 1971, D-Glucose suppression of tyrosine aminotransferase in rat-hepatoma cells grown in culture, *Eur. J. Biochem.* **24**:140.

MIYAKE, Y., GAYLOR, J. L., AND MORRIS, H. P., 1974, Abnormal microsomal cytochromes and electron transport in Morris hepatomas, *J. Biol. Chem.* **249**:1980.

MOTT, G. E., PITOT, H. C., AND GOLDFARB, S., 1974, Evidence of bile acid synthesis by transplantable hepatomas, *Cancer Res.* **34**:1688.

MOYER, G. H., AND PITOT, H. C., 1973, Protein turnover in microsomal subfractions of liver and Morris hepatomas 7800 and 9618A, *Cancer Res.* **33**:1316.

MUELLER, G. C., 1965, The role of RNA and protein synthesis in estrogen action, in: *Mechanisms of Hormone Action* (P. Karlson, ed.), pp. 228–245, Academic Press, New York.

MURTY, C. N., VERNEY, E., AND SIDRANSKY, H., 1974, Studies of initiation factors in protein synthesis of host liver and transplantable hepatoma, *Cancer Res.* **34**:410.

NORTHUP, S. J., BARTHEL, J. S., BROWN, H. D., CHATTOPADHYAY, S. K., AND MORRIS, H. P., 1972, Guanyl cyclase activity in Morris hepatoma 7787, 7795, 7800 and 9816A-2, *Missouri State Med.* **69**:934.

OKADA, F., 1968, Replicating units (replicons) of DNA in cultured mammalian cells, *Biophys. J.* **8**:650.

O'MALLEY, B. W., 1971, Mechanisms of action of steroid hormones, *New Eng. J. Med.* **284**:370.

ONO, T., POTTER, V. R., PITOT, H. C., AND MORRIS, H. P., 1963, Metabolic adaptations in rat hepatomas. III. Glucose-6-phosphate dehydrogenase and pyrimidine reductases, *Cancer Res.* **23**:385.

OTTEN, J., JOHNSON, G. S., AND PASTAN, I., 1972, Regulation of cell growth by cyclic adenosine 3′,5′-monophosphate—Effect of cell density and agents which alter cell growth on cyclic adenosine 3′,5′-monophosphate levels in fibroblasts, *J. Biol. Chem.* **247**:7082.

PAINTER, R. B., AND SCHAEFFER, A. W., 1969, Rate of synthesis along replicons of different kinds of mammalian cells, *J. Mol. Biol.* **45**:467.

PALMITER, R. D., 1973, Rate of ovalbumin messenger ribonucleic acid synthesis in the oviduct of estrogen-primed chicks, *J. Biol. Chem.* **248**:8260.

PALMITER, R. D., CATLIN, G. H., AND COX, R. F., 1973, Chromatin-associated receptors for estrogen, progesterone, and dihydrotestosterone and the induction of egg white protein synthesis in chick magnum, *Cell Differ.* **2**:163.

PASTAN, I., AND PERLMAN, R., 1970, Cyclic adenosine monophosphate in bacteria, *Science* **169**:339.

PEDERSON, T., 1974, Gene activiation in eukaryotes: Are nuclear acidic proteins the cause or the effect? *Proc. Natl. Acad. Sci. U.S.A.* **71**:617.

PENMAN, S., ROSBASH, M., AND PENMAN, M., 1970, Messenger and heterogenous nuclear RNA in HeLa cells in differential inhibition by cordycepin, *Proc. Natl. Acad. Sci. U.S.A.* **67**:1878.

PERAINO, C., AND PITOT, H. C., 1964, Studies on the induction and repression of enzymes in rat liver, II. Carbohydrate repression of dietary and hormonal induction of threonine dehydrase and ornithine-δ-transaminase, *J. Biol. Chem.*, **239**:4308.

PITOT, H. C., 1963, Substrate and hormonal interactions in the regulation of enzyme levels in rat hepatomas, in: *Advances in Enzyme Regulation*, Vol. I (G. Weber, ed.), pp. 309–319, Pergamon Press, Oxford.

PITOT, H. C., 1964, Altered template stability, the molecular mask of malignancy? *Perspect. Biol. Med.* **8**:50.

PITOT, H. C., 1969, The endoplasmic reticulum and phenotypic variability in normal and neoplastic liver, *A.M.A. Arch. Pathol.* **87**:202.

PITOT, H. C., 1971, The role of intracellular membranes in the regulation of genetic expression, in: *Oncology 1970* (R. L. Clark, ed.), pp. 648–655, Yearbook Medical Publishers, Chicago.

PITOT, H. C., AND MORRIS, H. P., 1961, Metabolic adaptations in rat hepatomas. II. Tryptophan pyrrolase and tyrosine α-ketoglutarate transaminase, *Cancer Res.* **21**:1009.

PITOT, H. C., AND YATVIN, M. B., 1973, Interrelationships of mammalian hormones and enzyme levels in vivo, *Physiol. Rev.* **53**:228.

PITOT, H. C., POTTER, V. R., AND MORRIS, H. P., 1961, Metabolic adaptations in rat hepatomas. I. The effect of dietary protein on some inducible enzymes in liver and hepatoma 5123C, *Cancer Res.* **21**:1001.

PITOT, H. C., PERAINO, C., MORSE, P. A., AND POTTER, V. R., 1963, Hepatomas in tissue culture compared with adapting liver in vivo, *J. Natl. Cancer Inst. Monogr.* **13**:229.

PITOT, H. C., PERAINO, C., LAMAR, C., AND KENNAN, A. L., 1965, Template stability of some enzymes in rat liver and hepatoma, *Proc. Natl. Acad. Sci. U.S.A.* **54**:895.

PITOT, H. C., IWASAKI, Y., INOUE, H., KASPER, C., AND MOHRENWEISER, M., 1972, Regulation of the levels of multiple forms of serine dehydratase and tyrosine aminotransferase in rat tissues, *Gann Monogr.* **13**:191.

PITOT, H. C., SHIRES, T., MOYER, G., AND GARRETT, C. T., 1974, Phenotypic variability as a manifestation of translational control in hepatocellular carcinomas, in: *Molecular Biology of Cancer* (H. Busch, ed.), pp. 523–534, Academic Press, New York.

POTTER, V. R., GEBERT, R. A., PITOT, H. C., PERAINO, C., LAMAR, C., LESHER, S., AND MORRIS, H. P., 1966, Systematic oscillations in metabolic activity in rat and in hepatomas. I. Morris hepatoma No. 7793, *Cancer Res.* **26:**1547.

QUATRECASAS, P., 1974, Hormone–receptor interaction and the plasma membrane, *Hosp. Pract.*, July, p. 73.

RAPIN, A. M. C., AND BURGER, M. N., 1974, Tumor cell surfaces: general alterations detected by agglutinins, *Adv. Cancer Res.* **20:**1.

RASMUSSEN, H., ARNAUD, C., AND HAWKER, C., 1964, Actinomycin D and the response to parathyroid hormone, *Science* **144:**1019.

RECHCIGL, M., 1971a, *Enzyme Synthesis and Degradation in Mammalian Systems*, Karger, New York.

RECHCIGL, M., 1971b, Intracellular protein turnover and the roles of synthesis and degradation in regulation of enzyme levels, in: *Enzyme Synthesis and Degradation in Mammalian Systems* (M. Rechcigl, ed.), pp. 237–310, Karger, New York.

RHOADS, R. E., McKNIGHT, G. S., AND SCHIMKE, R. T., 1973, Quantitative measurement of ovalbumin messenger ribonucleic acid activity, *J. Biol. Chem.* **248:**2031.

ROGERS, L. A., MORRIS, H. P., AND FOUTS, J. R., 1967, The effects of phenobarbital on drug metabolic enzyme activity, *J. Pharmacol Exp. Ther.* **157:**227.

ROSS, M. H., AND BRAS, G., 1965, Tumor incidence patterns and nutrition in the rat, *J. Nutr.* **87:**245.

RUBIN, H., 1972, Inhibition of DNA synthesis in animal cells by ethylene diamine tetraacetate, and its reversal by zinc, *Proc. Natl. Acad. Sci. U.S.A.* **69:**712.

RUTTER, W. J., KEMP, J. D., BRADSHAW, W. S., CLARK, W. R., RONZIO, R. A., AND SANDERS, T. G., 1968, Regulation of specific protein synthesis in cytodifferentiation, *J. Cell. Physiol.* **72:**(Suppl. 1).

SABATINI, D. D., AND BLOBEL, G., 1970, Controlled proteolysis of nascent polypeptides in rat liver cell fractions. II. Location of the polypeptides in rough microsomes, *J. Cell Biol.* **45:**146.

SABATIN, D. D., TASHIRO, Y., AND PALADE, G. E., 1966, On the attachment of ribosomes to microsomal membranes, *J. Mol. Biol.* **19:**503.

SABINE, J. R., ABRAHAM, S., AND CHAIKOFF, I. L., 1966, Lack of feedback control of fatty acid synthesis in a transplantable hepatoma, *Biochim. Biophys. Acta* **116:**407.

SABINE, J. R., ABRAHAM, S., AND CHAIKOFF, I. L., 1967, Control of lipid metabolism in hepatomas: Insensitivity of rate of fatty acid and cholesterol synthesis by mouse hepatoma BW7756 to fasting and to feedback control, *Cancer Res.* **27:**793.

SABINE, J. R., ABRAHAM, S., AND MORRIS, H. P., 1968, Defective dietary control of fatty acid metabolism in four transplantable rat hepatomas: Numbers 5123C, 7793, 7795, and 7800, *Cancer Res.* **28:**46.

SARMA, D. S. R., REID, I. M., AND SIDRANSKY, H., 1969, The selective effect of actinomycin D on free polyribosomes of mouse liver, *Biochim. Biophys. Res. Commun.* **36:**582.

SATO, S., MATSUSHIMA, T., AND SUGIMURA, T., 1969, Hexokinase isozyme patterns of experimental hepatomas of rats, *Cancer Res.* **29:**1437.

SAUNDERS, G. F., SHIRAKAWA, S., SAUNDERS, P. P., ARRIGHI, F. E., AND HUS, T. C., 1972, Populations of repeated DNA sequences in the human genome, *J. Mol. Biol.* **63:**323.

SCHAPIRA, F., 1970, Isozymes et cancer, *Pathol.-Biol.* **18:**309.

SCHIMKE, R. T., SWEENEY, E. W., AND BERLIN, C. M., 1965, The roles of synthesis and degradation in the control of rat liver tryptophan pyrrolase, *J. Biol. Chem.* **240:**322.

SCHORR, I., HINSHAW, H. T., COOPER, M. A., MAHAFFEE, D. AND NEY, R. L., 1972, Adenyl cyclase hormone responses of certain human endocrine tumors, *J. Clin. Endocr.* **34:**447.

SCHULTZ, G. A., 1974, The stability of messenger RNA containing polyadenylic acid sequences in rabbit blastocysts, *Exp. Cell Res.* **86:**190.

SCHUMM, D. E., AND WEBB, T. E., 1974, Modified messenger ribonucleic acid release from isolated hepatic nuclei after inhibition of polyadenylate formation, *Biochem. J.* **139:**191.

SCHUMM, D. E., McNAMARA, D. J., AND WEBB, T. E., 1973, Cytoplasmic proteins regulating messenger RNA release from nuclei, *Nature New Biol.* **245:**201.

SEED, R. W., AND GOLDBERG, I. H., 1963, Biosynthesis of thyroglobulin: Relationship to RNA-template and precursor protein, *Proc. Natl. Acad. Sci. U.S.A.* **50:**275.

SELLERS, L., AND GRANNER, D., 1974, Regulation of tyrosine aminotransferase activity in two liver-derived permanent cell lines, *J. Cell Biol.* **16:**337.

SHARMA, R. K., AND BRUSH, J. S., 1974, Metabolic regulation of steroidogenesis in adrenal cortico carcinoma cells of the rat: Effect of adrenocorticotropin and adenosine cyclic 3′,5′-monophosphate on the incorporation of (20S)-20 hydroxy (7α-^{3}H) cholesterol into deoxycorticosterone and corticosterone, *Biochem. Biophys. Res. Commun.* **56**:256.

SHEPPARD, J. R., 1972, Difference in the cyclic adenosine 3′ 5′ monophosphate levels in normal and transformed cell, *Nature New Biol.* **236**:14.

SHIRES, T. K., PITOT, H. C., AND KAUFFMAN, F. A., 1974, The membron: A functional hypothesis for the translational regulation of genetic expression, in *Biomembranes*, Vol. 5 (L. A. Manson, ed.), pp. 81–145, Plenum Press, New York.

SHUSTER, L., AND JICK, H., 1966, The turnover of microsomal proteins in the livers of phenobarbital-treated mice, *J. Biol. Chem.* **241**:5361.

SINGER, R. H., AND PENMAN, S. 1972, Stability of HeLa cell mRNA in actinomycin, *Nature (London)* **240**:100.

SIPERSTEIN, M. D., AND FAGAN, V. M., 1964, Deletion of the cholesterol-negative feedback system in liver tumors, *Cancer Res.* **24**:1108.

SIPERSTEIN, M. D., AND LUBY, L. J., 1969, in: *Fish in Research* (O. W. Neuhaus and J. E. Halver, eds.), pp. 87–102, Academic Press, New York.

SIPERSTEIN, M. D., FAGAN, V. M., AND MORRIS, H. P., 1966, Further studies on the deletion of the cholesterol feedback system in hepatomas, *Cancer Res.* **26**:7.

SIPERSTEIN, M. D., GUDE, A. M., AND MORRIS, H. P., 1971, Loss of feedback control of hydroxymethyl-glutaryl co-enzyme A reductase in hepatomas, *Proc. Natl. Acad. Sci. U.S.A.* **86**:315.

SMITH, S. J., JACOB, S. T., LIU, D. K., DUCEMAN, P., AND VESELL, E. S., 1974, Further studies on post-transcriptional stabilization of ribosomal precursor ribonucleic acid by phenobarbital, *Mol. Pharmacol.* **10**:248.

SOLING, H. D., KAPLAN, J., ERBSTOESSER, M., AND PITOT, H. C., 1969, The role of hormones in glucose repression in rat liver, in: *Advances in Enzyme Regulation*, Vol. 7 (G. Weber, ed.), pp. 171–182, Pergamon Press, New York.

SPIRIN, A. S., 1969, Informosomes, *Eur. J. Biochem.* **10**:20.

SPORN, M. B., AND DINGMAN, C. W., 1966, Studies on chromatin. II. Effects of carcinogens and hormones on rat liver chromatin, *Cancer Res.* **26**:2488.

STANCEL, G. M., LEUNG, K. M. T., AND GORSKI, J., 1973, Estrogen receptors in the rat uterus: Relationship between cytoplasmic and nuclear forms of the estrogen binding proteins, *Biochemistry* **12**:2137.

STEIN, G. S., SPELSBERG, T. C. AND KLEINSMITH, L. J., 1974, Nonhistone chromosomal proteins and gene regulation, *Science* **183**:817.

STEWART, G. A., AND FARBER, E., 1967, Reformation of functional liver polyribosomes from ribosome monomers in the absence of RNA synthesis, *Science* **157**:67.

SUDILOVSKY, O., PESTANA, A., HINDERAKER, P. M., AND PITOT, H. C., 1971, Cyclic adenosine 3′,5′-monophosphate levels during glucose repression in rat liver, *Science* **174**:142.

SUGIMURA, T., IKEDA, K., HIROTA, K., HOZUMI, M., AND MORRIS, H. P., 1966, Chemical, enzymatic and cytochrome assays of microsomal fraction of hepatomas of different growth rates, *Cancer Res.* **26**:1711.

SUGINO, A., AND OKAZAKI, R., 1973, RNA-linked DNA fragments *in vitro*, *Proc. Natl. Acad. Sci. U.S.A.* **70**:88.

TASCA, R. J., AND HILLMAN, N., 1970, Effects of actinomycin D and cycloheximide on RNA and protein synthesis in cleavage stage mouse embryos, *Nature (London)* **225**:1022.

TATA, J. R., 1969, The action of thyroid hormones, *Gen. Comp. Endocrinol. Suppl.* **2**:385.

TATA, J. R., ERNSTER, L., LINDBERG, O., ARRHENIUS, E., PEDERSEN, S., AND HEDMAN, R., 1963, The action of thyroid hormones at the cell level, *Biochem. J.* **86**:408.

TAYLOR, C. B., AND GOULD, R. G., 1950, Effect of dietary cholesterol on rate of cholesterol synthesis in the intact animal measured by means of radioactive carbon, *Circulation* **2**:467.

TAYLOR, J. H., 1973, Replication of DNA in mammalian chromosomes: Isolation of replicating segments, *Proc. Natl. Acad. Sci. U.S.A.* **70**:1083.

TEEL, R. W., AND HALL, R. G., 1973, Effect of dibutyryl cyclic AMP on the restoration of contact inhibition in tumor cells and its relationship to cell density and the cell cycle, *Exp. Cell Res.* **76**:390.

TERMAN, S. A., 1970, Relative effect of transcription-level and translation-level control of protein synthesis during early development of the sea urchin, *Proc. Natl. Acad. Sci. U.S.A.* **65**:985.

THOMPSON, E. D., TOMPKINS, G. M., AND CURRAN, J. F., 1966, Induction of tyrosine α-ketoglutarate transaminase by steroid hormones in a newly established tissue culture cell line, *Proc. Natl. Acad. Sci. U.S.A.* **56**:296.

TILGHMAN, F. M., HANSON, R. W., RESHEF, L., HOPGOOD, M. F., AND BALLARD, F. J., 1974, Rapid loss of translatable messenger RNA of phosphoenolpyruvate carboxykinase during glucose repression in liver, *Proc. Natl. Acad. Sci. U.S.A.* **71**:1304.

TREADOW, B. R., AND KHAIRALLAH, E. A., 1972, Regulation of phosphoenolpyruvate carboxykinase during starvation and glucose repression, *Nature New Biol.* **239**:131.

TROTTER, N. L., 1961, The effect of partial hepatectomy on subcutaneously transplanted hepatomas in mice, *Cancer Res.* **21**:778.

TRYFIATES, G. P., SHULER, J. K., HEFNER, M. H., AND MORRIS, H. P., 1974, Effect of B₆ deficiency on hepatoma 7794A growth rate: Activities of tyrosine transaminase and serine dehydratase before and after induction by hydrocortisone, *Eur. J. Cancer* **10**:147.

UENOYAMA, K., AND ONO, T., 1973, Post-transcriptional regulation of catalase synthesis in rat liver and hepatoma: Factors activating and inhibiting catalase synthesis, *J. Mol. Biol.* **74**:439.

VAN DER MEULEN, N., ABRAHAM, A. D., AND SEKERIS, C. E., 1972, Role of the nuclear cortisol binding protein in the control of transcription of thymocyte nuclei by cortison, *FEBS Letters* **25**:116.

VARANDANI, P. T., SHROYER, L. A., AND NASZ, M. A., 1972, Sequential degradation of insulin by rat liver homogenates, *Proc. Natl. Acad. Sci. U.S.A.* **69**:1681.

VENKATESAN, N., ARCOS, J. C., AND ARGUS, M. F., 1970, Amino acid induction and carbohydrate repression of dimethylnitrosamine demethylase in rat liver, *Cancer Res.* **30**:2563.

WATANABE, M., POTTER, V. R., AND MORRIS, H. P., 1970, Benzpyrene hydroxylase activity and its induction by methylcholanthrene in Morris hepatomas in host livers, in adult livers and in rat liver during development, *Cancer Res.* **30**:263.

WATSON, J. A., 1973, Cholesterol metabolism in HTC cells, in: *Tumor Lipids* (R. Wood, ed.), pp. 34–53, American Oil Chemist's Society Press.

WIENHOUSE, S., 1973, Isozyme patterns of hepatomas and tumor progression, *Neoplasma* **20**:559.

WEINHOUSE, S., AND ONO, T., 1972, *Isozymes and Enzyme Regulation in Cancer*, Gann Monograph, Vol. 13, University of Tokyo Press, Tokyo.

WEINHOUSE, S., LANGAN, J., AND SHATTON, J. A., 1973, Fatty acids as metabolic fuels of cancer cells, in: *Tumor Lipids* (R. Wood, ed.), pp. 14–20, American Oil Chemist's Society Press.

WHITLOCK, J. P., KAURMAN, R., AND BASERGA, R., 1968, Changes in thymidine kinase and α-amylase activity during isoproternenol-stimulated DNA synthesis in mouse salivary gland, *Cancer Res.* **28**:2211.

WILLIAMS, D. J., AND RABIN, B. R., 1969, The effects of aflatoxin B₁ and steroid hormones on polysome binding to microsomal membranes as measured by the activity of an enzyme catalysing disulphide interchange, *FEBS Letters* **4**:103.

WILLINGHAM, M. E., AND PASTAN, I., 1974, Cyclic AMP mediates the concanavalin A agglutinability of mouse fibroblasts, *J. Cell Biol.* **63**:288.

WILSON, J. D., 1972, The role of bile acids in the overall regulation of steroid metabolism, *Arch Int. Med.* **130**:493.

WILSON, S. H., AND HOAGLAND, M. B., 1967, Physiology of rat-liver polysomes—The stability of messenger ribonucleic acid and ribosomes, *Biochem. J.* **103**:556.

WILSON, S. H., HILL, H. Z., AND HOAGLAND, M. B., 1967, Physiology of rat-liver polysomes: Protein synthesis by stable polysomes, *Biochem. J.* **103**:567.

WISE, G. E., AND PRESCOTT, D. M., 1973, Initiation and continuation of DNA replication are not associated with the nuclear envelope in mammalian cells, *Proc. Natl. Acad. Sci. U.S.A.* **70**:714.

WOOL, I. G., AND MUNRO, A. J., 1963, An influence of insulin on the synthesis of a rapidly labeled RNA by isolated rat diaphragm, *Proc. Natl. Acad. Sci. U.S.A.* **450**:918.

WU, C., AND MORRIS, H. P., 1970, Responsiveness of glutamine-metabolizing enzymes in Morris hepatomas to metabolic modulations, *Cancer Res.* **30**:2675.

WU, C., BAUER, J. M., AND MORRIS, H. P., 1971, Responsiveness of two urea cycle enzymes in Morris hepatomas to metabolic modulations, *Cancer Res.* **31**:12.

WU, F. C., ELGIN, F. C. R., AND HOOD, L. E., 1973, Non-histone chromosomal proteins of rat tissues: A comparative study by gel electrophoresis, *Biochemistry* **12**:2792.

YAMADA, M., AND HANAOKA, F., 1973, Periodic changes in the association of mammalian DNA with the membrane during the cell cycle, *Nature New Biol.* **243:**227.

YAMAMOTO, K. R., AND ALBERTS, B. M., 1972, *In vitro* conversion of estradiol-receptor protein to its nuclear form: dependence on hormone and DNA, *Proc. Natl. Acad. Sci. U.S.A.* **69:**2105.

ZUCKERMAN, N. H., NARDELLA, P., MORRIS, H. P., AND ELWOOD, H. C., 1970, Lack of adaptation in lipogenesis by hepatomas 9098, 7794A and 9618A, *J. Natl. Cancer Inst.* **44:**79.

7

Genetics of Tumor Cells

SANDRA R. WOLMAN AND ALLAN A. HORLAND

1. Introduction: Structural Genetic Change as a Basis for Malignancy

The attributes of cell behavior and morphology which are recognizable as "cancer" are transmissible from a cell to its progeny. The set of alterations in a particular tumor cell is, in general, permanent and stable and inherited by the descendants of that tumor cell. For these reasons, it is appropriate to think that a change in the form or content of the cell's genetic material is responsible for the change to a malignant state. The permanence and transmissibility of cancer cell characteristics are best explained by structural alteration of the DNA in genes or chromosomes.

The DNA and chromosomes of tumor cells are often demonstrably different from those of normal cells. However, the changes are not uniform from tumor to tumor and there are many instances where no presently detectable abnormality in the genetic material is evident within tumor cells. Genetic changes could be necessary and intrinsic in tumor development or, alternatively, frequent but nonnecessary concomitants of tumor generation. Even if genetic change is not necessary in the etiology of cancer, questions still arise as to the role of genetic alteration in tumor evolution.

The conditions we define as genetic structural changes range from single-gene mutations to gross chromosomal alterations. Single-gene mutations include base substitutions resulting in either missense or nonsense mutants. Base-pair losses or gains can lead to a number of types of mutations including frameshifts, deletions, and duplications. The insertion of foreign genes into the host cell chromosome in viral transformation constitutes a larger structural change. Gross mutations include losses and gains of chromosomes, rearrangements and translocations of

SANDRA R. WOLMAN and ALLAN A. HORLAND • Department of Pathology, New York University, School of Medicine, New York, N.Y. Supported in part by PHS Grant CA 13821.

chromosomal material, and changes in ploidy. Point mutations which result in numerical instability (dysjunctional errors) or loss of morphological integrity of chromosomes (increased breakage and recombination) could be an important source of these larger mutations.

The possibility is raised frequently that interaction of an exogenous agent with a specific protein or RNA, or with a specific intracellular membrane or organelle, could result in a permanent change in gene expression. Such regulation of the manifestation of genetic potential is called "epigenetic" and is exemplified by differentiation. During the development of an organism, the differentiation of morphology and function of individual cells is not accompanied by alteration in their nucleic acids or chromosomes. In our discussion of the development of cancer, epigenetic alterations which induce functional changes in gene activity will not be considered as genetic alterations.

In this chapter, we will review some theories of tumor pathogenesis in terms of their implicit or explicit dependence on genetic alteration. Both spontaneous and inducible experimental malignancies provide examples against which theories can be evaluated. Methods for examining DNA and gene products will be discussed briefly with some pertinent results of comparisons between normal and tumor cells. The use of tissue culture systems as models for tumorigenesis will be considered, as will problems of cellular expression of genetic information. We will concentrate on the conflicts in interpretation of the role of cytogenetic alteration in tumor cells. Finally, we will attempt to integrate many of the observations into a cohesive pattern which shows that tumor development is dependent on structural alteration of genetic information.

2. Tumor Pathogenesis

2.1. Somatic Mutation

The thesis that a single chromosomal or genic mutational event is the specific change responsible for tumorigenesis has become known as the "somatic mutation theory." It fixes the basis for both initiation and propagation of cancer cell behavior in the molecular organization of the genome. Therefore, in a single step it accounts for the heritability and permanence of the malignant change. Von Hansemann (1890) and Boveri were among the first to suggest that an abnormal chromatin complex was a significant characteristic of malignant cells. In 1902, Boveri reported that abnormal cells arose from normal sea urchin eggs by abnormal cell division. He postulated that cancer cells could arise similarly from normal cells. The resultant altered "chromatin complex" would be sufficiently abnormal to derange the cell's behavior without interfering with its ability to replicate or to transmit the abnormality to its progeny. Boveri (1914) perceived this abnormality to be responsible for continued multiplication of tumor cells and clearly thought of it as a single step: "the abnormal mitosis which starts a tumor."

However, a single-step hypothesis is inadequate to explain many of the observations on human and experimental animal malignancies. There is usually a

prolonged delay between the "insult," when it can be identified, and the
appearance of tumors. Often, in animals treated with chemical carcinogens, repeated application or exposure to two or more different types of injury is required for production of tumors. MacKenzie and Rous (1941) described two stages in the development of coal-tar tumors in rabbits; tumors appeared after wounding of the carcinogen-treated skin. Similar observations led Berenblum (1954) to propose a two-step model consisting of "initiation" and "promotion" to explain the events necessary in malignant change. The first step, initiation, is a "specific, sudden, irreversible change in a normal cell" brought about by a carcinogen, which clearly could be interpreted as mutational. The second or promoting step is slower, less specific, and probably reversible and induces proliferation and possibly delayed maturation of the altered "initiated" cell.

Other investigators (Farber, 1972; Boutwell, 1974) have found it necessary to postulate more than two steps in tumorigenesis. Farber recently proposed a multistep sequence from the normal to the malignant cell in which initiation is followed by a second, genetically altered, proliferative state. In his experiments on chemical induction of malignant liver tumors, visible intermediate hyperplastic stages were identified. The hyperplastic hepatic nodules which developed after carcinogen ingestion contained damaged DNA. Thus there was evidence for mutation at a proliferative, nonmalignant stage. Farber suggested that further changes lead to a third stage of abnormal proliferation which is reversible in some experimental systems. Therefore, a final step in the sequence is that which results in irreversible cancer. This theory implies that genetic change is necessary but not sufficient for tumorigenesis.

Another essential aspect of Boveri's theory is that since much of the genetic information of the cell could be unaltered by the "tumor" mutations, specialized functions of the somatic cell from which it arose could still be expressed. The potentially infinite variability which could be generated among tumor cells is seen in the wide variety of observed phenotypes, some of which are highly differentiated and accumulate or secrete special cell products. In fact, enough of the genetic information is usually preserved so that the pathological basis for identification of a tumor depends on its morphological (and sometimes biochemical) resemblance to the tissue of origin.

It is not surprising that Boveri's theory has not been able to accommodate the complete range of phenomena discovered since it first appeared. His concept of somatic mutation is insufficient to account for many of the observations but nevertheless provides a basis for more comprehensive theories of cancer. DNA alteration as an efficient means for preserving and perpetuating new information remains the most logical mechanism for initiation of cancer.

2.2. Other Models Based on Mutation

In considering the relation of mutation to tumorigenesis, the small group of human tumors which are clearly genetically determined and inherited, such as polyposis of the colon or retinoblastoma, are an important source of information.

Knudson (Vol. 1) suggests that in these tumor syndromes the first step is an inherited (germinal) mutation which is therefore present in all cells of the individual. The second step in an afflicted individual is a somatic mutation that occurs with a frequency dependent on the spontaneous mutation rate [which for some deleterious human genes is of the order of 1 in 100,000 per organism generation (Neel, 1972) and is estimated for all types of mutation to be approximately 1 in a million per cell generation (Ohno, 1969)]. For example, considering the number of cells available in the retina, the development of a tumor is highly probable in an individual carrying the gene for retinoblastoma.

If the double-mutation model is valid for all tumors, then the development of a noninherited tumor would depend on the occurrence of two somatic mutations in the same cell. The incidence of sequential or cumulative mutations per cell is expected to increase with age, which is consistent with the increasing incidence of malignancy in human populations with age. Inherited tumors in man are characterized by early age of onset and multiplicity (Knudson, 1973). By contrast, the frequency of noninherited tumors is low enough so that multiple primary tumors in a given individual are rare.

Observations from another group of human disease syndromes may also have a bearing on the relationship of structural genetic changes to cancer. These autosomal recessive syndromes, Fanconi's anemia, Bloom's syndrome, xeroderma pigmentosum, and ataxia-telangiectasia, constitute a diverse set of diseases whose clinical symptoms include anemias, skeletal structural defects, skin disorders, and immune deficiency. One common feature of these syndromes is chromosomal instability (German, 1972, 1973). The chromosomes of cells from individuals with these diseases show evidence of increased breakage and recombination (Swift and Hirschhorn, 1966; German et al., 1970; Hecht et al., 1966; Sawitsky et al., 1966) (Fig. 1). In addition, in xeroderma pigmentosum and Fanconi's anemia there is evidence of defective DNA repair (Setlow et al., 1969; Poon et al., 1974). These patients almost invariably die from a malignancy in their second or third decade, if they survive the direct effects of the syndrome in infancy and childhood. If the in vitro observations of chromosome breakage and rearrangement are representative of cell divisions in vivo, then we must assume that innumerable mutational events occur throughout the life span of such patients. The initial mutation results in a highly variable population of cells from which new genetic combinations advantageous to the development of tumors may be selected.

The increased incidence of malignant disease with age should be examined in the context of a recently developed model for aging. Lemone Yielding (1974) has suggested that, with time, mutations accumulate preferentially in the "inactive" portions of the genome. If repair were possible only during limited periods of the cell cycle—i.e., during DNA replication—then errors would collect preferentially in cells with highly differentiated functions and infrequent cell divisions. An important but unsubstantiated assumption in this theory is that many of the regulatory genes for chromosome condensation, stimulus to cell division, and control of the mitotic apparatus are located in the inactive regions of the genome.

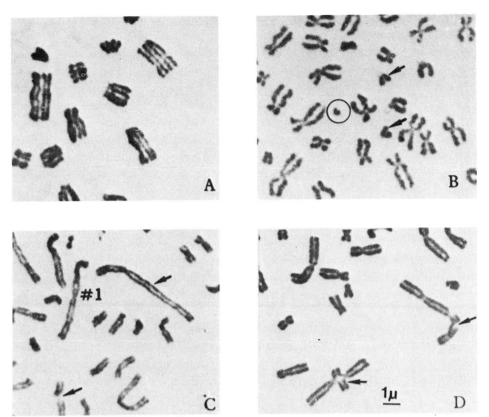

FIGURE 1. Portions taken from four metaphase spreads following 72-h lymphocyte culture of blood from a 6-yr-old male with Fanconi's anemia, showing various chromosomal abnormalities. (A) Endoreduplication with 46 *pairs* of chromosomes. (B) A deleted G-group chromosome (circled) resembling the Ph' (Philadelphia) chromosome. Arrows indicate two normal-sized G chromosomes. (C) A long "marker" chromosome (arrow) with one of the No. 1 chromosomes indicated for comparison. A pericentric break is also present (arrow). (D) Additional examples of breakage (arrows) and recombination resulting in a complex interchange. Reprinted from Pochedly, C., Collipp, P. J., Wolman, S. R., Suwansirikul, S., and Rezvani, I., 1971, Fanconi's anemia with growth hormone deficiency *J. Pediat. 79*:93–96.

The expected result of this model for aging is that a population of cells would accumulate damaged DNA due to differential repair, and this would result in decreased or lost mitotic efficiency. However, the same events which result in aging and cell death for most of a population could produce alterations leading toward a malignant state for a few cells. The occasional mutation which results in loss of a regulator gene that acts as a constraint on cell division would confer a relative proliferative advantage on the cell containing the mutation.

There is chromosomal evidence from human populations that mitotic efficiency decreases with age. Older individuals show a marked increase in aneuploid cells in lymphocyte cultures, usually in the form of loss of the second sex chromosome (Jacobs *et al.*, 1963). Phase III, the declining phase of cell growth in human fibroblast culture, has been equated with aging (Hayflick, 1965) and is also associated with increased chromosomal aberrations, both numerical and structural (Saksela and Moorhead, 1963; Yoshida and Makino, 1963). These aging cultures are also far more rapidly transformed by an oncogenic virus than are cultures in the rapidly dividing logarithmic growth phase (Todaro *et al.*, 1963*a*). There is some evidence that aging cultures show decreased ability to repair damaged DNA (Hart and Setlow, 1974). More important, experiments with various forms of irradiation have shown exact correspondence between shortening of the life span and induction of chromosome aberrations (Curtis and Crowley, 1963). Thus there is evidence for decreased mitotic efficiency and cumulative increase in at least one form of mutation (chromosome aberration) in aging cells, either of which may increase susceptibility to, or be a prerequisite for, the next step in neoplastic transformation.

The models of tumor generation we have discussed are etiological primarily at the level of the individual cells. The probability of, if not the requirement for, structural genetic change is explicit in at least one of the steps. Additional steps involving tumor-discarding or protective mechanisms such as immune surveillance are considered in Farber's (1972) Knudson's (Vol. 1) models. However, the ability to respond with immune defenses or to metabolize exogenous agents depends to some extent on the genetic constitution of the host. The responsible gene loci, like any others, are also subject to structural alteration. The complex relationship of mutation with the development of tumors is evident not only at the cellular level but also in terms of the whole organism.

2.3. Differentiation

An alternative model of tumor pathogenesis, which does not appear to depend on somatic mutation, opposes cellular differentiation to the development of malignancy. Differentiation, the expression of specialized characteristics or metabolic activity, is often accompanied by slowing or cessation of cell division in a tissue. Some degree of loss of differentiated function is characteristic of malignant cells. In many tumors, loss of differentiation is so extreme that it is impossible to distinguish the cell or tissue of origin on morphological grounds. An actively dividing cell with a short life cycle will have relatively less time for production of specialized metabolities, if it is assumed that such production does not occur during DNA synthesis and mitosis (Grobstein, 1959). This assumption has been supported by experiments *in vitro* showing increased collagen synthesis in stationary (nondividing) fibroblasts (Goldberg and Green, 1964) and central nervous system (CNS) protein production accompanying cessation of cell proliferation (Pfeiffer *et al.*, 1970). However, many counter examples can be cited. The work of Manner (1971) and Priest and Davies (1969) indicates that collagen synthesis occurs more rapidly in proliferating than in stationary cells. A positive correlation between cell proliferation and protein production has also been demonstrated with albumin synthesis by rat hepatoma cells (Ohanian *et al.*, 1969) and with elaboration of globulins by plasmacyte tumors (Byars and Kidson, 1970;

Cowan and Milstein, 1972). No correlation, either positive or negative, is found in the evidence of constant steroid synthesis during both logarithmic and stationary phases of cell growth (Yasumura *et al.*, 1966). It is therefore clear that the expression of differentiated function coexists in many situations with rapid cell division.

Tumor cells express alteration or loss of normal gene products but, with the exception of some viral and transplantation antigens (Klein *et al.*, 1960), have not demonstrated acquisition of new genetic information. Surface antigens such as carcinoembryonic antigen, and proteins such as α-fetoprotein, or the Regan isozyme, a fetal form of alkaline phosphatase, are elaborated by some tumors but are also found in undifferentiated, normal fetal cells. Not only in specific cell products but also in some aspects of behavior, malignant cells show resemblance to undifferentiated or fetal cells. The prime characteristic of tumor cells, invasion, is normal cellular behavior at certain times in development. The invasion of primitive germ cells into mesodermal ridges and other aspects of fetal development, the growth of the placenta, and even the behavior of mature inflammatory cells could all be characterized as invasive. These observations support an interpretation that malignancy corresponds to lack of differentiation.

If differentiation and neoplasia are truly opposing processes, then induction of differentiation should reverse the growth of tumors. Experimental support for this point of view is discussed in detail in Chapter 1 of this volume. Further examples drawn from work with hybridized cells in tissue culture will be discussed later in this chapter. The underlying implication of the differentiation theory is that the vital change in tumor cells is not in the basic genetic information but in the control of expression of this information and that the change is therefore epigenetic (Markert, 1968) and potentially reversible (Pierce, 1967; Braun, 1969). Reversibility of tumor expression has been associated with altered differentiation in experiments with "flat" revertants of virus-transformed cells (Pollack *et al.*, 1970), with malignant melanoma cells treated with 5-bromodeoxyuridine (Silagi and Bruce, 1970), and with hybrid cells (Harris *et al.*, 1969). These experiments could also support the interpretation that, with appropriate selective influences, genetically altered malignant cells might be removed from a cell population, leaving only reverse mutants or nonpropagating cells.

2.4. Experimental Models: Chemical, Viral, and Irradiation

The theories of cancer causation which have been advanced draw from observations on both spontaneous and experimental malignancies. Investigations in cancer research extend from epidemiological studies on the relationship of hot tea drinking to esophageal tumors (Brunning, 1974) to artificial experimental models for demonstration of the mutagenicity of many chemical compounds (Ames, 1972). In the former, an identifiable environmental variable is considered in relation to a specific type of cancer in a natural population. The latter is illustrated by a system in which man-made chemicals are mixed with mammalian liver enzymes and effects are measured in terms of the behavior of bacterial cultures—hardly a "natural" system. Nevertheless, the questions asked in a controlled, although artificial, system may be simpler and the answers more precise. Experimental systems based on known carcinogenic agents may reveal common modes of action or points of attack within the cell by these agents which will help to answer our questions about a genetic basis for malignancy.

Thus experiments with chemical carcinogens provide an invaluable tool for investigation of tumors. In some cases, a single dose of such a compound is capable of eliciting tumor formation (Huggins and Fukunishi, 1963). Many systems, both *in vivo* and *in vitro*, are being used to examine the earliest events in the interaction between a carcinogen and a host cell and to separate and to identify the subsequent steps in cellular alterations.

Many of the known chemical carcinogens are potential mutagens. The mutagenicity of these chemical compounds has been amply demonstrated in bacterial, yeast, and, more recently, a variety of mammalian systems (Miller and Miller, 1971). The basic similarity of DNA from all species appears to justify the extrapolation that mutagens in lower organisms should be regarded as potentially dangerous to man (Drake and Flamm, 1972). The types of assay range from elegant to relatively insensitive—from the demonstration of frameshift mutations in bacteria to the detection of chromosome aberrations in treated mammalian cells. However, within some series of closely related chemicals, such as the acridines, mutagenesis and carcinogenesis correlate poorly (Dulbecco, 1964; Burdette, 1955). Furthermore, a few potent mutagens (such as nitrogen mustard) apparently are not carcinogenic in experimental animals (Van Duuren and Sivak, 1968; Van Duuren, 1969). Many carcinogens are highly reactive chemicals which would be expected to react with many macromolecules within the cell, including proteins and RNA as well as DNA. Most of the reactions are probably irrelevant to the process of carcinogenesis.

When lack of correlation between carcinogenicity and mutagenicity is observed, it probably depends on differences in metabolism, electrophilic reactivity, or permeability of the chemical between the two test systems. In some experiments, a poor understanding of the chemical nature of the active or "ultimate" form of the carcinogen is responsible for discrepancies which a host-mediated assay can resolve (Legator and Malling, 1971). Further, the genetic variability of host cells in their capacity to generate or metabolize and degrade the carcinogen could give misleading results. A clinical example illustrating this type of variability is the connection demonstrated recently between aryl hydrocarbon hydroxylase (AHH) inducibility and lung cancer (Kellermann *et al.*, 1973). AHH is an enzyme which metabolizes aromatic hydrocarbons found in cigarette smoke; genetic variability divides people into three classes of high, intermediate, and low inducibility of the enzyme. Cells from lung cancer patients were found to have higher inducibility than those from control patient populations. Almost every chemical carcinogen can be shown to act as a mutational agent in some biological system, and, conversely, many mutagens are now assumed to be potential carcinogens. A defect in this assumption is that many mutagens are clearly not carcinogens (Berenblum, 1972). Nevertheless, mutagenic modification provides the most succinct explanation for preservation of necessary information during the prolonged period between application of a carcinogen and appearance of a tumor (Farber, 1972).

Certain viruses are regularly associated with and responsible for the development of malignant tumors. Systems of viral oncogenesis (some of which are discussed in detail in previous volumes) should be examined to determine whether a structural change in the genome is a crucial component in tumor induction. If an oncogenic DNA virus is integrated into the host genome and replicates with it, the virus constitutes, of itself, a structural genetic alteration. Acquisition of new viral genes and disruption of sequence within the host genome are implied. In addition, there may be other host cell alterations (mutations?) or genetic preconditions before the virus is permitted to enter the cell, or to break and enter the DNA chain. Huebner *et al.* (1963) demonstrated that virus-specific tumor antigens (T antigens) are present in host cells infected with an oncogenic DNA virus, polyoma or SV40. The demonstration of these antigens was the earliest proof that a portion of the viral genome is present in the host cell, is transmitted regularly at cell division, and is directing synthesis of a gene product. Westphal and Dulbecco (1968) used techniques of nucleic acid hybridization to demonstrate the presence of multiple copies of SV40 DNA within the host cell genome.

There is evidence that not only DNA viruses but also RNA viruses are carried in the chromosomes of the host cell. The murine leukemia viruses (MuLV) are located in the chromosome and there is Mendelian segregation of virus and antigens with cell division (Rowe, 1973). RNA-dependent DNA polymerase (reverse transcriptase) provides a mechanism by which information from RNA tumor viruses can be transcribed and carried in the host cell DNA.

Once present, an oncogenic virus may act by rearranging, activating, or damaging host cell genes in order to effect the transformation to a tumor cell. Many viruses are chromosome-breaking agents both *in vivo* and *in vitro*, although the damage inflicted by infectious viruses such as measles (Nichols, 1963), chicken pox (Aula, 1963) and herpes (Hampar and Ellison, 1961) has not been related to either transformation or tumorigenesis. Several of the oncogenic viruses induce rapid sequential alterations in the number and morphology of chromosomes of infected cells (Vogt and Dulbecco, 1963; Wolman *et al.*, 1964; Moorhead and Saksela, 1965). After infection with SV40, some cells go through more than one cycle of DNA replication without mitosis, resulting in polyploidy (Hirai *et al.*, 1974). However, the relationship between virus infection, chromosome damage, and oncogenesis is unclear. Experiments with adenovirus have indicated that chromosome damage is affected to a comparable extent by tumorigenic and nontumorigenic strains of the same virus (Stich, 1973). Some tumors resulting from oncogenic virus infection are karyotypically normal; these include Rous sarcoma virus tumors (Nichols, 1963, 1966), polyoma tumors (Hellström *et al.*, 1963), and mouse mammary tumors (Tjio and Ostergren, 1958).

Other physical and chemical agents have been associated with carcinogenesis, and many are amenable to the development of experimental models. One of the oldest and best known is ionizing radiation. Malignancy associated with the handling of radioactive materials can be documented as far back as the sixteenth century, with Pierre Curie representing one of the first examples in modern times. Examples of malignancy related to radiation exposure can be drawn from epidemiological studies of populations exposed to atomic bomb explosions (Lewis, 1957; National Academy of Sciences, 1956) and rates of cancer among radium-dial workers (Martland, 1931) and radiologists (March, 1961). The incidence of malignancy in uranium and other radioactive-mineral miners (Wanebo *et al.*, 1968) and many others exposed to industrial radiation hazards remains a serious concern, especially with increases in the use of nuclear sources of power.

A number of animal models have been developed to study situations analogous to accidental radiation exposure to humans. Radiation-induced leukemias in mice (Furth and Furth, 1936), lung tumors in baboons following inhalation of plutonium oxide (Metivier *et al.*, 1972), and bone tumors in dogs fed strontium-90 (Pool *et al.*, 1973) are all lesions which closely approximate those seen in radiation-exposed human populations.

One direct result of irradiation is chromosome damage, with breakage, rearrangement, and interference with mitotic separation. The degree of chromosome damage is proportional to the dose of radiation received. Muller (1928) pointed out that X-ray treatments cause both chromosome aberrations and gene mutations; later, a linear relationship was demonstrated between the two forms of mutation (Caldecott, 1961). Chromosome damage is now used as a basis for the assessment of radiation exposure (Dolphin and Lloyd, 1974). In summary, radiation, like the chemical and viral carcinogens, has been shown to interact with and alter the DNA of exposed cells.

3. Approaches to Study of the Genetic Material of Tumor Cells

If structural genetic change is a basis for malignancy, then we should expect to find tangible and measurable alterations in the DNA of tumor cells. Physical and chemical techniques are available for the direct examination of DNA. Malignant cells are characterized by altered expression of genetic information; therefore, we can also examine the genome indirectly by looking at gene products. Many methods depend on the availability of single cells or uniform populations of cells which can be manipulated. Therefore, techniques of tissue culture and cell hybridization are valuable in the study of cell genetics. Finally, there is a vast amount of data on the visible alterations of DNA in the chromosomes of tumor cells, which will be discussed in Section 4.

3.1. Direct Analysis of DNA

DNA may be examined directly by a combination of physical and chemical methods. Several basic steps are usually involved (Brookes and Lawley, 1971).

First, DNA must be isolated from whole cells and purified from other macromolecules and then broken down into oligonucleotides, nucleosides, or bases by
chemical or enzymatic means. Separation, identification, and evaluation of the
degradation products may depend on differential centrifugation, chromatography, electrophoresis, or spectroscopy.

DNA exposed to chemical carcinogens shows evidence of structural alterations.
As examples, chemically modified DNA is frequently more resistant to degradation methods than is normal DNA, and chromatographic separation is altered in
DNA subfractions bound to carcinogen (Brookes and Heidelberger, 1969).
Breaks in DNA result from exposure to the mutagenic alkylating agents. A small
number of alkylations are sufficient to sensitize the DNA to a nuclease, which then
causes single-stranded breaks at or near the site of alkylation (Strauss and
Robbins, 1968). Fractions of DNA of varying molecular weights resulting from
these breaks can be detected by band centrifugation. Similarly, techniques of light
scattering, viscosity, or sedimentation may be used to distinguish the intermediates formed by the exposure of DNA to carcinogenic agents (Brookes and
Lawley, 1971).

Direct visualization of DNA by electron micrography can also provide evidence
of carcinogen-induced alterations. Strand dissociations, breaks, and crosslinkages
of DNA treated *in vitro* have been seen after brief exposure to β-propiolactone
(Kubinski and Szybalski, 1974).

However, these techniques have several major limitations. The demonstration
of interaction between carcinogen and DNA *in vitro* need not be relevant to the
changes *in vivo* that are necessary for carcinogenesis. At present, there is no way to
relate the two experimentally. More important, direct analysis is sensitive to
changes in DNA in the range of about 1 part per 1000, whereas changes in as few
as 1 in many millions of nucleotides may give rise to a grossly detectable expression
of mutation (Strauss, 1971). Therefore, at present, the direct analysis of cellular
DNA has contributed to our understanding of carcinogenesis only to the extent
that many chemical carcinogens have been shown to interact directly with the
genetic material.

Quantitative nucleic acid cytochemistry based on the Feulgen reaction provides
another method by which the genetic information contained in eukaryotic cells
may be examined. Robert Feulgen, in 1918, observed that mild acid treatment of
DNA leaves a semidegraded product which reacts quantitatively with aldehyde
indicators. The Feulgen reaction may be used to produce either a color reaction or
a fluorescent compound (Kasten, 1964). Since the reaction is quantitative as well as
DNA specific, it provides means to compare the DNA of normal and tumor cells.

Quantitative histochemical analysis of DNA in nuclei of stained cells has been
accomplished using optical ultramicrospectrographic techniques (Caspersson
and Lomakka, 1962). Total nucleotide content in individual cells can be determined by UV absorption at 256 nm and the DNA content of Feulgen-stained cells
measured at 546 nm. This technique has been used to demonstrate quantitative
differences in DNA from normal and leukemic cell populations (Gahrton and
Foley, 1966). Microdensitometer measurements of Feulgen-stained nuclei have

been used to classify tumors by nucleic acid content (Atkin, 1964). A more sophisticated method uses fluorescent Feulgen-stained cells in suspension, flowing across an argon-ion-laser beam and reradiating energy which is measured for each cell by a pulse height analyzer. Thus the amount of DNA in large numbers of individual cells may be measured rapidly. This technique permits the collection and storage of data on the nucleic acid content of up to 50,000 individual cells per minute (Van Dilla *et al.*, 1969).

The DNA of normal (nonmalignant) cells measured by these techniques is consistent with results from other methods: germ cells show half the DNA content of somatic cells, and liver cells, a percentage of which are normally tetraploid, show two populations, one having twice the DNA of the other (Leuchtenberger *et al.*, 1954; Kasten, 1970). However, the interpretation of data on the DNA content of abnormal cells is more difficult.

Analyses of a particular experimental model by different methods illustrate some of the problems. One example of the transition from a normal to a neoplastic cell is represented by the response of liver cells to a carcinogen. The liver cells are rendered "premalignant" after treatment only in the sense that malignancies will develop in these livers with greatly increased frequency. It is not clear in what proportion or to what extent these cells are altered in other respects. Liver cell populations have been examined following treatment with the carcinogen N-2-fluorenylacetamide (FAA). By chromosomal analysis, the "premalignant" population is essentially unaltered, except that the numbers of tetraploid cells are reduced (Becker *et al.*, 1971). By contrast, Kasten (1970) has shown considerable variability in the DNA contents of individual cells after comparable treatment with the carcinogen dimethylaminoazobenzene (DAB). Thus, while chromosome studies fail to show the presence of abnormal cells, the cytochemical studies fail to indicate whether the abnormal cells are capable of division. Clearly, the application of more than one method to a single experimental system would be desirable. For example, in heteroploid lines growing in tissue culture the abnormal DNA content per cell remains surprisingly constant despite the variability of chromosome number per cell (Kraemer *et al.*, 1971). The combination of nucleic acid chemistry and cytogenetics is more informative than is either method used alone.

Measurement by DNA microfluorometry of fluorescent Feulgen-stained cells is not yet free of technical problems (Yataganas *et al.*, 1975). Nevertheless, it is a powerful means for exploring quantitative changes in DNA or of ploidy in malignancy and in various altered states of cell growth in ways that are presently not feasible using conventional cytogenetic techniques.

Methods of nucleic acid hybridization provide a new and precise means of studying differences between the DNA of malignant and nonmalignant cells. Close binding (annealing) occurs between structurally similar nucleotide chains. The hybridized product can be identified by density gradient centrifugation. Specific RNA or DNA, either naturally derived or prepared with polymerases *in vitro*, can be labeled with radioactive isotopes. The radioactive label then serves as a marker to identify and quantify comparable sequences of nucleotides between the prepared DNA or RNA and segments of nucleotide chains from different cells. Spiegelman *et al.* (1973) have used reverse transcriptase (RNA-directed DNA polymerase) from several murine tumors to create isotope-labeled DNAs. These DNA probes have been used to demonstrate homologies between murine and human breast tumors and between a murine leukemia virus and human leukemias and sarcomas. Their results offer strong support for a viral etiology in several human cancers.

By modifications of annealing methods and the use of RNA polymerase, differences in transcription products of DNA can be demonstrated. A comparison of several types of lymphoid cells indicated that highly repetitive sequences in RNA products were more frequent in acute leukemia cells, less so in chronic leukemia cells, and least frequent in cultured lymphoblastoid, presumably normal, cells (Sawada *et al.*, 1973). It is clear that annealing methods have only begun to be exploited as a means for investigation of the genomes of neoplastic cells.

Direct examination of the DNA of mammalian somatic cells by a variety of physical and chemical methods has demonstrated differences betweeen benign and malignant cell populations. However, these differences are relatively gross and have not been correlated with specific or localized alterations in DNA base-pair composition that may be relevant to malignant characteristics. At the present time, we rely much more heavily on indirect but more precise methods for the study of gene structure and function in benign and malignant cells.

3.2. Abnormalities of Gene Expression

Examination of the protein products of a cell or group of cells is an indirect approach to evaluation of the cell genome. The formation of new products is indicative either of new DNA sequences or of activation of previously repressed sites. Qualitative alteration in a product may reflect changes in base sequences as a result of mutation. A point mutation can be advantageous, neutral, or deleterious with respect to cell survival. We are limited in our ability to estimate true mutation frequency at structural (protein-producing) gene loci. We are far more limited in our ability to identify and detect changes in genes which regulate the functions of other genes or are responsible for purely intracellular functions.

Relatively few "new" cellular products have been identified in tumor cells. One group, the viral antigens, are dependent on the introduction and integration of viral DNA into the host genome (Huebner and Todaro, 1969). Their presence does not necessarily imply any further change in the host genome. The antigenicity of many chemically induced malignancies is evidence of alteration in cell-surface constituents. Transplantation antigens have been demonstrated in 3-methycholanthrene-induced sarcomas (Prehn and Main, 1957; Klein *et al.*, 1960) and a host of other chemically induced malignancies (Klein and Klein, 1962). The antigens of a given tumor are common to all cells of that tumor and there is little cross-reactivity with antigens of other tumors, even those induced by the same chemical. There is little or no loss of antigenicity even with prolonged passage

(Old *et al.*, 1962). Whether these "new" antigens in tumors actually represent new genetic mutations is unclear (Boyse, 1972).

Several of the products characteristic of tumor cells are also found in normal cells, usually at an earlier (fetal) stage of development of the organism. These include cell-surface antigens such as carcinoembryonic antigen (CEA) (Gold *et al.*, 1968), serum proteins such as α-fetoprotein (APF) (Abelev, 1971), and fetal forms of enzymes of which the Regan isozyme (fetal alkaline phosphatase) is an example (Nathanson and Fishman, 1971). The implications of production of fetal substances and the possibilities of gene derepression in explaining carcinogenesis are discussed at length in Chapters 2 and 3. Since the proteins produced by tumor cells do not differ structurally from those of the normal fetal cells, the altered expression of these products which are already encoded in the genome must involve regulation and repression sites. As mentioned above, our ability to detect mutations at these sites is severely restricted.

Point mutations may be used as a basis for mutagenicity tests in mammalian cell systems. Structural alteration in a normal cellular product is evidence of mutation; detection of structural alteration may depend on electrophoretic properties, antigenic differences, etc. Mutants of enzymes such as thymidine kinase (TK) or hypoxanthine guanine phosphoribosyltransferase (HEPRT) can be selected in cell culture by restrictive media and then analyzed (Kit *et al.*, 1966; Littlefield, 1963). A population of cells exposed to a chemical can then be evaluated in terms of the types and frequencies of mutations induced. Dependence on cloning ability of the treated cells has restricted these assays to near-diploid cells with high plating efficiency, and much work has been done with Chinese hamster cell lines (Chu *et al.*, 1969). However, the availability of human diploid, lymphoblastoid lines now makes it possible to test the mutagenicity of chemical compounds directly in human cells (Sato *et al.*, 1972).

Such assays need not be restricted to mutation at a single locus. New techniques of gel electrophoresis are available for detection of a battery of protein enzymes, many of which show polymorphic forms and rare variants. Approximately one-third of all point mutations have been estimated to give rise to proteins with altered electrophoretic mobility (Shaw, 1965). Examples of structural-deletion and regulatory mutants have been detected by examination of the protein products of cultured lymphoblastoid cells after treatment with a chemical mutagen (Povey *et al.*, 1973). These techniques could be applied to clones of tumor cells, cultured *in vitro*, and are potentially valuable as a means to demonstrate increased mutation rates or genetic instability.

3.3. Analogy of Transformation in Vitro

Cultured cells and somatic cell hybrids *in vitro* are new and powerful tools for the study of biological processes. Under controlled conditions (temperature, nutrients, etc.), cells may be studied singly and in aggregate and alterations in morphology, behavior, and response to additives may be isolated far more easily than in the whole animal. The phenomenon known as "transformation *in vitro*" is analogous to malignant alteration of cells *in vivo* in several ways. Transformation usually consists of altered morphology, increase in growth rate and in culture saturation density, altered cell-to-cell relationship (loss of contact inhibition), aneuploid chromosome constitution, ability to grow at greater dilution (cloning efficiency) or at lower serum concentration, and changes in cell surface properties (altered antigenicity, agglutinability with plant lectins, etc.). Correlations can be made between each of these alterations in cells growing *in vitro* and observations on the behavior of tumors and tumor cells. More important, many transformed cell lines give rise to tumors when inoculated into a suitable host animal.

The analogy is a useful one; in particular, the tissue culture environment allows us to isolate and examine interactions between cells and carcinogens and to monitor successive alterations. However, transformation *in vitro* is not synonymous with "carcinogenesis *in vitro*"; many "transformed" cells are not malignant when inoculated into animals (Todaro *et al.*, 1963*b*). Extensive evolution occurs in some cell lines with prolonged cultivation *in vitro*. There is experimental evidence that morphological transformation and acquisition of malignancy occur at separate points in time (Vogt and Dulbecco, 1963; Defendi, 1966; Sivak and Van Duuren, 1968; DiPaolo and Donovan, 1967) and tumorigenicity of a cell line may be lost as well as gained *in vitro* (Foley *et al.*, 1965). Some of the discrepancy probably depends on the suitability of the inoculated animal host and on its immune defenses. Moreover, the absence of morphological transformation does not guarantee nontumorigenicity of a cell line (Defendi *et al.*, 1963). It is clear, therefore, that the analogy drawn between transformed cells and tumor cells is not completely reliable; it is further weakened when only one or two of the criteria mentioned above are used to define "transformation" and it does not support the sweeping application to animal and human cancers of conclusions drawn from observations *in vitro*.

3.4. Cell Hybridization

The technique of somatic cell hybridization between and within species has created entirely new means for investigating the genomes of somatic cells. Hybrid cells have been produced from crosses between normal diploid cells, virus-transformed cells, and lines with variable properties which developed with prolonged cultivation *in vitro*. In these experiments, chromosome markers from the parental lines provide the evidence that fusion has occurred. It has become clear that most hybrid lines evolve rapidly and do not retain the full chromosomal complement from both parental donors. Of particular interest are the results of crosses between tumorigenic and nontumorigenic cell types. Most of the early fusion experiments resulted in highly malignant cells (Barski *et al.*, 1961; Defendi *et al.*, 1967; Gershon and Sachs, 1963; Scaletta and Ephrussi, 1965). The hybrid clones displayed many of the *in vitro* characteristics of the more malignant of the parent lines, and were at least as malignant in animal inoculations when immune reactions did not interfere with tumor growth.

By contrast, experiments by Harris *et al.* (1969) have demonstrated suppression of malignancy in hybrid cells. One parental line (A-9) they used was derived from mouse fibroblasts, had been grown for long periods *in vitro*, had been characterized with respect to several surface antigens and metabolic markers, and was essentially nontumorigenic. This line was hybridized with a series of three highly tumorigenic ascites cell lines: the first originated as a mouse mammary carcinoma and is known as the Ehrlich ascites tumor; the second, designated SEWA, began as an osteogenic sarcoma induced by polyoma virus; and the third, MSWBS, was a methycholanthrene-induced sarcoma. Within the first months after fusion, the hybrid lines were poor tumor inducers, with high chromosome numbers per cell. The few tumors which were obtained, relatively late after inoculation of A-9 × Ehrlich hybrid cells, had, however, lost approximately one-third of the chromosomes found in the original hybrid. Many of the chromosomes lost were markers from the A-9 parent. Later experiments confirmed these observations on suppression of malignancy using different fibroblast lines as the nontumorigenic parents, hybridized with other types of tumorigenic cells. Segregant sublines could also be obtained from nontumorigenic hybrids after variable periods of time in culture; these sublines had lower chromosome numbers and were occasionally highly malignant when inoculated into suitable animal hosts. When fusion between Ehrlich tumor cells and diploid fibroblasts resulted in malignant hybrids (Bregula *et al.*, 1971), tumorigenicity was attributed to chromosome losses from the hybrid cells *in vitro* prior to animal inoculation.

Suppression of malignancy in some hybrid lines while both parental sets of chromosomes are retained, and recurrence of malignant expression with chromosome segregation and loss, led to the suggestion that "malignancy behaves as a recessive trait" (Ephrussi, 1972). One possible interpretation is that malignancy results from a genetic deletion which is complemented in hybrids by genes from the nonmalignant parent line (Wiener *et al.*, 1971). Others who have observed similar phenomena suggest that suppression of malignancy should be "understood as the sum of several factors, not as a simple character of cells" (Murayama-Okabayashi *et al.*, 1971). In any event, one may question the use of the terms "recessive" and "dominant," which have very precise genetic meanings, to describe a complex phenotype which is surely determined by more than one pair of genes.

These findings with hybrid cells are reminiscent of those of the "flat" revertant cells described by Pollack *et al.* (1968). These large, slowly growing, contact-inhibited cells obtained by fluorodeoxyuridine (FUdR) treatment of virus-transformed malignant cells appeared to have many of the growth characteristics of "normal" cells. However, populations of "flat" cells were characterized by high chromosome numbers (Pollack *et al.*, 1970). As with the hybrids, highly malignant segregants with lower chromosome numbers inevitably appeared from the "flat" revertants.

Explanations based on repressor genes (Comings, 1973) and on gene dosage* phenomena have been invoked to account for the masking of malignancy in

---

* Gene dosage effect reflects the quantitative action of different alleles on the phenotypic expression of the corresponding character. The extent of the effect correlates with the frequency of the allele in the genotype (Rieger *et al.*, 1968). Therefore, in a nondiploid cell, differences in phenotype may relate to abnormal ratios of alleles rather than to structural alteration within these alleles.

hybrids. Many different specific genes may determine the results of the different crosses. For example, Grundner *et al.* (1971) suggested that decreased expression of membrane antigens, which was demonstrable in the fusions with Ehrlich tumor cells described above, was related to suppression of malignancy. Another interesting possibility was put forward by Rothschild and Black (1970) based on expression of thymidine kinase (TK) in SV40-transformed cells. They suggested that deficiency of a salvage-pathway enzyme (such as TK), which might not be expressed in a normal cell, could be a rate-limiting step in tumor cell metabolism and thereby limit the expression of malignancy in hybrid cells.

Ephrussi (1972) has drawn a parallel between the suppression of malignancy and the suppression of certain differentiated functions in hybrid cells, and has raised the possibility that both depend on epigenetic phenomena. Regulation of differentiated functions in the normal diploid cells of the intact animal is clearly epigenetic. Nevertheless, the genes responsible for these functions may be mutated as well as regulated: what Ephrussi calls the "determined state" is inherited. In hybrid cells, alterations in tumorigenic capacity and in expression of differentiated functions are accompanied by large changes in the numbers of chromosomes per cell. In addition to loss or gain of specific genes, there is probably alteration in the number of alleles coding for specific functions. The term "epigenetic" refers specifically to regulation of genetic potential, especially during the developmental process (Rieger *et al.*, 1968). It is an extension of the formal meaning to describe events as "epigenetic" which, in these hybrid cells, appear to be always mediated by alteration in gene or chromosome dosage. Segregation of chromosomes within hybridized cells, especially in interspecific crosses, provides a powerful means for investigation of gene localization and expression.

The techniques available for examining the genetic material of cells directly or indirectly have expanded enormously in recent years. Methods for isolating and examining mammalian cells growing in controlled environments, and for fusing cells and retaining portions of the genome, have made it possible to perform experiments that for reasons of time, complexity, or humanity are impossible in the intact animal. Clearly, one area to focus on is the identification and regulation of genes which express or control the behavior of malignant cells.

4. Cytogenetic Studies

4.1. Alterations in Human and Animal Tumors

At the present time, examination and analysis of metaphase chromosomes is probably the most widely used method for the evaluation of genetic material. Early studies of chromosome patterns in malignant tumors were hampered by two technical problems—the need for an adequate number of mitotic cells and the requirement for single-cell suspensions for visualization of metaphase chromosomes. The earliest studies of tumor cells were based on examination of histological sections of metaphase cells, which limited the precision of karyotypic analysis. Better visualization of metaphases was possible using specialized types of malignant tissue, such as ascites tumors of rodents; these highly mitotic, malignant neoplasms have been adapted to grow as cell suspensions in the peritoneal cavity.

In 1951, Makino and Kano began a series of studies on an azo-dye-induced ascites sarcoma of rats later characterized by Makino (1956) as showing a "high frequency of definite chromosome patterns specific to the kind of tumor and differing from those of ordinary tissue cells." The chromosome patterns were abnormal in terms of the number of chromosomes per cell and the presence of structurally altered chromosomes. In contrast, a histologically similar tumor, induced in like manner, was composed of cells which were predominantly diploid and thus similar in chromosome pattern to nonmalignant somatic cells (Yoshida, 1952). This diploid tumor, however, did show greater variability of chromosome number about the mode and increased chromosome breakage compared to a population of nonmalignant cells. At approximately the same time, Levan and Hauschka (1953) investigated the Ehrlich ascites tumor of mice, a malignancy not induced by a carcinogen. They found that most of the cells were aneuploid with a characteristic chromosome pattern for each tumor, with both numerical and morphological aberrations, in much the same way that patterns were present in the chromosomally abnormal tumors described by Makino.

These early studies illustrate two major points: (1) that some malignant cells show no apparent chromosomal changes from normal cells, other than an increased breakage and variability in chromosome number, and (2) that chromosome changes when present in malignant cells are usually related from cell to cell within a given tumor and show similar numerical and morphological aberrations.

The first human tumor cells to be karyotyped adequately were also from malignant effusions (Hansen-Melander et al., 1956; Koller, 1956). These tumors were invariably aneuploid. Marked variation was seen in the dividing cells, which included a high frequency of mitotic abnormalities; and rapid evolution of chromosome pattern in the cell population was observed with time. On the other hand, cell populations from benign human effusions always showed a well-defined diploid mode and few chromosomal variants (Sandberg and Hossfeld, 1970). Therefore, the results of early studies of human tumors differed from those of animals in that no diploid human tumors were found.

A tumor may be characterized by its "modal" karyotype, i.e., the chromosome number and morphological arrangement shown by the largest fraction of cells in a given tumor. This modal pattern may become altered in the course of time through acquisition, loss, or alteration in morphology of a relatively small number of chromosomes. The manner in which the observed chromosomal changes proceed is consistent with the hypothesis that all cells of a given tumor stem from a common ancestor cell which differs from its neighbors not only because of its malignant potential but also because of its capacity for karyotypic evolution. This is known as the "stem-line concept" (Makino, 1956), which accords well with the various mutation theories of carcinogenesis and with the clonal selection theory of tumor growth and evolution.

Structurally abnormal chromosomes, if sufficiently different from any members
of the normal set, are known as "marker" chromosomes, and are frequently used to identify or to tag and follow a population of tumor cells. Numerical alterations usually involve an increase in chromosome number. Presumably this occurs because the loss of genetic material could allow expression of haploid genes, many of which are disadvantageous to cell growth or lethal. An increase in chromosome number, on the other hand, would permit expression of new combinations of genes and chromosomes (Ohno, 1971).

The collection and interpretation of cytogenetic data from solid tumors have been impeded by a number of serious technical obstacles. Many tumors have relatively low mitotic rates and it is therefore difficult to obtain sufficient numbers of cells for cytogenetic analysis. Tumor growth is often associated with necrosis both within the tumor and in the surrounding tissues. A large, apparently solid tumor sometimes consists only of a rim of viable tumor tissue surrounding a large mass of necrotic material. Mitotic cells growing in such a marginal environment may harbor artifacts that have no bearing on their being malignant. Furthermore, since almost all solid tumors grow in a stroma of fibrous and vascular supporting tissue, cell suspensions from such tumors can be "contaminated" by nonmalignant stromal cells. The inflammatory cells which surround and infiltrate some tumors are another potential source of contamination.

Nevertheless, the number and the quality of malignant metaphase cells available for examination have increased greatly over the past 20 years. Mitotic arresting agents, such as colchicine and vinblastine, increase the yield of metaphase mitoses. These agents are given to tumor-bearing animals prior to sacrifice or can be added to cell suspensions after removal of a tumor from the animal. However, if the dosage of mitotic arresting agents is not carefully controlled, altered and distorted chromosomal morphology may result from the exposure. Proteolytic and other digestive enzymes, such as trypsin and hyaluronidase, and various types of mechanical separation aid in the preparation of single-cell suspensions and are important in separating tumor from stromal cells. Since mitotic cells lack a nuclear membrane and appear relatively more fragile than nonmitotic cells, they may be more vulnerable to damage by the suspensory techniques. The use of hypotonic solutions for swelling of the cells (Hsu, 1952; Tjio and Levan, 1956), which contributes greatly to the improved visual quality of metaphase chromosomes, carries the same hazard. The possibility that certain kinds of mitoses are more subject to damage than others cannot be ruled out.

Recent major advances in cytogenetics have resulted from the development of methods for chromosomal banding. There are essentially two new techniques; one depends primarily on staining with the fluorescent acridine dyes, quinacrine or quinacrine mustard (Caspersson et al., 1969), and the other is based on a variety of treatments including heat, alkaline denaturation, or enzyme digestion, applied to chromosome preparations prior to staining with Giemsa (Arrighi and Hsu, 1971; Sumner et al., 1971; Drets and Shaw, 1971; Dutrillaux and Lejeune, 1971; Patil et al., 1971; Seabright, 1972). These techniques demonstrate intrachromosomal patterns which are constant for a given species (Caspersson et al.,

1970a; Rowley and Bodmer, 1971; Francke and Nesbitt, 1971; Miller *et al.*, 1971; Wolman *et al.*, 1972); accurate identification of individual chromosomes and regions within chromosomes is now possible. Other important applications of banding include the characterization of structurally or numerically abnormal chromosomes (Shaw and Chen, 1974) and identification of the species of origin of chromosomes in hybrid cells.

Because of difficulties in direct tumor analysis, many tumors are cultured *in vitro* for variable periods of time prior to cytogenetic analysis. In tissue cultures, ample nutritional support for cell growth, direct controlled exposure to mitotic arresting agents, and simple methods for cell suspension all contribute to cytogenetic preparations of high quality. However, cytogenetic instability is common in cells growing in tissue culture. The altered metabolic environment may exert strong selective pressures which result in rapid evolution of karyotypic patterns. Therefore, the chief drawback to the cytogenetic analysis of tumor cells in tissue culture is that the chromosomes may no longer accurately reflect the populations *in vivo* from which they were derived. In fact, all of the techniques used to study the chromosomes of solid tumors are limited by methodological drawbacks which interfere with the interpretation of chromosomal changes. Despite these limitations, considerable information has been gathered on the chromosomal patterns of solid tumors and of tumor cells growing in tissue culture.

Most spontaneous human solid tumors have shown extensive chromosome aberrations. The modal chromosome number in a typical series of tumors ranges from about 35 (hypodiploid) to over 130 (hypertetraploid), the majority being in the hypotetraploid range (Sandberg and Hossfeld, 1970; Sandberg, 1974). With few exceptions, no consistent relationships have been apparent in the karyotypes of even histologically similar tumors (Spriggs *et al.*, 1962). Only rarely have human malignant solid tumors shown a predominantly diploid mode. The few reported cases have included several uncommon childhood malignancies such as nephroblastoma (three cases) (Cox, 1966) and neuroblastoma (one case) (Miles, 1967a), and rare examples of the more common varieties of adult tumors such as carcinoma of the breast (two cases) and adenocarcinoma of the endometrium (two cases) (Miles, 1967b; Toews *et al.*, 1968). Chromosome preparations for all of these cases were obtained by a direct method; therefore, the possibility exists that, because of technical artifact, only benign stromal cells were examined (Sandberg and Hossfeld, 1970).

Observations of nonsolid human tumors, particularly the acute leukemias, have shown that approximately half have diploid karyotypes with no apparent chromosomal abnormalities, while the other half are aneuploid with well-characterized modal patterns (Fitzgerald *et al.*, 1973; Trujillo *et al.*, 1974). The karyotypic examination of malignant blood-forming cells from the bone marrow elucidates a special situation which will be touched upon briefly here. A more extensive treatment may be found in Nowell's chapter in Volume 1 of this series.

In 1960, Nowell and Hungerford reported the discovery of a specific marker chromosome, the Philadelphia chromosome (Ph'), found only in the bone marrow cells of patients with chronic myelogenous leukemia (CML), which appeared to result from a partial deletion of one of the smallest acrocentric chromosomes. By fluorescent banding, the abnormal chromosome was identified as a G22 (Caspersson *et al.*, 1970*b*).* The Ph′ chromosome may be found in approximately 90% of patients with CML (Rundles, 1972). Recent studies in a small number of cases have demonstrated that the structural abnormality resulting in the Ph′ consists of a translocation of chromosomal material rather than a deletion as had been previously thought. Material comprising about half of the long arms of the G22 chromosome is translocated to the ends of the C9 chromosome in most of the cases studied (Rowley, 1973) and to the A2 or F19 chromosome in a few cases (Hayata *et al.*, 1973; Gahrton *et al.*, 1974). If one of a pair of identical twins develops CML, the abnormal chromosome is present only in the affected twin (Jacobs *et al.*, 1966; Goh *et al.*, 1967). Thus the Ph′ abnormality may be interpreted as an acquired somatic cell mutation in the bone marrow, with preferential survival and proliferation of the mutant cell clone.

CML patients whose marrow is Ph′ positive have a longer survival and show a better response to therapy than Ph′-negative patients (Whang *et al.*, 1968). The disease often shows a long quiescent phase which is typically followed by a phase of rapid deterioration. The phase of rapid deterioration is called the "blastic crisis" because of the appearance in the general circulation of very immature "blast" cells from the bone marrow, which have the capacity to set up foci of independent growth and proliferation in various organs. The cytogenetic picture often changes during blastic crisis from the diploid karyotype, normal save for the presence of the Ph′, to one characterized by the development of many aneuploid stem lines and sublines which vary from case to case in the manner seen in solid tumors (Whang *et al.*, 1968; Goh, 1974). In this phase, the Ph′ does not disappear and lines can often be found showing two or more small marker chromosomes identical in morphology with the Ph′. The clinical behavior of this disease has caused many recent observers to view CML as a type of "premalignant" state which has an extremely high risk of becoming a truly malignant acute leukemia recognizable as the "blastic crisis" (Pedersen, 1973). If CML does represent a type of premalignancy, then the Ph′ chromosome may be seen in the context of other premalignant states, some of which are also associated with specific marker chromosomes, as will be discussed subsequently.

It is obvious that human tumors can be neither transplanted nor induced for purposes of study. Therefore, data relevant to slow changes in stem-line karyotypes over the course of time, and changes in chromosome pattern and cell behavior as results of exposure to specific carcinogens, are derived mainly from animal experiments. One of the ways in which tumors of laboratory animals differ from human tumors is that they are often studied as transplants in inbred and therefore genetically more uniform populations. Human tumors, on the other

* The autosomes of the human karyotype are divided into morphological groups designated by letters A through G and arranged in order of descending size, with the No. 1 pair as the largest and the No. 22 pair as the smallest chromosomes. The sex chromosomes, X and Y, are similar in size and morphology to members of groups C and G, respectively.

hand, are usually not connected to known carcinogenic stimuli and occur in an outbred, genetically heterogeneous population.

4.2. Diploid Tumors

One of the striking differences between human and animal malignant solid tumors, as mentioned above, is that diploid tumors are fairly common in experimental animals yet very rare in humans (Bayreuther, 1960; Nowell *et al.*, 1967; Ohno, 1971; Koller, 1972). Their rarity in humans may be related to differences in genetic homogeneity. The RNA viruses in animals usually give rise to diploid tumors such as the Bittner mouse mammary tumor (Tjio and Ostergren, 1958) and the primary Rous sarcomas in rats (Mitelman, 1971). Many of the chemically induced rat hepatomas are diploid, although the same agents regularly induce markedly aneuploid tumors as well (Nowell *et al.*, 1967; Becker *et al.*, 1971, 1973).

The existence of diploid tumors clearly suggests that chromosome aberrations are not a necessary concomitant of the malignant state. However, these tumors may contain structural abnormalities not evident with the usual methods of chromosome staining. With the advent of fluorescent and other differential intrachromosomal banding techniques, a more extensive examination of the normal karyotype has become possible. The term "diploid" frequently conveys the meaning that the chromosomal material of a cell is normal. However, with available methods of intrachromosomal pattern recognition, it is now possible to recognize abnormal "diploid" cells. For example, a recent study using banding techniques has shown a structural rearrangement in cells of a diploid rat tumor (9121), a Morris hepatoma, which had been carried by transplantation for several years (Wolman *et al.*, 1973*a*) (Fig. 2). It is reasonable to expect that still newer methods of examination will be developed to demonstrate other types of chromosome alteration and further decrease the number of apparently chromosomally normal, diploid tumors.

Another important point with regard to the cytogenetics of tumor cells is demonstrated by a hepatoma (7800) that displays no identifiable deviation from normal banding patterns (Wolman *et al.*, 1973*a*). Yet examination of this tumor population revealed that more than 25% of the cells contained a nondiploid number of chromosomes. This level of variability is typical of most tumor cell populations and may be a reflection of genetic instability. Earlier studies of diploid tumors also emphasized that variation in chromosome number is far greater than that found in normal tissues (Tjio and Ostergren, 1958; Hellström *et al.*, 1963).

No diploid metastatic tumors have been reported (Sandberg and Hossfeld, 1973). Under certain circumstances, primary diploid tumors may evolve into aneuploid tumors with transplantation. Evolution to an aneuploid pattern is frequently coupled with less morphological differentiation and more rapid or more independent growth of the tumor. These observations suggest the possibility that diploid and nearly diploid tumors may represent a different or possibly

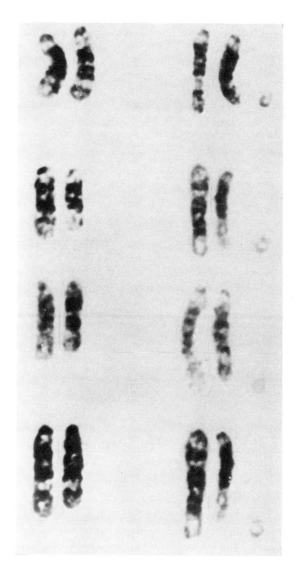

FIGURE 2. G-banded No. 2 chromosomes and small telocentric chromosomes of the 9121 tumor. Left: No. 2 chromosomes from four cells having a diploid (42) complement of chromosomes. Right: No. 2 chromosomes plus small telocentric chromosomes from four cells with 43 chromosomes. Note asymmetry of size and subterminal differences in banding pattern between the No. 2 chromosomes. No other deviations from the normal rat banding pattern were found.

incomplete stage in the expression of malignancy. If the ability to metastasize is correlated with aneuploidy, the type of chromosomal instability which is typical of "diploid" tumors could very well be a prerequisite for the development of full tumor potential.

4.3. Ploidy

Many solid tumors, whether human or nonhuman, stabilize at a hypotetraploid mode. Hypotetraploid modes are also characteristic of many transformed cells and lines permanently adapted to growth *in vitro*. In several experimental systems, one of the immediate effects of an oncogen is to increase the proportion of tetraploid cells in the treated population. In an extensive review of virus-induced chromosome aberrations, Bartsch (1970) has noted that induction of numerical alterations is mainly restricted to the oncogenic viruses, and several examples of tetraploidy induced by Rous, polyoma, and SV40 virus exposure are cited. Delayed induction of polyploidy has been found with adenovirus 12 (Stich and Yohn, 1965). Many of the studies with chemical carcinogens have concentrated on the demonstration of structural rather than numerical alterations in chromosomes. However, polyploidy and tetraploidy were found in human cells treated with sulfhydryl compounds (Jackson and Lindahl-Kiessling, 1964), and marked increases in tetraploidy have been observed in populations of diploid rat fibroblasts treated with chemical carcinogens (Wolman et al., 1975). Defendi and his associates have analyzed the significance of polyploidy in transformation by an oncogenic virus. They have found that after infection with SV40 a portion of the cell population undergoes two cycles of DNA replication without cell division, resulting in tetraploidy (Lehman and Defendi, 1970; Lehman et al., 1971). They also have indirect evidence that the polyploid cells may be the source of the transformed cells; populations with greater numbers of tetraploid cells give rise to transformed colonies more frequently (Hirai et al., 1974).

A sudden increase in ploidy can occur in a single step, either by interference with cell division after completion of chromosome replication or by fusion of two nuclei in a single cytoplasmic membrane. Increased proportions of hyperploid cells are frequently observed after sudden alterations in conditions for growth of cultured cells (i.e., subculturing into a new medium, transfer from ascitic growth to culture in vitro). Increases in ploidy have also been associated with rapid evolution in many other experimental situations (Levan and Biesele, 1958; Hsu and Somers, 1961; Horibata and Harris, 1970; Moriwaki et al., 1971), and tetraploidy has been implicated in the emergence of immunoresistant tumor lines (Sinkovics et al., 1970).

Polyploidy has been described as a means for adaptation to a rapidly changing environment (Dobzhansky, 1951). Naturally occurring hyperploids in the plant world appear under conditions of environmental stress (alpine and arctic regions) and appear to have "high survival value" (Swanson et al., 1967). Polyploid plants show a higher tolerance to irradiation than do diploids (Sparrow and Gunckel, 1955). Polyploids of different parental strains (hybrids) have considerable adaptive value, presumably due to the environmental tolerance of both parents. Another observed consequence of polyploidy in plants is abnormal segregation of chromosomes (Sybenga, 1972). Since polyploid or hyperploid cells are common in animal tumors and appear to be induced by carcinogen treatment, it is possible that, like plant cells, they are more adaptable and better able to withstand environmental alteration than are diploid cells.

Abnormal chromosome segregation also results from hyperploidy in animal cells. In a recent study of spontaneous tetraploids arising from rodent cells in tissue culture, approximately 30% of the mitoses observed were tripolar (Pera, personal communication). A tetraploid line carried by Martin and Sprague (1969) continued to produce diploid daughter cells. In terms of tumor development, the sudden acquisition of extra chromosomes by a cell, followed by abnormal segregation, permits considerable latitude in terms of new combinations of genes and chromosomes. In the presence of a full diploid complement, additional individual chromosomes may be lost, without expression of cellular lethality. Variations in gene dosage are to be expected. In both these respects, polyploids are comparable to somatic cell hybrids. The hyperploid cell is able to generate greater genetic variability than the diploid cell and is potentially able to tolerate and survive more variable environmental conditions.

No uniformity of pattern has emerged from chromosomal studies of tumors. Some tumors are basically diploid, with a small proportion of numerically aberrant cells. Others show morphological alterations or evidence of structural instability, while many tumors show extensive numerical and morphological changes. Nevertheless, the significance of chromosomal alterations in tumors should not be discounted because of their lack of consistency.

5. Evolution of Tumors

5.1. Premalignant and Proliferative States

The attempt to evaluate genetic alterations in tumor cells is hampered by the lack of a rigorous and generally applicable definition of a tumor cell. In any discussion of malignancy, one of the most difficult problems is to define the boundary between "premalignant" and "malignant." A tumor which invades locally, and metastasizes and kills the animal which bears it, is clearly malignant and is usually recognizable by a host of morphological and metabolic features. However, the transition from the normal to the neoplastic cell may consist of many steps. There are recognizable altered or proliferative states in the course of development of particular tumors, and these intermediates may represent vital steps in the evolution to a cancer cell. The term "precancerous" has been applied to some cellular states which are distinguished from the normal and the clearly malignant, but its meaning is neither well defined nor consistent.

Carcinogenesis in the rat liver during prolonged feeding with a chemical carcinogen is an experimental example in which transitional states may be identified. Over a period of several months, there is usually a proliferative phase during which hepatic nodules are formed and a picture akin to cirrhosis is sometimes seen. Some of these nodules disappear, while cells within other nodules apparently go on to develop into true malignant hepatomas (Teebor and Becker, 1971). It is possible that the hyperplastic nodule may result from nonspecific hepatic injury. What is not clear is whether some nodule cells are irrevocably committed to developing into cancer cells. Alternatively, they may be altered cells which must depend on another set of specific conditions or events in order to survive or to develop into malignant cells.

Other precancerous states may not be recognizably marked by morphological alteration from the normal cell. Is every cell from a patient with Fanconi's anemia to be considered precancerous because of its vulnerability to chromosome damage or because of the likelihood of his developing a tumor? Is the retina a "precancerous" tissue in an individual carrying the gene for retinoblastoma? If we know that a single exposure to a chemical is capable of eliciting a cancer, are all the cells which interact with that chemical "premalignant?"

In all these examples, we know that a special population of cells is vulnerable, whether we are able to identify that population by its biochemistry, its history, its cytogenetic aberrations, or its morphology. The vulnerability and the transition to malignancy are separable. Only a few cells from each of these populations actually do eventually give rise to a population of malignant cells. It is even possible that the changes which characterize the bulk of a premalignant population are not at all typical of the few cells which do progress to malignancy. Such changes might even mask the true premalignant changes. Nevertheless, we cannot ignore the potential information to be gained from examination of these populations.

5.2. Temporal Relationship of Chromosome Damage to Tumor Development

Evidence of genetic alteration that precedes tumor development is found in many cytogenetic studies. In this context, we have already mentioned the chromosomal instability syndromes in man, and there are several reports indicating that other systemic chromosome aberrations are associated with increased incidence of malignant disease (Wald et al., 1961; MacSween, 1965; Mamunes et al., 1961; Jackson et al., 1965; Gilman et al., 1970). The observed linkage among radiation exposure, chromosome damage, and carcinogenesis has also been discussed.

The sequence in time between chromosome damage and other effects of oncogenic agents emphasizes the significance of mutational damage. Links between chromosome abnormalities and the earliest observable stages of human cancer have been studied in a variety of systems. Chromosome alterations have been demonstrated in the earliest cell divisions after exposure of human cells to an oncogenic virus, SV40, *in vitro*, long before other effects attributable to viral transformation could be recognized (Wolman et al., 1964). Exposure of mammalian cells in culture to nontoxic levels of chemical carcinogens such as diepoxybutane, dimethylcarbamoylchloride, or benz[a]pyrene results in visible chromosome damage within 1–7 days of treatment (Wolman et al., 1975) (Fig. 3). It is important to establish whether these early changes are predictive and can be associated reliably with the later appearance of phenotypic transformation.

In a study of carcinoma of the uterine cervix, Granberg (1971) showed that, in general, wide variation of chromosome numbers and karyotypes was characteristic of preinvasive lesions (carcinoma *in situ*). Invasive tumors, on the other hand, seldom have more than one stem line (Atkin, 1967). In addition, a tendency toward reduction in the proportion of chromosomes of the B, D, and G groups was found in these tumors, and perhaps an excess of C group chromosomes. Similarly, in studies of chromosome abnormalities of neoplasms of the colon which included benign, "premalignant," and malignant tumors, Lubs and Kotler

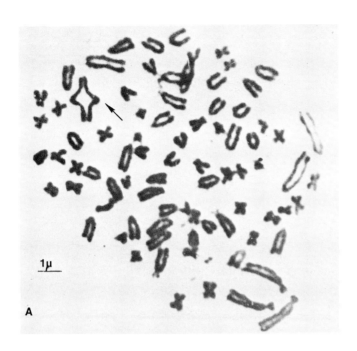

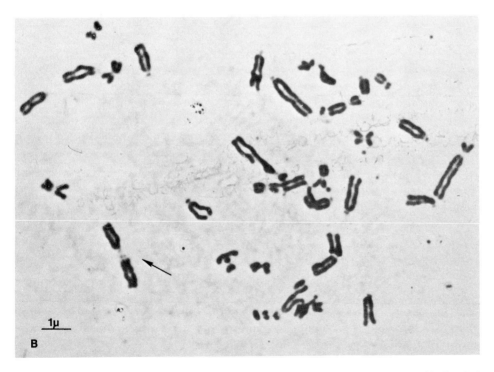

FIGURE 3. Metaphase preparations from diploid rat fibroblast cultures treated *in vitro* with chemical carcinogens. The treated populations showed statistically significant increases in several types of chromosome aberrations (A) 0.04 μg/ml diepoxybutane for 7 days. The cell is hypotetraploid and contains an exchange figure (arrow). (B) 9.0 μg/ml of dimethylcarbamoylchloride for 1 day. Breaks, exchanges, and fragments are common and a centromeric association (arrow) is noted.

(1967) showed that the premalignant lesions (villous adenomas) exhibited wide variation of chromosome number and were characterized by the absence of either predominant cell lines or marker chromosomes. In contrast, malignant tumors (adenocarcinomas) not only were aneuploid but also contained at least one distinct stem-cell line. Even lesions which are considered to have a very low or nonexistent malignant potential (adenomas without atypia) were composed of cells which were not normal in chromosome constitution, but were predominantly pseudo-diploid, commonly with 47 or 48 chromosomes per cell (Enterline and Arvan, 1967).

In bladder tumors, Lamb (1967) demonstrated an abrupt change in chromosome number in invasive disease as opposed to carcinoma *in situ*. In his study, all noninvasive tumors had near-diploid modes, whereas most of the invasive tumors were nondiploid. There was also a relationship between chromosome number and histological appearance, with the more differentiated tumors having a more nearly diploid mode. Furthermore, with loss of differentiation there was also a decrease in the percentage of cells having chromosome counts at the modal number.

Chromosome changes thought to be indicative of early malignancy have also been observed in ovarian tumors. A benign ovarian tumor (cystic adenoma) which has a low malignant potential was found to have chromosome abnormalities consistent with the stem-line concept of clonal evolution (Fraccaro *et al.*, 1968). Porter *et al.* (1969) demonstrated markedly aneuploid cells in a similar tumor, which they felt were suggestive of early malignant change because such a degree of aneuploidy had previously been reported only in frankly malignant cells. In addition to the work on solid tumors described above, chromosome changes associated with what may be the early stages of malignant processes have been studied in diseases of the hematopoietic system. As mentioned above, the Ph′ chromosome of chronic myelogenous leukemia is considered by some observers to be an alteration marking a "premalignant" event. Consistent chromosome changes have also been reported in polycythemia vera (Reeves *et al.*, 1972), in that an abnormal F20 chromosome, missing approximately half to two-thirds of its long arms, can be demonstrated in about 15% of cases (Lawler *et al.*, 1970). Myelofibrosis is often characterized by aneuploidy (characteristically triploidy for the C8 chromosome) (de la Chapelle *et al.*, 1972). These last two diseases are considered premalignant in the somewhat different sense that patients suffering from them are at increased risk for developing acute leukemia.

It is, of course, possible to interpret the so-called precancerous characteristics and the eventual cancers as independent consequences of an initial event rather than as sequential. If we believe, however, that neoplastic change depends on more than one event, then intermediate stages should occur, and we are dependent on observations of these stages to perceive the significant features of cellular evolution. Examination of precancerous cell populations may not only help to identify steps in the sequence but may also serve to isolate vulnerable points where the sequence can be stopped or reversed.

There is considerable evidence that tumors are clonal—i.e., derived from a single cell of origin. Much of this evidence comes from observations of chromosome patterns. In most cases, the cells of an individual tumor show a well-defined modal number of chromosomes, and while there are variations around the mode, and often subpopulations of cells at multiples of the mode, these only emphasize the "stem-line" nature of the modal cell. A distinctive or marker chromosome is frequently present in many or all cells of a tumor (Atkin and Baker, 1966). The concept that an unusual morphological entity would have arisen more than once is less acceptable than that the tumor cells were derived from a single cell carrying the abnormality.

Uniformity of gene product has sometimes been used as evidence for a unicellular origin of tumors. Many tumors of lymphoid or plasma cells appear to be monoclonal based on the homogeneity of the immunoglobulin produced or demonstrable on the surface of the tumor cells (Preud'homme and Seligman, 1972; Mårtensson, 1963). Much of the evidence for clonality is based on demonstration of uniformity of glucose-6-phosphate dehydrogenase (G6PD) expression. The gene for G6PD is X linked; its product has no known selective value in tumor cells. Two forms of the enzyme, called A and B, are recognizable by their different electrophoretic mobilities. Because of the random inactivation of one of the X chromosomes, each cell from a heterozygote female will express only one form of the enzyme. Its presence can be demonstrated quantitatively in very small amounts of tissue and even in single cells. Whereas the heterozygote individual from whom a tumor is derived shows both A and B types of enzyme in her normal tissues, single tumors from such individuals, whether benign or malignant, have shown either the A or the B form of the enzyme. Studies on uterine fibroid tumors (Linder and Gartler, 1965), leukemias (Fialkow, 1972), warts (Murray *et al.*, 1971), and Burkitt's lymphoma (Fialkow *et al.*, 1970) indicate that the same X chromosome is expressed in all cells of a given tumor and therefore support the probability of a single cell of origin. However, using similar techniques of G6PD cellular expression, Gartler *et al.* (1966) have demonstrated that trichoepitheliomas (hereditary benign epithelial tumors probably of hair-follicle origin) frequently show a mixed phenotype, as do hereditary neurofibromas (Fialkow, 1971). With the exception of these hereditary tumors, the biochemical evidence supports a clonal origin of tumor growth.

The chromosomal evidence is, in some respects, unreliable. Chromosome patterns observed within a tumor at a given point in time may have little to do with the original cell(s) of that tumor. Rapid selection of a cell type (or karyotype) advantageous for growth can result in the uniformity observed within a population of malignant cells. In a series of hepatic tumors induced in the rat by ingestion of the chemical carcinogen FAA, approximately half of the primary tumors were diploid and half were hypotetraploid (Becker *et al.*, 1973). The successive transplant generations showed very rapid chromosomal evolution in some cases.

One aneuploid primary tumor gave rise to two widely differing sublines in the first transplant generation (the modal chromosome number of one subline was 60, the other 100) which have been carried separately and have remained fairly stable through 35 transplantations. The diploid tumors gradually became hyperdiploid (mode of 45) over ten transplant generations. One of them suddenly, at the sixteenth transplant, showed an increase in chromosomal rearrangement, with a number of new marker chromosomes which could be identified in the majority of metaphase cells (Fig. 4). There was simultaneously a marked increase in the growth rate of the tumor.

Levan (1973) has observed that tumors of rats induced by either Rous sarcoma virus or the chemical carcinogen 7,12-dimethylbenz[α]anthracene (DMBA) generally show a diploid chromosome pattern when first examined. With time and repeated transplantation, new, distinctive, and apparently stable chromosome

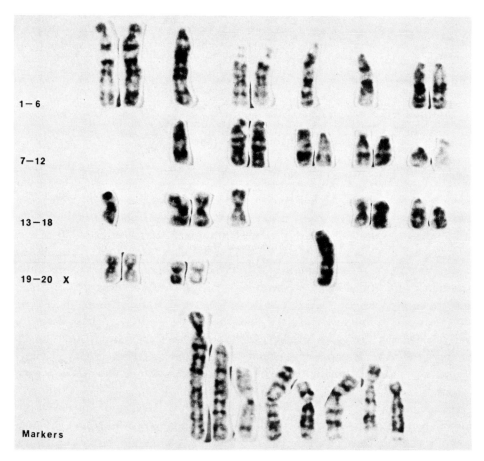

FIGURE 4. G-banded karyotype of a pseudodiploid, rapidly growing subline from a diploid rat hepatoma. There is extensive rearrangement of the karyotype with formation of marker chromosomes.

patterns are obtained. By contrast, a report by Chen and Shaw (1973) showed a set of relatively unstable chromosome aberrations (ring forms, dicentrics, etc.) in a human melanoma, which persisted even after the tumor cells were cultured *in* *vitro* for several months. The retention of these unstable forms despite their potential lethality indicates a surprising absence of chromosomal evolution. Neither diploidy nor karyotypic instability is a reliable indicator of patterns of chromosome evolution in tumors. Since many tumors (expecially human malignancies) are not studied early in their life histories, their uniformity of chromosome patterns may be more a reflection of selective influences than of clonal origins.

The importance of selective influences is supported by recent observations on marker chromosomes in certain mouse lymphomas. The lymphoma L-1210 (V) is a pseudodiploid tumor with a large submetacentric marker chromosome (Hutchison *et al.*, 1966). A number of sublines have been adapted to grow *in vitro* in the presence of thiol supplements (mercaptoethanol, cysteine, etc.) (Broome and Jeng, 1973). Some of these sublines rapidly (in 2–6 wk) lost the marker chromosome, while remaining pseudodiploid. In one case, after prolonged cultivation *in vitro* the marker reappeared. In each case, the subline when stable showed the presence or absence of the marker in more than 95% of the cells (Wolman *et al.*, 1973b). More important, the presence or absence of the marker could be correlated in each subline with an antigenic component, θ, of the cell surface (Table 1). Similar evolution *in vivo* could provide a source of variation among tumor cells, with obvious implications for immunoselection.

Neither the persistence of chromosome pattern during transplantation or passage *in vitro* nor the uniformity of pattern within a tumor cell population at a given point in time guarantees that that pattern was present at the inception of the

TABLE 1

Relation of θ Antigen to Chromosomal Marker in L-1210(V) Sublines

Cell type	Days in culture	θ	Percent marker
ME	50	−	100
ME	161	−	100
ME	175	+	50
A-1	90(30)[a]	+	0
A-2	41(30)	±[b]	19
A-3	43(30)	−	100
A-5	103(30)	−	100
AC-1	50(16)	−	100
AC-2	70(64)	−	95
AC-4	140(40)	+	0
AC-ME-60	200+(60)	−	80

[a] The number in parentheses refers to the number of days of growth in thiol-containing medium.
[b] Discrepancy between two tests.

tumor. Karyotypic evolution may, however, give considerable information about the cellular evolution and behavior of a particular tumor.

6. Chromosomal Localization of "Cancer" Genes

The lack of uniformity in and occasional complete absence of chromosome abnormalities in tumor cells have led many observers to discount their significance in tumor etiology. Others, unwilling to ignore such a common characteristic of malignant cells, have suggested that chromosome changes may play some role in the evolution of tumors and are not simply a by-product of the causative event(s). Yet, in looking at mutations as a class, the large (or chromosomal) mutation is more likely to have a large effect in modifying cell behavior than is the point mutation (Drake and Flamm, 1972). This is relevant only for somatic cells since the point mutation is far less likely to be lethal to the organism.

The suggestion made by Boveri (1914) that certain chromosomes inhibit while others promote cell division was ignored for many years. Boveri proposed that benign tumors might have gained chromosomes that promote division while malignant tumors "besides this positive quality would also be characterized by the lack of certain other chromosomes." This view of malignancy as dependent on the presence or absence or relative dosage effect of certain chromosomal sites has been revived recently in a number of forms and supported by a wide variety of experimental evidence.

A specific chromosomal imbalance was reported by Gofman et al. (1967) in several lines of human cells in culture. The cell lines analyzed, which were derived from both benign and malignant tissues (HeLa, Detroit 98, HEp-2, WISH, etc.) but were tumorlike in growth characteristics, were shown to have a relative increase in the E16 chromosomes. There is recent evidence that many human cell lines may actually have been derived from a single source, HeLa, by cross-contamination (Gartler, 1968; Nelson-Rees et al., 1974). At the time of Gofman's study, the E16 was one of the few members of the human chromosome set which could be identified definitely on morphological grounds. With the advent of special stains and banding procedures, definitive identification of each chromosome in the karyotype is now available for many species. Gofman's suggestion with respect to the E16 chromosome in the human has not been supported and in fact no general specific increase or decrease in chromosomal components of tumor cells has been demonstrated.

There is, however, evidence to implicate certain chromosomal sites in a few particular kinds of human tumors. The first specific and consistent association was, of course, Nowell and Hungerford's (1960) observation of deletion in a G-group chromosome associated with chronic myelogenous leukemia—the Philadelphia chromosome. With fluorescent banding the deleted chromosome was identified as a G22; and Rowley (1973) has shown that this alteration is not a deletion but a translocation, as discussed earlier. Another report links polycythemia vera with an F20 deletion (Reeves *et al.*, 1972). A loss or partial loss of the G22 appears to characterize a large group of meningeal tumors studied by Mark *et al.* (1972) and Zankl and Zang (1972). In fact, Levan and his collaborators (Levan, 1973) have been able to demonstrate consistent aspects of chromosome patterns in a number of human tumors, including gliomas which are characterized by losses in C and D groups (Mark, 1971; Mitelman *et al.*, 1972), cervical carcinomas which show losses in D and increases in C groups (Granberg, 1971), and Burkitt's lymphomas in which abnormal banding of D14 was found (Manolov and Manolova, 1972). Each of these patterns appears to be tumor specific.

There is evidence in animal systems for agent-specific patterns. Earlier work in Levan's laboratories on transplantable animal tumors indicated that specific selection for chromosome alterations was occurring. They had studied sarcomas induced by Rous sarcoma virus (RSV) and by the chemical carcinogen DMBA. These malignancies were generally diploid when first examined but became aneuploid on repeated transplantation. A different but characteristic pattern of chromosome selection was found with each agent. The RSV tumors acquired a medium-sized telocentric and two subtelocentric chromosomes; the DMBA tumors acquired a large telocentric and a metacentric chromosome (Mitelman *et al.*, 1972). Independent observations in other laboratories on rat leukemias induced with DMBA gave results similar to those with the DMBA-induced sarcomas (Kurita *et al.*, 1968). Levan (1973) concluded therefore that nonrandom karyotypic alterations in these animal tumors were determined by the particular oncogenic agents rather than by tissue specificity.

The work of several investigators studying hamster cells *in vitro* and *in vivo* suggests that particular chromosomes in the hamster carry factors important in the expression or suppression of malignancy. Hitotsumachi *et al.* (1971, 1972) studied hamster cells treated *in vitro* by polyoma virus or dimethylnitrosamine, and analyzed the chromosomes of the transformed clones. They found a preferential increase of group 5 hamster chromosomes and a relative decrease in the chromosomes of groups 6 and 7 in their transformed colonies. Benedict *et al.* (1975) evaluated the chromosome patterns of tumors induced *in vivo* in hamsters by inoculation of cultured cells transformed by the chemical 1β-D-arabinofuranosylcytosine (araC). The tumors showed preferential retention and relative loss of the same types of hamster chromosomes found in the transformation experiments *in vitro*. These hamster experiments, in contrast to those discussed earlier, show specificity neither for the tissue from which the tumor derives nor for the inducing agent, but only for the species.

Other analyses of human tissues, however, appear to reaffirm the significance of tissue specificity in the determination of dominant tumor karyotypes. In ataxia-telangiectasia, a chromosome breakage syndrome with high incidence of lymphoid neoplasia, several investigators have reported persistence of and apparent selection for clones of cells bearing breaks or translocations of one of the D14 chromosomes (Hecht *et al.*, 1973). Sandberg and Sakurai (1973) have noted a curious tendency to retain the Y chromosome in leukemia cells of older males and there is evidence that the Y chromosome is retained in solid tumors as well (Litton *et al.*, 1972). In addition, the Y chromosome uniformly persists in those females who have gonadoblastic tumors (Teter and Boczkowski, 1967; Segall *et al.*, 1973).

A cohesive pattern may be emerging from the complex, apparently tissue-specific chromosome patterns of human tumors. The human tumors examined thus far show selection for cells with abnormalities in only a few chromosomes: duplications and deficiencies of C8 chromosomes are common in some leukemias and gastrointestinal polyps; structural aberrations of D14 are found in ataxia-telangiectasia and Burkitt's lymphoma; deletions and rearrangements involving G22 are found in meningiomas and cells from chronic myelogenous leukemia. Evolution of specific patterns of chromosome changes may point to the location of particular genes important in tumor growth and development. As suggested below, these observations are particularly important because they point to a way of reconciling the conflicting perceptions of the role of chromosome changes in the etiology and behavior of tumors.

7. Conclusion: A Multistep Model

We have oriented this discussion to the premise that cancer is a disease based on somatic mutation. We suggest that just as there is more than one type of tumor, there is also more than one pathway for arriving at the state we recognize as tumor. Many different normal or mutated genes may be responsible for the modified behavior of malignant cells. Rather than postulating specific "cancer" genes, we prefer to think that alterations in many genes (some of which are expressed in all cells, and some of which are expressed only in specialized cells) may result in cellular behavior relevant to cancer. These alterations may be sequential and are probably cumulative, but it is not at all clear that there is only one "final common pathway"—that is, that the same genes or same sequence of genic events are responsible for the development of cancer in all cells.

Great similarities are observed among tumors developing from a common organ site or cell type, especially when the tumors are induced by a specific agent. The mutations significant in tumorigenesis are more likely to involve cell regulatory functions than specific differentiated functions. Since many mutations produce missense or nonsense genes, the expected result to the cell is loss of regulatory function. The types of gene change to be expected are those relevant to the phenotypes of tumor cells: control of cell division, rate of cell division, repair of DNA, formation and regulation of surface components and antigens, loss of rate-limiting metabolic regulators—in sum, alterations which confer a relative growth or survival advantage on the cell. In particular, we would expect that at least one of the genes vital to tumor transformation is concerned with regulation of orderly mitotic division, since one of the reliable characteristics of malignant tumors is their genetic variability. Insufficient emphasis has been given to this great variability within tumor cell populations. The possibilities for selection of new "advantageous" cell types may be accounted for by changes in the external as well as the internal milieu.

In order for these altered genes to be inherited, we suggest that they must be structurally altered—by base-pair substitution, insertion, duplication, or loss. Alternatively, a permanent alteration in activity state could be mediated by rearrangement of chromosomal locations or structural alteration of operator or repressor sites. The control and expression of differentiated functions raise many questions about an epigenetic rather than a genetic basis for malignancy. However, the ability to differentiate and the control and regulatory genes which permit cell specialization are inherited from one generation (of people) to the next. The fact that there are normal sequences of cell differentiations should only emphasize that the intracellular chemicals that control these sequences are subject to abnormal as well as normal influences, some of which result in permanent loss or derangement of function. When the results of a disturbance are invariably associated with chromosome dosage alterations, it is reasonable to conclude that the intracellular chemical affected is DNA, even though the same function is mediated by epigenetic events in normal differentiation.

Obviously such gene mutations do not require visible chromosome alterations, as is evident from the frequent finding of "diploid" tumors. It has become clear that in many tumors chromosome alterations characterize a late stage in the evolution of the tumor. It is equally clear, however, that the development of many tumors may be mediated by chromosome alterations. In these cases (the chromosome instability syndromes in man, the chromosome-damaging effects of oncogenic viruses, irradiation, and chemical carcinogens), the initial damage appears to be nonspecific. A genetically more variable population is created, and with increased variability there is an increase in the probability that a proliferative state will arise (either by alteration in gene dosage or from phenomena of chromosome rearrangement and gene activation). Thus the visibly altered chromosome patterns we find evolving in tumor cells may constitute markers for the locations of particular genes relevant to tumor cell functions.

The situation is further complicated in that "malignancy" has no sharp boundaries but depends, in its definition, to some extent on the observer and the system being observed. Transformation is sometimes referred to as "carcinogenesis *in vitro*"—yet transformed cells do not always give rise to tumors. "Diploid" tumors are transplantable, yet do not metastasize. Carcinoma *in situ* of the uterine cervix is morphologically malignant but noninvasive and has a peak incidence 10 years earlier than invasive malignancy at the same site. These different degrees on the overall scale of malignancy may be taken as examples of the many stages that are possible in the evolution from a normal to a fully malignant cell.

In summary, the nonuniform nature of the disease(s) called cancer must be stressed. Different sequences of genetic alterations are likely to be involved in the initiation and perpetuation of different tumors. Consequently, initiation may be nothing more than the creation of a genetically variable population. The fixation and perpetuation of an abnormal proliferative state may depend on selection or further mutation. The resulting malignant behavior is highly variable and depends on the sequence of evolution in that particular clone of cells. However, the retention of great genetic variability within the tumor cell population is a guarantee that the tumor is better able to survive alterations in the environment than the more homogeneous population of host cells.

ACKNOWLEDGMENTS

We are grateful to Edward Goldstein, Henry Rothschild, Andrew Sivak, Timo Vesikari, and especially Eric Wolman for their helpful comments and criticisms of this manuscript.

8. References

ABELEV, G. I., 1971, Alpha-fetoprotein in ontogenesis and its association with malignant tumors, *Adv. Canc. Res.* **14:**295–358.

AMES, B. N., 1972, A bacterial system for detecting mutagens and carcinogens, in: *Mutagenic Effects of Environmental Contaminants* (H. E. Sutton and M. I. Harris, eds.), pp. 57–66, Academic Press, New York.

ARRIGHI, F. E., AND HSU, T. C., 1971, Localization of heterochromatin in human chromosomes, *Cytogenetics* **10:**81–86.

ATKIN, N. B., 1964, Nuclear size in carcinoma of the cervix: Its relation to DNA content and to prognosis, *Cancer* **17:**1391–1399.

ATKIN, N. B., 1967, A carcinoma of the cervix uteri with hypodiploid and hypotetraploid stem-lines, *Eur. J. Cancer* **3:**289–291.

ATKIN, N. B., AND BAKER, M. C., 1966, Chromosome abnormalities as primary events in human malignant disease: Evidence from marker chromosomes, *J. Natl. Cancer Inst. U.S.A.* **36:**539–557.

AULA, P., 1963, Chromosome breaks in leukocytes of chickenpox patients, *Hereditas* **49:**451–453.

BARSKI, G., SORIEUL, S., AND CORNEFERT, FR., 1961, "Hybrid" type cells in combined cultures of two different mammalian cell strains, *J. Natl. Cancer Inst. U.S.A.* **26:**1269–1277.

BARTSCH, H. D., 1970, Virus-induced chromosomal alterations in mammals and man, in: *Chemical Mutagenesis in Mammals and Man* (F. Vogel, and G. Röhrborn, eds.), pp. 420–432, Springer, New York.

BAYREUTHER, K., 1960, Chromosomes in primary neoplastic growth, *Nature (London)* **186:**6–9.

BECKER, F. F., FOX, R. A., KLEIN, K. M., AND WOLMAN, S. R., 1971, Chromosome patterns in rat hepatocytes during N-2-fluorenylacetamide carcinogenesis, *J. Natl. Cancer Inst. U.S.A.* **46:**1261–1269.

BECKER, F. F., KLEIN, K. M., WOLMAN, S. R., ASOFSKY, R., AND SELL, S., 1973, Characterization of primary hepatocellular carcinomas and initial transplant generations, *Cancer Res.* **33:**3330–3338.

BENEDICT, W. F., RUCKER, N., MARK, C., AND KOURI, R. E., 1975, Correlation between the balance of specific chromosomes and the expression of malignancy in hamster cells, *J. Natl. Cancer Inst. U.S.A.* **54:**157–162.

BERENBLUM, I., 1954, A speculative review: The probable nature of promoting action and its significance in the understanding of the mechanism of carcinogenesis, *Cancer Res.* **14:**471–477.

BERENBLUM, I., 1972, Possible relationships between mutagenesis and carcinogenesis, in: *Mutagenic Effects of Environmental Contaminants* (E. H. Sutton and M. I. Harris, eds.), pp. 177–183, Academic Press, New York.

BOUTWELL, R. K., 1974, The function and mechanism of promoters of carcinogenesis, *Chemical Rubber Co. Crit. Rev. Toxicol.* **2:**419–443.

BOVERI, T., 1914, *Zur Frage der Entstehung maligner Tumoren*, Fisher, Jena. (English translation: Boveri, M., 1929, *The Origin of Malignant Tumors*, Williams and Wilkins, Baltimore.)

BOYSE, E. A., 1972, Immuno-genetics in the study of cell surfaces: Some implications for morphogenesis and cancer, in: *Current Research in Oncology, 1972* (C. B. Anfinsen, M. Potter, and A. N. Schechter, eds.), pp. 57–94, Academic Press, New York.

BRAUN, A. C., 1969, *The Cancer Problem: A Critical Analysis and Modern Synthesis*, Columbia University Press, New York.

BREGULA, U., KLEIN, G., AND HARRIS, H., 1971, The analysis of malignancy by cell fusion. II. Hybrids between Ehrlich cells and normal diploid cells, *J. Cell Sci.* **8:**673–680.

BROOKES, P., AND HEIDELBERGER, C., 1969, Isolation and degradation of DNA from cells treated with tritium-labeled 7,12–dimethylbenz(alpha)anthracene: Studies on the nature of the binding of this carcinogen to DNA, *Cancer Res.* **29:**157–165.

BROOKES, P., AND LAWLEY, P. D., 1971, Effects on DNA, chemical methods, in: *Chemical Mutagens*, Vol. I (A. Hollaender, ed.), pp. 121–144, Plenum Press, New York.

BROOME, J. D., AND JENG, M. W., 1973, Promotion of replication in lymphoid cells by specific thiols and disulfides *in vitro*: Effects on mouse lymphoma cells in comparison with splenic lymphocytes, *J. Exp. Med.* **138:**574–592.

BRUNNING, D. A., 1974, Oesophageal cancer and hot tea, *Lancet* **1:**272.

BURDETTE, W. J., 1955, The significance of mutation in relation to the origin of tumors: A review, *Cancer Res.* **15:**201–226.

BYARS, N., AND KIDSON, C., 1970, Programmed synthesis and export of immunoglobulin by synchronized myeloma cells, *Nature (London)* **226:**648–650.

CALDECOTT, R. S., 1961, Seedling height, oxygen availability, storage, and temperature: Their relation to radiation-induced genetic and seedling injury in barley, in: *Effects of Ionizing Radiation on Seeds*, pp. 3–24, International Atomic Energy Agency, Vienna.

CASPERSSON, T. O., AND LOMAKKA, G. M., 1962, Scanning microscopy techniques for high resolution quantitative cytochemistry, *Ann. N.Y. Acad. Sci.* **97:**449–463.

CASPERSSON, T., ZECH, L., MODEST, E. J., FOLEY, G. E., WAGH, U., AND SIMONSSON, E., 1969, Chemical differentiation with fluorescent alkylating agents in *Vicia faba* metaphase chromosomes, *Exp. Cell Res.* **58:**128–140.

CASPERSSON, T., ZECH, L., JOHANSSON, C., AND MODEST, E. J., 1970a, Identification of human chromosomes by DNA-binding fluorescent agents, *Chromosoma* **30:**215–227.

CASPERSSON, T., GAHRTON, G., LINDSTEN, J., AND ZECH, L., 1970b, Identification of the Philadelphia chromosome as a number 22 by quinacrine mustard fluorescence analysis, *Exp. Cell Res.* **63:**238–240.

CHEN, T. R., AND SHAW, M. W., 1973, Stable chromosome changes in a human malignant melanoma, *Cancer Res.* **33:**2042–2047.

CHU, E. H. Y., BRIMER, P., JACOBSON, K. B., AND MERRIAM, E. V., 1969, Mammalian cell genetics. I. Selection and characterization of mutations auxotrophic for L-glutamine or resistant to 8-azaguanine in Chinese hamster cells *in vitro*, *Genetics* **62:**359–377.

COMINGS, D. E., 1973, A general theory of carcinogenesis, *Proc. Natl. Acad. Sci. U.S.A.* **70:**3324–3328.

COWAN, N. J., AND MILSTEIN, C., 1972, Automatic monitoring of biochemical parameters in tissue culture: Studies on synchronously growing mouse myeloma cells, *Biochem. J.* **128:**445–454.

COX, D., 1966, Chromosome constitution of nephroblastomas, *Cancer* **19:**1217–1224.

CURTIS, H., AND CROWLEY, C., 1963, Chromosome aberrations in liver cells in relation to the somatic mutation theory of aging, *Radiat. Res.* **19:**337–344.

DEFENDI, V., 1966, Transformation *in vitro* of mammalian cells by polyoma and simian 40 viruses, *Prog. Exp. Tumor Res.* **8:**125–188.

DEFENDI, V., LEHMAN, J., AND KRAEMER, P., 1963, "Morphologically normal" hamster cells with malignant properties, *Virology* **19:**592–598.

DEFENDI, V., EPHRUSSI, B., KOPROWSKI, H., AND YOSHIDA, M. C., 1967, Properties of hybrids between polyoma-transformed and normal mouse cells, *Proc. Natl. Acad. Sci. U.S.A.* **57:**299–305.

DE LA CHAPELLE, A., SCHRÖDER, J., AND VUOPIO, P., 1972, 8-Trisomy in the bone marrow: Report of two cases, *Clin. Genet.* **3:**470–476.

DiPAOLO, J. A., AND DONOVAN, P. J., 1967, Properties of Syrian hamster cells transformed in the presence of carcinogenic hydrocarbons, *Exp. Cell Res.* **48:**361–377.

DOBZHANSKY, T., 1951, *Genetics and the Origin of Species*, 3rd ed., Columbia University Press, New York.

DOLPHIN, G. W., AND LLOYD, D. C., 1974, The significance of radiation-induced chromosome abnormalities in radiological protection, *J. Med. Genet.* **11:**181–189.

DRAKE, J. W., AND FLAMM, W. G., 1972, The molecular basis of mutation, in: *Mutagenic Effects of Environmental Contaminants*, (H. E. Sutton and M. I. Harris, eds.), pp. 15–26, Academic Press, New York.

DRETS, M. O., AND SHAW, M. W., 1971, Specific banding patterns of human chromosomes, *Proc. Natl. Acad. Sci. U.S.A.* **68:**2073–2077.

DULBECCO, R., 1964, Summary of 1964 biology research conference, *J. Cell. Comp. Physiol.* **64:**181–186 (Suppl. 1).

DUTRILLAUX, B., AND LEJEUNE, J., 1971, Sur une nouvelle technique d'analyse du caryotype humain, *C. R. Acad. Sci. Ser. D* **272:**2638–2640.

ENTERLINE, H. O., AND ARVAN, D. A., 1967, Chromosome constitution of adenoma and adenocarcinoma of the colon, *Cancer* **20:**1746–1759.

EPHRUSSI, B., 1972, *Hybridization of Somatic Cells*, Princeton University Press, Princeton, N.J.

FARBER, E., 1972, Chemical carcinogenesis, in: *Current Research in Oncology, 1972* (C. B. Anfinsen, M. Potter, and A. N. Schechter, eds.), pp. 95–124, Academic Press, New York.

FIALKOW, P. J., 1971, Single or multiple cell origin for tumors? *New Engl. J. Med.* **285:**1198–1199.

FIALKOW, P. J., 1972, Use of genetic markers to study cellular origin and development of tumors in human females, *Adv. Cancer Res.* **15:**191–226.

FIALKOW, P. J., KLEIN, G., GARTLER, S. M., AND CLIFFORD, P., 1970, Clonal origin for individual Burkitt tumors, *Lancet* **1:**384–386.

FITZGERALD, P. H., CROSSEN, P. E., AND HAMER, J. W., 1973, Abnormal karyotypic clones in human acute leukemia: Their nature and clinical significance, *Cancer* **31:**1069–1077.

FOLEY, G. E., HANDLER, A. H., LYNCH, P. M., WOLMAN, S. R., STULBERG, C. S., AND EAGLE, H., 1965, Loss of neoplastic properties *in vitro*. II. Observations of KB sublines, *Cancer Res.* **25:**1254–1261.

FRACCARO, M., MANNINI, A., TIEPOLO, L., GERLI, M., AND ZARA, C., 1968, Karyotypic clonal evolution in a cystic adenoma of the ovary, *Lancet* **1:**613–614.

FRANCKE, U., AND NESBITT, M., 1971, Identification of the mouse chromosomes by quinacrine mustard staining, *Cytogenetics* **10:**365–366.

FURTH, J., AND FURTH, O. B., 1936, Neoplastic diseases produced in mice by general irradiation with X-rays, *Am. J. Cancer* **28:**54–65.

GAHRTON, G., AND FOLEY, G. E., 1966, Cytochemical population analysis of the DNA, RNA and protein content of human leukemia cells, *Acta Med. Scand.* **180:**485–496.

GAHRTON, G., ZECH, L., AND LINDSTEN, J., 1974, A new variant translocation (19 g+, 22 g−) in chronic myelocytic leukemia, *Exp. Cell Res.* **86:**214–216.

GARTLER, S. M., 1968, Apparent HeLa cell contamination of human heteroploid cell lines, *Nature (London)* **217:**750–751.

GARTLER, S. M., ZIPRKOWSKI, L., KRAKOWSKI, A., EZRA, R., SZEINBERG, A., AND ADAM, A., 1966, Glucose-6-phosphate dehydrogenase mosaicism as a tracer in the study of hereditary multiple trichoepithelioma, *Am. J. Hum. Genet.* **18:**282–287.

GERMAN, J., 1972, Genes which increase chromosomal instability in somatic cells and predispose to cancer, in: *Progress in Medical Genetics*, Vol. VIII (A. G. Steinberg and A. G. Bearn, eds.), pp. 61–101, Grune and Stratton, New York.

GERMAN, J., 1973, Oncogenic implication of chromosomal instability, in: *Medical Genetics* (V. A. McKusick and R. Claiborne, eds.), pp. 39–50, HP Publishing Co., New York.

GERMAN, J., GILLERAN, T., LAROCK, J., AND REGAN, J. D., 1970, Mutant clones amidst normal cells in cultures of xeroderma pigmentosum skin, *Am. J. Hum. Genet.* **22:**10a.

GERSHON, D., AND SACHS, L., 1963, Properties of a somatic hybrid between mouse cells with different genotypes, *Nature (London)* **198:**912–913.

GILMAN, P. A., JACKSON, D. P., AND GUILD, H. G., 1970, Congenital agranulocytosis, prolonged survival and terminal acute leukemia, *Blood* **36:**576–585.

GOFMAN, J. W., MINKLER, J. L., AND TANDY, R. K., 1967, *A Specific Common Chromosomal Pathway for the Origin of Human Malignancy*, Lawrence Radiation Laboratory Reports (UCRL-50356), University of California, Livermore.

GOH, K. O., 1974, Additional Philadelphia chromosomes in acute blastic crisis of chronic myelocytic leukemia: Possible mechanism of producing additional chromosomal abnormalities, *Am. J. Med. Sci.* **267:**229–240.

GOH, K., SWISHER, S. N., AND HERMAN, E. C., 1967, Chronic myelocytic leukemia and identical twins, *Arch. Intern. Med.* **120:**214–219.

GOLD, P., GOLD, M., AND FREEDMAN, S. O., 1968, Cellular location of carcinoembryonic antigens of the human digestive system, *Cancer Res.* **28:**1331–1334.

GOLDBERG, B., AND GREEN, H., 1964, An analysis of collagen secretion by established mouse fibroblast lines, *J. Cell Biol.* **22:**227–258.

GRANBERG, I., 1971, Chromosomes in preinvasive, micro-invasive and invasive cervical carcinoma, *Hereditas* **68:**165–218.

GROBSTEIN, C., 1959, Differentiation of vertebrate cells, in: *The Cell*, Vol. I (J. Brachet and A. E. Mirsky, eds.), pp. 437–496, Academic Press, New York.

GRUNDER, G., FENYÖ, E. M., KLEIN, G., KLEIN, E., BREGULA, U., AND HARRIS, H., 1971, Surface antigen expression in malignant sublines derived from hybrid cells of low malignancy, *Exp. Cell Res.* **68:**315–322.

HAMPAR, B., AND ELLISON, S. A., 1961, Chromosomal aberrations induced by an animal virus, *Nature (London)* **192:**145–147.

HANSEN-MELANDER, E., KULLANDER, S., AND MELANDER, Y., 1956, Chromosome analysis of a human ovarian cystocarcinoma in the ascites form, *J. Natl. Cancer Inst. U.S.A.* **16:**1067–1081.

HARRIS, H., MILLER, O. J., KLEIN, G., WORST, P., AND TACHIBANA, T., 1969, Suppression of malignancy by cell fusion, *Nature (London)* **223:**363–368.

HART, R. W., AND SETLOW, R. B., 1974, Correlation between deoxyribonucleic acid excision-repair and life-span in a number of mammalian species, *Proc. Natl. Acad. Sci. U.S.A.* **71:**2169–2173.

HAYATA, I., KAKATI, S., AND SANDBERG, A. A., 1973, A new translocation related to the Philadelphia chromosome, *Lancet* **2:**1385.

HAYFLICK, L., 1965, The limited *in vitro* lifetime of human diploid cell strains, *Exp. Cell Res.* **37:**614–636.

HECHT, F., KOLER, R. D., RIGAS, D. A., DAHNKE, G. S., CASE, M. P., TISDALE, V., AND MILLER, R. W., 1966, Leukemia and lymphocytes in ataxia-telangiectasia, *Lancet* **2:**1193.

HECHT, F., MCCAW, B. K., AND KOLER, R. D., 1973, Ataxia-telangiectasia: Clonal growth of translocation lymphocytes, *New Engl. J. Med.* **289:**286–291.

HELLSTRÖM, K. E., HELLSTRÖM, I., AND SJOGREN, H. O., 1963, Further studies on karyotypes of a variety of primary and transplanted mouse polyoma tumors, *J. Natl. Cancer Inst. U.S.A.* **31:**1239–1253.

HIRAI, K., CAMPBELL, G., AND DEFENDI, V., 1974, Changes of regulation of host DNA synthesis and viral DNA integration in SV40-infected cells, in: *Control of Proliferation in Animal Cells*, pp. 151–166, Cold Spring Harbor Laboratory, Cold Spring Harbor, N.Y.

HITOTSUMACHI, S., RABINOWITZ, Z., AND SACHS, L., 1971, Chromosomal control of reversion in transformed cells, *Nature (London)* **231:**511–514.

HITOTSUMACHI, S., RABINOWITZ, Z., AND SACHS, L., 1972, Chromosomal control of chemical carcinogenesis, *Int. J. Cancer* **9:**305–315.

HORIBATA, K., AND HARRIS, A. W., 1970, Mouse myelomas and lymphomas in culture, *Exp. Cell Res.* **60:**61–77.

HSU, T. C., 1952, Mammalian chromosomes *in vitro*. I. The karyotype of man, *J. Hered.* **52:**167–172.

HSU, T. C., AND SOMERS, C. E., 1961, Effects of 5-bromodeoxyuridine on mammalian chromosomes, *Proc. Natl. Acad. Sci. U.S.A.* **47:**396–403.

HUEBNER, R. J., AND TODARO, G. J., 1969, Oncogenes of RNA tumor viruses as determinants of cancer, *Proc. Natl. Acad. Sci. U.S.A.* **64:**1087–1094.

HUEBNER, R. J., ROWE, W. P., TURNER, H. C., AND LANE, W. T., 1963, Specific adenovirus complement-fixing antigens in virus-free hamster and rat tumors, *Proc. Natl. Acad. Sci. U.S.A.* **50:**379–389.

HUGGINS, C., AND FUKUNISHI, R., 1963, Mammary and peritoneal tumors induced by intraperitoneal administration of 7,12-dimethylbenz(alpha)anthracene in newborn and adult rats, *Cancer Res.* **23:**785–789.

HUTCHISON, D. J., ITTENSOHN, O. L., AND BJERREGAARD, M. R., 1966, Growth of L1210 mouse leukemia cells *in vitro*, *Exp. Cell Res.* **42:**157–170.

JACKSON, A. W., MULDAL, S., OCKEY, C. H., AND O'CONNER, P. J., 1965, Carcinoma of male breast in association with the Klinefelter syndrome, *Br. Med. J.* **1:**223–225.

JACKSON, J. F., AND LINDAHL-KIESSLING, K., 1964, Action of sulfhydryl compounds on human leukocyte mitoses *in vitro*, *Exp. Cell Res.* **34:**515–524.

JACOBS, E. M., LUCE, J. K., AND CAILLEAU, R., 1966, Chromosome abnormalities in human cancer: Report of a patient with chronic myelocytic leukemia and his nonleukemic monozygotic twin, *Cancer* **19:**869–876.

JACOBS, P. A., BRUNTON, M., COURT BROWN, W. M., DOLL, R., AND GOLDSTEIN, H., 1963, Change of human chromosome count distributions with age: Evidence for a sex difference, *Nature (London)* **197:**1080–1081.

KASTEN, F. H., 1964, The Feulgen reaction—An enigma in cytochemistry, *Acta Histochem.* **17**:88–99.

KASTEN, F. H., 1970, The potential of quantitative cytochemistry in tumor and virus research, in: *Introduction to Quantitative Cytochemistry*, Vol. II (G. L. Wied and G. F. Bahr, eds.), pp. 263-296, Academic Press, New York.

KELLERMANN, G., SHAW, C. R., AND LUYTEN-KELLERMAN, M., 1973, Aryl hydrocarbon hydroxylase inducibility and bronchogenic carcinoma, *New Engl. J. Med.* **289**:934–937.

KIT, S., DUBBS, D. R., AND FREARSON, P. M., 1966, HeLa cells resistant to bromodeoxyuridine and deficient in thymidine kinase activity, *Int. J. Cancer* **1**:19–30.

KLEIN, G., AND KLEIN, E., 1962, Antigenic properties of other experimental tumors, *Cold Spring Harbor Symp. Quant. Biol.* **27**:463–470.

KLEIN, G., SJOGREN, H. O., KLEIN, E., AND HELLSTRÖM, K. E., 1960, Demonstration of resistance against methylcholanthrene induced sarcomas in the primary autochthonous host, *Cancer Res.* **20**:1561–1572.

KNUDSON, A. G., 1973, Mutation and human cancer, *Adv. Cancer Res.* **17**:317–352.

KOLLER, P. C., 1956, Cytological variability in human carcinomatosis, *Ann. N.Y. Acad. Sci.* **63**:793–816.

KOLLER, P. C., 1972, *Recent Results in Cancer Research*, Vol. 38: *The Role of Chromosomes in Cancer Biology*, Springer, New York.

KRAEMER, P. M., PETERSON, D. F., AND VAN DILLA, M. A., 1971, DNA constancy in heteroploidy and the stem line theory of tumors, *Science* **174**:714–717.

KUBINSKI, H., AND SZYBALSKI, E. H., 1974, Effects of beta-propiolactone on the conformation of DNA, *Am. Assoc. Cancer Res. Proc.* **15**:49.

KURITA, Y., SUGIYAMA, T., AND NISHIZUKA, Y., 1968, Cytogenetic studies on rat leukemia induced by pulse doses of 7,12-dimethylbenz(alpha)anthracene, *Cancer Res.* **28**:1738–1752.

LAMB, D., 1967, Correlation of chromosome counts with histological appearances and prognosis in transitional-cell carcinoma of the bladder, *Br. Med. J.* **1**:273–277.

LAWLER, S. D., MILLARD, R. E., AND KAY, H. E. M., 1970, Further cytogenetical investigations in polycythaemia vera, *Eur. J. Cancer* **6**:223–233.

LEGATOR, M. S., AND MALLING, H. V., 1971, The host-mediated assay. A practical procedure for evaluating potential mutagenic agents in mammals, in: *Chemical Mutagens*, Vol. 2 (A. Hollaender, ed.), pp. 569–589, Plenum Press, New York.

LEHMAN, J. M., AND DEFENDI, V., 1970, Changes in deoxyribonucleic acid synthesis regulation in Chinese hamster cells infected with simian virus 40, *J. Virol.* **6**:738–749.

LEHMAN, J. M., MAUEL, J., AND DEFENDI, V., 1971, Regulation of DNA synthesis in macrophages infected with simian virus 40, *Exp. Cell Res.* **67**:230–233.

LEMONE YIELDING, K., 1974, A model for aging based on differential repair of somatic mutational damage, *Perspect. Biol. Med.* **17**:201–207.

LEUCHTENBERGER, C., LEUCHTENBERGER, R., AND DAVIS, A. M., 1954, A microspectrophotometric study of the desoxyribose nucleic acid (DNA) content in cells of normal and malignant human tissues, *Am. J. Pathol.* **30**:65–85.

LEVAN, A., 1973, Chromosome patterns in tumors, *Nobel Symp.* **23**:217–229.

LEVAN, A., AND BIESELE, J. J., 1958, Role of chromosomes in carcinogenesis, as studied in serial tissue culture of mammalian cells, *Ann. N.Y. Acad. Sci.* **71**:1022–1053.

LEVAN, A., AND HAUSCHKA, T. S., 1953, Endomitotic reduplication mechanisms in ascites tumors of the mouse, *J. Natl. Cancer Inst. U.S.A.* **14**:1–42.

LEWIS, E. B., 1957, Leukemia and ionizing radiation *Science* **125**:965–972.

LINDER, D., AND GARTLER, S. M., 1965, Glucose-6-phosphate dehydrogenase mosaicism, utilization as a cell marker in the study of leiomyomas, *Science*, **150**:67–69.

LITTLEFIELD, J. W., 1963, The inosinic acid pyrophosphorylase activity of mouse fibroblasts partially resistant to 8-azaguanine, *Proc. Natl. Acad. Sci. U.S.A.* **50**:568–575.

LITTON, L. E., HOLLANDER, D. H., BORGAONKAR, D. S., AND FROST, J. K., 1972, Y chromatin of interphase cancer cells: A preliminary study, *Acta Cytol.* **16**:404–407.

LUBS, H. A., AND KOTLER, S., 1967, The prognostic significance of chromosome abnormalities in colon tumors, *Ann. Intern. Med.* **67**:328–336.

MACKENZIE, I., AND ROUS, P., 1941, The experimental disclosure of latent neoplastic changes in tarred skin. *J. Exp. Med.* **73**:391–415.

MACSWEEN, R. N. M., 1965, Reticulum-cell sarcoma and rheumatoid arthritis in a patient with XY/XXY/XXXY Klinefelter's syndrome and normal intelligence, *Lancet*, **1**:460–461.

MAKINO, S., 1956, Further evidence favoring the concept of the stem cell in ascites tumors of rats, *Ann. N.Y. Acad. Sci.* **63**:818–830.

MAMUNES, P., LAPIDUS, P. H., ABBOTT, J. A., AND ROATH, S., 1961, Acute leukemia and Klinefelter's syndrome, *Lancet* **2**:26–27.

MANNER, G., 1971, Cell division and collagen synthesis in cultured fibroblasts, *Exp. Cell Res.* **65**:49–60.

MANOLOV, G., AND MANOLOVA, Y., 1972, Marker band in one chromosome 14 from Burkitt lymphomas, *Nature (London)* **237**:33–34.

MARCH, H. C., 1961, Leukemia in radiologists, ten years later, *Am. J. Med. Sci.* **242**:137–147.

MARK, J., 1971, Chromosomal characteristics of neurogenic tumors in adults, *Hereditas* **68**:61–100.

MARK, J., LEVAN, G., AND MITELMAN, F., 1972, Identification by fluorescence of the G chromosome lost in human meningiomas, *Hereditas* **71**:163–168.

MARKERT, C. L., 1968, Neoplasia, a disease of cell differentiation, *Cancer Res.* **28**:1908–1914.

MÅRTENSSON, L., 1963, On "a key point of modern biochemical genetics," *Lancet* **1**:946–947.

MARTIN, G. M., AND SPRAGUE, C. A., 1969, Parasexual cycle in cultivated human somatic cells, *Science* **166**:761–763.

MARTLAND, H. S., 1931, The occurrence of malignancy in radioactive persons: A general review of data gathered in the study of the radium dial painters, with special reference to the occurrence of osteogenic sarcoma and the inter-relationship of certain blood diseases, *Am. J. Cancer* **15**:2435–2516.

METIVIER, H., NOLIBE, D., MASSE, R., AND LAFUMA, J., 1972, Cancers provoqués chez le Singe Babouin (*Papio papio*) par inhalation de PuO$_2$, *C. R. Acad. Sci. Ser. D* **275**:3069–3071.

MILES, C. P., 1967a, Chromosome analysis of solid tumors. I. Twenty-eight nonepithelial tumors, *Cancer* **20**:1253–1273.

MILES, C. P., 1967b, Chromosome analysis of solid tumors. II. Twenty-six epithelial tumors, *Cancer* **20**:1274–1287.

MILLER, E. C., AND MILLER, J. A., 1971, The mutagenicity of chemical carcinogens: Correlations, problems, and interpretations, in: *Chemical Mutagens*, Vol. I (A. Hollaender, ed.), pp. 83–119, Plenum Press, New York.

MILLER, O. J., MILLER, D. A., KOURI, R. E., ALLDERDICE, P. W., DEV, V. G., GREWAL, M. S., AND HUTTON, J. J., 1971, Identification of the mouse karyotype by quinacrine fluorescence, and tentative assignment of seven linkage groups, *Proc. Natl. Acad. Sci. U.S.A.* **68**:1530–1533.

MITELMAN, F., 1971, The chromosomes of fifty primary Rous rat sarcomas, *Hereditas* **69**:155–186.

MITELMAN, F., MARK, J., LEVAN, G., AND LEVAN, A., 1972, Tumor etiology and chromosome pattern, *Science* **176**:1340–1341.

MOORHEAD, P. S., AND SAKSELA, E., 1965, The sequence of chromosome aberrations during SV40 transformation of a human diploid cell, *Hereditas* **52**:271–284.

MORIWAKI, K., IMAI, H. T., YAMASHITA, J., AND YOSIDA, T. H., 1971, Ploidy fluctuations of mouse plasma-cell neoplasm MSPC-1 during serial transplantation, *J. Natl. Cancer Inst. U.S.A.* **47**:623–637.

MULLER, H. J., 1928, Measurement of gene mutation rate in *Drosophila*, its high variability, and its dependence upon temperature, *Genetics* **13**:279–357.

MURAYAMA-OKABAYASHI, F., OKADA, Y., AND TACHIBANA, T., 1971, A series of hybrid cells containing different ratios of parental chromosomes formed by two steps of artificial fusion, *Proc. Natl. Acad. Sci. U.S.A.* **68**:38–42.

MURRAY, R. F., HOBBS, J., AND PAYNE, B., 1971, Possible clonal origin of common warts (verruca vulgaris), *Nature (London)* **232**:51–52.

NATHANSON, L., AND FISHMAN, W. H., 1971, New observations on the Regan isoenzyme of alkaline phosphatase in cancer patients, *Cancer* **27**:1388–1397.

National Academy of Sciences–National Research Council, 1956, *The Biological Effects of Atomic Radiation*, Summary Reports, Washington, D.C.

NEEL, J. V., 1972, The detection of increased mutation rates in human populations, in: *Mutagenic Effects of Environmental Contaminants* (H. E. Sutton and M. I. Harris, eds.), pp. 99–119, Academic Press, New York.

NELSON-REES, W. A., FLANDERMEYER, R. R., AND HAWTHORNE, P. K., 1974, Banded marker chromosomes as indicators of intraspecies cellular contamination, *Science* **187**:1093–1096.

NICHOLS, W. W., 1963, Relationships of viruses, chromosomes and carcinogenesis, *Hereditas* **50**:53–80.

NICHOLS, W. W., 1966, The role of viruses in the etiology of chromosomal abnormalities, *Am. J. Hum. Genet.* **18**:81–92.

NOWELL, P. C., AND HUNGERFORD, D. A., 1960, A minute chromosome in human chronic granulocytic leukemia, *Science* **132**:1497.

NOWELL, P. C., MORRIS, H. P., AND POTTER, V. R., 1967, Chromosomes of "minimal deviation" hepatomas and some other transplantable rat tumors, *Cancer Res.* **27**:1565–1579.

OHANIAN, S. H., TAUBMAN, S. B., AND THORBECKE, G. J., 1969, Rates of albumin and transferrin synthesis *in vitro* in rat hepatoma-derived H₄II-EC₃ cells, *J. Natl. Cancer Inst. U.S.A.* **43**:397–406.

OHNO, S., 1969, The spontaneous mutation rate revisited, and the possible principle of polymorphism generating more polymorphism, *Can. J. Genet. Cytol.* **11**:457–467.

OHNO, S., 1971, Genetic implication of karyological instability of malignant somatic cells, *Physiol. Rev.* **51**:496–526.

OLD, L. J., BOYSE, E. A., CLARKE, D. A., AND CARSWELL, E. A., 1962, Antigenic properties of chemically induced tumors, *Ann. N.Y. Acad. Sci.* **101**:80–106.

PATIL, S. R., MERRICK, S., AND LUBS, H. A., 1971, Identification of each human chromosome with a modified "Giemsa" stain, *Science* **173**:821–822.

PEDERSEN, B., 1973, The blastic crisis of chronic myeloid leukemia, acute transformation of a pre-leukaemic condition, *Br. J. Haematol.* **25**:141–145.

PERA, F., 1974, personal communication, Anatom. Institut der Universität Bonn, West Germany.

PFEIFFER, S. E., HERSCHMAN, H. R., LIGHTBODY, J., AND SATO, G., 1970, Synthesis by a clonal line of rat glial cells of a protein unique to the nervous system, *J. Cell. Physiol.* **75**:329–340.

PIERCE, G. B., 1967, Teratocarcinoma: Model for a developmental concept of cancer, *Curr. Top. Dev. Biol.* **2**:223–246.

POLLACK, R. E., GREEN, H., AND TODARO, G. J., 1968, Growth control in cultured cells: Selection of sublines with increased sensitivity to contact inhibition and decreased tumor-producing ability, *Proc. Natl. Acad. Sci. U.S.A.* **60**:126–133.

POLLACK, R., WOLMAN, S., AND VOGEL, A., 1970, Reversion of virus-transformed cell lines: Hyperploidy accompanies retention of viral genes, *Nature (London)* **228**:938, 967–970.

POOL, R. R., WILLIAMS, R. J. R., AND GOLDMAN, M., 1973, Induction of tumor involving bone in beagles fed toxic levels of strontium 90, *Am. J. Roentgenol.* **118**:900–908.

POON, P. K., O'BRIEN, R. L., AND PARKER, J. W., 1974, Defective DNA repair in Fanconi's anaemia, *Nature (London)* **250**:223–225.

PORTER, I. H., BENEDICT, W. F., BROWN, C. D., AND PAUL, B., 1969, Recent advances in molecular pathology: A review. Some aspects of chromosome changes in cancer, *Exp. Mol. Pathol.* **11**:340–367.

POVEY, S., GARDINER, S. E., WATSON, B., MOWBRAY, S., HARRIS, H., ARTHUR, E., STEEL, C. M., BLENKINSOP, C., AND EVANS, H. J., 1973, Genetic studies on human lymphoblastoid lines; isozyme analysis on cell lines from forty-one different individuals and on mutants produced following exposure to a chemical mutagen, *Ann. Hum. Genet.* **36**:247–266.

PREHN, R. T., AND MAIN, J. M., 1957, Immunity to methylcholanthrene-induced sarcomas, *J. Natl. Cancer Inst. U.S.A.* **18**:769–778.

PREUD'HOMME, J. L., AND SELIGMAN, M., 1972, Surface bound immunoglobulins as a cell marker in human lymphoproliferative diseases, *Blood* **40**:777–794.

PRIEST, R. E., AND DAVIES, L. M., 1969, Cellular proliferation and synthesis of collagen, *Lab. Invest.* **21**:138–142.

REEVES, B. R., LOBB, D. S., AND LAWLER, S. D., 1972, Identity of the abnormal F-group chromosome associated with polycythaemia vera, *Humangenetik* **14**:159–161.

RIEGER, R., MICHAELIS, A., AND GREEN, M. M., 1968, *A Glossary of Genetics and Cytogenetics*, Springer, New York.

ROTHSCHILD, H., AND BLACK, P. H., 1970, Effect of loss of thymidine kinase activity on the tumorigenicity of clones of SV40-transformed hamster cells, *Proc. Natl. Acad. Sci. U.S.A.* **67**:1042–1049.

ROWE, W. P., 1973, Genetic factors in the natural history of murine leukemia virus infection: G. H. A. Clowes memorial lecture, *Cancer Res.* **33**:3061–3068.

ROWLEY, J. D., 1973, A new consistent chromosomal abnormality in chronic myelogenous leukemia identified by quinacrine fluorescence and Giemsa staining, *Nature (London)* **234**:290–293.

ROWLEY, J. D., AND BODMER, W. F., 1971, Relationship of centromeric heterochromatin to fluorescence banding patterns of metaphase chromosomes in the mouse, *Nature (London)* **231**:503–506.

RUNDLES, R. W., 1972, Chronic granulocytic leukemia, in: *Hematology* (W. J. Williams, E. Beutler, A. J. Erslev, and R. W. Rundles, eds.), pp. 680–695, McGraw-Hill, New York.

SAKSELA, E., AND MOORHEAD, P. S., 1963, Aneuploidy in the degenerative phase of serial cultivation of human cell strains, *Proc. Natl. Acad. Sci. U.S.A.* **50**:390–395.

SANDBERG, A. A., 1974, Chromosome changes in human malignant tumors, an evaluation, in: *Recent Results in Cancer Research*, Vol. 44: *Special Topics in Carcinogenesis* (E. Grundmann, ed.), pp. 75–85, Springer, New York.

SANDBERG, A. A., AND HOSSFELD, D. K., 1970, Chromosomal abnormalities in human neoplasia, *Ann. Rev. Med.* **21**:379–408.

SANDBERG, A. A., AND HOSSFELD, D. K., 1973, Chromosomes in the pathogenesis of human cancer and leukemia, in: *Cancer Medicine* (J. F. Holland and E. Frei, eds.), pp. 165–177, Lea and Febiger, Philadelphia.

SANDBERG, A. A., AND SAKURAI, M., 1973, The missing Y chromosome and human leukaemia, *Lancet* **1**:375.

SATO, K., SLESINSKI, R. S., AND LITTLEFIELD, J. W., 1972, Chemical mutagenesis at the phosphoribosyl-transferase locus in cultured human lymphoblasts, *Proc. Natl. Acad. Sci. U.S.A.* **69**:1224–1248.

SAWADA, H., GILMORE, V. H., AND SAUNDERS, G. F., 1973, Transcription from chromatins of human lymphocytic leukemia cells and normal lymphocytes, *Cancer Res.* **33**:428–434.

SAWITSKY, A., BLOOM, D., AND GERMAN, J., 1966, Chromosomal breakage and acute leukemia in congenital telangiectatic erythema and stunted growth, *Ann. Intern. Med.* **65**:487–495.

SCALETTA, L. J., AND EPHRUSSI, B., 1965, Hybridization of normal and neoplastic cells *in vitro, Nature (London)* **205**:1169.

SEABRIGHT, M., 1972, The use of proteolytic enzymes for the mapping of structural rearrangements in the chromosomes of man, *Chromosoma* **36**:204–210.

SEGALL, M., SHAPIRO, L. R., FREEDMAN, W., AND BOONE, J. A., 1973, X0/XY gonadal dysgenesis and gonadoblastoma in childhood, *Obstet. Gynecol.* **41**:536–541.

SETLOW, R. B., REGAN, J. D., GERMAN, J., AND CARRIER, W. L., 1969, Evidence that xeroderma pigmentosum cells do not perform the first step in the repair of ultraviolet damage to their DNA, *Proc. Natl. Acad. Sci. U.S.A.* **64**:1035–1041.

SHAW, C. R., 1965, Electrophoretic variation in enzymes, *Science* **149**:936–943.

SHAW, M. W., AND CHEN, T. R., 1974, The application of banding techniques to tumor chromosomes, in: *Chromosomes and Cancer* (J. German, ed.), Wiley, New York.

SILAGI, S., AND BRUCE, S. A., 1970, Suppression of malignancy and differentiation in melanotic melanoma cells, *Proc. Natl. Acad. Sci. U.S.A.* **66**:72–78.

SINKOVICS, J. G., DREWINKO, B., AND THORNELL, E., 1970, Immunoresistant tetraploid lymphoma cells, *Lancet* **1**:139–140.

SIVAK, A., AND VAN DUUREN, B. L., 1968, Studies with carcinogens and tumor-promoting agents in cell culture, *Exp. Cell Res.* **49**:572–583.

SPARROW, A. H., AND GUNCKEL, J. E., 1955, The effects on plants of chronic exposure to gamma radiation from radiocobalt, in: *Proceedings of the International Conference on the Peaceful Uses of Atomic Energy*, Vol. 12, pp. 52–59, United Nations, Geneva.

SPIEGELMAN, S., AXEL, A., BAXT, W., GULATI, S. C., HEHLMANN, R., KUFE, D., AND SCHLOM, J., 1973, Molecular evidence for a viral etiology of human cancer, in: *Seventh National Cancer Conference Proceeding* (S. L. Arje, coordinator), pp. 21–41, Lippincott, Philadelphia.

SPRIGGS, A. I., BODDINGTON, M. M., AND CLARKE, C. M., 1962, Chromosomes of human cancer cells, *Br. Med. J.* **2**:1431–1435.

STICH, H. F., 1973, Oncogenic and nononcogenic mutants of adenovirus 12: Induction of chromosome aberrations and cell divisions, *Prog. Exp. Tumor Res.* **18**:260–272.

STICH, H. F., AND YOHN, D. S., 1965, Viruses and mammalian chromosomes. V. Chromosome aberrations in tumors of Syrian hamsters induced by adenovirus type 12, *J. Natl. Cancer Inst. U.S.A.* **35**:603–615.

STRAUSS, B. S., 1971, Physical-chemical methods for the detection of the effect of mutagens on DNA, in: *Chemical Mutagens*, Vol. I (A. Hollaender, ed.), pp. 145–174, Plenum Press, New York.

STRAUSS, B. S., AND ROBBINS, M., 1968, DNA methylated *in vitro* by a monofunctional alkylating agent as a substrate for a specific nuclease from *Micrococcus lysodeikticus, Biochim. Biophys. Acta* **161**:68–75.

SUMNER, A. T., EVANS, H. J., AND BUCKLAND, R. A., 1971, New techniques for distinguishing between human chromosomes, *Nature New Biol.* **232**:31–32.

SWANSON, C. P., MERZ, T., AND YOUNG, W. J., 1967, Variation: Sources and consequences involving chromosomal numbers, in: *Cytogenetics*, pp. 125–143, Prentice-Hall, Englewood Cliffs, N.J.

SWIFT, M. R., AND HIRSCHHORN, K., 1966, Fanconi's anemia: Inherited susceptibility to chromosome breakage in various tissues, *Ann. Intern. Med.* **65**:496–503.

SYBENGA, J., 1972, Numerical variants, in: *General Cytogenetics*, pp. 213–281, American Elsevier, New York.

TEEBOR, G., AND BECKER, F. F., 1971, Regression and persistence of hyperplastic hepatic nodules induced by *N*-2-fluorenylacetamide and their relationship to hepatocarcinogenesis, *Cancer Res.* **31**:1–3.

TETER, J., AND BOCZKOWSKI, K., 1967, Occurrence of tumors in dysgenetic gonads, *Cancer* **20:**1301–1310.

TJIO, J. H., AND LEVAN, A., 1956, The chromosome number of man, *Hereditas* **42:**1–6.

TJIO, J. H., AND OSTERGREN, G., 1958, The chromosomes of primary mammary carcinomas in milk virus strains of the mouse, *Hereditas* **44:**451–465.

TODARO, G. J., WOLMAN, S. R., AND GREEN, H., 1963a, Rapid transformation of human fibroblasts with low growth potential into established cell lines by SV-40, *J. Cell. Comp. Physiol.* **62:**257–265.

TODARO, G. J., NILAUSEN, K., AND GREEN, H., 1963b, Growth properties of polyoma virus-induced hamster tumor cells, *Cancer Res.* **23:**825–832.

TOEWS, H. A., KATAYAMA, K. P., MASUKAWA, T. M., AND LEWISON, E. F., 1968, Chromosomes of benign and malignant lesions of the breast, *Cancer* **22:**1296–1307.

TRUJILLO, J. M., CORK, A., HART, J. S., GEORGE, S. L., AND FREIREICH, E. J., 1974, Clinical implications of aneuploid cytogenetic profiles in adult acute leukemia, *Cancer* **33:**824–831.

VAN DILLA, M. A., TRUJILLO, T. T., MULLANEY, P. F., AND COULTER, J. R., 1969, Cell microfluorometry, a method for rapid fluorescence measurement, *Science* **163:**1213–1214.

VAN DUUREN, B. L., 1969, The interaction of some mutagenic and carcinogenic agents with nucleic acids, in: *Physico-chemical Mechanisms of Carcinogenesis* (E. D. Bergmann and B. Pullman, eds.), pp. 149–158, Israeli Acad. Sci. Humanities.

VAN DUUREN, B. L., AND SIVAK, A., 1968, Tumor-promoting agents from *Croton tiglium L.* and their mode of action, *Cancer Res.* **28:**2349–2356.

VOGT, M., AND DULBECCO, R., 1963, Steps in the neoplastic transformation of hamster embryo cells by polyoma virus, *Proc. Natl. Acad. Sci. U.S.A.* **49:**171–179.

VON HANSEMANN, D., 1890, Über asymmetrische Zellteilung in Epithelkrebsen und deren biologische Bedeutung, *Virchow's Arch. Pathol. Anat.* **119:**299–326.

WALD, N., BORGES, W. H., LI, C. C., TURNER, J. H., AND HARNOIS, M. C., 1961, Leukaemia associated with mongolism, *Lancet* **1:**1228.

WANEBO, C. K., JOHNSON, K. G., SATO, K., AND THORSLUND, T. W., 1968, Lung cancer following atomic radiation, *Am. Rev. Resp. Dis.* **98:**778–787.

WESTPHAL, H., AND DULBECCO, R., 1968, Viral DNA in polyoma and SV-40 transformed cell lines, *Proc. Natl. Acad. Sci. U.S.A.* **59:**1158–1165.

WHANG, J. P., CANELLOS, G. P., CARBONE, P. P., AND TJIO, J. H., 1968, Clinical implications of cytogenetic variants in chronic myelocytic leukemia (CML), *Blood* **32:**755–766.

WIENER, F., KLEIN, G., AND HARRIS, H., 1971, The analysis of malignancy by cell fusion. III. Hybrids between diploid fibroblasts and other tumor cells, *J. Cell Sci.* **8:**681–692.

WOLMAN, S. R., HIRSCHHORN, K., AND TODARO, G. J., 1964, Early chromosomal changes in SV-40 infected human fibroblast cultures, *Cytogenetics* **3:**45–61.

WOLMAN, S. R., PHILLIPS, T. F., AND BECKER, F. F., 1972, Fluorescent banding patterns of rat chromosomes in normal and primary hepatocellular carcinomas, *Science* **175:**1267–1269.

WOLMAN, S. R., HORLAND, A. A., AND BECKER, F. F., 1973a, Altered karyotypes of transplantable "diploid" tumors, *J. Natl. Cancer Inst.* **51:**1909–1914.

WOLMAN, S. R., JENG, M., AND BROOME, J. D., 1973b, Selection for structural and karyotypic variants of a mouse lymphoma by 2-mercaptoethanol *in vitro*, *Genetics* **74:**s298–s299.

WOLMAN, S. R., BRAMSON, S., McMORROW, L. M., AND SIVAK, A., 1975, Chromosome damage induced by chemical carcinogens in cultured rat embryo fibroblasts, in preparation.

YASUMURA, Y., BUONASSISI, V., AND SATO, G., 1966, Clonal analysis of differentiated function in animal cell cultures. I. Possible correlated maintenance of differentiated function and the diploid karyotype, *Cancer Res.* **26:**529–535.

YATAGANAS, X., MITOMO, Y., TRAGANOS, F., STRIFE, A., AND CLARKSON, B., 1975, Evaluation of a Feulgen-type reaction in suspension using flow microfluorimetry and a cell separation technique, *Acta Cytol.* **19:**71–78.

YOSHIDA, M. C., AND MAKINO, S., 1963, A chromosome study of non-treated and an irradiated human *in vitro* cell line, *Jpn. J. Hum. Genet.* **8:**39–45.

YOSHIDA, T., 1952, Studies on an ascites (reticulo-endothelial cell?) sarcoma of the rat, *J. Natl. Cancer Inst. U.S.A.* **12:**947–969.

ZANKL, H., AND ZANG, K. D., 1972, Cytological and cytogenetical studies on brain tumors, *Humangenetik* **14:**167–169.

Growth of Tumors

8

Cell Division and Tumor Growth

CHARLES LIGHTDALE AND MARTIN LIPKIN

1. Introduction

In a benign or malignant tumor, cells have escaped from restrictions and controls imposed on their normal growth. The morphological description of tumor growth is based on the kinds of cells that comprise the tumor. Defining how these cells grow is the goal of cell kinetics. The growth process develops from a dynamic, frequently changing, and complex series of events. Cell kinetics provides a "motion picture" type of analysis of what has taken place during growth and complements histology. Further, and most important, it adds a useful dimension to biochemical measurements which attempt to describe regulatory control processes that guide cells through their stages of proliferation and differentiation. Thus, an understanding of the proliferation kinetics of cells has a useful role in defining the expression of neoplastic transformation and the response of cells to therapy.

2. Measurement of Tumor Growth

The simplest means of assessing tumor growth is to make direct serial measurements of tumor size, which can be done in certain experimental and human tumors. In solid tumors, size and weight are the directly measurable parameters. In dispersed or nonsolid tumors, estimates of actual cell numbers can be obtained.

CHARLES LIGHTDALE and MARTIN LIPKIN•Memorial Sloan-Kettering Cancer Center, New York, N.Y.

For example, in the Ehrlich ascites tumor in mice, the number of tumor cells may be quantitated by aspiration and indicator dilution techniques. In solid tumors, estimates of size can sometimes be obtained by external measurement using vernier calipers. Ways of expressing and utilizing the data obtained have varied. They have included measurements of greatest diameter, mean diameter, tumor area using two dimensions, and tumor volume as the product of three dimensions (Lala, 1971). Among these measurements, tumor volume is an important parameter, expressing cell proliferation and tumor growth; however, determining volume or weight from linear measurements poses a practical problem. In an experimental transplantable tumor system in rats, Steel *et al.* (1966) used caliper measurements of the greatest and smallest superficial dimensions. The product of the two measurements termed "tumor area" was actually the area of the rectangle enclosing the tumor. The animals were sacrificed and the tumors removed and weighed. A curve relating tumor weight to "tumor area" was then constructed and used to interpret measurements for the particular tumor involved. Provided that the tumor in question did not change its average shape or growth characteristics, the technique was free from systematic error. The curve, which conformed to a two-thirds power law, could also be used to interpret measurements of other tumors, provided that skin thickness and tumor geometry were similar.

3. Growth Curves

Relating tumor weight to time, using superficial measurements and a calibration curve to determine weight, provides a "growth curve." Usually with weight plotted vertically and time horizontally on semilogarithmic scales, growth curves are convex upwards and flatten out with time. In other words, in most cases the specific growth rate decreases with time (Steel, 1973).

In some situations, however, conventional growth curves form straight lines on a semilog plot. This is exponential growth, the simplest situation. Growth rate as a fraction of tumor size is constant, and the logarithm of tumor volume increases linearly with time. Volume doubling times can be easily calculated from such curves:

$$\text{Specific growth rate} = k = 1/V \cdot dV/dt$$

$$V = V_0\, e^{kt}$$

$$\log V = \log V_0 + kt$$

The growth constant k is equal to $0.693/Td$, where Td is the volume doubling time.

Exponential growth occurs in some cell cultures, ascites tumors, mouse leukemias, and certain transplantable tumor systems in rats. In these situations, a "generation time" is equal to population doubling time, the time for the cell population to increase by a factor of 2.

In other cases, however, tumor growth is smooth but not exponential. Growth
curves can then be fitted with various mathematical functions within the statistical
uncertainty of the measurements. Many attempts have been made to relate a
mathematical expression of growth to most situations in order to delineate a past
history or predict future growth of a tumor. Laird (1969) proposed a modified
exponential law of growth in which successive doublings occur at increasingly
longer intervals. The increase in doubling times is more rapid than explained by
an exponential law, and is better represented by a Gompertz function.

Three parameters are utilized, W_0, initial tumor size, A_0 initial specific
growth rate for the period of observation, and α, the rate of exponential decay of
A_0:

$$W_t = W_0 e[A_0(1-e^{-\alpha t})/\alpha]$$

W_t is tumor size at time t (Laird, 1969). This Gompertz function describes an
asymmetrical type of sigmoidal growth on a linear scale. The inflection point, the
point of maximum growth rate, occurs when the volume is 37% of the final
plateau volume. Laird (1965) and McCredie et al. (1965) demonstrated the
applicability of the Gompertz function to many experimental tumors. Their
computations fit experimental tumor growth better than the previously used
more simple functions.

Dethlefsen et al. (1968) pointed out, however, that in many experiments the
inflection point in the Gompertz curve is not reached before the death of the
animal. In addition, the calculated plateau values for tumor volume may be larger
than the animal by several orders of magnitude. Thus, as Steel (1973) noted, it is
doubtful whether in many cases the Gompertz function has much biological
significance.

Mendelsohn suggested a different equation, which, like the Gompertz formula
uses three parameters:

$$dV/dt = kV^b$$

V is tumor volume, dV/dt is the growth rate, k is a growth constant, and the
exponent b defines the mode of growth (Mendelsohn, 1963; Dethlefsen et al.,
1968). This approach is based on the supposition that tumors can grow in many
ways, exponentially, cube root, linearly, or otherwise, and attempts to fit the data
with a function that allows for this flexibility in behavior. To make an appropriate
estimate of the exponent b, Mendelsohn and colleagues used a computer to
generate a curve that best fit their data. They used this technique to study the C3H
mouse mammary tumor, and found that the average mode of growth was close to
the cube root mode (Mendelsohn, 1963; Mendelsohn and Dethlefsen, 1968;
Dethlefsen et al., 1968).

While Mendelsohn and his colleagues felt their methods provided an additional
tool for the analysis of tumor growth, they have warned against the overinterpre-
tation of tumor growth curves. They emphasize the need for reliable measurements of sufficient number and over a sufficient time (Dethlefsen et al., 1968). The
relative merit of their approach versus the equally complex Gompertz function is

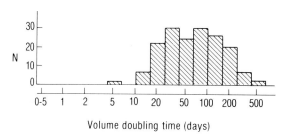

FIGURE 1. Histogram showing the distribution of volume doubling times of a wide variety of primary and secondary human tumors. The wide range of growth rates extends from a doubling time as short as a week to over a year, with the median in the region of 2 months. Redrawn from Steel (1973).

not yet established. As Steel (1973) and Dethlefsen *et al.* (1968) point out, errors are introduced when extrapolations are extended far beyond the measured data. This is mainly because as tumor size changes the equation of tumor growth often changes as well. Spontaneous tumors usually grow in a disorderly, nonsteady, individual manner, making analysis even more difficult than in experimental animal systems.

Spontaneous neoplasms in seven dogs and a cat were studied by Owen and Steel (1969). In most cases, the measurements were made on X-rays of lung metastases. The volume doubling times ranged from 7 to 150 days. Measurements of growth rate have rarely been made in human tumors, which when inoperable are often difficult to measure accurately. Lung tumors or metastases that can be followed by X-ray are the most frequently measured. A few breast, bone, colon, and rectal tumors have also been serially measured. The data obtained on lung tumors show a marked variation. Methods used to measure pulmonary lesions seen on X-ray pictures usually involved a simple vernier caliper or transparent plastic ruler. Tumor volume can be computed as $\pi/6$ times the cube of the mean diameter. Some of these human tumors have a volume doubling time as short as weeks, others over a year, with a median of approximately 2 months (Fig. 1). In some situations in man, lung metastases have shown growth that is essentially exponential over long periods. For the most part, however, human tumors grow differently from experimental transplanted tumors in animals. Steel (1973) compared the volume doubling times of 24 well-studied experimental tumor types with human data. Only three of the experimental animal tumors had a doubling time longer than 14 days, and only 5% of the group of human tumors had a doubling time shorter than 14 days.

4. Cell Kinetics

Clearly, to explain the slow growth of human tumors requires an evaluation of the individual cells comprising these tumors. Possibilities are that some cells are dividing at a slower rate, are partially entering a nondividing dormant state, or are being lost. Understanding tumor growth is based on analyzing these cellular events, and cell kinetic techniques provide an approach to this analysis. The key to the study of cell kinetics is the availability of markers of cell division, which can be used as tools to obtain information about the life history of cells.

The stathmokinetic technique involves the counting of mitotic figures, the most direct means of marking a cell division. The rate of cell production is assumed to be proportional to the number of cells observed in mitosis. An unknown factor, however, is the duration of the mitoses observed. To overcome the uncertainty of mitosis duration, the stathmokinetic method employs agents that have the relatively specific action of producing metaphase arrest, such as colchicine or *Vinca* alkaloids. A dose is selected that blocks all dividing cells during mitosis without disturbing the progression of cells into division. Cell birth rate can then be calculated from the rate of the accumulation of cells in metaphase (Lala, 1971).

The mitotic index or fraction of cells in mitosis in a steady-state situation can be calculated from the equation

$$I_m(t) = I_m(o)[1 + t/t_m]$$

$I_m(t)$ is the mitotic index at time t after a complete mitotic blocking, $I_m(o)$ is the initial mitotic index, and t_m is the mitotic time. From this, mitotic time can be calculated as

$$t_m = I_m(o) \cdot t/[I_m(t) - I_m(o)]$$

and during exponential growth

$$t_m = I_m(o) \cdot t/ln2[I_m(t) - I_m(o)]$$

Knowing mitotic index and mitotic time in any tissue permits calculation of cell birth rate:

$$k_b(\text{birth rate}) = I_m \text{ (fraction of cells in mitosis)}/t_m \text{ (duration of mitosis)}$$

There are many practical difficulties in using metaphase arrest measurements *in vivo*. The stathmokinetic technique has largely been superseded by techniques utilizing the tritium-labeled nucleoside thymidine. The development of this agent marked a new era in the study of cellular kinetics.

4.2. Tritiated Thymidine

Thymidine, a specific precursor for DNA, was successfully synthesized and labeled with tritium in 1957. Thymidine is incorporated into the nuclei of cells which are actively synthesizing new DNA, and the β-particles emitted by decay of tritium can be used to expose a silver grain photographic emulsion to produce a microautoradiograph. The cells that were synthesizing DNA when exposed to tritiated thymidine become permanently tagged because of the high stability of nuclear DNA. When cells divide, the tritium marker is diluted but still carried by the daughter cells.

4.3. Cell Birth Rate

Cell birth rate can be calculated using tritiated thymidine in a manner similar to that described above in stathmokinetic studies. Shortly after injection, the proportion of cells tagged with radiolabeled thymidine is counted to obtain a "labeling index." Birth rate is derived by dividing the labeling index by the duration of DNA synthesis. A correction must be made, however, for expanding cell populations where the distribution of all ages is not uniform (age density distribution). This relates to the fact that in a growing population of cells there is an increased probability of finding cells undergoing DNA synthesis (Steel *et al.*, 1966).

4.4. Turnover Time

"Turnover time" is the reciprocal of the birth rate. Steel (1975) describes this as the time within which the existing rate of cell production would yield a number of cells equal to the original cell population. A similar concept is the "potential doubling time," the time in which the cell number would double if all cells were conserved and new cells proliferated at the same speed (Mendelsohn and Dethlefsen, 1968).

4.5. Intermitotic Time

While it was suspected for some time that DNA synthesis might occur during the interphase between mitoses, this was shown conclusively in the early 1950s using radiolabeled precursors and cytophotometric measurements. Thus, while mitosis is a marker of cell division, the interphase is the focus for understanding the period of DNA synthesis and many aspects of the kinetics of cellular proliferation.

4.6. Labeled Mitoses Technique

The most direct way of determining the intermitotic time of proliferating cells is the fraction or percent labeled mitoses curve introduced by Quastler and Sherman (1959). The technique is widely used and can yield much information about the cell cycle and its components. Tritiated thymidine administered to mammals by intravenous or intraperitoneal routes is incorporated into both normal tissue and tumors only during a brief period (Fig. 2). This allows a pulse label which is short compared to the time required for DNA synthesis. It can be taken as a virtually instantaneous label, forming a cell cohort that is initially synchronous. It is then further assumed that if DNA synthesis occurs cell division will follow. This has been found to be the case in most tissues and tumors. A third assumption is that the dose of radiation used will not harm the cell or affect cell division. Radiation limits have been established by trial. Fourth, it is assumed that essentially all cells in the DNA synthetic phase will be labeled, which seems to be true. A fifth assumption is that there is no significant reutilization of labeled breakdown products, which may not be completely true (Lala, 1971). Other assumptions used in analyzing labeled mitoses curves will be discussed below.

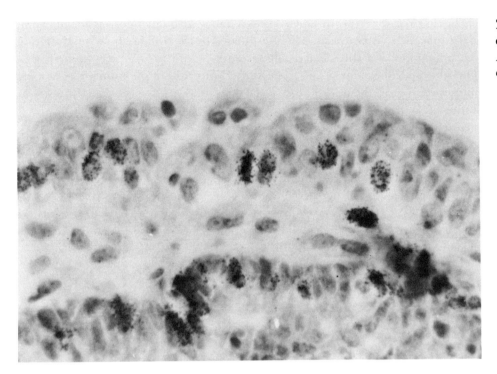

FIGURE 2. Microautoradiograph of an expanding colonic neoplasm of mouse after administration of 1,2-dimethylhydrazine showing epithelial cells labeled with [³H]TdR.

After the labeled thymidine is administered, specimens of tissue are taken at set intervals and microautoradiographs are prepared. There is an initial period when no cells in mitosis are labeled, since these mitotic cells were not synthesizing DNA when the thymidine pulse arrived. Shortly, however, usually within the first two hours, a large number of labeled cells will be observed in mitosis, and then again after a few hours most mitotic figures will become labeled (Fig. 3).

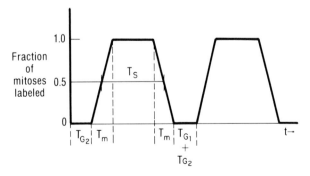

FIGURE 3. Labeled mitoses curve after a pulse injection of [³H]TdR as a function of time, for an ideal steady-state population of identical cells moving uniformly through the cell cycle.

The time required for the labeled cells to move through mitosis is an indication of the time of DNA synthesis. This is estimated by the distance between the rising and falling limbs of the labeled mitoses curve or the area under the first peak (Quastler and Sherman, 1959). The second increase in the number of labeled mitoses represents the next period of cell division. The time between the peaks of counts of labeled mitoses is therefore the intermitotic period. A commonly used method is to measure the 50% level of the first and second rising limbs of the curve to get a somewhat more precise value for intermitotic time.

The sharpness of the peaks reflects the synchrony of the original labeled cell cohort. Since all cells will not initially have taken the same time to synthesize DNA, even the first peak will not be completely sharp, and the second peak may be blurred beyond recognition by loss of synchrony in synthetic time. If a second peak is observed, the sharpness of the second peak in relation to the first indicates the amount of spread in intermitotic time.

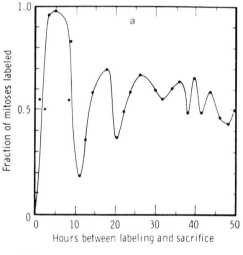

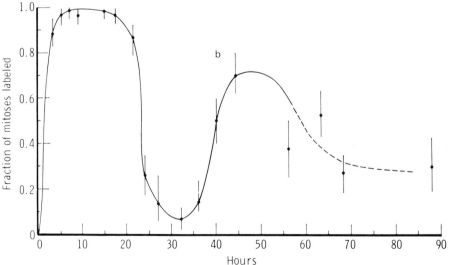

FIGURE 4. Experimental determination of labeled mitoses curves after tritiated thymidine injection into (a) intestine of newborn hamster and (b) normal colon of man.

In order to extract more information from labeled mitoses curves, simulated curves to fit the observed data and mathematical models have been employed. Based on work of Howard and Pelc (1953), the intermitotic time has been divided into stages. The G_1 or first gap is observed after mitosis and before DNA synthesis; the S or DNA synthetic phase follows G_1; the G_2 or second gap comes after DNA synthesis and occurs before mitosis, which is called the M or mitotic phase. The M phase can also be defined as the point in the cycle where one G_2 cell becomes two G_1 cells.

In an idealized situation with a uniform population of proliferating cells, the percentage of labeled mitoses plotted against time would produce periodic trapezoid-shaped curves (Fig. 3). Such waves are never actually seen because of variability in the cell population (Fig. 4). Complex mathematical models have been constructed and computers have been used to fashion model curves by several investigators, including Barrett (1966), Fried (1970), Steel and Hanes (1971), Steel (1972), and Takahashi *et al.* (1971). If a curve fits the experimental data, cycle phase times can be estimated. Steel (1973) and Lipkin and Deschner (1968) have noted that such a curve is acceptable as consistent with the data, but is recognized to be not the only possible analysis. It has been pointed out that there is little evidence to support any assumed form for the distribution of phase durations. Another problem is that cells with long intermitotic times are poorly recognized, since they are seen less in mitosis, and calculated distributions can be an unreliable means of indicating the proportions of these cells (Lala, 1971). However, sophisticated mathematical treatments are not always needed, and median, minimum, and maximum cycle phase times can often be easily measured from labeled mitoses curves.

4.8. Grain Count Halving

If not enough mitotic figures occur to obtain a labeled mitoses curve, the grain count halving technique has been used to estimate cell cycle parameters. As extensively discussed by Fried (1972), the essentials of this technique involve counting grains on interphase cells in microautoradiographs and assuming this number to be halved at mitosis. The technique is subject to a number of possible errors, for which correction factors have been devised. In general, there is a tendency for overestimating cell cycle times, but in some situations the halving procedure may be useful.

4.9. Continuous Labeling

Other methods have been used to gain insight into the stages of the cell cycle. Microspectrophotometric estimates of DNA in the nuclei of individual cells have been employed. There have also been other applications of autoradiographic techniques, for example, continuous labeling with tritiated thymidine. The tagged thymidine is given *in vivo* by continuous infusion or by repeated injections at intervals shorter than the S phase. It is most often used on tissue culture preparations where labeled nucleoside is left in the medium. All the cells must be actively proliferating, so that all the mitotic figures are labeled. Specific cycle times can be calculated. S phase can be estimated by counting at a short interval after tritiated thymidine is administered, the "flash labeling index." Alternatively, in continuous labeling experiments, S phase can be obtained by counting grain saturation in an average cell, or more roughly from the rate of increase in labeling index. In this technique, there is the risk of radiation dosage affecting cell kinetics (Mendelsohn, 1965; Wimber, 1963).

4.10. Double Labeling

The time required for DNA synthesis can also be measured by double-labeling thymidine with two different isotopes, ^3H and ^{14}C. The energy emitted by the β-particles from ^3H is lower than that from ^{14}C. If a thick emulsion is used in making autoradiographs, the exposed silver grains from the two isotopes can be distinguished at different levels. Wimber (1963) and Lala (1968) used this technique in a variety of experiments, combining *in vivo* and *in vitro* labeling to study the flux of cells into and out of DNA synthesis. While reliable S-phase times can be estimated, there seems to be no advantage over labeled mitoses experiments which estimate all cycle phases.

4.11. Combined Methods

Another means of obtaining information on the components of the cell cycle is to combine the use of stathmokinetic and labeling methods. In this way, continuous labeling with [^3H]thymidine, in the presence of a mitotic arrest agent in tissue culture, allows an accumulation of labeled cells in mitosis. Cells synthesize DNA and move into mitosis but do not return to G_1. A plateau is observed when all G_1 cells have moved into S. It must be assumed that the mitotic block is complete and that there is no degeneration of cells arrested in metaphase (Puck and Steffen, 1963; Lala, 1971).

In relating tumor growth to cell proliferation, factors other than the characteristics of the dividing cells or intermitotic time must be considered. First, all the cells in the tumor will not be dividing, and second, many of the tumor cells will be lost. The nondividing cells can be of several types. At some point, cells that were dividing may reach a mature, sterile, or vegetative state, where they continue to survive but not proliferate. Another type of nondividing cell, however, is in a resting state, retaining the ability to proliferate when the proper stimulus is received. These cells are in a "G_0" phase. Other cells may not actually be in a resting state, but their proliferation may be inhibited by factors such as a lack of sufficient nutrients. Most of these cells will have G_1 DNA content, although in some tissues, such as epidermis and esophagus, some cells have been shown to enter a resting state after DNA synthesis and are in the G_2 phase. In any case, the percentage of cells in a tumor that are proliferating can vary a great deal between tumors and in the same tumor as it ages.

5. Growth Fraction

Mendelsohn (1960, 1962) has proposed the concept of "growth fraction" to indicate the proportion of proliferating tumor cells. "Proliferative index" has also been used to express this concept, which is important in understanding tumor growth. There is no way to histologically distinguish those cells which have the ability to proliferate. The usual method of estimating growth fraction utilizes labeled mitoses techniques. The growth fraction denotes the fraction of proliferating cells in the whole population of cells.

Steel (1973) has pointed out that a major problem in estimating the growth fraction in this manner is that cells with very long intermitotic times will be misclassified as nondividing cells. However, the growth fraction concept is still useful if this bias is not overlooked and it is recognized that it is an estimate based on assumptions made in creating a mathematical model. Combination of tritium labeling and mitotic arrest techniques may also be useful in differentiating a long G_1 from the G_0 phase. Bresciani (1968) has introduced a concept of "distribution ratio" directly related to growth fraction, and representing the ratio of the "newborn cells" remaining in the cycling stage to those losing their ability to proliferate after each cycle. Unlimited growth occurs when the "d ratio" is greater than 1.

6. Clonogenic Cells

It must also be noted that all cycling cells are not the same. Some will have a limited capacity to divide, for example, over only several generations. Other cells have the potential to produce an unlimited line of descendents. These are the so-called stem cells or clonogenic cells, because each cell has the ability to form an isolated clone. Both proliferating cells and cells in a G_0 state may have clonogenic potential. Unfortunately, there is at present no technique that has been able to define those tumor cells which are clonogenic (Steel, 1973). This represents a marked limitation in ability to completely define cell proliferation in any tumor system.

7. Cell Loss

While intermitotic time and growth fraction are the major determinants of the input to tumor growth, the output or cell loss factor must be considered to complete the dynamic picture. In some situations, cell loss becomes a major factor in determining growth rate.

The primary way to measure the overall rate of cell loss is from the discrepancy between the potential doubling time calculated from thymidine labeling and measurements of tumor growth rate. Steel has proposed the expression of cell loss as a factor ϕ, the ratio of cell loss to birth rate, indicating the effect of cell loss on production. This quantitates the loss of growth potential by the tumor (Steel, 1967). Mathematical expressions accounting for cell loss have been reviewed by Steel (1968) and Lala (1971). Cells may be lost by a variety of means, including cell death, exfoliation, migration, or metastases. Cell death in tumors may be caused by disorganized cellular architecture, with cells unable to receive essential metabolites. Areas of necrosis in tumors may cause death of adjacent cells by diffusion of cytotoxic materials. Abnormal mitoses may produce cells incapable of survival. Information on the mode of cell loss can be obtained by combining data from repeated labeling experiments with knowledge of cell cycle durations, growth fractions, and rate of overall cell loss. Models assuming different possibilities can then be constructed and best-fit curves found.

8. Growth Coefficient

We have recently developed a kinetic parameter to measure the fraction of proliferating cells retained in expanding neoplasms. In precancerous colonic growth in man, epithelial cells undergo malignant transformation with increasing frequency as the size of the excrescences increases. Further, during transformation some of the cells acquire new properties that enable them to accumulate in increasing numbers in the expanding lesions. Therefore, it is of particular interest to monitor the number of proliferating cells retained in these expanding neoplasms, for the development of malignancy will be related to that portion of the proliferating cell population. In a recent study of an individual with inherited adenomatosis of the colon and rectum, the birth rate of cells (k_b) and growth rate of lesions (k_g) were measured in cells per hour per cell. The *growth coefficient* (k_g/k_b) indicated that one-fourth of the cells born had developed properties enabling them to be retained in expanding colonic polyps and three-fourths of the new cells were extruded.

9. Experimental and Human Tumors

In practical terms, a wide number of different kinetic situations have been found to exist among different natural and experimental tumors. The goal of an ideal kinetic study is to measure and describe all the parameters that define growth. Several models have been proposed on the basis of combining the major possibilities, and these have been reviewed by Mendelsohn and Dethlefsen (1968).

In normal tissues with steady-state or constant cell renewal, such as hematopoietic or intestinal tissue, there is a movement of cells from a stem-cell component through a proliferating stage to a mature-cell stage which is finally lost (Lipkin, 1971). In a well-differentiated carcinoma, the process is similar except, of course, that an excess of cell production over cell loss causes growth. On the other extreme is an undifferentiated tumor, in which normal cell production has stopped and all cell loss is by necrosis and death. In another situation, all cells produced may be conserved in a simple expanding population. There is a continuous spectrum with respect to these properties.

In many human tumors, unlike experimental transplantable tumors, ascites tumors, or cell cultures, the growth fraction is quite low, generally less than 50%. In many tumors, slow growth is also the result of a close competition between cell production and cell loss. In many aging tumors, an increasing number of cells can enter a G_0 phase, and cell populations become less homogeneous (Steel, 1973). While a reduction of intermitotic time is a potential factor in slowing growth rate, this has not been found to occur in several different tumors. Tannock (1968) has shown in an experimental system, the mouse mammary tumor, that intermitotic time stayed in the same range as proliferating cells migrated from a region close to a blood vessel to one near a necrotic area. This work suggests that growth fraction and cell loss are usually the most important influences on solid tumor growth rate. This is not uniformly the case, however. For example, in mouse ascites tumors, the mitotic cell cycle time does increase with age, along with a decline in growth fraction. Increase in cell loss is significant here only in a late stage (Frindel et al., 1969).

A number of kinetic experiments have been performed to study tissues during the induction of neoplasia and to compare spontaneous tumors and normal tissues. In many situations, intermitotic time decreases during carcinogenesis, but this seems to be a nonspecific effect. Probably more important, the growth fraction in most cases increases. Again, human solid tumors are characterized by slow growth, sometimes proliferating less rapidly than some of the normal renewing tissues. One of the most important features of human tumors seems to be a very large rate of cell loss.

Cell kinetic studies relating exposure of tumors to therapeutic agents have led to new understanding of this area. For example, it has been shown that radiation causes a G_2 arrest in cells, most of which recover. While those cells continue to proliferate, many are doomed after subsequent cycles. Unlike normal tissues, some tumor cells have been found to have a prolonged intermitotic time after recovery from G_2 block, mainly due to a lengthening of the G_1 phase (Steel, 1973; Hermens and Barendsen, 1967; Mendelsohn, 1967).

The spleen colony and the L-1210 mouse leukemia models have been extensively studied for kinetic changes after chemotherapy. Much has been learned about the effects of various drugs. For example, in the leukemia model, chemotherapeutic agents toxic to cells in S phase have been found to be very effective, and follow first-order kinetics in their cytotoxicity. These S-phase-specific agents, however, are less effective in solid tumors where fewer clonogenic cells enter S phase per unit time (Skipper and Schnabel, 1973). Clarkson *et al.* (1965) have pointed out the difficulty in treating human cancers where some tumor cells are proliferating more slowly than some normal tissues. Thus rapidly dividing cells of the intestinal epithelium and bone marrow are subject to "toxic" damage by agents which may not at all affect dormant tumor cells with proliferative potential.

Such cell kinetic information should be useful in the design of improved combined therapeutic approaches to cancer (Simpson, Herren and Lloyd, 1970). As suggested by Steel (1973), the major goal of tumor kinetic studies, perhaps, has become a better definition of the clonogenic cell, its relation to the neoplastic stem cell, and its vulnerability to therapeutic agents.

10. References

BARRETT, J. C., 1966, A mathematical model of the mitotic cycle and its application to the interpretation of percentage labelled mitoses data, *J. Natl. Cancer Inst.* **37**:443–450.

BRESCIANI, F., 1968, Cell proliferation in cancer, *Eur. J. Cancer* **4**:343–366.

CLARKSON, B., OTA, R., OKAHITO, T., AND O'CONNOR, A., 1965, Kinetics of proliferation of cancer cells in neoplastic effusions in man, *Cancer* **18**:1189–1213.

DETHLEFSEN, L. A., PREWITT, J. M. S., AND MENDELSOHN, M. L., 1968, Analysis of tumor growth curves, *J. Natl. Cancer Inst.* **40**:389–405.

FRIED, J., 1970, A mathematical model to aid in the interpretation of radioactive tracer data from proliferating cell populations, *Math. Biosci.* **8**:379–396.

FRIED, J., 1972, Proposal for the determination of generation time variability and dormancy of proliferating cell populations by a modification of the grain-count halving method, *J. Theor. Biol.* **34**:535–555.

FRINDEL, E., VALLERON, A., VASSORT, F., AND TUBIANA, M., 1969, Proliferation kinetics of an experimental ascites tumor of the mouse, *Cell Tissue Kinet.* **2**:51–65.

HERMENS, A. F., AND BARENDSEN, G. W., 1967, Cellular proliferation patterns in an experimental rhabdomyosarcoma in the rat, *Eur. J. Cancer* **3**:361–369.

HOWARD, A., AND PELC, S. R., 1953, Synthesis of deoxyribonucleic acid in normal and irradiated cells and its relation to chromosome breakage, *Heredity Suppl.* **6**:261–273.

LAIRD, A. K., 1965, Dynamics of tumor growth, *Br. J. Cancer* **19**:278–291.

LAIRD, A. K., 1969, Dynamics of growth in tumors and in normal organisms, *Natl. Cancer Inst. Monog.* **30**:15–29.

LALA, P. K., 1968, Measurement of S period in growing cell populations by a graphic analysis of double labeling with ^{3}H- and ^{14}C-thymidine, *Exp. Cell Res.* **50**:459–563.

LALA, P. K., 1971, Studies on tumor cell population kinetics, in: *Methods in Cancer Research*, Vol. 6, (H. Busch, ed.), pp. 4–93, Academic Press, New York.

LIPKIN, M., 1971, The proliferative cycle of mammalian cells, in: *The Cell Cycle and Cancer* (R. Baserga, ed.), pp. 1–26, Dekker, New York.

LIPKIN, M., AND DESCHNER, E., 1968, Comparative analysis of cell proliferation in the gastrointestinal tract of newborn hamsters, *Exp. Cell Res.* **49**:1–12.

MCCREDIE, J. A., INCH, W. R., KRUUV, J., AND WATSON, T. A., 1965, The rate of tumor growth in animals, *Growth* **29**:331–347.

MENDELSOHN, M. L., 1960, The growth fraction: A new concept applied to tumors, *Science* **132**:1496.

MENDELSOHN, M. L., 1962, Autoradiographic analysis of cell proliferation in spontaneous breast cancer of C3H mouse. III. The growth fraction, *J. Natl. Cancer Inst.* **28**:1015–1029.

MENDELSOHN, M. L., 1963, Cell proliferation and tumor growth, in: *Cell Proliferation* (L. F., Lammerton and R. J. M. Fry, eds.), pp. 190–212, Blackwell, Oxford.

MENDELSOHN, M. L., 1965, The kinetics of tumor cell proliferation, in: *Cellular Radiation Biology* (University of Texas, M. D. Anderson Hospital and Tumor Institute), pp. 498–513, Williams and Wilkins, Baltimore.

MENDELSOHN, M. L., 1967, Radiation effects in tumors, in: *Radiation Research* (G. Silini, ed.), pp. 659–675, North-Holland, Amsterdam.

MENDELSOHN, M. L., AND DETHLEFSEN, L. A., 1968, Tumor growth and cellular kinetics, in: *The Proliferation and Spread of Neoplastic Cells* (University of Texas, M. D. Anderson Hospital and Tumor Institute), pp. 197–212, Williams and Wilkins, Baltimore.

OWEN, L. N., AND STEEL, G. G., 1969, The growth and cell population kinetics of spontaneous tumors in domestic animals, *Br. J. Cancer* **23**:493–509.

PUCK, T. AND STEFFEN, J., 1963, Life cycle analysis of mammalian cells, *I. Biophysical Journal* **3**:379–397.

QUASTLER, H., AND SHERMAN, F. G., 1959, Cell population kinetics in the intestinal epithelium of the mouse, *Exp. Cell Res.* **17**:420–438.

SIMPSON-HERREN, L., AND LLOYD, H. H., 1970, Kinetic parameters and growth curves for experimental tumor systems, *Cancer Chemother. Rep.* **54**:143–174.

SKIPPER, H. E., AND SCHNABEL, F. M., 1973, Quantitative and cytokinetic studies in experimental tumor models, in: *Cancer Medicine* (J. F. Holland and E. Frei, eds.), pp. 629–650, Lea and Febiger, Philadelphia.

STEEL, G. G., 1967, Cell loss as a factor in the growth rate of human tumors, *Eur. J. Cancer* **3**:381–387.

STEEL, G. G., 1968, Cell loss from experimental tumors, *Cell Tissue Kinet.* **1**:193–207.

STEEL, G. G., 1972, The cell cycle in tumors: An examination of data gained by the technique of labelled mitoses, *Cell Tissue Kinet.* **5**:87–100.

STEEL, G. G., 1973, Cytokinetics of neoplasia, in: *Cancer Medicine* (J. F. Holland and E. Frei, eds.), pp. 125–140, Lea and Febiger, Philadelphia.

STEEL, G. G., AND HANES, S., 1971, The technique of labelled mitoses: Analysis by automatic curve fitting, *Cell Tissue Kinet.* **4**:93–105.

STEEL, G. G., ADAMS, K., AND BARRETT, J. C., 1966, Analysis of the Cell population kinetics of transplanted tumors of widely-differing growth rate, *Br. J. Cancer* **20**:784–800.

TAKAHASHI, M., HOGG, J. D., JR., AND MENDELSOHN, M. L., 1971, The automatic analyses of FLM curves, *Cell Tissue Kinet.* **4**:505–518.

TANNOCK, I. F., 1968, The relation between cell proliferation and the vascular system in a transplanted mouse mammary tumor, *Br. J. Cancer* **22**:258–273.

WIMBER, D., 1963, Methods for studying cell proliferation with emphasis on DNA labels, in: *Cell Proliferation* (L. F. Lammerton, and R. J. M. Fry, eds.), pp. 1–17, Blackwell, Oxford.

9

Stimulation

JOSEPH LOBUE AND MILAN POTMESIL

1. Introduction

Two distinctly different types of stimulatory phenomena are discussed in this chapter, cell proliferation as triggered or enhanced by humoral stimulators and stimulation of the spread of tumor metastases. Humoral stimulators of hematopoiesis and tissue growth represent important components of complex, interrelated, and remarkably versatile systems governed by mechanisms that are not completely understood. Consequently, our selection of topics has had to be somewhat discriminatory and is limited for the most part to those agents which have been implicated, at least to some extent, in stimulation of neoplastic as well as normal cell growth.

Thrombopoietin (reviewed by Odell, 1972, 1973), which undoubtedly plays an important role in normal homeostatic control of platelet production but for which there is little concrete information regarding stimulation of cell proliferation, is not considered. Other factors for which insufficient documentation is available, such as the granulopoietic stimulators described by Bierman (1964) ("leukopoietin-G") and Delmonte (1968) ("renal granulopoietic factor"), or which are considered to be of immunological significance (e.g., lymphokines like "lymphopoietin"; Metcalf, 1958) have also been omitted from discussion. Finally, radiation and chemotherapeutic drugs, which under specific conditions produce

JOSEPH LOBUE AND MILAN POTMESIL • Laboratory of Experimental Hematology, Department of Biology, Graduate School of Arts and Science, New York University, New York, N.Y., and the Cancer and Radiobiological Research Laboratory, The City of New York Health and Hospitals Corporation, and Department of Biology, New York University, New York, N.Y. Preparation of this chapter and the original work reported were supported by research and training grants from the National Cancer Institute (1-R01-CA12815-03, 1-R01-CA12076-04), the National Heart and Lung Institute (5-R01-HL03357-17, 5-T01-HL05645-10) of the USPHS, and The National Leukemia Association, Inc.

adverse effects characterized by enhanced proliferation in normal renewal tissues, are also not included in this chapter, as these will be discussed in a subsequent volume by Potmesil and LoBue.

2. Stimulation of Cell Proliferation

2.1. Steroids and Other Hormones

A detailed consideration of hormonal effects on cellular reproduction may be found in Epifanova (1967) and elsewhere in this volume. Treatment of this topic will be restricted here to recent studies of hormonal stimulation of hematopoietic stem cell proliferation. For definitions and abbreviations used in this chapter, see Table 1.

A series of investigations by Byron (1971, 1972a,b) in mice has unequivocally established, using cytocidal doses of [^{3}H]TdR ("thymidine suicide") or hydroxyurea as an indicator of change in the kinetic state of these stem cells, that both testosterone hydrogen succinate and 5-β-dihydrotestosterone are capable of stimulating G_0-state or prolonged G_1-state colony-forming units (CFU-s) into active DNA synthesis *in vitro*. Phosphodiesterase activation has been found to have no effect on the stimulatory response to these hormones, which strongly suggests that the adenyl cyclase system and cyclic nucleotides do not mediate this type of steroid action. Moreover, since the culture system employed was plasma and serum free, it would appear that the androgenic steroid effects are direct and independent of any "plasma macromolecules" (Byron, 1970, 1975a).

In vivo studies by Byron (1970) have established that androgenic steroids (testosterone propionate, 5-β-dihydrotestosterone, and 19-nortestosterone phenylpropionate) also act to stimulate CFU-s proliferation in the intact mouse and that this effect is erythropoietin independent, a conclusion anticipated as a result of earlier-cited experiments using plasma- and serum-free *in vitro* systems.

TABLE 1

Abridged Classification of Hematopoietic Stem Cells

Cell type	Designations	Assay methods
Primary hematopoietic multi-potential stem cell	CFU-s[a], CFU, CFC	Spleen colonization (Lajtha, 1970)
Secondary "committed" granulocytic stem cell	CFU-c[a], AFC, CFC	Agar culture (Stohlman *et al.*, 1974)
Secondary "committed" erythroid stem cell	ERC[a], CFU-E	Plasma clot culture (Axelrad *et al.*, 1974)

[a] These are the designations used in the text.

Administration of testosterone propionate and 5-β-dihydrotestosterone to mice also increased the number of both femoral CFU-s and CFU-c and enhanced CFU-s regeneration following sublethal irradiation (Byron and Testa; and Whiting, in Byron, 1975a). Prostaglandin E_2 has been found to trigger murine CFU-s into active DNA synthesis in a wide range of dose levels (Feher and Gidali, 1974), and imidazole inhibition of phosphodiesterase activity is without effect on this type of stimulation. Once again, this suggests that prostaglandin action is direct and does not involve any secondary messenger system.

In summary, recent studies by Byron and others (reviewed by Byron, 1975a) have established that androgenic steroids, prostaglandins, and a number of other agents, e.g., β_1-adrenergic and cholinergic receptor site stimulators (Byron, 1975b), are capable of triggering "quiescent" hematopoietic stem cells into active proliferative cycle. As emphasized by Byron (1975a), future research should be aimed at determining which of these substances, if any, are actually physiological regulators and how these agents might be of practical use in manipulating stem-cell proliferation so that hematological responses to therapeutic or toxic agents might be favorably altered. Since stem cells probably represent the primary target cells for development of neoplastic disease, solutions to such problems could be of potential practical significance.

2.2. Erythropoietin

2.2.1. Erythropoietin and Erythropoietin-Responsive Cell

There is overwhelming evidence that the glycoprotein hormone erythropoietin (Ep) exerts its effect predominantly on erythropoietin-responsive stem cells (ERC) to engender, among other things, a series of biochemical processes leading to the formation of hemoglobin. Thus, as Gordon (1973) has so aptly stated, "Ep is a unique agent. It specifically causes differentiation of a hematopoietic precursor cell, the Ep-responsive cell (ERC), into the earliest recognizable members of the nucleated erythroid cell line. . . . Thus it constitutes an excellent tool for investigating molecular events associated with and resulting in formation of a unique product—hemoglobin." For critical, authoritative, and exhaustive literature reviews, see Krantz and Jacobson (1970) and Gordon (1973).

Molecular events associated with Ep effects on adult hematopoietic tissue include antecedent RNA synthesis (of unspecified nuclear RNA, ribosomal-precursor RNA, tRNA, and globin messenger), DNA synthesis, genesis of an iron uptake mechanism, stromal formation, and heme synthesis. In the older literature, there were scattered and somewhat inconclusive reports that Ep may stimulate proliferation within the developing erythron and that this agent may have a nonspecific growth-promoting effect in nonhemic normal and neoplastic tissues. These latter findings have been criticized on the grounds that stimulation of nonerythroid tissue may have resulted not from Ep itself but rather from associated contaminants (Gordon, 1973).

In recent literature, there is a strong indication that Ep stimulates cell multiplication within the ERC compartment. Reissmann and Samorapoompichit (1970) tested this direct effect of Ep using a sophisticated experimental design. The effect of Ep treatment on erythropoiesis was examined in MF1 female mice in which both the CFU-s and the erythroblast population were eliminated. CFU-s numbers in these animals were essentially reduced to zero by gastric tubal instillation of myleran and erythroblasts were eliminated by polycythemia, induced by exposure to low atmospheric pressure and maintained by hypertransfusion. Their results conclusively established that polycythemic mice devoid of both CFU-s and erythroblasts and primed with 6 U Ep for as long as 8 days responded to a test dose of 1 U Ep with greatly enhanced erythropoiesis, as compared with CFU-s-deficient polycythemic or nonpolycythemic mice not primed with the hormone. This was interpreted as indicating a direct stimulatory effect of Ep on the intermediate, erythroid committed stem cell (ERC) which presumably had not been eliminated by prior treatments. These investigators also confirmed the well-established fact that Ep induces erythroid differentiation, and the data further suggested that ERC (or potential ERC; see Lajtha, 1970, 1972) are required to undergo several maturing divisions before they develop "responsiveness" to Ep.

2.2.2. Erythropoietin and Murine Erythroblastic RLV-A Disease; Phenylhydrazine "Therapy"; Erythropoietin "Therapy"

Studies have been conducted on the potential therapeutic role of Ep in the management, through stimulation of maturation, of the anemia of myeloproliferative diseases in an animal model system, murine RLV-A disease. RLV-A disease is a virtually induced (Fredrickson et al., 1972) preleukemic erythroblastosis of BALB/c mice characterized by development of hepatosplenomegaly and fatal anemia (LoBue et al., 1972, 1974). Although a hemolytic component exists (Morse et al., 1973), the anemia results primarily from a failure of adequate erythroid maturation. This, in turn, leads to a massive accumulation of stem cells and erythroid precursors in the liver, spleen, and other organs. In spite of the severe progressive anemia, plasma Ep levels are inappropriately low (Ebert et al., 1972; Camiscoli et al., 1972), a phenomenon which seems to be due to increased clearance of the hormone, and which counteracts its enhanced production (OKunewick and Erhard, 1974). Both bleeding and administration of phenylhydrazine (PHZ) significantly elevate Ep levels in these mice (LoBue et al., 1974). Moreover, it has been demonstrated that the maturation block of RLV-A can be overcome by PHZ-induced hemolytic anemia or by single courses of treatment with Ep. Both of these procedures result in marked reticulocytosis and pronounced increases in the circulating red cell mass with temporary alleviation of anemia (LoBue et al., 1974). This is shown in Figs. 1 and 2. To determine if treatment by PHZ, through endogenous Ep, or exogenous Ep itself would be of any value in management of the anemia in RLV-A disease, experiments described in the following part of this section were conducted (LoBue et al., 1975).

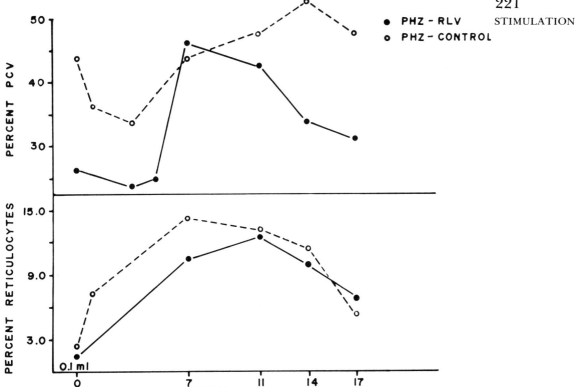

FIGURE 1. Average reticulocyte percentages and packed red cell volumes (PCV) in three RLV-A anemic and two control male BALB/c mice following a single injection of 0.1 ml of 1% PHZ solution.

a. Phenylhydrazine "Therapy." BALB/c mice 4 wk old, six of each sex, were inoculated intraperitoneally with 0.1 ml of undiluted viremic plasma obtained from mice bearing an RLV-induced transplantable leukemia (Fredrickson *et al.*, 1972). The progression of the virally induced anemia was monitored by periodic reticulocyte counts using Brecher's (1949) "new methylene blue" technique, microhematocrits, and differential leukocyte counts. As individual mice became frankly anemic (i.e., hematocrits dropped to about 30%), PHZ "therapy" was initiated. Treatment initially consisted of giving these anemic mice 0.1 ml of a 1% phenylhydrazine HCl solution in saline intraperitoneally; thereafter, the therapy was directed by hematocrit values. Three male and three female virus-treated mice served as controls of viral potency. The results of treatment of male mice with PHZ are presented in Fig. 3. Following onset of anemia, all male controls were dead within about 1 month, or within about 3–4 months following the inoculation of virus. In sharp contrast to control mice, the six males treated with PHZ responded after an initial hemolytic reaction by enhanced erythropoiesis, as indicated by reticulocytosis and gradual elevation in hematocrit values. Response to PHZ in two of the six mice has continued to be highly satisfactory. At present, almost 17 months after initiation of "therapy," or 19 months after viral inoculation and 16 months after death of the last control mouse, anemia has been controlled and surviving mice continue to respond well. Four treated male mice have died;

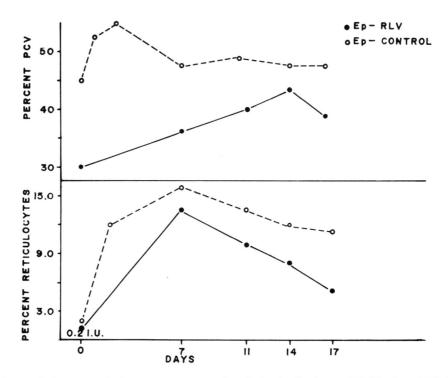

FIGURE 2. Average reticulocyte percentages and packed red cell volumes (PCV) in three RLV-A anemic and two control male BALB/c mice following a single injection of 0.2 U Ep.

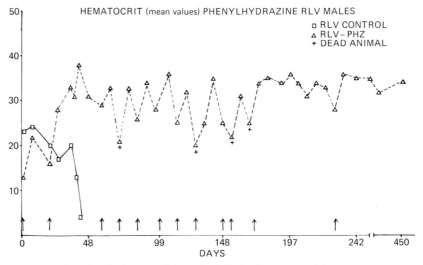

FIGURE 3. Alterations in hematocrit in male RLV-A mice treated with PHZ in "therapy" trials. Arrows indicate PHZ injections, and it may be noted that no PHZ injections have been administered for the last several months. Abscissa indicates days after onset of therapy, not time after inoculation of virus.

however, their survival time exceeded by $3\frac{1}{2}$–$5\frac{1}{2}$ months that of untreated controls.

b. Erythropoietin "Therapy." BALB/c mice 4 wk old, seven of each sex, were inoculated with viremic plasma and the development of anemia was monitored as described above. As soon as animals became anemic, treatment with Ep (Sheep, Step III, Connaught Laboratories, Toronto, Canada) was initiated. For the first several months of treatment, three successive injections of 0.2 U Ep were administered at each bout of therapy. However, this dose seemed to worsen the anemia in some recipients and the dosage was reduced to a single injection of 0.2 U Ep per bout. Three male and three female virus-treated mice served as controls of viral potency. Data obtained for males in this trial are given in Fig. 4. Similar data were obtained for females. It may be seen that in responders Ep "therapy" markedly ameliorated the anemia of RLV-A disease. At present, survival time of these mice has already exceeded that of untreated controls by about 9 months. However, therapeutic response of mice initially treated with high doses of Ep (0.6 U Ep per bout) was not satisfactory, and seven out of 14 mice have died. Five out of seven remaining responders are continuously under control, with 0.2 U Ep applied per bout. Thus chronic administration of Ep to RLV-A anemic mice—if a proper dosage is used—controls anemia and results in a significant prolongation of life.

In conclusion, PHZ therapy trials showed that endogenously generated Ep could be an important factor in control of RLV-A anemia. As expected, severely anemic mice, in relapse, sometimes had considerable difficulty in handling the additional anemic stress imposed by PHZ (LoBue *et al.*, 1974). Unfortunately, duration of PHZ-induced remission is highly variable and this precludes the

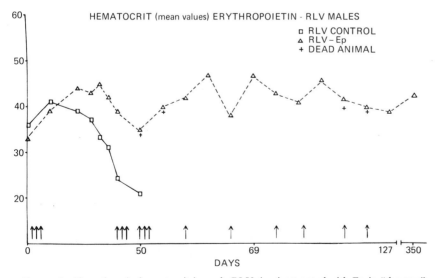

FIGURE 4. Alterations in hematocrit in male RLV-A mice treated with Ep in "therapy" trials. Arrows indicate Ep injections, and it may be noted that no Ep injections have been administered for the last several months. Abscissa as in Fig. 3.

possibility that the administration of PHZ can always be optimally spaced for every experimental subject. This is especially true in the early phases of "therapy." Three of the mice that died manifested abnormal peripheral leukocyte counts and abnormal morphology of leukocytes in the last blood samples taken. Two animals were found to have a massive peripheral lymphocytosis reminiscent of lymphatic leukemia and one had a peripheral blood picture suggestive of monomyelocytic leukemia. These results are not surprising, since development of frank leukemia after RLV infection is known to occur in those mice which survive the erythroblastic phase of the disease (Rauscher, 1962; Boiron et al., 1965; Pluznik et al., 1966).

As indicated earlier, RLV-A-infected BALB/c mice manifest inappropriately low plasma levels of Ep in spite of progressive and ultimately fatal anemia. However, RLV-A anemic mice subjected to the additional anemic stress imposed by phlebotomy or PHZ hemolysis respond with increased appearance of this hormone in the plasma (LoBue et al., 1974). Since PHZ induces the enhanced production of endogenous Ep and since this is undoubtedly the mechanism whereby erythropoiesis is stimulated in PHZ "therapy" trials, an attempt was made to "treat" the anemia of RLV-A disease with exogenous Ep. The data obtained suggest that such an approach offers considerable promise. The failures experienced could have been due to Ep "overdose" in susceptible mice. Ep, under certain circumstances, is known to exacerbate RLV disease (LoBue et al., 1974). Thus, properly administered, erythropoietin may have potential therapeutic value in the management of anemia in myeloproliferative diseases in which responsive stem cells and erythroid precursors are available but Ep plasma levels are ineffectively low.

2.3. Humoral Stimulators of Granulocytopoiesis

Two reviews discuss, in considerable detail, experiments exploring the regulation of myelopoiesis in vivo and in vitro (Stohlman et al., 1974) and the colony-stimulating factor (Metcalf, 1973); therefore, only brief reference will be made to humoral stimulators of granulopoiesis under normal conditions. However, various implications with regard to the leukemias will be stressed.

2.3.1. Colony-Stimulating Factor; Diffusible Granulopoietic Stimulator; Antichalones; Leukocytosis-Inducing Factor

The progenitor cell of the granulocytic series [colony-forming unit in culture (CFU-c), also designated in the literature as colony-forming cell (CFC) [review by Metcalf and Moore, 1971] can be identified by its ability to form colonies in vitro in semisolid culture medium or liquid suspension culture. In murine systems, colony-stimulating factor (CSF) is responsible for the initiation and sustenance of this colony growth (Pluznik and Sachs, 1965; Bradley and Metcalf, 1966; Metcalf and Foster, 1967). Human as well as other nonrodent mammalian hematopoietic cell suspensions are capable of significant autostimulation (Iscove et al., 1971; Moore and Williams 1972a), which is most likely explained by the production of

CSF by cells exhibiting autostimulation (Stohlman *et al.*, 1974). CSF, capable of

stimulating the growth not only of granulocyte but also of macrophage colonies
(Paran and Sachs, 1969), is ubiquitous in its distribution in the rodent and is also
present in man in normal as well as leukemic urine, serum, and many tissues
including hematopoietic (Robinson *et al.*, 1969; reviewed by Metcalf, 1973, and by
Stohlman *et al.*, 1974). CSF was prepared in concentrated and partially purified
form, and has been shown to be a glycoprotein with a molecular weight of 45,000
(Stanley and Metcalf, 1969, 1971; Stanley *et al.*, 1970). Murine CSF and normal
and leukemic human CSF have basic biochemical similarities, but there are a
number of differences in certain biochemical properties within and among
species. This might account for the fact that CSF from some sources favors
macrophage and that from others granulocytic differentiation (Stohlman *et al.*,
1974). Murine CSF is ineffective as a stimulating agent for human CFU-c, whereas
CSF of human origin provides effective stimulation for culture growth of both
human and murine hematopoietic tissues. This can be achieved by adding
peripheral blood or bone marrow leukocytes to cultures either as a feeder layer or
as a component of conditioned medium (Robinson and Pike, 1970; Iscove *et al.*,
1971). Peripheral blood leukocytes obtained from patients with acute myeloblastic
leukemia in relapse and used as a source of CSF failed in some experiments to
stimulate colony growth of normal or leukemic CFU-c (Greenberg *et al.*, 1971;
Robinson *et al.*, 1971). In other experiments, this stimulation was effective (Moore
et al., 1973). The apparent discrepancy between experimental results is discussed
in Section 2.3.2.

There is a considerable lack of certainty in the literature regarding the cell type
which provides CSF. Originally it was suggested that granulocytes were the source
(Robinson and Kurnick, 1972), but further experiments have indicated that a
major source of CSF is the monocyte (Moore and Williams, 1972*b*; Chervenick
and LoBuglio, 1972; Golde *et al.*, 1972). The ubiquitous presence of CSF is well
established and suggests that the cells providing this factor are distributed
throughout the body. The monocyte–macrophage system, or fibroblasts and the
collagen–vascular system, might be a prime candidate (Stohlman *et al.*, 1974).
Experimental data also indicate that erythrocyte hemolysate influences the
activity of CSF (Bradley *et al.*, 1971; Heit *et al.*, 1974). The additive stimulatory
effect of erythrocyte lysate and CSF may represent a situation in which either a
precursor of the CFU-c becomes sensitive to CSF, or the more mature cell type
regains its capacity to respond to CSF (Van den Engh, 1974). Injected or infused
CSF may also exert a stimulatory effect on granulocytopoiesis *in vivo* (Bradley *et
al.*, 1969; Metcalf and Stanley, 1971). The growth of colonies *in vitro* may be
affected by two types of inhibitors present in mouse and human serum, in urine,
and in media conditioned by a variety of tissues (reviewed by Stohlman *et al.*,
1974). Serum levels of CSF are relatively low in normal mice (Robinson *et al.*, 1967)
and even lower in germ-free mice than in conventional mice (Metcalf *et al.*, 1967),
but increase after X-irradiation (Hall, 1969; Morley *et al.*, 1971) or administration
of endotoxin (Metcalf, 1971; Quesenberry *et al.*, 1972; Chervenick, 1972),
pertussis vaccine (Shadduck *et al.*, 1971), poly(I)-poly(C) (McNeill and Killen,

1971), antineutrophilic serum (Shadduck and Negabhushanom, 1971; Quesenberry *et al.*, 1972), or other substances. Increased levels of CSF have also been reported in the serum and urine of man and experimental animals following infection (Foster *et al.*, 1968), in man after surgery (Weiner and Robinson, 1971), in leukemic animals (Robinson *et al.*, 1967), and in patients with leukemia (Robinson and Pike, 1970). Increased quantities of CSF induced by endotoxin *in vivo* have the potential to stimulate the growth of granulocytic CFU-c *in vitro*, whereas endotoxin added directly to unstimulated granulocytic CFU-c, or to CFU-c stimulated by a conditioned medium does not enhance colony growth (Chervenick, 1972; Quesenberry *et al.*, 1972). However, this does not apply to all endotoxin preparations (McNeill, 1970). Experimental data suggest that the host's own bacterial flora may control the serum level of CSF via intermittent endotoxemia, induced for instance by radiation injury of the gastrointestinal tract (Morley *et al.*, 1971). Elevated levels of CSF in turn may represent the primary determinant of granulocyte production and release (Quesenberry *et al.*, 1972). It has been established, however, that tolerance to many endotoxin-mediated effects can be developed and this may be overcome only by an increased dose of endotoxin (Stohlman *et al.*, 1974). There are several conjectural explanations of the mechanism by which endotoxin might increase CSF levels: CSF may merely represent a metabolite of endotoxin rather than a separate humoral agent; endotoxin-induced neutropenia may trigger the production and release of CSF; CSF may normally be produced at a constant rate, but bound and neutralized by neutrophils, remaining unbound in plasma at endotoxin-induced neutropenic stage. Endotoxin may also act through an antigen–antibody reaction and/or through complement activation resulting in injury to peripheral granulocytes and release of CSF (Quesenberry *et al.*, 1972). It certainly could be hypothesized that CSF is an important regulator of myelopoiesis, but unfortunately there is no direct evidence that CSF is responsible for CFU-c differentiation *in vivo*. Furthermore, the mechanisms involved in regulatory processes associated with the production of CSF are not clearly understood (Stohlman *et al.*, 1974), and factors other than CSF may be present and influence the growth of CFU-c in tested systems.

A humoral substance present in body fluids of irradiated or endotoxin-treated mice, diffusible granulopoietic stimulator (DGS), stimulates the growth of myeloblasts and promyelocytes in Millipore membrane diffusion chambers implanted intraperitoneally (Rothstein *et al.*, 1971). There are indications that DGS represents only one component of some wider humoral control mechanisms governing granulocyte production (Rothstein *et al.*, 1971, 1973; Boecker *et al.*, 1971). The DGS activity is separable from serum CSF activity. Thus CSF acting *in vitro* and *in vivo* and DGS acting *in vivo* appear to be different substances affecting the production of granulocytes (Rothstein *et al.*, 1973). The existence of DGS has not yet been confirmed by other investigators. Preirradiation of the chamber host enhances the number of granulocytic diffusion-chamber progenitor cells (Boyum *et al.*, 1972*a,b*). The enhancing effect of irradiation of the host may depend on stimulation by some released humoral agent(s), or lack of an inhibitory factor, but participation of other factors, e.g., "trophic" function of materials released from dead cells, cannot be eliminated. It has been suggested that the enhancing effect can be explained either by reduction of chalone, a humoral substance preventing the entry of granulocytic precursors into DNA synthesis, or by an increased concentration of antichalone, a substance with an opposite action, in irradiated animals.

The concept of humoral principles ("antisubstances") antagonistic to the action of mitosis-inhibiting chalones, and presumed to be directly associated with them in the dual feedback control of cell production and functional tissue mass, has generated wide theoretical interest (Forscher and Houck, 1973) but, to date, little experimental support. Probably the most systematic investigations of the "antichalone concept" have been carried out by Rytömaa and Kiviniemi (1967, 1968a,b). These investigators have presented results which they interpret as indicating the existence of "granulocytic antichalone" in the sera of Sprague-Dawley male rats subjected to serial "leukophoresis." In 664 in vitro tests, "leukophoresis serum" was found to enhance DNA synthesis in myeloid cells as judged by [³H]TdR incorporation but had no effect on total cell numbers. Analysis of variance of experimental data suggested that no stimulation of maturation rate was produced by leukophoresis serum since interactions between serum–effect and incubation time–effect were not found to be significant. The authors conclude from these data that the increased appearance of [³H]TdR-labeled mature granulocytes was the result of a specific direct effect of granulocytic antichalone contained within the leukophoresis serum, which stimulated "resting" granulocytic precursors (G_0 or prolonged G_1 cells) into DNA synthesis and subsequent division. Such an interpretation is difficult to accept in view of the finding that in spite of a 170% increase in mature granulocyte labeling no absolute increase in the number of these cells was observed.

Rytömaa and Kiviniemi (1968a) have found that granulocytic chalone, but not antichalone, can be extracted from intact or homogenized leukocyte suspensions. This suggests that antichalone may not originate in circulating granulocytes. Preliminary results of partial purification of leukophoresis serum on Sephadex columns suggest a chemically undefined substance of molecular weight 30,000–35,000 as the active principle corresponding to granulocytic. In accordance with the dual control concept, antichalone concentrations were elevated in leukophoresis serum whereas granulocytic chalone levels were reduced.

As an alternative to the active participation of specific antichalones in direct stimulation of cell division, Fell (1973) has proposed that lysosomal hydrolases released either as a result of tissue death or through physiological stimulation may act indirectly as stimulators of cell proliferation by destruction of inhibitory chalones. Also, direct primary effects of lysosomal enzymes on induction of cell replication have been strongly implicated in some (e.g., lymphoid blastogenesis; for review, see Johnson and Rubin, 1970) but not all systems (e.g., liver regeneration; Becker and Lane, 1966). Therefore, it follows that the possible involvement of lysosomal hydrolases should be considered in any experiment designed to test for the participation of antichalones in the humoral control of tissue mass (see also Section 2.4).

Leukocytosis-inducing factor (LIF) (Gordon *et al.*, 1960, 1964), neutrophilia-inducing activity (Boggs *et al.*, 1968), and neutrophil-releasing activity (Stohlman *et al.*, 1974) may all be an identical protein that produces leukocytosis by discharge of granulocytes from their sites of "storage." The mechanism by which LIF acts is unknown, but it has been suggested that the substance interacts directly with sinusoids rather than granulocytes (Stohlman *et al.*, 1974). There is some evidence that LIF enhances blood flow rate through the bone marrow (Dornfest *et al.*, 1962). According to studies using both endotoxin stimulation and induced endotoxin tolerance, this activity is separable from the activity of CSF or DGS (Quesenbery *et al.*, in Stohlman *et al.*, 1974; Rothstein *et al.*, 1973). This has been confirmed in isolated rat hind leg perfusion experiments (Broxmeyer *et al.*, 1974).

2.3.2. Normal and Leukemic Granulocytic Colony-Forming Units and Colony-Stimulating Cells

The cell that gives rise to a granulocytic colony *in vitro*, CFU-c, has been reported to differ in density (Worton *et al.*, 1969; Haskill *et al.*, 1970), velocity sedimentation rate (Worton *et al.*, 1969), and proliferation characteristics (Iscove *et al.*, 1971; Metcalf, 1972) from the bone marrow pluripotential stem cell (CFU-s). Results of other experiments indicate that there are no strict boundaries between these two cell types (Dicke *et al.*, 1971), but rather a spectrum of differentiation, and various degrees of "stemness." It has also been suggested that only progenitor cells which have achieved a certain level of differentiation are capable of growth *in vitro* as granulocytic CFU-c (Stohlman *et al.*, 1974). From morphological studies, two cell types stand out as potential candidates for the granulocytic CFU-c, transitional lymphoid cells and blast cells, presumably myeloblasts (Moore *et al.*, 1972). Spontaneous colony formation, with no exogenous CSF added, has been observed in human bone marrow and peripheral blood cultures (Pike and Robinson, 1970; Iscove *et al.*, 1971; Moore *et al.*, 1972) as well as in cultures of animal origin (Moore and Williams, 1972*a*). Since colony formation of human granulocytes is most effectively stimulated by feeder layers of human peripheral leukocytes (Pike and Robinson, 1970) and by conditioned media prepared from cultured leukocytes or spleen cells (Iscove *et al.*, 1971; Paran *et al.*, 1970), a conclusion has been reached that spontaneous colony formation was due to the formation and release of CSF by the colony-stimulating cells (CSC). These cells were studied in human (Chervenick and LoBuglio, 1972; Golde and Cline, 1972) and in monkey (Moore and Williams, 1972*b*) peripheral blood. CSC and CFU-c coexist in human bone marrow, and the growth of granulocytic colonies *in vitro* depends on the concentration of cells of both types in the culture (Haskill *et al.*, 1972). All studies conducted thus far have concluded that CSF production is a property of cells with glass adherence. A nonadherent cell population separated from normal human bone marrow was more dependent for colony formation in cultures on added CSF than an unseparated cell suspension (Messner *et al.*, 1973). CSC separated from CFU-c by density gradient centrifugation and adherence columns, have a light to intermediate density and active adherence properties; morphologically, they resemble monocytes. The CSF produced by these cells is antigenically cross-reactive with human urine CSF (Moore *et al.*, 1973).

Formation of granulocytic colonies has been tested in several clinical disorders such as chronic neutropenic states, acquired neutropenias, and cyclic neutropenia, in clinical studies of bone marrow transplantation, in patients manifesting a preleukemic state (reviewed by Stohlman *et al.*, 1974), and in patients with acute or chronic myelocytic leukemia. Spontaneous colony formation *in vitro* due to endogenous formation of CSF by CSC was observed in patients with acute and chronic myelocytic leukemia in remission at relatively low concentrations of cultivated bone marrow or peripheral blood leukocytes, whereas in untreated acute forms high cell concentrations were necessary (Moore, 1973). Quantitative reconstitution procedures revealed that in acute leukemia CSC are abnormal in number or in CSF productive capacity (Messner *et al.*, 1973). This observation has been substantiated by numerous investigators. Moore *et al.* (1973) found that blood and bone marrow leukocytes of patients with acute myelocytic leukemia in relapse, and chronic myelocytic leukemia in acute transformation phase were characterized either by a complete lack of colony formation *in vitro* or by formation of small aggregates ("clusters") of poorly differentiated cells. The formation of "clusters" may represent a few abortive divisions or faulty differentiation of CFU-c. Remission is associated with a return to normal conditions; i.e., "cluster" formation is replaced mostly by normal colony formation. The extent of defective proliferation of leukemic CFU-c as reported by different authors (Paran *et al.*, 1970; Robinson and Pike, 1970; Iscove *et al.*, 1971) is difficult to compare because of the diverse criteria applied in their respective studies (Stohlman *et al.*, 1974); however, restoration of normal colony-forming capacity by CSF derived from normal peripheral leukocytes, splenic tissue, or human embryonic kidney tissue was uniformly achieved. In contrast, blood leukocytes from patients with acute myelocytic leukemia did not stimulate *in vitro* colony growth of normal or leukemic human bone marrow target cells (Paran *et al.*, 1970; Robinson and Pike, 1970; Robinson *et al.*, 1971). In another study, however, normal stimulatory capacity was found with leukocytic feeder layers prepared from the peripheral blood of some untreated patients with acute leukemia (Moore *et al.*, 1973). The stimulatory capacity of leukemic feeder layers did not correlate with the extent of spontaneous colony formation, nor was a correlation found between clinical status and the stimulatory effects of leukemic peripheral blood. This, if true, indicates that defective CSF production by presumably abnormal CSC progeny of leukemic monocytes is not the sole cause of impaired colony formation in acute myelocytic leukemias. The presence of CSF in the serum and urine of patients with this disorder has been widely documented (reviewed by Stohlman *et al.*, 1974), but systematic studies correlating the clinical course with the serum level of CSF, comparing serum and urinary levels, and relating these levels to intercurrent infections are lacking.

CFU-c in peripheral blood and bone marrow of leukemic patients in relapse have an abnormally light buoyant density and a low "suiciding" index after incubation with [^{3}H]TdR (Moore *et al.*, 1973). Complete remission is associated with restoration of normal CFU-c and with the return of their normal capacity to proliferate and differentiate. It has been suggested that this indicates a reemergence of the normal stem-cell population which remained dormant during relapse, presumably confined to G_0 phase. Studies of Aye *et al.* (1974) suggest a rather considerable variation of CSC and CFU-c populations in individual patients with acute myelocytic leukemia. The reviewed experimental results indicate that not only are CSC, a possible source of CSF, in an insufficient supply in leukemic peripheral blood and bone marrow during the relapse, but also the response of CFU-c to stimuli is altered. In the absence of marker chromosomes, however, it is difficult to prove whether this defect concerns primarily the differentiation and proliferation of normal, leukemic or both granulocytic cell subpopulations.

In chronic granulocytic leukemia, *in vitro* growth of differentiated granulocytic colonies from peripheral blood and bone marrow has been observed. CFU-c, almost all of them descendants of a Ph'-positive leukemic cell precursor, are capable of giving rise to colonies with morphologically normal differentiated cells. CFU-c are significantly increased in the peripheral blood of untreated patients (Paran *et al.*, 1970; Chervenick *et al.*, 1971; Shadduck and Nankin, 1971; Moore *et al.*, 1973), whereas in treated patients with normalized counts of peripheral blood leukocytes CFU-c are reduced or absent (Moore *et al.*, 1973; Goldman *et al.*, 1974). There is no relationship between the number of myeloblasts in the peripheral blood and the number of granulocytic colonies observed in a particular experiment. The relative increase in CFU-c in the bone marrow of untreated patients appears to be only two- to threefold as compared with normal bone marrow, but the absolute increase is much higher as the total myeloid mass of untreated patients is greatly enlarged (Goldman *et al.*, 1974). After treatment and reduction of the total leukocyte count, CFU-c appear to be normal in number in the bone marrow (Moore *et al.*, 1973; Goldman *et al.*, 1974). Peripheral blood leukocytes of untreated patients are a very poor source of CSF (Goldman *et al.*, 1974), and this conflicts with the data of Moore *et al.* (1973), who reported good feeder layer activity of these leukocytes. However, the target cells (CFU-c) used in these experiments were of different origin (human vs. murine). Peripheral blood leukocytes from patients with a normalized peripheral blood count after therapy have normal CSF activity. The finding that the peripheral blood of untreated patients does not provide CSF can be explained, according to Goldman *et al.* (1974), as a consequence of suppression of CSF production by the large number of granulocytes. An alternative explanation is that two distinct monocyte populations are the source of CSF: one, defective in CSF production, predominates in the peripheral blood before treatment; the other, indistinguishable from the normal monocyte population and efficient in CSF production, proliferates after treatment.

2.4.1. Growth-Stimulating Factor

In earlier histological studies, growth-stimulating effects of tumors on adjoining normal tissue were intimated (Merwin and Algire, 1956; Argyris and Argyris, 1962; Argyris, 1965), and this suggestion seems to be supported by observations made in mixed cultures of neoplastic and normal tissue (Ludford and Barlow, 1944; Randive and Bhide, 1962). In these latter experiments, tissue cultures derived from different types of tumors showed different degrees of stimulatory effects on explants of normal tissue. The possibility that such stimulatory phenomena are the result of some diffusible agent have been examined. Growth-stimulating substances have been demonstrated in medium harvested from tissue cultures of cells injected with Rous sarcoma virus (Rubin, 1970), normal murine mammary cell cultures, cultures of mouse mammary adenocarcinomas (Nair and DeOme, 1972, 1973*a,b*), and cultures of cell lines derived from human neoplasms (Rounds, 1970). These substances were designated either as the overgrowth-stimulating factor (OSF; Rubin, 1970) or the growth-stimulating factor (GSF; Nair and DeOme, 1973*a*). Rubin (1970) made the interesting observation that the growth of chick embryo cells in cultures containing predominantly cells uninfected with Rous sarcoma virus (RSV) does not diminish with increased cell density. This suggests that those few transformed RSV-infected cells may release a material responsible for stimulating uninfected crowded cells to overgrow. To test this substance, media removed from cultures of RSV-infected cells were added to uninfected cultures of chick embryo cells in which growth had been inhibited by crowding. Following addition of media, [^{3}H]TdR incorporation was increased 3–6 times over control cultures, mitotic indices were doubled, and cell numbers increased twofold over those in untreated cultures. OSF activity was detectable in culture media by 4–5 days after infection with RSV, increased a hundredfold by 6–7 days, and maintained this level for another 3 days. The OSF may be detected in old, uninfected cultures, but the time of appearance is considerably delayed and levels are low. Removal of RSV from culture media by sedimentation at 75,000 *g* for 2 hr or treatment of media with neutralizing antibody had no effect on OSF activity. This indicates that neither whole viral particles nor their envelope antigen possesses OSF activity. Chemically, the OSF appears to be a thermolabile protein and its activity may be mimicked by both trypsin and pronase, which suggests that the OSF may be a proteolytic enzyme.

A soluble fraction stimulating the growth of density-inhibited mouse embryo cells in cultures has been derived from spontaneous mouse mammary tumors (Nair and DeOme, 1973*b*). A comparable preparation was obtained from the normal mouse mammary gland and from the kidney of tumor-bearing mice, although not from the kidney of tumor-free virgin mice. The stimulatory effect of the soluble fraction does not seem to be related to mouse mammary tumor virus carried by the donor mice. The GSF, present in the soluble fraction, can be concentrated by dialysis or precipitated by 60% saturated ammonium sulfate. The ammonium sulfate precipitate can be further separated by Sephadex G100 column chromatography. The precipitability of GSF is similar to the preparation of OSF from the culture media of cells infected with RSV (Rubin, 1970), and thus it seems that GSF is a protein or a mixture of proteins (Nair and DeOme, 1973b). Stimulation of DNA synthesis induced by GSF in tissue cultures is not comparable to the action of serum added to density-inhibited cell cultures (Nair; Nair and DeOme, in Nair and DeOme, 1973b).

Precise chemical identity and biochemical function of the GSF are not known, and therefore it cannot be ruled out that the GSF may be a surface-active lysosomal protease (Nair and DeOme, 1973b). These are found in altered concentrations in certain tumor cells (e.g., see Schnebli, 1972; Bosmann, 1972) and are known to induce growth in "contact-inhibited" confluent culture systems. Burger (1970) observed that as little as 0.007% crystalline trypsin stimulated cell growth in density-inhibited cultures of 3T3 mouse fibroblasts. Although this growth-promoting effect was prevented by addition of the trypsin inhibitor ovomucoid, the phenomenon was not limited to trypsin alone since both pronase and ficin were able to initiate cell reproduction in inhibited plateau-phase cultures of 3T3 cells. Only a brief exposure (45 min) to 0.0005% protease was needed to evoke mitotic activity, which became apparent 48 h after application of the stimulus. Similarly, Sefton and Rubin (1970) reported increased [³H]TdR incorporation and elevated labeling and mitotic indices after the exposure of density-inhibited chick embryo cell cultures to 3 μg/ml of crystalline trypsin. Soybean inhibitor abolished this effect but did not influence pronase stimulatory activity. Regarding protease inhibitors, Schnebli and Burger (1972) and Schnebli (1974) have conclusively demonstrated inhibition of tumor cell growth in culture by treatment with inhibitors of proteolytic enzyme activity.

2.4.2. Epidermal-Epithelial Growth Factor

Levi-Montalcini and Cohen (1960) and Cohen (1960) observed that administration of partially purified extracts of nerve growth factor (NGF) from murine submaxillary glands to newborn mice resulted in early opening of their eyelids and precocious eruption of the teeth. Several years later, Cohen (1962) isolated from the submaxillary gland of adult Swiss-Webster mice a heat-stable protein, distinct from NGF and from parotin, possessing the ability to accelerate tooth eruption and eyelid opening in neonatal mice and rats. This active polypeptide was originally designated "tooth–lid factor" and was isolated in a homogeneous form. Chemical characterization revealed an approximate minimal molecular weight of 15,000, inactivation by chymotrypsin and bacterial proteinase, absence of lysine and phenylalanine, and an isoelectric pH of 4.2. Subsequently, Cohen and Elliott (1963) and Cohen (1964, 1965) were able to demonstrate that accelerated eyelid opening was due to enhanced epidermal growth. When 5 μg/ml of isolated active protein was added to cultures containing 3-mm-thick explants of back or anterior shank skin isolated from 7-day chick embryos, marked epidermal thickening was produced. [³H]TdR autoradiographic analysis indicated that the stimulating protein, EGF, enhanced cell proliferation in the basal layer of the skin.

In addition to effects on tooth eruption, eyelid opening, and skin proliferation in the neonate and embryo, EGF has also been reported to stimulate growth in a number of cultured normal epithelial tissues from young adult rats (Jones, 1966). Turkington (1969a) demonstrated that 0.5 μg/ml of highly purified EGF increased DNA synthesis, mitotic indices, and [³H]TdR labeling indices in incubated explants obtained from a spontaneous mammary adenocarcinoma, and he suggested that this stimulatory effect triggers quiscent neoplastic cells (cells in G_0 or prolonged G_1) into S phase. EGF also stimulates DNA and RNA synthesis and DNA polymerase activity and increases labeling and mitotic indices in normal mouse mammary gland tissue (Turkington, 1969b). However, the role EGF plays in the control of mammary epithelial cell replication and in the growth of spontaneous mammary carcinomas requires further elucidation. Turkington et al. (1971) have directed their attention to the functional role of the submaxillary gland in EGF physiology and the species distribution of this polypeptide. They used a direct demonstration of EGF in situ in tissue sections by rabbit anti-EGF antibodies conjugated with fluorescein isothiocyanate and estimated the rate of EGF synthesis by first incubating submaxillary gland explants with [¹⁴C]protein hydrolysates and [¹⁴C]leucine, and then extracting and determining the [¹⁴C]EGF. It was found that EGF was actively synthesized and stored within the submaxillary gland of mice in tubular cells; that treatment of female mice with testosterone considerably increased the normally reduced levels of EGF in the submaxillary gland, apparently by enhancing the number of tubular cells. Although EGF was found in submaxillary glands of mouse, rat and rabbit, it was not present in bull, pig, rhesus monkey, or man. As indicated by Turkington et al. (1971), this failure to detect EGF in some species does not necessarily prove its absence. In these instances, the chemical form of EGF may have been different enough to render conventional extraction procedures ineffective and also to prevent cross-reactivity with anti-murine-EGF antibodies.

2.4.3. Nerve Growth Factor

Nerve growth factor was first extracted from murine sarcomas (for review, see Angeletti et al., 1973). NGF, essential for growth and development of the sympathetic nervous system, is a protein of about 40,000 mol wt. The amino acid sequence of NGF has been determined and it has been established that the molecule is composed of three subunits but that only one subunit of these is required for biological activity. Murine submaxillary gland and snake venom are the best sources of NGF, but the microsomal fractions of heart, spleen, and kidney also possess NGF activity. NGF is known to increase glucose utilization, stimulate de novo mRNA synthesis, enhance polysome formation and protein synthesis, increase production of adrenergic neurotransmitters, and stimulate de novo formation of neurotubular subunits in target tissues. Levi-Montalcini (1975) has recently emphasized most strenuously the specificity of action of the NGF as a unique stimulator of growth and development of embryonic sensory and sympathetic neurons.

JOSEPH
LOBUE AND
MILAN
POTMESIL

3. Stimulation of the Incidence of Neoplastic Metastases

3.1. Clinical Studies: Stimulation by Irradiation

Stimulatory effects of therapeutic irradiation of normal tissues on the dissemination and growth of metastases in irradiated loci have been claimed in some clinical studies (Patterson and Russell, 1959, Dao and Kovaric, 1962; Bond, 1967). However, adverse effects of irradiation on metastatic development have been definitely demonstrated experimentally in the lungs (Dao and Yogo, 1967; Fisher and Fisher, 1969; Brown, 1973a; Van den Brenk et al., 1971. 1973b), liver (Koike et al., 1963; Fisher and Fisher, 1969; Van den Brenk and Kelly, 1973), and kidney (Van den Brenk and Kelly, 1973). More than 50 years of attention have been given to the possibility of enhanced metastatic processes in patients receiving radiotherapy for breast and lung cancer, or postoperative radiotherapy for breast cancer, or prophylactic lung irradiation in circumstances in which the existence of undetected pulmonary metastasis is high; e.g., in patients with testicular carcinoma, Wilms' tumor, osteosarcoma, or other types of sarcoma. In patients with lung metastases of Wilms' tumor, whole lung irradiation combined with actinomycin D provides a better chance for control of the disease than irradiation of radiographically visible nodules (Hussey et al., 1971; Monson et al., 1972; Cassady et al., 1973). Multiple drug therapy combined with radiation to known sites of sarcoma and testicular carcinoma involvement and to both entire lungs may offer longer complete remission than would result from radiation alone (Wharam et al., 1974). Extensive data on postoperative management of patients with breast cancer have been presented (for review, see Fisher et al., 1971), and a number of communications have either confirmed or denied the aforementioned possibility. Patterson and Russell (1959) suggested that prophylactic radiotherapy for breast cancer, with liver lying in the path of radiation beams, increased the incidence of liver metastases. Another clinical observation indicated that postoperative radiotherapy for breast cancer increased the incidence and rate of development of metastases in neighboring organs (Bond, 1967). In a later study on postoperative radiotherapy of lung cancer, Patterson and Russell (1962) commented that, in terms of overall results, the prophylactic irradiation applied was of little value. Interestingly enough, the incidence of metastases after prophylactic irradiation was higher not only in an organ neighboring the field of radiation (liver) but also in a distant organ (brain). Two clinical studies using comparable postoperative irradiation techniques produced divergent results. Dao and Kovaric (1962) described an increased incidence of pulmonary and skin metastases in women with breast cancer who had received postoperative irradiation of lung fields as compared with operated-on but unirradiated patients. Chu et al. (1967) reported higher 5-year survival rates in patients irradiated after surgery for breast cancer, and results of a widely based clinical trial (Fisher et al., 1971) indicated that the use of postoperative irradiation has decreased regional occurrences of breast cancer. However, the incidence of metastases in the respiratory and digestive systems was higher than that for unirradiated patients. Analyses of

tive and radiation techniques as well as differences among investigated tumors.
The uncertainty concerning the significance of the stimulatory effect of
radiotherapy on dissemination and growth of metastases reflects the rather
inadequate criteria proposed for clinical trials, which do not permit more definite
conclusions.

3.2. Experimental Studies

3.2.1. Stimulation by Irradiation

Numerous experimental investigations have been performed with various tumors
to obtain information regarding the effect of irradiation on the incidence of
metastases. Experiments with rats (Dao and Yogo, 1967; Fisher and Fisher, 1969;
Van den Brenk and Sharpington, 1972; Van den Brenk et al., 1973a,b) and mice
(Brown, 1973a; Withers and Milas, 1973) have indicated that lung irradiation
increased the number of pulmonary "metastases" arising from intravenously
injected tumor cells, or from tumor cells disseminated from solid tumors located
in the calf-muscle region (Van den Brenk et al., 1973b). Enhanced production of
macrocolonies in preirradiated lungs was demonstrated with injected cell suspensions isolated from isogeneic or allogeneic mouse or rat sarcomas and mouse
mammary carcinomas. The efficiency of this phenomenon is higher in young
experimental animals, is related to the dose of preirradiation, and is transitional in
nature. Its maximum is reached several hours, days, or weeks after irradiation,
and thereafter decreases gradually. Stimulation of colony formation in lungs by
irradiation is strictly a local phenomenon and is not affected by irradiation of
thymus, spleen, or other tissues. Loss of immunological competence is probably
not responsible for enhanced numbers of colonies in irradiated lungs since
stimulatory effects of local irradiation on clonogenic efficiency have been reported
not only in allogeneic but also in syngeneic systems, in which immunological
incompatibility between tumors and hosts should be considered as insignificant.
In rats immunized by allogeneic tumor cells, the number of lung macrocolonies
induced by intravenous application of tumor cells was very low. This was not
significantly changed by whole-body irradiation of older rats, but increased in rats
of weanling age and was also moderately increased by antilymphocytic serum
(ALS). The results were interpreted as indicating that whole body irradiation and
treatment with ALS may increase clonogenic efficiency in rats hyperimmunized
against injected tumor cells by some mechanism other than the suppression of
immunological responses.

3.2.2. Inflammation and Anti-inflammation Agents

The induction rate of macrocolonies in the lungs by intravenously injected
allogeneic tumor cells is relatively low in untreated rats and can be greatly
increased by induced acute inflammation. Acute inflammatory reactions were

induced by cellulose sulfate, extracts of normal rat lung homogenate, or condensation products of p-methoxyphenethylmethylamine with formaldehyde (Van den Brenk *et al.*, 1974*b*). All these substances cause cellular damage with release of biogenic amines and bradykinin and induce local and systemic reactions characteristic of inflammation. Application of pharmacological mediators of inflammation such as histamine, 5-hydroxytryptamine, bradykinin, and of prostaglandins alone did not increase the incidence of lung colonies. Inflammation induced by cellulose sulfate did not prevent the actions of tumor–host immunity established in the same rat against allogeneic tumor cells. The two processes, inflammation and immunity, appeared to act independently. It was also shown that induced inflammatory reaction stimulated the growth of subcutaneously transplanted xenogeneic carcinoma (Van den Brenk and Upfill, 1958). The anti-inflammatory corticosteroids cortisone, hydrocortisone, dexamethasone, and mepyramine administered in high doses caused a five- to tenfold reduction in the number of "metastatic" colonies in lung and kidney following an intravenous injection of tumor cells in unirradiated and whole-body-irradiated rats or in rats with local irradiation of the lung tissue. An anti-inflammatory drug, phenylbutazone, exercised an effect comparable to that of corticosteroids, whereas the mineralocorticosteroids aldosterone and 11-desoxycorticosterone failed to influence the number of colonies. Steroid therapy also decreased growth and spread of tumor cells implanted into the leg muscle of rats (Van den Brenk *et al.*, 1974*a*) and dexamethasone inhibited the stimulatory effect of cellulose sulfate on "metastatic" colony formation in adrenalectomized rats (Van den Brenk *et al.*, 1974*b*).

3.2.3. Thromboplastin and Anticoagulants

Stimulation of the growth of transplanted murine tumors by a predominance of lethally irradiated cells added to the inoculum of viable cells is a well-recognized phenomenon (Révész, 1956). Hewitt *et al.* (1973) have demonstrated that admixture of lethally irradiated tumor cells to viable tumor cells of the same origin increases their clonogenic efficiency and reduces both the latent period of tumor growth and the time necessary for the growing tumor to reach a specific size. A similar effect was obtained when erythrocytes were added to viable tumor cells (Yatvin *et al.*, 1973; Peters and Hewitt, 1974). An association between the growth of tumors or their readiness to metastasize and the process of coagulation has been repeatedly suggested and experimentally substantiated. The accumulated evidence indicates that the coagulation mechanism (Fisher and Fisher, 1961; Wood *et al.*, 1961; Hagmar, 1970), or, more specifically, the formation and stabilization of fibrin (O'Meara, 1958; Cliffton and Agostino, 1964; Ketcham *et al.*, 1971) enhance the seeding of metastatic cells, their survival, and growth. Incorporation of viable tumor cells in fibrin clots before implantation or an admixture of brain extracts to viable cells significantly delayed the disappearance of these cells labeled with [^{125}I]UdR. It was also demonstrated that lethally irradiated lymphoid and bone marrow cells, ineffective in enhancing the "take" of viable tumor cells, were almost totally free of thromboplastin activity. On the contrary, lethally irradiated cells of solid sarcomas and carcinomas exhibiting stimulatory effects on viable tumor cells showed thromboplastin activity (Peters and Hewitt, 1974). Subsequently, Peters and Hewitt (1974) advanced a hypothesis suggesting that the thromboplastin activity exerted by lethally irradiated tumor cells was directly related to the enhancement of the clonogenic efficiency of transplanted viable cells. A fibrin lattice is formed during the coagulation process initiated by released thromboplastin. This lattice surrounds viable cells and provides optimal conditions for their seeding, survival, and proliferation (Grossi et al., 1960; Hewitt et al., 1973; Peters and Hewitt, 1974), for "stromification" of the growing tumor, and for growth of regenerating blood vessels (Stearns, 1940a,b; O'Meara in Peters and Hewitt, 1974). This hypothesis seems to be further supported by several other observations, e.g., that brain extracts and erythrocyte lysates used in experiments are a source of thromboplastin (Quick et al., 1954), or that whole body irradiation, stimulatory to the metastatic spread of experimental tumors, increases the rate of synthesis of fibrinogen (John and Miller, 1968). Treatment with the anticoagulant warfarin reduced the number of lung metastases resulting from an implanted tumor or injected tumor cells (Ryan et al., 1968, 1969; Brown, 1973b), but negative results have also been reported (Higashi and Heidelberger, 1971). Several mechanisms may participate in reduction of the number of bloodborne metastases (reviewed by Brown, 1973b), but analysis of experimental data demonstrates that warfarin does not kill tumor cells directly and does not inhibit cell division. The data support, although they do not prove, the hypothesis postulating the reduction in bloodborne metastases as an effect of anticoagulation, in preventing the formation of adequate thrombi and attachment of tumor cells to the capillary endothelium. The number of pulmonary metastases that developed following an intravenous inoculation of Walker 256 tumor cells were substantially decreased when human fibrinolysin was applied prior to the inoculation (Grossi et al., 1960). However, anticoagulant treatment of rats with heparin had no detectable effect on the incidence of tumor colonies in the lungs (Van den Brenk et al., 1974b). Also, cellulose sulfate, used as an inducer of acute inflammatory reaction in these experiments (see Section 3.2.2), causes marked prolongation of blood clotting time and increases fibrinolytic activity of the blood (Rothschild, 1968). Rather unexpectedly, the incidence of lung metastases was substantially enhanced by this drug (Van den Brenk et al., 1974b). A fibrinogen-depleting agent, a purified enzyme fraction of viper venom, failed to inhibit the stimulatory effect of lethally irradiated cells added to the inoculum as a potential source of thromboplastin. This was determined by the rate of loss of [^{125}I]UdR-labeled viable tumor cells from the site of the inoculum (Peters and Hewitt, 1974). The fibrinolytic enzyme system and the physiology of fibrinolysis, however, are complex phenomena with numerous factors participating. For example, differences in fibrinolytic activity between micro- and macrocirculation or a slowly established equilibrium between fibrinogen levels of intravascular and extravascular pools (Wintrobe et al., 1974) may explain, at least partially, described negative experimental results.

3.3. Possible Mechanisms Involved

Preirradiation of receptor sites such as skin and subcutaneous tissue, soft tissue of an extremity or brain tissue, inhibited growth of subsequent tumor implants. This so-called tumor-bed effect has been reviewed by Fisher and Fisher (1969). Irradiation of other receptors such as lung, liver, and kidney prior to intravascular injection of tumor cells resulted in enhancement of colony formation in these organs (Koike *et al.*, 1963; Fisher and Fisher, 1969; Van den Brenk and Kelly, 1973; Van den Brenk *et al.*, 1971, 1973*b*). The mechanism responsible for these adverse effects of radiation on metastatic formation of tumor colonies is not fully understood. An increased incidence of lung colonies after irradiation of the lungs has been interpreted as inactivation of the local macrophage scavenging system or reduced clearance of tumor cells from the lungs caused by postradiational dilatation of capillaries and increased permeability leading to decreased blood-flow velocity (Brown, 1973*a*). However, some experimental data do not support these conclusions. For example, no evidence of inactivated macrophages was found after local irradiation of the lung with appropriate doses, and immediate trapping and retention of injected tumor cells took place in both unirradiated and irradiated lungs (Shaeffer *et al.*, 1973; Van den Brenk *et al.*, 1973*b*).

Inflammation leads to rapid regenerative growth of the stroma, including blood vessels, and provides a comparable growth-promoting stimulus for both seeded "metastatic" and grafted cancer cells. The time of maximal inflammatory changes in irradiated lung tissue coincides with the highest colony-forming capacity; when the inflammatory reaction subsides and reparative fibrosis starts, the efficiency of colony formation decreases (Fidler and Leidman, 1972). Attenuation and delay of acute inflammation by steroids result in reduced colony formation (Van den Brenk *et al.*, 1973*b*, 1974*a,b*). It is postulated that changes associated with reparative cell proliferation play a substantial role in "takes" and growth of metastatic cells. The increase in concentration of growth-stimulating substance (GSS) as a result of radiation damage of normal tissue can act locally *in vivo* and may have a growth-promoting effect on seeded tumor cells (Van den Brenk and Sharpington, 1972; Van den Brenk *et al.*, 1973*a*, 1974*b*). A diffusible GSS was obtained from inflammatory exudates induced in rats and seemed to be heat stable and inactivated by ribonuclease and trypsin (Menkin, 1961). Van den Brenk *et al.* (1974*b*) suggested that the capacity of different types of tumors to produce GSS may vary widely and may influence the changes of survival and proliferation of seeded cells. GSS is also considered to be present in high concentrations in rapidly growing organs of young animals. This might account for the difference in the production of metastatic macrocolonies in preirradiated lungs between weanling and adult rats (Van den Brenk and Sharpington, 1972; Van den Brenk *et al.*, 1973*b*). Growth promoting factors which may be similar or identical to GSS are discussed in Section 2.4.

The present understanding of the stimulatory effect provided by lethally irradiated tumor cells may be summarized as follows: the addition of these cells to the inocula of viable cells provides a source of thromboplastin; when released from damaged cells, thromboplastin triggers the coagulation reaction, leading to the formation of a fibrin lattice which would be expected to provide optimal conditions for cell survival and proliferation (Peters and Hewitt, 1974). Release of thromboplastin can also be associated with radiation or mechanical damage and surgical trauma to normal tissues. Injury to normal tissues might damage endothelium in capillaries and arterioles, with the formation of stable fibrin at the time when tumor cells are arrested in blood vessels. This would offer tumor cells a better opportunity to invade surrounding tissues as compared with the reversible platelet–protein aggregations which are mostly formed around attached tumor cells in undamaged organs (Jones et al., 1971). Studies with $[^{125}I]$UdR-labeled tumor cells have indicated that there is higher retention of cells in irradiated than in normal lungs, this difference being evident in the early phase of cell attachment to endothelial surfaces (Van den Brenk et al., 1974a). Release of tissue thromboplastin not only induces fibrin clot formation but also may enhance the clonogenic efficiency of seeded tumor cells. The different links in one complex process leading to enhanced metastases may be represented by tissue damage with reactive inflammation, accompanied by regenerative cellular proliferation, and damage of endothelium in blood vessels; activation of the coagulation system, attachment of isolated tumor cells or cell clusters to endothelial surfaces, and their surrounding by a fibrin meshwork; and stimulation of tumor-cell motion and proliferation. Such a cascade phenomenon could occur not only in preirradiated organs but also in traumatized liver and other organs or tissues (Fisher and Fisher, 1959, 1963; review by Ferris et al., 1973) and, at least partially, in organs with local reactive changes induced by whole body irradiation or ALS (Van den Brenk et al., 1973b).

4. Conclusion

A vast variety of humoral substances have been described in the literature, each with claims of involvement in stimulatory processes that lead to the enhancement of cell proliferation or maturation in specific target tissues. Some of these substances also seem to be implicated in stimulatory effects on neoplasms. There is unquestionable evidence that the glycoprotein hormone erythropoietin induces differentiation of the erythropoietin-responsive cell ERC, a committed bone marrow stem cell, leading to the formation of hemoglobin. Erythropoietin also induces differentiation of accumulated erythroid precursors in mice with erythroblastic RLV-A disease, and this leads to a remission in the course of the disease. The experimental evidence that the humoral colony-stimulating factor (CSF) enhances proliferation and differentiation of the committed granulocytic stem cell (CFU-c) also seems to be well established. However, the relationship between CSF and endotoxin effects, antichalones, or diffusible granulocytopoietic stimulator DGS is still unclear. The existence of a leukocytosis-inducing factor UF has been verified experimentally in several species, but, likewise, its relation to CSF and regulation of granulopoiesis is not yet fully understood. The link between CSF, colony-stimulating cells (CSC) which release this factor, and CFU-c has been investigated in granulocytic leukemias and it has been suggested that CSC are abnormal in number or in CSF productive capacity in this disease. There may be two distinct cell populations of CSC, one defective and the other normal or indistinguishable from normal, and it could be proliferation of the latter which occurs during the remission of leukemia. In addition, leukemic patients appear to possess defective CFU-c. Nonhematopoietic growth-stimulating substances represent a group of factors with growth stimulatory effects on target tissues *in situ*, such as neoplasms, epithelial tissue, and sympathetic nervous system, or on explants and cell cultures of neoplastic and embryonic tissue. The precise chemical identity of these stimulators and the mechanism by which they act are not known with certainty, and it cannot be excluded that some of these substances are identical to lysosomal enzymes. One of these, the growth-stimulating factor, might also be involved at some specific stage of metastatic "seeding" of tumor cells in target organs.

In experimental animals, preirradiation of the lung enhances, in this organ, the development of tumor foci arising from either intravenously injected tumor cells or tumor cells disseminated from implanted solid tumors. The mechanisms responsible for radiation-stimulated metastatic formation of tumor colonies may include tissue damage with reactive inflammation and damage of endothelium in blood vessels, activation of the coagulation system, attachment of isolated tumor cells or cell clusters to endothelial surfaces, their surrounding by a fibrin meshwork, and stimulation of tumor-cell motion and proliferation. All of these may represent different links in one complex process leading to enhanced metastases not only in preirradiated lungs but also in traumatized liver. However, uncertainty prevails in clinical medicine concerning the significance of the stimulatory effects of radiotherapy on dissemination and growth of metastases.

ACKNOWLEDGMENTS

The authors wish to acknowledge the technical and secretarial help of Amando Ronquillo and Blanche Ciotti in the preparation of the manuscript.

5. References

ANGELETTI, R. H., ANGELETTI, P. U., AND LEVI-MONTALCINI, R., 1973, The nerve growth factor, in: *Humoral Control of Growth and Differentiation*, Vol. I (J. LoBue and A. S. Gordon, eds.), Academic Press, New York.

ARGYRIS, T. S., 1965, The growth promoting effects of tumors on tissues, in: *Advances in Biology of Skin*, Vol. 6 (N. Montagna, ed.), Pergamon Press, New York.

ARGYRIS, T. S., AND ARGYRIS, B. F., 1962, Differential response of skin epithelium to growth-promoting effects of subcutaneously transplanted tumor, *Cancer Res.* **22**:73.

AXELRAD, A. A., McLEOD, D. L., AND SHREEVE, M. M., 1974, Properties of cells that produce erythrocytic colonies in plasma cultures, in: *Second International Conference on Hemopoiesis in Culture* (W. Robinson, ed.), Grune and Stratton, New York.

AYE, M. T., NIHO, Y., TILL, J. E., AND MCCULLOCH, E. A., 1974, Studies of leukemic cell populations in culture, *Blood* **44**:205.

BECKER, F. F., AND LANE, B. P., 1966, Regeneration of the mammalian liver. IV. Evidence on the role of cytoplasmic alterations in preparation for mitosis, *Am. J. Pathol.* **49**:227.

BIERMAN, H. R., 1964, Characteristics of leukopoietin-G, *Ann. N.Y. Acad. Sci.* **113**:753.

BOECKER, W. R., BOYUM, A., CARSTEN, A. L., AND CRONKITE, E. P., 1971, Human bone marrow (HBM) and blood (HPB) stem cell kinetics, *Blood* **38**:819.

BOGGS, D. R., CHERVENICK, P. A., MARSH, J. C., CARTWRIGHT, G. E., AND WINTROBE, M. M., 1968, Neutrophil releasing activity in plasma of dogs injected with endotoxin, *J. Lab. Clin. Med.* **72**:177.

BOIRON, M., LEVY, J.-P., LASNERET, J., OPPENHEIM, S., AND BERNARD, J., 1965, Pathogenesis of Rauscher leukemia, *J. Natl. Cancer Inst.* **35**:865.

BOND, W. H., 1967, The influence of various treatments on survival rates in cancer of the breast, in: *The Treatment of Carcinoma of the Breast* (A. S. Jarrett, ed.), Excerpta Medica, London.

BOSMANN, H. B., 1972, Elevated glycosidase and proteolytic enzymes in cells transformed by RNA-tumor virus, *Biochim. Biophys. Acta* **264**:339.

BOYUM, A., BOECKER, W., CARSTEN, A. L., AND CRONKITE, E. P., 1972a, Proliferation of human bone marrow cells in diffusion chambers implanted into normal or irradiated mice, *Blood* **40**:163.

BOYUM, A., CARSTEN, A., LAERUM, O. D., AND CRONKITE, E. P., 1972b, Kinetics of cell proliferation of murine bone marrow cells cultured in diffusion chambers: Effect of hypoxia, bleeding, erythropoietin injections, polycythemia, and irradiation of the host, *Blood* **40**:174.

BRADLEY, T. R., AND METCALF, D., 1966, The growth of bone marrow cells in vitro, *Aust. J. Exp. Biol. Med.* **44**:287.

BRADLEY, T. R., METCALF, D., SUMMER, M., AND STANLEY, E. R., 1969, Characteristics of in vitro colony formation by cells from hematopoietic tissues, *Hemic Cells in Vitro* **4**:22.

BRADLEY, T. R., TELFER, P. A., AND FRY, P., 1971, Effect of erythrocytes on mouse bone marrow colony development in vitro, *Blood* **38**:353.

BRECHER, G., 1949, New methylene blue as a reticulocyte stain, *Am. J. Clin. Pathol.* **19**:895.

BROWN, J. M., 1973a, The effect of lung irradiation on the incidence of pulmonary metastases in mice, *Br. J. Radiol.* **46**:613.

BROWN, J. M., 1973b, A study of the mechanism by which anticoagulation with warfarin inhibits blood-borne metastases, *Cancer Res.* **33**:1217.

BROXMEYER, H., VANZANT, G., ZUCALI, J. R., LOBUE, J., AND GORDON, A. S., 1974, Mechanisms of leukocyte production and release. XII. A comparative assay of the leukocytosis-inducing factor (LIF) and the colony-stimulating factor (CSF), *Proc. Soc. Exp. Biol. Med.* **145**:1262.

BURGER, M. M., 1970, Proteolytic enzymes initiating cell division and escape from contact inhibition of growth, *Nature (London)* **227**:170.

BYRON, J. W., 1970, Effect of steroids on the cycling of haemopoietic stem cells, *Nature (London)* **228**:1204.

BYRON, J. W., 1971, Effect of steroids and dibutyryl cyclic AMP on the sensitivity of haemopoietic stem cells to ^{3}H-thymidine in vitro, *Nature (London)* **234**:39.

BYRON, J. W., 1972a, Evidence for a β-adrenergic receptor initiating DNA synthesis in haemopoietic stem cells, *Exp. Cell Res.* **71**:228.

BYRON, J. W., 1972b, Comparison of the action of ^{3}H-thymidine and hydroxyurea on testosterone-treated haemopoietic stem cells, *Blood* **40**:198.

BYRON, J. W., 1975a, Manipulation of the cell cycle of the hemopoietic stem cell: A review summary, *Exp. Hematol.* (in press).

BYRON, J. W., 1975b, Cholinergic mechanisms and the hemopoietic stem cell, in: *Proceedings of the Second International Symposium on Erythropoiesis*, Tokyo University Press, Tokyo (in press).

CAMISCOLI, J. F., LOBUE, J., GORDON, A. S., ALEXANDER, P., SCHULTZ, E. F., WEITZ-HAMBURGER, A., AND FREDRICKSON, T. N., 1972, Absence of plasma erythropoietin in mice with anemia induced by Rauscher leukemia virus, *Cancer Res.* **32**:2843.

CASSADY, J. R., PEFFP, M., FILLER, R. M., JAFFE, N., AND HELLMAN, S., 1973, Considerations in the radiation therapy of Wilms' tumor, *Cancer* **32**:598.

CHERVENICK, P. A., 1972, Effect of endotoxin and postendotoxin plasma on in vitro granulopoiesis, *J. Lab. Clin. Med.* **79**:1014.

CHERVENICK, P. A., AND LOBUGLIO, A. F., 1972, Human blood monocytes: Stimulators of granulocyte and mononuclear colony formation in vitro, *Science* **178**:164.

CHERVENICK, P. A., ELLIS, L. D., PAN, S. F., AND LAWSON, A. L., 1971, Human leukemic cells: In vitro growth of colonies containing the Philadelphia (Ph) chromosome, *Science* **174**:1134.

CHU, F. C. H., LUCAS, J. C., JR., FARROW, J. H., AND NICKSON, J. J., 1967, Does prophylactic radiation therapy given for cancer of the breast predispose to metastases? *Am. J. Roentgenol.* **99**:987.

CLIFFTON, E. E., AND AGOSTINO, D., 1964, Effect of inhibitors of fibrinolytic enzymes on development of pulmonary metastases, *J. Natl. Cancer Inst.* **33**:753.

COHEN, S., 1960, Purification of nerve-growth promoting protein from the mouse salivary gland and its neuro-cytotoxic antiserum, *Proc. Natl. Acad. Sci.* **46**:302.

COHEN, S., 1962, Isolation of a mouse submaxillary gland protein accelerating incisor eruption and eyelid opening in the new-born animal, *J. Biol. Chem.* **237**:1555.

COHEN, S., 1964, Isolation and biological effects of an epidermal growth-stimulating protein, in: *Metabolic Control Mechanisms in Animal Cells* (W. Rutter, ed.), National Cancer Institute Monograph 13, D.H.E.W., Washington, D.C.

COHEN, S., 1965, The stimulation of epidermal proliferation by a specific protein (EGF), *Dev. Biol.* **12**:394.

COHEN, S., AND ELLIOTT, G. A., 1963, The stimulation of epidermal keratinization by a protein isolated from the submaxillary gland of the mouse, *J. Invest. Dermatol.* **40**:1.

DAO, T. L., AND KOVARIC, J., 1962, Incidence of pulmonary and skin metastases in women with breast cancer who received post-operative irradiation, *Surgery* **52**:203.

DAO, T. L., AND YOGO, H., 1967, Enhancement of pulmonary metastases by X irradiation in rats bearing mammary cancer, *Cancer* **20**:2020.

DELMONTE, L., 1968, Differential spleen colony bioassay for granulopoietic factor (GPF) and endotoxin, *Exp. Hematol.* **16**:14.

DICKE, K. A., PLATENBURG, M. G. E., AND VAN BEKKUM, D. W., 1971, Colony formation in agar: *In vitro* assay for haemopoietic stem cells, *Cell Tissue Kinet.* **4**:463.

DORNFEST, B. S., LOBUE, J., HANDLER, E. S., GORDON, A. S., AND QUASTLER, H., 1962, Mechanisms of leukocyte production and release. I. Factors influencing leukocyte release from isolated perfused rat femora, *Acta Haematol.* **28**:42.

EBERT, P. S., MAESTRI, N. E., AND CHIRIGOS, M. A., 1972, Erythropoietic responses of mice to infection with Rauscher leukemia virus, *Cancer Res.* **32**:41.

EPIFANOVA, O. I., 1967, *Hormones and the Reproduction of Cells*, Israel Program of Scientific Translations, Jerusalem.

FEHER, I., AND GIDALI, J., 1974, Prostaglandin E_2 as a stimulator of stem cell proliferation, *Nature (London)* **247**:550.

FELL, H. B., 1973, Commentary on "Epidermal chalone: Cell cycle specificity of two epidermal growth inhibitors" by K. Elgjo, *Natl. Cancer Inst. Monogr.* **38**:77.

FERRIS, P., MOLOMUT, N., AND LOBUE, J., 1973, Trauma and tumor growth with special emphasis on wound stress and "wound hormones," in: *Humoral Control of Growth and Differentiation* (J. LoBue and A. S. Gordon, eds.), Academic Press, New York.

FIDLER, I. J., AND LEIDMAN, J., 1972, Enhancement of experimental metastasis by x-ray: A possible mechanism, *J. Med.* **3**:172.

FISHER, B., AND FISHER, E. R., 1959, Experimental studies of factors influencing hepatic metastases. III. Effect of surgical trauma with special reference to liver injury, *Ann. Surg.* **150**:731.

FISHER, B., AND FISHER, E. R., 1961, Anticoagulants and tumor cell lodgement, *Cancer Res.* **27**:421.

FISHER, E. R., AND FISHER, B., 1963, Experimental studies of factors influencing metastases. XIII. Effect of hepatic trauma in parabiotic pairs, *Cancer Res.* **23**:896.

FISHER, E. R., AND FISHER, B., 1969, Effects of X irradiation on parameters of tumor growth, histology, and ultrastructure, *Cancer* **24**:39.

FISHER, B., SLACK, N. H., CAVANAUGH, P. J., GARDNER, B., AND RAVDIN, R. G., 1971, Post-operative radiotherapy in the treatment of breast cancer: Results of the NSABP Clinical Trial, *Ann. Surg.* **172**:711.

FORSCHER, B. K., AND HOUCK, J. C. (eds.), 1973, *"Chalones": Concepts and Current Researches*, National Cancer Institute Monograph 38, D.H.E.W., Washington.

FOSTER, R., METCALF, D., ROBINSON, W. A., AND BRADLEY, T. R., 1968, Bone marrow colony stimulating activity in human sera: Results of two independent surveys in Buffalo and Melbourne, *Br. J. Haematol.* **15**:147.

FREDRICKSON, T. N., LOBUE, J., ALEXANDER, P., JR., SCHULTZ, E. F., AND GORDON, A. S., 1972, A transplantable leukemia from mice inoculated with Rauscher leukemia virus, *J. Natl. Cancer Inst.* **48**:1597.

GOLDE, D. W., AND CLINE, M. J., 1972, Identification of the colony stimulating cell in human peripheral blood, *J. Clin. Invest.* **51**:2981.

GOLDE, D. W., FINLEY, T. N., AND CLINE, M. J., 1972, Production of colony stimulating factor by human macrophages, *Lancet* **2**:1397.

GOLDMAN, J. M., TH'NG, K. H., AND LOWENTHAL, R. M., 1974, *In vitro* colony forming cells and colony stimulating factor in chronic granulocytic leukaemia, *Br. J. Cancer* **30**:1.

GORDON, A. S., 1973, Erythropoietin, *Vitam. Horm. (N.Y.)* **31**:105.

GORDON, A. S., NERI, R. O., SIEGEL, C. D., DORNFEST, B. S., HANDLER, E. S., LoBUE, J., AND EISLER, M., 1960, Evidence for a circulating leukocytosis-inducing factor (LIF), *Acta Haematol.* **23**:323.

GORDON, A. S., HANDLER, E. S., SIEGEL, C. D., DORNFEST, B. S., AND LoBUE, J., 1964, Plasma factors influencing leukocyte release in rats, *Ann. N.Y. Acad. Sci.* **113**:766.

GREENBERG, P. L., NICHOLS, W. C., AND LEHRIER, S. L., 1971, Granulopoiesis in acute myeloid leukemia and preleukemia *New Engl. J. Med.* **284**:1225.

GROSSI, C. E., AGOSTINO, D., AND CLIFFTON, E. E., 1960, The effect of human fibrinolysin on pulmonary metastases of Walker 256 carcinosarcoma, *Cancer Res.* **20**:605.

HAGMAR, B., 1970, Experimental tumor metastases and blood coagulability, *Acta Pathol. Microb. Scand.* **211**:1.

HALL, B. M., 1969, The effects of whole body irradiation on serum colony-stimulating factor and *in vitro* colony forming cells in the bone marrow, *Br. J. Haematol.* **17**:553.

HASKILL, J. S., MCNEILL, T. A., AND MOORE, M. A. S., 1970, Density distribution analysis of *in vivo* and *in vitro* colony forming cells in bone marrow, *J. Cell Physiol.* **75**:167.

HASKILL, J. S., MCKNIGHT, R. D., AND GALBRAITH, P. R., 1972, Cell–cell interaction *in vitro*: Studies by density separation of colony forming, stimulating and inhibiting cells from human, *Blood* **40**:394.

HEIT, W., KERN, P., KUBANEK, B., AND HEIMPEL, H., 1974, Some factors influencing granulocytic colony formation *in vitro* by human white blood cells, *Blood* **44**:511.

HEWITT, H. B., BLAKE, E. R., AND PORTER, E. H., 1973, The effect of lethally irradiated cells on the transplantability of murine tumors, *Br. J. Cancer* **28**:123.

HIGASHI, H., AND HEIDELBERGER, C., 1971, Lack of effect of warfarin (N-S-C-59813) alone or in combination with 5-fluorouracil (NSC-19893) on primary and metatastic L1210 leukemia and adenocarcinoma 755, *Cancer Chem. Rep. Part I* **55**:29.

HUSSEY, B. H., CASTRO, G. R., SULLIVAN, M. P., AND SATOW, W. W., 1971, Radiation therapy in management of Wilms' tumor, *Radiology* **101**:663.

ISCOVE, N. N., SENN, J. S., TILL, J. E., AND MCCULLOCH, E. A., 1971, Colony formation by normal and leukaemic human marrow cells in culture: Effect of conditioned medium from human leukocytes, *Blood* **31**:1.

JOHN, D. W., AND MILLER, L. L., 1968, Effect of whole body x-irradiation of rats on net synthesis of albumin, fibrinogen, α_1-acid glycoprotein and α_2-globulin (acute phase globulin) by the isolated perfused rat liver, *J. Biol. Chem.* **243**:268.

JOHNSON, L. I., AND RUBIN, A. D., 1970, Lymphocyte growth and proliferation in culture, in: *Regulation of Hematopoiesis* (A. S. Gordon, ed.), Appleton-Century-Crofts, New York.

JONES, D. S., WALLACE, A. C., AND FRASER, E. E., 1971, Sequence of events in experimental metastases of Walker 256 tumor: Light, immuno-fluorescent, and electron microscopic observations, *J. Natl. Cancer Inst.* **46**:493.

JONES, R. O., 1966, The *in vitro* effect of epithelial growth factor on rat organ cultures, *Exp. Cell Res.* **43**:645.

KETCHAM, A. S., SUGARBAKER, E. V., RYAN, J. J., AND ORME, S. K., 1971, Clotting factors and metastasis formation, *Am. J. Roentgenol.* **111**:42.

KOIKE, A., NAKAZATO, H., AND MOORE, G. E., 1963, The fate of Ehrlich cells injected into the portal system, *Cancer* **16**:716.

KRANTZ, S. B., AND JACOBSON, L. O., 1970, *Erythropoietin and the Regulation of Erythropoiesis*, University of Chicago Press, Chicago.

LAJTHA, L. G., 1970, Stem cell kinetics, in: *Regulation of Hematopoiesis* (A. S. Gordon, ed.), Appleton-Century-Crofts, New York.

LAJTHA, L. G., 1972, Kinetics of proliferation and differentiation in hemopoiesis, in: *Regulation of Erythropoiesis* (A. S. Gordon, M. Condorelli, and C. Peschle, eds.), Il Ponte, Milan.

LEVI-MONTALCINI, R., 1975, Nerve growth factor, Letter to editor, *Science* **187**:113.

LEVI-MONTALCINI, R., AND COHEN, S., 1960, Effect of extract of the mouse submaxillary salivary gland on the sympathetic system of mammals, *Ann. N.Y. Acad. Sci.* **85**:324.

LoBUE, J., ALEXANDER, P., JR., FREDRICKSON, T. N., SCHULTZ, E. F., GORDON, A. S., AND JOHNSON, L. I., 1972, Erythrokinetics in normal and disease states: Virally-induced murine erythroblastosis: A model system, in: *Regulation of Erythropoiesis* (A. S. Gordon, M. Condorelli, and C. Peschle, eds.), Il Ponte, Milan.

LoBue, J., Gordon, A. S., Weitz-Hamberger, A., Ferdinand, P., Camiscoli, J. F., Fredrickson, T. N., and Hardy, W. D., Jr., 1974, Erythroid differentiation in murine erythroleukemia, in: *Control of Proliferation in Animal Cells* (B. Clarkson and R. Baserga, eds.), Cold Spring Harbor Laboratory, Cold Spring Harbor, N.Y.

LoBue, J., Fredrickson, T. N., Gallicchio, V., Ronquillo, A., and Gordon, A. S., 1975, Exogenous and endogenous erythropoietin in the treatment of the fatal anemia of RLV disease, in: *Proceedings of the Second International Symposium on Erythropoiesis*, Tokyo University Press, Tokyo (in press).

Ludford, R. J., and Barlow, H., 1944, The influence of malignant cells upon the growth of fibroblasts *in vitro, Cancer Res.* **4:**694.

McNeill, T. A., 1970, Antigenic stimulation of bone marrow colony forming cells. 1. Effect of antigens on normal bone marrow cells *in vitro, Immunology* **18:**39.

McNeill, T. A., and Killen, M., 1971, The effect of synthetic double-stranded polyribonucleotides on haemopoietic colony forming cells *in vivo, Immunology* **21:**751.

Menkin, V., 1961, Studies of the growth promoting factor of exudates in reference (a) to its effect on the development of spontaneous neoplasms in tumour susceptible mice; (b) to its presence in rabbit exudate; (c) in its comparative growth potential in organs of immature and adult animals, *Pathol. Biol.* **9:**861.

Merwin, R. M., and Algire, G. H., 1956, The role of graft and host vessels in vascularization of grafts of normal and neoplastic tissue, *J. Natl. Cancer Inst.* **17:**23.

Messner, H. A., Till, J. E., and McCulloch, E. A., 1973, Interacting cell populations affecting granulopoietic colony formation by normal and leukemic human marrow cells, *Blood* **42:**701.

Metcalf, D., 1958, The thymic lymphocytosis-stimulating factor, *Ann. N.Y. Acad. Sci.* **73:**113.

Metcalf, D., 1971, Acute antigen-induced elevation of serum colony stimulating factor (CSF) levels, *Immunology* **21:**427.

Metcalf, D., 1972, Studies on colony formation *in vitro* by mouse hematopoietic cells, *Proc. Soc. Exp. Biol. Med.* **139:**511.

Metcalf, D., 1973, The colony stimulating factor, in: *Humoral Control of Growth and Differentiation,* Vol. I, (J. LoBue and A. S. Gordon, eds.), Academic Press, New York.

Metcalf, D., and Foster, R., Jr., 1967, Behavior on transfer of serum stimulated bone marrow colonies, *Proc. Soc. Exp. Biol. Med.* **126:**758.

Metcalf, D., and Moore, M. A. S., 1971, *Haemopoietic Cells,* North-Holland, Amsterdam.

Metcalf, D., and Stanley, E. R., 1971, Haematological effects in mice of partially purified colony stimulating factor (CSF) prepared from human urine, *Br. J. Haematol.* **21:**481.

Metcalf, D., Foster, R., and Pollard, M., 1967, Colony stimulating activity of serum from germfree normal and leukemic mice, *J. Cell. Physiol.* **70:**131.

Monson, K. J., Brand, W. N., and Boggs, J. D., 1972, Results of small-field irradiation of apparent solitary metastasis from Wilms' tumor, *Radiology* **104:**157.

Moore, M. A. S., 1973, *In vitro* colony formation by normal and leukemic human hematopoietic cells: Characterization of the colony-forming cells, *J. Natl. Cancer Inst.* **50:**603.

Moore, M. A. S., and Williams, N., 1972a, Physical separation of *in vitro* colony forming cells from colony stimulating cells in blood and bone marrow, *J. Cell. Physiol.* **80:**195.

Moore, M. A. S., and Williams, N., 1972b, Characterization of the colony stimulating cell, in: *In Vitro Culture of Hemopoietic Cells* (D. W. van Bekkum and K. A. Dicke, eds.), Radiobiological Institute, TNO, Rijswijk.

Moore, M. A. S., Williams, N., and Metcalf, D., 1972, Purification and characterization of the *in vitro* colony forming cells in monkey hemopoietic tissue, *J. Cell. Physiol.* **79:**283.

Moore, M. A. S., Williams, N., and Metcalf, D., 1973, *In vitro* colony formation by normal and leukemic human hematopoietic cells: Interaction between colony forming and colony stimulating cells, *J. Natl. Cancer Inst.* **50:**591.

Morley, A., Rikard, K. A., Howard, D., and Stohlman, F., Jr., 1971, Studies on the regulation of granulopoiesis. IV. Possible humoral regulation, *Blood* **37:**14.

Morse, B. S., Giuliani, D., Giuliani, E. R., LoBue, J., and Fredrickson, T. N., 1973, Defective iron utilization in viral induced murine erythroblastosis, Program, Annual Meeting, American Society of Hematology.

Nair, B. K., and DeOme, K. B., 1972, Induction of DNA synthesis in density inhibited cultures of mouse embryo cells by a factor present in mouse mammary tumors, *in Vitro* **7:**272.

Nair, B. K., and DeOme, K. B., 1973a, A growth-stimulating factor released by cultured mouse mammary tumor cells, *Cancer Res.* **33:**2754.

NAIR, B. K., AND DEOME, K. B., 1973b, A growth-stimulating factor from solid mouse mammary tumors, *Cancer Res.* **33**:3222.

ODELL, T. T., JR., 1972, Regulation of the megakaryocyte–platelet system, in: *Regulation of Organ and Tissue Growth* (R. J. Goss, ed.), Academic Press, New York.

ODELL, T. T. JR., 1973, Humoral regulation of thrombopoiesis, in: *Humoral Control of Growth and Differentiation*, Vol. I (J. LoBue and A. S. Gordon, eds.), Academic Press, New York.

OKUNEWICK, J. P., AND ERHARD, P., 1974, Accelerated clearance of exogenously administered erythropoietin by mice with Rauscher viral leukemia, *Cancer Res.* **34**:917.

O'MEARA, R. A. Q., 1958, Coagulative properties of cancers, *J. Med. Sci.* **394**:474.

PARAN, M., AND SACHS, L., 1969, The continued requirement for inducer for development of macrophage and granulocyte colonies, *J. Cell. Physiol.* **73**:91.

PARAN, M., SACHS, L., BARAK, Y., AND RESNITZKY, P., 1970, *In vitro* induction of granulocyte differentiation in hematopoietic cells from leukemic and nonleukemic patients, *Proc. Natl. Acad. Sci.* **67**:1542.

PATTERSON, R., AND RUSSELL, M. H., 1959, Clinical trials in malignant disease. II, III. Breast cancer, *J. Fac. Radiol. London* **10**:130.

PATTERSON, R., AND RUSSELL, M. H., 1962, Clinical trials in malignant disease. IV. Lung cancer, *Clin. Radiol.* **13**:141.

PETERS, L. J., AND HEWITT, H. B., 1974, The influence of fibrin formation on the transplantability of murine tumour cells: Implications for the mechanism of the Révész effect, *Br. J. Cancer* **29**:279.

PIKE, B. L., AND ROBINSON, W. A., 1970, Human bone marrow colony growth in agar gel, *J. Cell, Physiol.* **76**:77.

PLUZNIK, D. H., AND SACHS, L., 1965, The cloning of normal mast cells in tissue cultures, *J. Cell Comp. Physiol.* **66**:319.

PLUZNIK, D. H., SACHS, L., AND RESNITZKY, P., 1966, The mechanism of leukemogenesis by Rauscher leukemia virus, *Natl. Cancer Inst. Monogr.* **22**:3.

QUESENBERRY, P., MORLEY, A., STOHLMAN, F., JR., RICKARD, K. A., HOWARD, D., AND SMITH, M., 1972, Effect of endotoxin on granulopoiesis and colony stimulating factor, *New Engl. J. Med.* **286**:227.

QUICK, A. J., GEORGATSOS, G. G., AND HUSSEY, C. V., 1954, Clotting activity of human erythrocytes: Theoretical and clinical implications, *Am. J. Med. Sci.* **228**:207.

RANDIVE, K. J., AND BHIDE, S. V., 1962, Tissue interactions between normal and malignant cells, in: *Biological Interactions in Normal and Neoplastic Growth* (M. J. Brennen and W. L. Simpson, eds.), Little, Brown, New York.

RAUSCHER, F. J., 1962, A virus-induced disease of mice characterized by erythrocytopoiesis and lymphoid leukemia, *J. Natl. Cancer Inst.* **29**:515.

REISSMANN, K. R., AND SAMORAPOOMPICHIT, S., 1970, Effect of erythropoietin on proliferation of erythroid stem cells in the absence of transplantable colony forming units, *Blood* **36**:287.

RÉVÉSZ, L., 1956, Effect of tumor cells killed by X-rays upon the growth of admixed viable cells, *Nature (London)* **178**:1391.

ROBINSON, W., AND KURNICK, J. E., 1972, Granulocyte colony formation *in vitro* by bone marrow from patients with granulocytopenia and aplastic anemia, in: *In Vitro Culture of Hemopoietic Cells* (D. W. van Bekkum and K. A. Dicke, eds.), Radiobiological Institute, TNO, Rijswijk.

ROBINSON, W. A., AND PIKE, B., 1970, Leukopoietic activity in human urine, *New Engl. J. Med.* **282**:1291.

ROBINSON, W. A., METCALF, D., AND BRADLEY, T. R., 1967, Stimulation by normal and leukemic mouse sera of colony formation *in vitro* by mouse bone marrow cells, *J. Cell. Physiol.* **69**:83.

ROBINSON, W., STANLEY, E. R., AND METCALF, D., 1969, Stimulation of bone marrow colony growth *in vitro* by human urine, *Blood* **33**:396.

ROBINSON, W. A., KURNICK, J. E., AND PIKE, B. L., 1971, Colony growth of human leukemic peripheral blood cells *in vitro*, *Blood* **38**:500.

ROTHSCHILD, A. M., 1968, Some pharmacodynamic properties of cellulose sulphate, a kininogen depleting agent in the rat, *Br. J. Pharmacol. Chemother.* **33**:501.

ROTHSTEIN, G., HÜGL, E. H., BISHOP, C. R., AND ATHENS, J. W., 1971, Stimulation of granulopoiesis by a diffusible factor *in vivo*, *J. Clin. Invest.* **50**:2004.

ROTHSTEIN, G., HÜGL, E. H., CHERVENICK, P. A., ATHENS, J. W., AND MACFARLANE, J., 1973, Humoral stimulators of granulocyte production, *Blood* **41**:73.

ROUNDS, D. E., 1970, Growth-modifying factor from cell lines of human malignant origin, *Cancer Res.* **30**:2847.

RUBIN, H., 1970, Overgrowth stimulating factor released from Rous sarcoma cells, *Science* **167**:1271.

RYAN, J. J., KETCHAM, A. S., AND WEXLER, H., 1968, Warfarin treatment of mice bearing autochthonous tumors: Effect of spontaneous metastases, *Science* **162**:1493.

RYAN, J. J., KETCHAM, A. S., AND WEXLER, H., 1969, Warfarin therapy as an adjunct to the surgical treatment of malignant tumors in mice, *Cancer Res.* **29**:2191.

RYTÖMAA, T., AND KIVINIEMI, K., 1967, Regulation system of blood cell production, in: *Control of Cellular Growth in Adult Organisms* (H. Teir and T. Rytömaa, eds.), Academic Press, New York.

RYTÖMAA, T., AND KIVINIEMI, K., 1968a, Control of granulocyte production. I. Chalone and antichalone, two specific humoral regulators, *Cell Tissue Kinet.* **1**:329.

RYTÖMAA, T., AND KIVINIEMI, K., 1968b, Control of granulocyte production. II. Mode of action of chalone and antichalone, *Cell Tissue Kinet.* **1**:341.

SCHNEBLI, H. P., 1972, A protease-like activity associated with malignant cells, *Schweiz. Med. Wochenschr.* **102**:1194.

SCHNEBLI, H. P., 1974, Growth inhibition of tumor cells by protease inhibitors: Consideration of the mechanisms involved, in: *Control of Proliferation in Animal Cells* (B. Clarkson and R. Baserga, eds.), Cold Spring Harbor Laboratory, Cold Spring Harbor, N.Y.

SCHNEBLI, H. P., AND BURGER, M. M., 1972, Selective inhibition of growth of transformed cells by protease inhibitors, *Proc. Natl. Acad. Sci.* **69**:3825.

SEFTON, B. M., AND RUBIN, H., 1970, Release from density dependent growth inhibition by proteolytic enzymes, *Nature (London)* **227**:843.

SHADDUCK, R. K., AND NANKIN, H. R., 1971, Cellular origin of granulocytic colonies in chronic myeloid leukemia, *Lancet* **2**:1097.

SHADDUCK, R. K., AND NEGABHUSHANOM, N. G., 1971, Granulocyte colony stimulating factor: Response to acute granulocytopenia, *Blood* **38**:559.

SHADDUCK, R. K., NUMSA, N. G., AND KREBS, J., 1971, Granulocyte colony stimulating factor. II. Relation to *in vivo* granulopoiesis, *J. Lab. Clin. Med.* **78**:53.

SHAEFFER, J., EL-MAHDI, A. M., AND CONSTABLE, W. C., 1973, Lung colony assays of murine mammary tumor cells irradiated *in vivo* and *in vitro*, *Radiology* **109**:703.

STANLEY, E. R., AND METCALF, D., 1969, Partial purification and some properties of the factor in normal and leukemic human urine stimulating mouse bone marrow colony growth *in vitro*, *Aust. J. Exp. Biol. Med. Sci.* **47**:467.

STANLEY, E. R., AND METCALF, D., 1971, The molecular weight of colony stimulating factor (CSF), *Proc. Soc. Exp. Biol. Med.* **137**:1029.

STANLEY, E. R., MCNEILL, T. A., AND CHAN, S. H., 1970, Antibody production to the factor in human urine stimulating colony formation *in vitro* by bone marrow cells, *Br. J. Haematol.* **18**:585.

STEARNS, M. L., 1940a, Studies on the development of connective tissue in transparent chambers in the rabbit's ear I, *Am. J. Anat.* **66**:133.

STEARNS, M. L., 1940b, Studies on the development of connective tissue in transparent chambers in the rabbit's ear II, *Am. J. Anat.* **67**:55.

STOHLMAN, F., JR., QUESENBERRY, P. J., AND TYLER, W. S., 1974, The regulation of myelopoiesis as approached with *in vivo* and *in vitro* techniques, in: *Progress in Hematology*, Grune and Stratton, New York.

TURKINGTON, R. W., 1969a, Stimulation of mammary carcinoma cell proliferation by epithelial growth factor *in vitro*, *Cancer Res.* **29**:1457.

TURKINGTON, R. W., 1969b, The role of epithelial growth factor in mammary gland development *in vitro*, *Exp. Cell Res.* **57**:79.

TURKINGTON, R. W., MALES, J. L., AND COHEN, S., 1971, Synthesis and storage of epithelial-epidermal growth factor in submaxillary gland, *Cancer Res.* **31**:252.

VAN DEN BRENK, H. A. S., AND KELLY, H., 1973, Stimulation of growth of metastases in local x-irradiation in kidney and liver, *Br. J. Cancer* **28**:349.

VAN DEN BRENK, H. A., S., AND SHARPINGTON, C., 1972, Effect of local x-irradiation of a primary sarcoma in the rat on dissemination and growth of metastases: Dose–response characteristics, *Br. J. Cancer* **25**:812.

VAN DEN BRENK, H. A. S., AND UPFILL, J., 1958, Heterologous growth of Ehrlich ascites tumor in histamine-depleted rats, *Aust. J. Sci.* **21**:20.

VAN DEN BRENK, H. A. S., MOORE, V., AND SHARPINGTON, C., 1971, Growth of metastases from primary sarcoma in the rat following whole body irradiation, *Br. J. Cancer* **25**:186.

VAN DEN BRENK, H. A. S., SHARPINGTON, C., AND ORTON, C., 1973a, Macrocolony assays in the rat of allogenic Y-P388 and W-256 tumor cells injected intravenously: Dependence of colony forming efficiency on age of host and immunity, *Br. J. Cancer* **27**:134.

VAN DEN BRENK, H. A. S., BURCH, W. M., ORTON, C., AND SHARPINGTON, C., 1973b, Stimulation of clonogenic growth of tumor cells and metastases in the lungs by local x-radiation, *Br. J. Cancer* **27**:291.

VAN DEN BRENK, H. A. S., KELLY, H., AND ORTON, C., 1974a, Reduction by anti-inflammatory corticosteroids of clonogenic growth of allogeneic tumour cells in normal and irradiated tissues of the rat, *Br. J. Cancer* **29**:365.

VAN DEN BRENK, H. A. S., STONE, M., KELLY, H., ORTON, C., AND SHARPINGTON, C., 1974b, Promotion of growth of tumor cells in acutely inflamed tissues, *Br. J. Cancer* **30**:246.

VAN DEN ENGH, G. J., 1974, Quantitative *in vitro* studies on stimulation of murine haemopoietic cells by colony stimulating factor, *Cell Tissue Kinet.* **7**:537.

WEINER, H. L., AND ROBINSON, W. A., 1971, Leukopoietic activity in human urine following operative procedures, *Proc. Soc. Exp. Biol. Med.* **136**:29.

WHARAM, M. D., PHILLIPS, T. L., AND JACOBS, E. M., 1974, Combination chemotherapy and whole lung irradiation for pulmonary metastases from sarcomas and germinal cell tumors of the testes, *Cancer* **34**:136.

WINTROBE, M. M., LEE, G. R., BOGGS, D. R., BITHELL, T. C., ATHENS, J. W., AND FOERSTER, G., 1974, *Clinical Hematology*, Lea and Febiger, Philadelphia.

WITHERS, H. R., AND MILAS, L., 1973, Influence of pre-irradiation of lung on development of artificial pulmonary metastases of fibrosarcoma in mice, *Cancer Res.* **33**:1931.

WOOD, S., JR., HOLYOKE, E. D., AND YARDLEY, J. H., 1961, Mechanism of metastasis production by blood-borne cancer cells, *Can. Cancer. Conf.* **4**:167.

WORTON, R. G., McCULLOCH, E. A., AND TILL, J. E., 1969, Physical separation of hemopoietic stem cells from cells forming colonies in culture, *J. Cell. Physiol.* **74**:171.

YATVIN, M. B., STONE, H. B., AND CLIFTON, K. H., 1973, Tumor growth stimulation in mice by radiation killed tumor cells and erythrocytes, in: *Fifth International Symposium on Cancer* (L. Leveri, ed.), University of Perugia Publications, Perugia, Italy.

10

Endocrine Factors and Tumor Growth

Kelly H. Clifton and Bhavani N. Sridharan

1. Endocrine Homeostasis and Carcinogenesis

1.1. Introduction

The sciences of endocrinology and cancer biology have developed hand in hand. Among the discoveries which followed the expansion of the experimental approach to medicine exemplified by Claude Bernard's definition of the concept of homeostasis within the internal milieu (see translation of 1865 text: Bernard, 1949) was the British surgeon Beatson's recognition of an association between the ovaries and breast cancer (Beatson, 1896).

Neither science flowered, however, until after the turn of the century. Both were in part spurred by the development and widespread utilization of standardized experimental animals. A nineteenth-century leader in infectious disease research achieved a second immortality by isolating a broadly transplantable mammary carcinoma from a genetically undefined mouse (Erhlich, 1906), and the Erhlich carcinoma is still propagated in one form or another in virtually every cancer research institute in the world. It was not until the introduction of highly inbred mouse strains by C. C. Little and associates in the 1920s and 1930s (Strong, 1942; Heston, 1949), however, that successful transplantation of virtually all tumors and many normal tissues became feasible. Similarly, following the

Kelley H. Clifton and Bhavani N. Sridharan • Radiobiology Research Laboratories, Department of Radiology, University of Wisconsin Medical School, Madison, Wisconsin.
Work in this laboratory is supported by grants No. DT-350 and CA-13881 from the American Cancer Society and the National Cancer Institute, respectively, and by Cancer Center Grant CA-14520, National Cancer Institute.

isolation and synthesis of epinephrine, increased progress in isolation and purification of other hormones was stimulated in part by the development and ready availability of many lines of laboratory rat—for example, the Long-Evans strain, in which the stages of the estrus cycle, so important to the isolation of ovarian hormones, were first defined (Long and Evans, 1922). An explosion of information on endocrine–cancer relationships ensued in the groups of Lacasagne (1939), Zondek (1941), Bittner (1946), Burrows (1949), Furth (1953), Gardner *et al.* (1953), Foulds (1954), Huggins (1957), DeOme *et al.* (1959), and many others. By the late 1950s, the broad biological concepts of hormonal influences in carcinogenesis and tumor growth had been defined. Research since that time has increased knowledge of the intricate details within this framework, and the bulk of this chapter will deal with these more recent findings. The following is a brief summary of the salient features of the framework drawn from many, but principally from the concept of hormone-dependent and autonomous neoplasia of Furth (1953, 1959), discussions with colleagues, and personal experience. We thus take no credit for the originality of the ideas summarized, but assume responsibility for any distortion of the concepts of others. In the remainder of the chapter, rather than attempt to deal with the actions of each hormone, or the endocrine relationships of neoplasms of each endocrine gland and hormone-responsive tissue, we have chosen examples to discuss in more detail, or several examples to illustrate a general point. Where possible, readers are referred to recent reviews.

1.2. Induction and Progression of Endocrine-Related Tumors

In the most naive sense, a tumor can be described as a local excess of cells, and all metazoans appear susceptible to tumor formation. Such a cellular excess may result from (1) a decrease in the cell cycle time, with the dividing cell life span held constant, (2) an increase in the number of divisions during the dividing cell life span, cell cycle time being constant, or (3) a combination of these (Clifton and Meyer, 1956). One or both occur during many normal or experimentally induced adaptive processes—e.g., in the hematopoietic system during adaptation to high altitude, in the uterine endometrium during the follicular phase, and in regenerating liver after partial hepatectomy. These do not normally result in tumor formation because the cells involved respond to growth regulatory mechanisms which change as the organism's physiological needs are met.

It follows that tumor formation may result *either* from a genotypic or phenotypic change in one or more cells which alters the response to growth regulatory factors *or* from a change in the balance of regulatory factors which results in the maintenance of a normal capacity to proliferate but at an abnormally high level for an abnormally long period of time. Of the known or postulated regulatory systems, the hormones are the most obvious.

In practice, neoplasms of the second type, comprised of "normal cells in an abnormal environment"—i.e., of cells which would not give rise to tumors in a balanced physiological milieu—have been seen primarily in cancer biology laboratories. Clinical oncologists deal for the most part with masses of cells which are already altered in their response to regulatory mechanisms. As such, they see but a part of the spectrum. Studies of endocrine-imbalance-induced neoplasms have been valuable in elucidating the steps from the normal to such fully malignant autonomous cells, and have revealed clues to their treatment and prevention. In this regard, it is of importance to note that the authors know of no evidence to indicate that the natural hormones possess carcinogenic actions which are unrelated to their normal stimulatory or inhibitory effects.

Hormone-dependent tumors have been defined by Furth (1959) as those which will grow only in the presence of hormone excess or deficiency—i.e., will not give rise to tumors when grafted in intact, otherwise untreated histocompatible animals. Such tumors arise in response to disruption of endocrine feedback systems which normally control cell numbers and are most usually dependent on the specific imbalance by which they were induced. They may locally invade in their primary host, and may metastasize when grafted in hormonally *conditioned* animals with that specific imbalance.

On repeated transplantation, or occasionally in the primary host, such tumors give rise to *autonomous* cells, i.e., to cells capable of tumor formation in normal, unconditioned histocompatible animals. Many such autonomous neoplasms retain *responsiveness* to the causative hormone imbalance, or to normal levels of a given hormone. Such responsiveness usually decreases with time, and *reversely responsive* variants may occasionally arise which grow better in untreated than in hormone-conditioned hosts.

The earliest known physiological changes during endocrine-dependent tumor formation and growth involve alterations in hormone sensitivity—e.g., a decrease in the estrogen levels optimal for growth of dependent mammotropic pituitary tumors (MtT) (Clifton and Furth, 1961) and the loss of a requirment for high thyrotropin-releasing hormone levels during induction of primary thyrotropic pituitary tumors (TtT) (Clifton, 1963; Clifton and Yatvin, 1974). Karyotopic abnormalities have also been described in primary and dependent estrogen-induced pituitary (Waelbroeck-VanGaver, 1969) and testicular (Hellstrom, 1961) tumors, but their significance to tumor induction and progression, if any, is unclear.

Dependent tumors of endocrine glands and of endocrine endorgans usually retain some of their specific functions, but this may differ among tumors of the same cell type of origin. As noted by Foulds (1954) in his classic studies of a unique series of hormone-responsive murine mammary carcinomas, changes in the specific functional characteristics, such as milk secretion, occur independently. During tumor progression, many endocrine gland tumors lose hormone-secretory capacity (Furth *et al.*, 1960). Others retain high secretory capacity although capable of rapid growth and of metastasizing in unconditioned hosts. Still others may change in the specific pattern of hormonally active compounds released (*cf.* Clifton, 1959). In steroid-secreting tumors, this change is often from the hormone type which is the endproduct of a long series of synthetic steps—e.g., an estrogen—to an intermediate compound in the synthetic chain with distinctly different physiological effects—e.g., a progestin or androgen. In hypophyseal neoplasms which initially secrete a predominance of one hormone with small amounts of a second, the ratio of the two products may become reversed. Finally, the capacity for production of a hormone not initially secreted and not intermediate in the synthesis of the original hormonal products may arise—e.g., the secretion of AtH by a transplantable pituitary tumor strain which initially secreted only mammotropin and somatotropin (*cf.* Furth *et al.*, 1973).

1.3. Hormones and Carcinogens

Hormonal interactions with chemical, viral and physical carcinogens are currently of broad experimental interest, and may be of great practical importance in relation to human cancer. On the basis of a review of mammotropin and experimental mammary carcinogenesis, it was clear by 1960 that

1. Specific hormones in *normal* levels may be necessary for the development of carcinomas secondary to an oncogenic virus, chemical carcinogen, or radiation. Once established, some of these tumors may continue to require normal hormone levels for growth or successful transplantation.
2. Specific hormones in *elevated* levels may increase the susceptibility to an oncogenic virus, may reduce the threshold carcinogenic dose of chemicals or radiation, may increase the tumor frequency, and may reduce tumor latency. Some tumors may retain responsiveness to elevated levels of the specific hormone (Clifton, 1961).

Since 1960, many details of the hypothalamic-hypophyseal control system have been elucidated, and hormone-binding sites, intracellular transport, and some mechanisms of action have been clarified. New exquisitely sensitive hormone assay techniques have become available, and more subtle endocrine interactions in carcinogenesis are now amenable to investigation.

1.4. The Hypothalamic–Hypophyseal–End–Organ Axes

The responsiveness of the anterior pituitary gland to external stimuli has long been recognized through observations of such events as the effects of light on reproductive cycles, the initiation and maintenance of lactation by suckling, and the effects of psychic stress on adrenocortical activity (for more detail on endocrine feedback systems in general, see Turner and Bagnara, 1971). The mediation of such effects and of internal end-organ hormone actions on the anterior pituitary is now largely attributed to a group of releasing or inhibiting hormones or "factors" produced in the hypothalamus. The nature and functions of these hypophysiotropins have been reviewed in detail (Meites, 1970; Guillemin, 1971; Blackwell and Guillemin, 1973; Furth *et al.*, 1973; Gual and Rosemberg, 1973; Schally *et al.*, 1973). Current knowledge of their structure and the

TABLE 1

Structure and Function of Hypophysiotropic Releasing Hormones (·RH) and Inhibiting Hormones (·IH)

Hypophysiotropin (synonym)	Structure (remarks)	Hormone(s) affected (synonyms)	References
A.RH (C.RH)	Ac-Ser-Tyr-Cys-Phe-His-(Asp-NH$_2$,Glu-NH$_2$)-Cys-(Pro,Val)-Lys-Gly-NH$_2$[a]	AtH (ACTH, adreno-corticotropin, corticotropin)	Schally and Bowers (1964)
L.RH (LH.RH)	(pyro)Glu-His-Trp-Ser-Tyr-Gly-Leu-Arg-Pro-Gly-NH$_2$	LH (luteinizing hormone, ICSH) FSH (follicle-stimulating hormone)	Baba et al. (1971) Matsuo et al. (1971a,b)
T.RH (TSH.RH)	(pyro)Glu-His-Pro-NH$_2$	TtH (thyrotropin, TSH)	Nair et al. (1970), Burgus et al. (1970)
M.IH (P.IH)	(small polypeptide, structure not known)	MtH (mammotropin, prolactin, LTH)	Talwalker et al. (1963) Meites and Nicoll (1966)
F.RH (FSH.RH)	(probably L.RH)	FSH	(see above)
M.RH (P.RH)	(postulated; T.RH?)	MtH	Nicoll et al. (1970), Tashjian et al. (1971)
S.RH (GH.RH)	Val-His-Leu-Ser-Ala-Glu-Glu-Lys-Glu-Ala[b]	StH (somatotropin, growth hormone)	Schally et al. (1971) Kastin et al. (1972)
S.IH (GH.IH)	(postulated; M.IH?)	StH	Krulich et al. (1968)

[a] From posterior pituitary; hypothalamic A.RH may be different; partial, tentative amino acid sequence.
[b] Releases bioactive but not immunoactive StH.

hormones they control is summarized in Table 1, which also contains the abbreviations of the hormone names to be used in this chapter.

These neural hormones are transported from the neuron cell bodies where they are synthesized through specialized axons and released into the proximal capillary bed of the unique hypophyseal portal system in the hypothalamus and the infundibular stalk. The blood from this capillary bed is collected into portal veins to be redistributed into the distal sinusoids within the anterior pituitary gland. There the "releasing hormones" (·RH) and the "inhibiting hormones" (·IH) stimulate or inhibit the synthesis and release of specific anterior pituitary hormones. The hypophysiotropins are distinct from antidiuretic and oxytocic hormones, which are similarly transported from the specialized secretory neurons through axons to the pars nervosa, where they are released into conventional capillaries to act at remote sites.

Neural control of hypophysiotropin secretion may be mediated by one or all of the nerve tracts which reach the hypothalamus from the limbic system, the globus pallidus, and the reticular formation of the midbrain. These effects may in turn be mediated via local release of catecholamines. For example, parenteral administration of a variety of agents which reduce brain catecholamine levels results in increased blood MtH levels, and treatment with L-dopa reduces M·IH levels (Meites, 1972b).

Humoral control of hypophysiotropin secretion is achieved by both "short-loop" and "long-loop" feedback—i.e., by inhibition or stimulation by their respective pituitary hormones, and by inhibition or stimulation by hormones from other endocrine glands. For example, secretion of FSH, LH, StH, AtH, and MtH is inhibited by high blood levels of these hormones, as a result of short-loop inhibition or stimulation of specific hypophysiotropin release (Fig. 1). Corticoids of the cortisone type inhibit A·RH and AtH release, and thyroxine and related hormones inhibit T·RH and TtH release by long-loop feedback (Fig. 2). Estrogens inhibit M·IH secretion and directly stimulate MtH release.

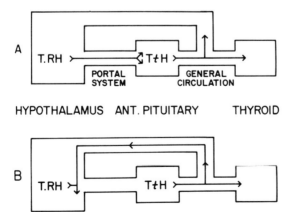

FIGURE 1. Short-loop feedback. (A) T.RH passes through hypothalamic-hypophyseal portal system and stimulates TtH secretion in pituitary. (B) TtH enters general circulation, reaches hypothalamus, and there inhibits T.RH release.

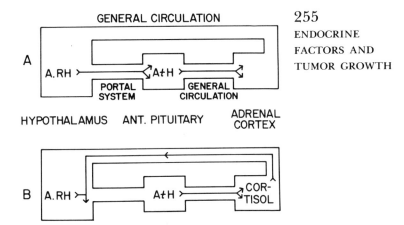

FIGURE 2. Long-loop feedback. (A) A.RH passes through portal system and stimulates AtH secretion in anterior pituitary. (B) AtH stimulates cortisol secretion in adrenal cortex, which reaches hypothalamus and inhibits A.RH secretion.

The regulatory effect of estrogens on L·RH and gonadotropin release is more complicated. The action of the preovulatory surge of estrogen from the ripening follicle on the hypothalamus and pituitary results in a surge of L·RH and brings about a surge of LH from the pituitary. The latter precipitates ovulation of the ripened follicle (McCann, 1970). In contrast, chronic maintenance of high estrogen levels inhibits secretion of both LH and FSH (Clifton and Meyer, 1956). Thyroid hormones also act directly on the anterior pituitary to inhibit TtH secretion (Sinha and Meites, 1965).

The dependence of the anterior pituitary gland on the stimulatory action of the releasing hormones is illustrated by the effect of interruption of the hypothalamic-hypophyseal portal veins by surgical section of the infundibular stalk, which interrupts the hypothalamic-hypophyseal portal veins, or by grafting of the anterior pituitary at sites remote from the hypothalamus. Under these conditions, the secretion of all the anterior pituitary hormones but MtH rapidly falls. In contrast, due to release from the damping effect of M·IH, MtH secretion is increased (Nikitovitch-Winer and Everett, 1958a; Meites, 1972b). Conversely, grafts of anterior pituitary tissue into some regions of the hypothalamus of hypophysectomized animals function normally (Nikitovitch-Winer and Everett, 1958b).

1.5. Hormone Transport and Target-Cell Effects

Within the endocrine system, the hypothalamic-hypophyseal system is unique in the existence of a specialized vascular delivery system for transport of hormones from the site of production to the site of action without dilution in the general circulation (Harris, 1948; Green and Harris, 1949). Within the CNS, the aromatic amines mediate excitation at the synapses by direct, extremely short-distance diffusion. When released in adequate amounts from specialized ganglia or the adrenal medulla, compounds of this group, such as epinephrine, also produce well-known hormonal effects on distant tissues. The best-known effects of the remaining hormones are brought about by secretions which have passed into the capillaries of the endocrine gland, thence entered the venous drainage, traversed the pulmonary circulation, and reached the endocrine end organ, much diluted, via the peripheral arterial system.

Within the blood, many hormones form temporary complexes with specific plasma proteins. The protein–hormone complex may serve to prolong hormone action by preventing its catabolism, and act as a reservoir which dampens rapid fluctuations in hormonal effects. The binding equilibria of related hormones may differ significantly. For example, thyroxine (T_4) is bound primarily to a specific α-globulin in the plasma, whereas triiodothyronine (T_3) occurs bound to both albumin and α-globulin (Turner and Bagnara, 1971). The rapid metabolic effects of injected T_3 as compared to the prolonged and delayed effects of T_4 may be in part related to this difference. Adrenocorticoids and gonadal steroids also display variations in plasma binding. Corticosteroid-binding protein tightly binds cortisol, corticosterone, and progesterone, and less firmly binds aldosterone and testosterone. Sex-steroid-binding protein binds both estradiol and testosterone (Baulieu *et al.*, 1970).

The specificity of the initial step in the action of a hormone depends on the presence of specific receptors on or within the responding cell. The receptors for the catecholamines and the larger peptide hormones—those of the pituitary and pancreatic islets, relaxin, and the gastrointestinal hormones—are all believed to be located on the plasma membrane, and the action of all is believed to involve stimulation or inhibition of the formation of adenosine-3′,5′-monophosphate (cAMP) or related cyclic nucleotides (Robison *et al.*, 1968). For example, the receptor protein for insulin is unidirectionally oriented toward the outer surface on fat cell membranes, and appears to be glycoprotein in nature (Cuatrecasas, 1973) (Fig. 3). In physiological concentrations, insulin decreases cAMP concentrations and has been shown to inhibit the activity of the enzyme adenyl cyclase,

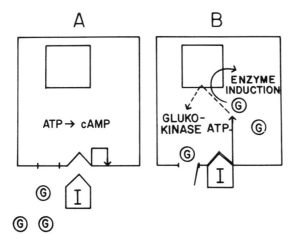

FIGURE 3. Postulated insulin action. (A) Insulin (I) and glucose (G) approach cell where adenyl cyclase is catalyzing cAMP formation. (B) As a result of insulin–plasma membrane receptor complex, glucose enters cell, cAMP formation is inhibited, glucokinase in induced, and other glucose-utilizing enzymes are induced by substrate.

which catalyzes the transformation of ATP into cAMP. (It is worthy of note that adenyl cyclase activity is stimulated in these cells by glucagon, AtH, and epinephrine.) Whether this effect on adenyl cyclase is a direct modulating action of the insulin–receptor complex, whether it is mediated via release of an intermediate messenger molecule which might produce other effects as well, or whether it is the result of a complex-induced conformational change in the plasma membrane is unknown (Cuatrecasas, 1973). The last possibility is attractive in that it might also offer a mechanism by which insulin brings about increased transport of glucose and amino acids into the cell (*cf*. Pitot and Yatvin, 1973).

In addition to affecting transport, the binding of insulin results in increased protein and RNA synthesis, glucose utilization, gluconeogenesis, glycogen formation, and lipid synthesis in the appropriate cell types. The insulin–receptor complex itself and its effects on adenyl cyclase do not directly induce the formation of all of the enzymes which catalyze these processes. For example, glycogen synthetase, glucokinase, phosphofructokinase, pyruvate kinase, and glucose-6-phosphate dehydrogenase are all increased by insulin, but only glucokinase is induced directly by its action. The others are either activated from an inactive form or are induced by their substrates (Pitot and Yatvin, 1973). The latter illustrates one mechanism by which the direct effects of a hormone on a limited number of intracellular sites—e.g., glucose transport and glucokinase—can be amplified to alter an entire metabolic process.

The differing actions of insulin on different cell types—e.g., glucose utilization in muscle cells and lipogenesis in fat cells—illustrate further that, given specific cellular hormone-binding sites, the effect of the hormone will depend on the differentiated state of the responding cell. Perhaps because of its ubiquity, and the severity of the sequelae of its excess or deficiency, insulin has not generally been considered in endocrine neoplasia. However, insulin is essential for, and may induce, mitoses in some cells (Lockwood *et al.*, 1967) and may play an essential role in tumor induction and growth.

In contrast to the large peptide hormones, steroid and thyroid hormones are taken into the target cells, and the cytosol of steroid-responsive cells contains hormone-specific receptor proteins. After the initial binding in the cytosol, steroids are transported to the nucleus, and there affect transcription (Britten and Davidson, 1969; O'Malley and Means, 1972). For example, specific estrogen receptors have been found in a variety of estrogen target tissues. On entry into the cell, the estrogen is first found bound to a cytoplasmic receptor protein which sediments on ultracentrifugation as an 8 S or 4 S unit, depending on the ionic strength of the medium (McGuire and Julian, 1971; Jensen *et al.*, 1972) (Fig. 4). The initial entry and binding are not temperature dependent, occurring rapidly at temperatures of less than 37°C. With time at 37°C, but not at lower temperatures, the estrogen is carried into the nucleus, where it occurs bound with protein in a 5 S estrogen–protein complex (Jensen *et al.*, 1972). The initial binding is conpetitively inhibited by a number of drugs which antagonize the uterine-growth-promoting actions of estrogens, e.g., ethomethoxytriphetol (MER-25), nafoxide, and clomiphene (Jensen *et al.*, 1972).

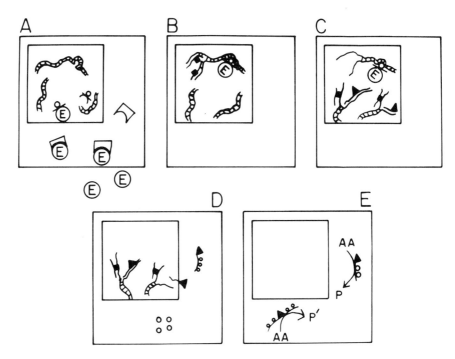

FIGURE 4. Estrogen action. (A) Estrogen (E) enters cytosol and combines with receptor protein, is transported to nucleus to combine with nuclear receptor. (B) Estrogen combines with estrogen operon and derepressor RNA molecules are synthesized. (C) Derepressor RNA molecules derepress enzyme operons. (D) mRNA molecules enter cytoplasm and bind with ribosomes. (E) New proteins (P and P′) are synthesized from amino acids (AA).

To account for the multiple actions of estrogens, it has been postulated that the estrogen–nuclear protein complex binds to the DNA of a specific estrogen operon which contains an operator locus and a group of functionally linked cistrons (Britten and Davidson, 1969; O'Malley and Means, 1972) (Fig. 4). The latter are postulated to code for a series of derepressor RNA molecules which in turn derepress genes for a battery of proteins. Once again, this postulate could account both for the differences in response of functionally different estrogen target cells and for amplification of hormone action. Its proof awaits further data.

It has been shown that the nuclear protein–estrogen complex stimulates the activity of nucleolar RNA polymerase *in vitro*. Estrogens also cause an acute increase in adenyl cyclase activity and cAMP levels in uterine tissue *in vivo*, although the latter effect may be mediated via catecholamines or, perhaps, estrogen-induced release of another hormone. Finally, in addition to an increase in a variety of enzymes (Pitot and Yatvin, 1973), estrogens stimulate the synthesis of "sex-specific" proteins. The synthesis of one type of these proteins is sensitive to actinomycin D, whereas synthesis of another, a nonhistone nuclear protein, is not (DeAngelo and Gorski, 1970; Barker, 1971).

Thyroid hormones are concentrated by several tissues, including the hypothalamus and anterior pituitary, and liver contains an apparently specific binding protein. As is well known, the primary intracellular site of T_3 and T_4 action appears to be on the mitochondrial enzymes which control oxygen utilization. In a variety of tissues including cultured human cells (Sterling *et al.*, 1973), T_4 is converted to T_3. The conversion process is intracellular, and is most rapid in those tissues with the highest metabolic rate. It has been suggested that this conversion is necessary for full hormone action.

In this discussion, the sites of action and results of exposure to insulin and to estrogen have been presented as models of peptide and steroid hormone action mechanisms, respectively. For further detail, readers are referred to the comprehensive reviews of Robison *et al.* (1968), Mueller (1971), Jensen *et al.* (1972), O'Malley and Means (1972), Pitot and Yatvin (1973), Cuatrecasas (1974), and King and Mainwaring (1974).

2. Mammary Growth and Oncogenesis: A Model of Hormone Effects

2.1. Introduction

Among Occidental women, breast cancer is the foremost malignant disease, and is the leading cause of death of American women 40–44 yr of age (Seidman, 1969). As a consequence, mammary tumors have been one of the most intensively investigated classes of neoplasms, and were among the first in which endocrine involvement was demonstrated and for which hormonal therapy was initiated. An appraisal of present knowledge of the role of hormones in the etiology and progression of breast cancer will be used below as a frame of reference for hormone action in neoplasia, to illustrate both general progress and areas of deficiency in information (see Currie, 1958; *Annual Clinical Conference on Cancer*, 1968; Forrest and Kunkler, 1968; Dao, 1972). In the following sections, emphasis will be placed on experimental findings, which, however, will be related to clinical problems and data as appropriate.

2.2. Normal Growth and Differentiation

The fetal mammary glands arise as epithelial downgrowths along the bilateral mammary ridges. Transitory growth and even secretion (the "witch's milk" of neonatal humans) may occur immediately after parturition, probably due to prenatal stimulation by mammotropic hormones of maternal and/or placental origin (Friesen, 1973; Parke, 1973). Thereafter, glands of immature animals are comprised primarily of branched ducts lined with a single layer of epithelium accompanied by basally located myoepithelial cells and surrounded by a basement membrane. Alveoli, when present, are clustered at the end of the smallest duct branches, and are similarly comprised of a single epithelial layer accompanied by basal myoepithelial cells and a basement membrane. Further ductal arborization occurs in response to the hormonal changes of puberty and full ductoalveolar development occurs with pregnancy. Nandi (1958) and Nandi and Bern (1960) found in hypophysectomized-ovariectomized female mice that a "cocktail" comprised of estrogen, progesterone, and MtH would support full ductoalveolar mammary growth. The addition of a glucocorticoid was required for milk secretion by the differentiated gland. In some strains, deoxycorticosterone could be substituted for progesterone, and StH for MtH. Beuving and Bern (1972) extended these findings to rats. When MtH-secreting pituitary tumors (MtT) were employed as indwelling hormone sources in adrenogonadectomized male rats, however, full ductoalveolar development was obtained in the absence of steroid hormone replacement (Clifton and Furth, 1960). In agreement with the above, addition of a glucocorticoid was required for milk secretion. The difference between these results could in part be due to species differences, but it seemed more likely to be due to differences in the levels of MtH obtainable by injection of heterospecific hormones. Talwalker and Meites (1961, 1964) have demonstrated that ductoalveolar development can be induced in adrenogonadectomized rats by multiple daily injections of heterospecific MtH and StH. The circulating half-life of MtH has been estimated by *in vitro* bioassay to be about 15 min (Turkington, 1972c). In contrast, radioimmunoassays of sera from MtT-bearing rats reveal steadily increasing MtH levels, which may reach more than a hundredfold normal when the MtT are large (Ito *et al.*, 1971; Clifton *et al.*, 1974).

The cumulative experimental evidence indicates that MtH is the primary stimulant of mammary growth and differentiation, and that in its absence other hormones have little or no effect (Furth and Clifton, 1966; Meites *et al.*, 1972). The latter play important supportive roles in mammary differentiation and function, however. Estrogens, for example, inhibit M·IH production and thus increase MtH secretion and directly stimulate the hypophyseal mammotropic cells to synthesize and release MtH. In addition, estrogens directly potentiate the action of the latter on the mammary cells. Nagasawa and Yanai (1971a) implanted estrogen-containing pellets in one mammary gland of ovariectomized rats which they later grafted with anterior pituitary to increase MtH levels. Only the gland containing the estrogen pellet was stimulated as measured by morphology and DNA content. As noted above, the direct action of estrogens on mammary cells depends on specific estrogen receptor protein(s) in the cytosol.

Progestins have no effect on MtH release (Gräf *et al.*, 1973; Robyn *et al.*, 1973). Mammary cells contain specific progestin-binding proteins, however, and progesterone potentiates alveolar differentiation in the presence of MtH (Nandi, 1958; Furth and Clifton, 1958; Meites, 1972a).

Lockwood *et al.* (1967) have performed a series of informative studies on the hormonal control of division and differentiation of mouse mammary cell suspensions in short-term culture. When suspensions are prepared from the glands of mid-pregnant mice—i.e., from glands which have been subjected to the physiological equivalent of Nandi's hormone "cocktail" *in vivo*—the presence of insulin alone in the medium brings about a wave of mitoses. Sera contain other agents which may substitute for insulin in inducing this first mitotic wave *in vitro* (Oka and Topper, 1972). Both MtH and insulin are essential for further division *in vitro* (Mukherjee *et al.*, 1973). The addition of insulin, MtH, and cortisol is required for the differentiative processes necessary to milk protein production—e.g., RNA synthesis, enzyme formation or activation, and the development of the rough endoplasmic reticulum (Lockwood *et al.*, 1967; Turkington *et al.*, 1973). Insulin is required throughout. Cortisol must be present before the first wave of mitosis, and MtH acts thereafter (Lockwood *et al.*, 1967; Turkington, 1972*a*). The polyamine peptide spermidine occurs in high concentration in lactating mammary glands. Oka (1974) has found that spermidine can substitute for cortisol in the induction of milk protein synthesis *in vitro*, and suggests that spermidine may mediate the steroid effect. It is noteworthy that neither estrogen nor progesterone is required for this differentiation *in vitro*.

As previously noted, the first step in insulin action on muscle and other cells is binding to specific sites on the responding cell membrane. Labeled MtH has also been found to bind to the plasma membranes of pregnant mouse mammary cells and rabbit mammary cells (Turkington, 1972*a*; Turkington *et al.*, 1973; Friesen *et al.*, 1973), and Birkinshaw and Falconer (1972) have demonstrated its localization on the basal membrane of alveolar cells *in vivo*. Labeled MtH bound to mouse mammary cells is competitively displaced by unlabeled MtH, less efficiently by placental lactogen and StH, and not at all by LH or TtH, and binding parallels the induction of casein production (Turkington, 1972*b*). Specific binding to mouse or rabbit mammary gland cells has been used as an assay for MtH concentrations (Turkington, 1972*b*; Shiu *et al.*, 1973). The first intracellular effect of MtH binding is induction of a cAMP-dependent protein kinase. Subsequently, proteins in the plasma membrane, ribosomes, and nuclei become phosphorylated, and casein is induced.

Cortisol, like estrogens and progestins, is believed to enter the cell and to be transported bound to specific proteins to the nucleus, where it affects transcription processes.

Thyroid hormone is not required for mammary growth and differentiation, but the state of thyroid function may indirectly alter mammary cell responsiveness to hormonal stimulation. T_3 and T_4 induce MtH release *in vitro* (Meites, 1973). Conversely, thyroid deficiency brings about an increase in T·RH release and TtH secretion. T·RH in turn increases secretion of MtH as well as TtH (Bowers *et al.*, 1971; Meites, 1973). Furthermore, in rats in which elevated TtH levels were experimentally induced, the growth response of mammary tissue to MtH was significantly increased (Mittra, 1974).

Whether StH plays a direct role in mammary growth under normal circumstances is not altogether clear. As noted, heterospecific StH can substitute for heterospecific MtH in some mammary-growth-promoting hormone mixtures. Furthermore, grafted MtT of the type used to induce mammary growth without steroids (Clifton and Furth, 1960) secrete StH as well as MtH (Ueda *et al.*, 1968), and some individual cells in these tumors may secrete both hormones (Ito *et al.*, 1972; Ueda *et al.*, 1973). Estrogen increases StH as well as MtH secretion (Meites, 1972*a*). However, purified heterospecific MtH and StH may have actions different than those of the native hormones *in vivo*. Finally, StH and MtH are known to have marked molecular similarity (Niall, 1972), which might lead to an overlap in activity under experimental circumstances.

Transplantation techniques and hormonal manipulation have been employed in studies of the interrelationships among the three functionally different mammary cells—ductal epithelium, alveolar epithelium, and myoepithelium. In inbred mice, normal mammary tissue is readily transplantable into mammary fat pads from which the glandular anlagen have been surgically excised at weaning (DeOme *et al.*, 1959; Daniel *et al.*, 1971). Such grafts give rise to glandular structures which may fill, but remain confined to the fat pad. Glandular growth has been observed after grafting of unselected mouse mammary tissue (Daniel *et al.*, 1971), of monolayer short-term cultures of mammary epithelium (Daniel and DeOme, 1965), and of selected segments of ductal tissue (Chew and Hoshino, 1970). Following implantation of the duct pieces, the basement membrane disappears and the cells disaggregate. Cylindrical or spheroidal multilayered mammary cell reaggregates are then observed, and a new basement membrane is re-formed within 3 days. Finally, a central lumen develops linked by the single epithelial layer typical of a normal mammary duct. These ducts grow and coalesce to yield a continuous single mammary tree (Chew and Hoshino, 1970). In the presence of elevated MtH levels from MtT, grafts of unselected monodispersed rat mammary cells placed in the interscapular white fat pads first give rise to single or clustered alveoluslike structures, and later to fully developed glands (Gould and Clifton, 1974). Daniel *et al.* (1971) serially transplanted mouse mammary tissue fragments to recipient mice with hormone balances which preferentially favored ductal with some alveolar growth (virgin, untreated females) or alveolar proliferation and differentiation (females with elevated MtH levels from extracranial grafts of pituitary tissue). Glands continuously stimulated by high MtH levels displayed a progressively diminishing capacity for alveolus formation. Those passed in virgin animals showed progressively diminished ductal growth, but retained the capacity to form alveoli in response to the elevated MtH of pregnancy and lactation. Daniel *et al.* (1971) concluded that the alveolar growth response in the latter case was the result of a cellular "reprogramming" in response to a new hormonal environment. Slemmer (1972) produced genotypically mosaic mammary glands by transplantation into F_1 hybrids of mixed mammary gland tissue from the two parent strains. After growth of the genotypically mosaic glands, fragments were reimplanted into recipients of both parent strains. Because of histocompatibility differences between the two parent strains, only those cells in the grafted mosaic gland which had originated from that particular parent strain would be expected to survive such transplantation. Several mosaics which gave rise to complete mammary glands in F_1 hybrids, when backgrafted to one parent strain would yield primary ductal growth. When grafted into the other parent strain, the same mosaic tissue gave rise only to alveolar growths. On the basis of these results, those of comparable studies with premalignant mammary growths, and the differential aging described by Daniel *et al.* (1971), Slemmer (1972) concluded that the normal mammary tissue of adult mice is comprised of three distinct and fixed cell types: ductal epithelium, alveolar

epithelium, and myoepithelium. Slemmer also concluded (see below) that each
cell type possesses differing neoplastic potential. It is not yet known whether these
important conclusions are generalizable to other species. Furthermore, the data
are equally consistent with the hypothesis that alveolar epithelium, and perhaps
myoepithelium, is derived by differentiation from ductal epithelium under
hormonal influence, but that the reverse process is uncommon or does not occur.

2.3. Experimental Mammary Carcinogenesis

In summarizing his classic studies, Bittner (1942, 1946) described three factors in
the etiology of the "spontaneous" mammary carcinoma of mice: genetic susceptibility, hormonal influence, and the "milk factor" (the mouse MTV, now recognized as an oncornavirus). The first two of these have been amply confirmed in
other species, but incontrovertible evidence for the participation of a virus has
been obtained only in mice.

The development of frank carcinoma in mice is preceded by the appearance of
premalignant hyperplastic alveolar nodules which form under the influence of
the MTV transmitted during nursing or a second related virus transmitted *in utero*
(DeOme *et al.*, 1970). The hormonal milieu of multiple pregnancies predisposes to
carcinoma formation (Lathrop and Loeb, 1913; Bittner, 1946), but, with the
exception of the unusual pregnancy-responsive tumors described by Foulds
(1954, 1956), once carcinomas have developed in mice they are either fully
autonomous or but marginally responsive to hormones.

Although benign fibroadenomas are the most common spontaneous mammary
neoplasm of rats, carcinomas can be induced experimentally. Hyperplastic
alveolar nodules were found to precede carcinoma development in dimethylbenzanthracene (DMBA) treated rats (Beuving and Bern, 1972), and such preneoplastic lesions may also occur in other species. Many breast tumors in rats, like those
in man, but unlike those in mice, retain hormone responsiveness.

Not long after their discovery, chronic treatment with purified or isolated
estrogens was reported to induce both pituitary tumors and mammary carcinomas in rats and mice (*cf.* Clifton, 1959; Russfield, 1966). Although multiple
hypophyseal implants were shown by Loeb and Kirtz (1939) and Mühlbock and
Boot (1959) to also increase mouse mammary carcinoma incidence, estrogens
continued to be considered the primary mammary-tumor-promoting hormone
class. This conclusion was strengthened by observations that growth stasis and/or
regression occurred in many rat mammary fibroadenomas (Huggins and
Mainzer, 1958) and induced carcinomas (Huggins *et al.*, 1959) after ovariectomy
or combined adrenogonadectomy.

More recent studies have progressively shifted the emphasis to the anterior
pituitary (*cf.* Meites, 1972b; Furth *et al.*, 1973). Nandi *et al.* (1960) found that either
heterospecific MtH or in some strains StH would, in the presence of estrogen and
progesterone, induce hyperplastic nodules and, ultimately, carcinomas in MTV-
infected mice. The effectiveness of StH in mammary maintenance and lactation

was restricted to mouse strains in which tumor incidence is high in nulliparous females (Nandi and Bern, 1960). Intact ovaries were essential for the genesis of hyperplastic nodules in the glands of DMBA-treated rats. Once established, however, such nodules persisted in ovariectomized animals (Beuving and Bern, 1972). The pivotal role of MtH in mammary carcinogenesis was emphasized by experiments in which grafted MtT were used as indwelling hormone sources. Such MtT grafts rendered adult mice of normally resistant strains susceptible to mammary carcinoma development following the injection of extracts containing MTV, and caused the rapid appearance of mammary carcinomas in rats treated with radiation or methylcholanthrene (*cf.* Furth, 1973). In the presence of elevated MtH levels, the effective dose of methylcholanthrene was reduced by an order of magnitude (Kim *et al.*, 1960). Since these studies, the elevation of MtH by other experimental procedures—i.e., injection of heterospecific hormones, placement of hypothalamic lesions which destroy the source of M·IH, as well as pituitary grafts—have been shown to potentiate mammary carcinoma induction by chemicals or MTV (Meites, 1972*b*; Bruni and Montemurro, 1971). Multiple pituitary grafts also increased the incidence of mammary adenomas and fibroadenomas in the absence of added carcinogens in a susceptible strain of rats (Welsch *et al.*, 1970). Conversely, suppression of MtH production by chronic administration of 2-bromo-α-ergocryptine suppressed hyperplastic nodule formation and carcinogenesis in MTV-infected mice (Welsch and Gribler, 1973). Although mammary carcinomas were rare in rats receiving no treatment other than grafts of MtT in earlier studies (*cf.* Clifton, 1961; Furth, 1973), Meites (1972*b*) recently reported their appearance in otherwise untreated W/Fu rats grafted with either of two strains of MtT. On transplantation, these carcinomas behaved as fully dependent neoplasms, growing only in the presence of elevated MtH from concurrently grafted MtT. Their growth in MtT-grafted rats was not prevented by adrenogonadectomy.

Although elevated MtH levels increase the incidence and growth rate of carcinogen-induced carcinomas, such tumors can be induced and grow in female rats in the presence of normal MtH titers (Nagasawa *et al.*, 1973). Tumor regression follows ovariectomy, adrenogonadectomy, hypophysectomy, depression of MtH by administration of L-dopa or ergocornine, or administration of specific antibodies to MtH (Huggins *et al.*, 1959; Kim *et al.*, 1960; Butler and Pearson, 1971; Meites, 1972*a*; Quadri *et al.*, 1973). Elevation of MtH levels by grafting of MtT reestablished growth of methylcholanthrene-induced carcinomas which had regressed after hypophysectomy *or* ovariectomy (Kim *et al.*, 1960). Similarly, injection of MtH stimulated the appearance of new carcinomas and regrowth of tumors which had regressed following adrenogonadectomy, hypophysectomy, or adrenogonadohypophysectomy of carcinogen-treated rats (Sterental *et al.*, 1963; Nagasawa and Yanai, 1970; Pearson *et al.*, 1972). Estrogen treatment did not cause carcinoma regrowth in hypophysectomized animals, nor did StH in adrenogonadectomized animals (Nagasawa and Yanai, 1970, Pearson *et al.*, 1972).

Although MtH plays a cardinal role in mammary oncogenesis and growth, its effectiveness is altered by the presence or absence of other hormones, and by the sequence of hormone and carcinogen stimulation. Functionally different mammary cell types may respond differently to the same hormones and may give rise to different types of neoplasms. Slemmer (1972) described transplantable premalignant mammary nodules from methylcholanthrene-treated or MTV-infected mice which were comprised primarily of ductal epithelium, primarily of alveolar epithelium, or primarily of multibranched structures which exhibited squamous metaplasia and which were believed to be of myoepithelial origin. The former two types progressed to carcinomas, whereas the latter gave rise to fibroadenomas. Cultures of cells from transplanted or primary mouse MTV-related mammary carcinomas have consistently yielded "spindle cells" which form characteristic "stranded" colonies *in vitro*, as well as one or more epithelial cell types. Cloned or selected lines of these spindle cells gave rise on inoculation in histocompatible mice to unique tumors displaying a "stranded" cell arrangement, whereas the epithelial cell lines yielded typical adenocarcinomas (Cohn and Clifton, 1971).

The earliest mammary neoplasms which develop following irradiation of otherwise untreated female rats are most usually adenocarcinomas, whereas those which appear late are most often fibroadenomas (Shellabarger *et al.*, 1957). In a recent study, the incidence of the late-appearing fibroadenomas in irradiated female rats was increased by the moderately elevated MtH levels from extracranial grafts of single pituitary glands. Carcinomas were less common, but occasionally occurred alone or within fibroadenomas. In other experiments in which MtH was more markedly increased by grafting irradiated rats with MtT, mammary carcinomas developed (Clifton *et al.*, 1974). Thus the nature as well as the incidence of the neoplasms resulting from a given carcinogenic agent may be altered by quantitative differences in MtH levels. These results may be related to the finding of Shellabarger and Soo (1973) that treatment of neonatal rats with either estrogen or testosterone decreased the mammary carcinoma response to DMBA, but increased the adenofibroma response. Ovarian weights were depressed, fewer follicles were present, and corpora lutea were absent in these neonatally treated animals.

Estrogen treatment of irradiated rats greatly increased the incidence of mammary carcinomas (Segaloff and Maxfield, 1971), probably both by stimulation of MtH release and by synergism of MtH action at the mammary cell level. The latter effect is illustrated by the experiment of Sinha *et al.* (1973), who found that ovariectomy caused rapid regression of mammary cancers in DMBA-treated rats with heightened MtH levels as a result of median eminence lesions, although it had no effect on the plasma MtH titers. Mammary tumors regrew in these animals after ovarian grafts. The physiological effects of the latter were primarily estrogenic.

In contrast, although estrogen in high doses causes a marked elevation in serum MtH levels, it inhibits induction and growth of DMBA-induced rat mammary carcinomas. This effect is apparently dependent on the ratio rather than the absolute quantities of the two hormones, in that the inhibition of tumor appearance and growth is overcome if MtH titers are further raised by injection of the hormone or by grafting of additional pituitary tissue (Nagasawa and Yanai, 1971*b*; Meites *et al.*, 1971).

Progesterone may also play synergistic and antagonistic roles in breast car-cinogenesis. In MTV-free hybrid mice bearing grafted pituitary tissue, chronic treatment with progesterone synergized with all estrogen levels tested in inducing mammary carcinomas (Boot *et al.*, 1973). Despite the fact that the highest estrogen dose employed alone resulted in the highest MtT induction in both the pituitary gland *in situ* and the pituitary graft, mammary tumor incidence was less than at lower estrogen doses. The added progesterone in conjunction with the highest estrogen dose reduced the MtH titers somewhat, and markedly reduced hyperp-lasia in the pituitary *in situ*, but not in the pituitary graft (Boot *et al.*, 1973). These latter results demonstrate antagonism by progesterone of the estrogen action on M·IH release by the hypothalamus, but not on the direct action of estrogen on the MtH-secreting cells of the grafted pituitary tissue.

Recent results yield some insight into the role of adrenocorticoids in breast carcinogenesis. After mammary carcinomas have developed, as noted above, adrenalectomy usually inhibits tumor growth or is without effect. In contrast, adrenalectomy soon after radiation exposure of rats grafted with an MtT strain which also secretes AtH caused rapid appearance of multiple mammary car-cinomas at a time when none was found in intact irradiated MtT-grafted animals (Clifton *et al.*, 1974). As noted above, glucocorticoids are essential to differentia-tion for milk secretion, and the mammary glands of the intact, MtT-bearing rats in this latter experiment were distended with milk. It is likely that secretory differentiation of a given mammary cell reduces or abolishes the capacity of that cell to proliferate. In the presence of both glucocorticoids and high MtH levels, many of the radiation-damaged epithelial cells may thus have been lost from the proliferative cell population. Accordingly, when differentiation was precluded by adrenalectomy, more of the altered cells may have retained proliferative capacity and contributed to carcinoma formation. The inhibition of the growth of established mammary carcinomas by adrenalectomy, when observed, is more probably related to the removal of an extragondal source of estrogen than to glucocorticoid deficiency.

The sequence of hormone and carcinogen exposure plays a critical role in the oncogenic response. Progesterone treatment initiated before DMBA exposure (Jabara *et al.*, 1973) or irradiation (Segaloff, 1973) had a protective effect. When given from 2 days after DMBA, progesterone increased tumor incidence. Both pregnancy (*cf.* MacMahon *et al.*, 1973) and experimental elevation of MtH levels by a variety of means (Meites, 1972*b*) *before* exposure to carcinogen reduced mammary carcinoma formation, although all these increased tumor incidence when initiated *after* carcinogen treatment. These results also suggest a differentia-tion-dependent change in carcinogen metabolism or a diversion to cells toward a less proliferative state. Hormone-carcinogen interactions in mammary growth and oncogenesis are summarized in Fig. 5.

Carcinogen-induced mammary carcinomas in rats have been used to advantage in studies of the mechanisms of estrogen effects which have yielded insight into tumor progression. Ten to twelve percent of such tumors do not regress after ovariectomy, do not contain estrogen-binding protein in their cytosol, and do not concentrate estrogen in complexed form in their nuclei (McGuire and Julian, 1971; Jensen *et al.*, 1972). In one such autonomous tumor, the defect in the early steps of estrogen metabolism appeared to be restricted to the cytosol receptor protein. When estrogen was incubated with cytosol and chromatin from the tumor, no estrogen–chromatin complex was formed. However, when receptor-rich cytosol from uterus was mixed with tumor chromatin, estrogen became complexed with the latter (McGuire *et al.*, 1972).

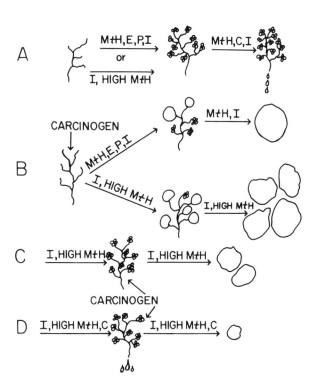

FIGURE 5. Hormone action on mammary cells. (A) Ductoalveolar growth stimulated by MtH, estrogen (E), progesterone (P), and insulin (I). Secretion occurs in presence of MtH, cortisol (C), and I. (B) When carcinogen is given before hormonal stimulation, nodules are formed which give rise to carcinomas under MtH stimulation. If high MtH levels are given, more nodules and carcinomas are formed. (C) If high MtH is given before carcinogen, fewer carcinomas are obtained. (D) If high MtH *and* C are given before carcinogen, carincoma induction is further suppressed.

2.4. Human Breast Cancer: Problems and Prospects

Elucidation of the hormonal mechanisms in initiation, progression, and control of mammary carcinomas promises to aid in identification of high-risk populations, in choice and improvement of therapy, and ultimately, perhaps, in reduction of risk. In the following, these aspects are briefly discussed in the light of results from experimental animals (see also *Annual Clinical Conference on Cancer*, 1968; MacMahon *et al.*, 1973; Murphy, 1973; Pasteels and Robyn, 1973).

The naturally occurring compound estriol may be considered an antiestrogen. Although it produces estrogenic effects, its potency is generally less than that of the other two natural estrogens, estradiol and estrone. When given in conjunction with the latter compounds, estriol reduces their effectiveness (MacMahon *et al.*, 1973), and has been shown to compete for cytoplasmic estrogen receptor sites (Wotiz *et al.*, 1968). An analysis of the estriol/(estradiol plus estrone) ratio has been suggested as a means of identifying patients with a high risk of breast cancer—i.e., it was suggested that a low estriol quotient predisposed to breast cancer while a high relative estriol concentration was protective (Lemon *et al.*, 1966; Lemon, 1969). Although this postulate is supported by the low estriol quotients in Caucasian woman, who are known to have a relatively high cancer incidence, and by the high quotient in Oriental populations, with low incidence, it has not received broad support in case-control studies within a Caucasian population (MacMahon *et al.*, 1973). Furthermore, the differences between Oriental and Caucasian populations include genetic, environmental, and sociological factors which may enter the cancer susceptibility equation.

Among those points of difference between Caucasian and Oriental populations which may potentially alter breast cancer susceptibility is diet, and particularly the intake of iodine. It has long been noted that the epidemiological distribution of breast cancer is similar to that of iodine-deficiency diseases, being highest in the "goiter belts" (Spencer, 1954; Bogardus and Finley, 1961; Eskin, 1970). Such deficiency is rare in Oriental populations, with a high seafood intake. Within the United States, the regional distributions of endemic goiter and high breast cancer mortality correlate remarkably well, and autopsy studies of a large series of breast cancer victims showed a disproportionate number of thyroid abnormalities, the preponderance of which were of long-standing types (Somers, 1955). Although results of thyroid function tests in breast cancer patients and controls have led to conflicting conclusions, several reports indicate that the prognosis of breast cancer patients with thyroid disease is poorer than that of euthyroid women (Bogardus and Finley, 1961; Backwinkel and Jackson, 1964; Moossa *et al.*, 1973).

A common feature of hypothyroid and many treated hyperthyroid cases is elevated TtH levels and, presumably, elevated T·RH. As noted, T·RH has been shown experimentally to stimulate MtH as well as TtH release. Although elevated MtH has not been uniformly demonstrated in women with breast cancer (Boyns *et al.*, 1973), Kwa *et al.* (1974) have reported elevated titers in members of families with high breast cancer rates. Reserpine and related drugs increase MtH titers by suppression of M·IH release (Meites *et al.*, 1972). Jick *et al.* (1974) have reported that women receiving chronic reserpine therapy suffer a 3.5-fold increase in breast cancer risk, but this finding awaits confirmation.

Mittra *et al.* (1974) were unable to detect greater basal MtH levels or increases in serum MtH in response to T·RH injections in mammary cancer patients with early or advanced disease. There were elevated basal TtH levels in such patients, however, and an exaggerated TtH release occurred in response to injected T·RH as compared to matched controls (Mittra and Haywood, 1974). In the light of the demonstration that TtH increases the sensibility of rat mammary epithelium to MtH (Mittra, 1974), it is clear that those conditions which bring about increased T·RH and TtH release may play a two-pronged role in breast cancer etiology—i.e., both stimulation of MtH release and potentiation of MtH action. It

will be of interest to see whether the incidence of breast cancer in the goiter belts
decreases as the first generations raised with iodized salt reach cancer age.

The state of thyroid function may also affect mammary carcinogenesis by way of altering steroid hormone production. In both hyperthyroid and hypothyroid patients, the ratio of urinary 17-hydroxycorticoids/urinary androgens (etiocholanolone and androsterone) is elevated—in the former case as a result of an increase in 17-hydroxycorticoid excretion, and in the latter as a result of a decrease in both, but a more marked decrease in urinary androgens (Sneddon *et al.*, 1968). In a large prospective study, Bulbrook *et al.* (1971) found that women with low etiocholanolone and androsterone excretion rates had a higher breast cancer incidence than those with higher androgen excretion rates. Furthermore, early breast cancer patients with high hydroxycorticoid/androgen excretion ratios had poorer prognoses than those with lower ratios (Hayward and Bulbrook, 1968). It is not yet clear how, or if, these findings in man relate to the mammary-carcinogenesis-enhancing effect of adrenal deficiency in MtT-bearing rats or to the protective effect of androgens in experimental mammary carcinogenesis. It is clear from both clinical and experimental data, however, that measurement of no single hormone species is likely to yield adequate data for identification of high-risk populations.

A procedure to identify those advanced breast cancer patients most apt to profit from endocrine ablation or hormone administration would be of great aid in guiding therapy. The lack of estrogen receptor protein was correlated with lack of response to ovariectomy in rat tumors. Jensen *et al.* (1972) found that 77% of the human tumors which contained estrogen receptor proteins responded to endocrine treatment, whereas only 4% of those without receptors responded favorably. This procedure, of course, measures but the first step in the estrogen response system. Procedures for a more complete analysis of the system, including nuclear protein–estrogen complexing ability, may yield more definitive information. Furthermore, the relationship between presence of absence of response to estrogen and responsiveness to MtH has not been clarified.

Hobbs *et al.* (1973) described a test for homone dependence based on the maintenance of histological integrity and persistence of dehydrogenase activity in slices of breast cancer tissues incubated with hormones. Of the 120 samples examined, 58 were not responsive to MtH alone, to MtH combined with estrogen or androgen, or to either steroid alone. Thirty-eight (32%) responded to MtH alone or in combination, and 24 (20%) to one or the other steroid. No clinical correlations have yet been determined.

The metabolic transformation, and consequent alteration of biological activity, of steroid hormones within target organs and neoplasms has recently been recognized (Adams and Wong, 1972; Griffiths *et al.*, 1972; Dao *et al.*, 1972). Steroid sulfation is believed to be one of the initial steps in such transformation. Dao and Libby (1972) and Dao (1973) investigated the capacity of breast cancer tissues from 109 postmenopausal women to sulfurylate dehydroepiandrosterone (DHEA) and estradiol, and correlated these capacities with the response to adrenalectomy. Cancer samples from 30 of these women contained no steroid sulfokinase activity, and all failed to respond to adrenalectomy. In 46 cases, the ability to sulfurylate estradiol was greater than the capacity for DHEA sulfation, and only 15% of these patients responded to adrenalectomy. In contrast, 24 of 33 (73%) patients whose cancer tissue showed DHEA sulfation equal to or greater than estradiol sulfation obtained objective remission following adrenalectomy. In a smaller series, steroid sulfokinase activity was measured in primary tumors at the time of mastectomy. Forty of 76 patients (53%) whose cancer either contained no sulfokinase or sulfated estradiol more efficiently than DHEA suffered recurrence. In contrast, all of the ten patients whose cancers sulfated DHEA more efficiently than estradiol had not had recurrence during the period of observation.

Although the role of steroid sulfation and of steroid transformation in the mammary cancer cell economy is not yet clearly defined, further studies in this area appear promising. For example, breast cancer tissues have been shown in various laboratories to convert DHEA and pregnenolone to Δ^{4-3}-ketosteroids, and to convert testosterone to estriol and to 16α-hydroxyestrone (Dao, 1973). It is thus possible that the gain of autonomy in some mammary cancers is the result of their capacity to synthesize the hormonally active steroids they require for growth from precursors which are not otherwise mammary cancer growth promoting (Adams and Wong, 1972; Dao et al., 1972; Griffiths et al., 1972).

Ovariectomy has been recommended as a prophylactic procedure only for premenopausal patients with proven axillary node involvement at the time of mastectomy, and Lewison (1970) also recommends that all breast cancer patients be advised to avoid estrogens. In premenopausal patients with advanced disease, approximately 25% respond to surgical or radiotherapeutic castration alone (Lewison, 1961), whereas about 40% of postmenopausal or ovariectomized premenopausal patients respond to adrenalectomy (Fracchia et al., 1970).

In cumulative series of 3000 advanced breast cancer patients on whom surgical or radiation hypophysectomies had been performed, 33–50% had previously responded to ovariectomy. Of the latter group, 90% responded to hypophysectomy, whereas only 10% of those who failed to respond to adrenogonadectomy improved after hypophysectomy (Miller, 1970). These results serve to emphasize the interrelationship of steroid and hypophyseal hormone actions. They illustrate further that removal of hypophyseal hormones has effects which exceed those of removal of steroids. As pointed out by Miller (1970), hypophysectomy as the first ablative procedure makes gonadectomy or adrenalectomy unnecessary, as it removes the source not only of MtH and StH but also of AtH and the gonadotropins.

The search for the medical equivalent of ablative therapy is rapidly expanding in two areas—the development of antiestrogens and of pharmacological agents which control MtH secretion. Antiestrogens are believed to act by competition with the natural estrogens at their site of action. The compounds dimethylstilbestrol, erythro MEA, cisclomiphene, and Parke-Davis CI-628 are all bound to estrogen receptors in human breast cancers (Korenman, 1972), and all counteract the uterine-growth-promoting effects of natural estrogens (i.e., are antiuterotropic). Following the demonstration that the release of the hypophysiotropins was controlled by catecholamines, L-dopa and the monoamine oxidase inhibitors pargyline, iproniazid, and similar compounds were found to markedly decrease serum MtH titers by increasing M·IH release (Meites, 1972a,b). As previously noted, drugs of the ergot family such as 2-bromo-α-ergotamine both increase M·IH release and directly inhibit MtH secretion (Meites, 1972a). It seems likely that further development of these two approaches will result in a single or combined specific drug regimen that will render endocrine ablation unnecessary (cf. Pasteels and Robyn, 1973).

The means by which surgical ablation of the hypophyseal stalk and thus of the hypothalamic-hypophyseal portal systems brings about therapeutic effects in advanced breast cancer (Turkington et al., 1971) are not clear. As noted by these investigators and in experimental animals, separation of the anterior pituitary from the immediate control by M·IH leads to increased serum MtH and a decrease in other tropic hormones, and thus would be expected to have deleterious effects. However, excesses of estrogen have been shown to antagonize relatively high levels of MtH in promoting tumor growth in rats. Perhaps in some mammary cancer cells or in some individuals with unique hormonal balances, excess MtH leads to an analogous paralysis of proliferation, or perhaps the decrease in another tropic hormone is the critical factor.

In postmenopausal women with metastatic disease, approximately 21% obtain objective remission with androgen therapy, whereas 36% respond to high levels of estrogen (Kennedy, 1970). As previously noted, the effect of high estrogen dosage is not due to inhibition of MtH secretion, but is rather dependent on an altered balance in the MtH/estrogen ratio. The action of androgens may be due in part to an inhibition of gonadotropin with consequent reduction in extragonadal estrogen production, and in part to a direct antagonism of the action of MtH and other hormones at the level of the tumor cell.

Finally, the most effective way short of ablative procedures for a young woman to reduce her risk of future breast cancer—albeit one which is unlikely to be widely followed for that specific purpose—is to carry a child to term as soon after menarche as possible. It has long been recognized that breast cancer in women—as opposed to mice—is a disease of the nulliparous, whereas cervical carcinoma is more common in the multiparous. In their classic review, MacMahon et al. (1973) summarized the dominant features of the pregnancy effect:

1. Breast cancer risk increases with increasing age at first full-term pregnancy. Those primaparous at age 18 or less have about one-third the risk of those primaparous at age 30 or of nulliparous women.
2. Risk increases with age at first birth, to exceed the risk of nulliparae in those first pregnant after age 30 or so.
3. The protective effect appears limited to the age at first birth, and is independent of subsequent pregnancies, or, to current knowledge, of lactation.
4. Protection is afforded only by full-term pregnancy.
5. Protection so gained persists throughout life.

MacMahon *et al.* conclude (1973, p. 22): "that the protection is afforded only by the first pregnancy and is not substantially modified by subsequent births suggests that the first full-term pregnancy has a 'trigger' effect, which either produces a permanent change in the factors responsible for the high risk or changes the breast tissue and makes it less susceptible to malignant transformation." The authors also point out the possible analogy to rats, in which pregnancy before carcinogen exposure is protective but after exposure is tumor promoting (Dao and Sunderland, 1959; Moon, 1969; McCormick and Moon, 1965). The marked difference from the effect of pregnancy in mice may be related to the presence of the MTV in the latter or to differences in hormone patterns during sexual cycles (Mühlbock and Boot, 1959).

MacMahon *et al.* (1973) also allude to the protective effect of the second half of pregnancy. During this period, the hormonal balance is characterized by a steady increase in circulating progestins, a marked increase in estrogens, of which, however, a major portion is estriol, and a progressive increase in the level of MtH, which reaches a maximum during the last month (Turner and Bagnara, 1971; MacMahon *et al.*, 1973; Robyn *et al.*, 1973). In addition, there are peptide hormones of placental origin including placental lactogen and chorionic gonadotropin. The total hormonal milieu is optimal for ductoalveolar growth and differentiation in the mammary gland. In view of the fact that permanent reduction in risk requires a full-term pregnancy, it seems that further detailed analysis of the physiological events of the second half of gestation with special reference to breast differentiation and/or permanent changes in hormone secretory patterns is desirable.

The embryological literature is filled with examples of abnormalities resulting from the lack of an inducing agent at the "right" time in development, even though the inducer may occur in abundance at later times. For most of human evolution, pregnancy soon after menarche was the rule rather than the exception. Thus pregnancy at a young age may be looked upon not as protective but rather as the normal sequence of events, and necessary for normal differentiation of either the breast, the endocrine system, or both.

Accordingly, postponement of the first pregnancy to the mid-20s or later can be construed as abnormal from an evolutionary standpoint. It may not be farfetched to suggest that, when more information is available, young women can be treated prophylactically soon after menarche with the critical hormonal sequence simulating pregnancy. Such treatment might be looked upon as the medical prevention of a societally induced cancer-predisposing abnormality of differentiation.

3. General Problems in Endocrine Oncogenesis

3.1. Introductory Remarks

The following discussion is restricted to examples selected to illustrate outstanding problems and recent insights in hormone-related neoplasia. Earlier results on tumorigenesis in endocrine glands and hormone-responsive organs have been detailed in the monograph of Russfield (1966), and in reviews of others (Furth, 1953; Gardner, 1953; Hertz, 1957; Kirschbaum, 1957; Noble, 1957; Clifton, 1959; Furth *et al.*, 1973).

3.2. The Initial Change

On close examination, virtually all experimental oncogenesis systems involve more than one step or phase—as exemplified by Berenblum's initiation–promotion hypothesis of chemical carcinogenesis (Berenblum and Shubik, 1947)—and tumors induced by endocrine imbalance are no exception. The final product of endocrine tumor progression, the autonomous tumor, is comprised of cells phenotypically, and probably genotypically, different from their normal ancestors. But what is the nature of the first recognizable step? Is it reversible or irreversible? Are there differences in the nature of the first recognizable step between those systems in which, as far as is known, tumor formation occurs as a result of endocrine imbalance alone and those in which both hormones and nonendocrine oncogenic agents are involved?

The earliest detected alterations during the progression of two types of pituitary tumors—MtT and TtT—both involve a decrease in the requirement for a stimulatory hormone. For example, the optimum estrogen dose for growth of primary MtT in rat pituitary tissue *in situ* or in grafts beneath the kidney capsule was ten- to a hundredfold the optimum for growth of intramuscular or subcapsular grafts of autonomous-responsive MtT. The optimal estrogen dose for growth of the early-generation transplants of dependent MtT varied with the tumor line. It either resembled that for the pituitary *in situ* or the autonomous tumor or was intermediate between them (Clifton and Furth, 1961).

As previously noted, estrogens play a dual role in the control of the mammotropic cells of the pituitary, acting both directly to stimulate proliferation and indirectly to inhibit hypothalamic M·IH release. As extracranial grafts of normal pituitary tissue placed remote from the hypothalamus responded to the different estrogen doses in the same fashion as the pituitary *in situ*, it is concluded that changes in the estrogen dose–response of grafted dependent MtT were due to alterations in response to the direct action of estrogen, and not mediated by effects on M·IH.

Thyroid hormones also play direct and hypothalamus-mediated roles in control of the pituitary thyrotropes. In contrast to MtT, the earliest recognized alteration during TtT progression involves a change in responsiveness to the hypothalamic-mediated effect. The dependent TtT which arise in pituitaries *in situ* in thyroidectomized mice are readily transplantable to extracranial sites in thyroid-deficient recipients (Furth *et al.*, 1973). However, pituitary tissue from either intact or recently radiothyroidectomized male mice did not give rise to TtT when grafted beneath the kidney capsules of thyroidectomized recipients, although TtT developed in the pituitary glands *in situ* in the host mice (Clifton, 1963).

Observations on changes in pituitary gland weight and radiolabeled precursor incorporation into pituitary DNA during TtT induction suggested a change in proliferative behavior of a fraction of the hypothyseal cells 200–250 days after radiothyroidectomy (Clifton, 1966). In a recent experiment (Clifton and Yatvin, 1974), groups of male donor mice were killed at intervals varying from 139 to 313 days after radiothyroidectomy, and their pituitaries were grafted beneath the kidney capsules of recently thyroidectomized recipient mice. All recipient animals were killed, and the grafts were weighed 510–511 days after radiothyroidectomy of the initial pituitary donors (Fig. 6). Thus the total term of exposure of the pituitary tissue to the thyroid–deficient state was the same in all groups. The variable was the portion of that time during which the tissue was in immediate circulatory connection with the hypothalamus.

In this study, TtT development clearly depended on retention of direct connection with the hypothalamus and thus, presumably, on high T·RH levels for 200 or more days after initiation of thyroid hormone deficiency (Fig. 6). Thereafter, altered thyrotropic cells were present which proliferated in thyroid-deficient hosts at extracranial sites where T·RH levels were presumably low or nil. In the light of the fact that growth of dependent TtT grafts can be prevented, and regression of small tumors brought about, by thyroid hormone replacement (*cf.* Furth *et al.*, 1973), these results indicate that the altered cells of primary dependent TtT have lost their requirement for high levels of T·RH as a prerequisite for proliferation, but that they retain sensitivity to the direct proliferation-suppressing action of thyroid hormone (Clifton and Yatvin, 1974).

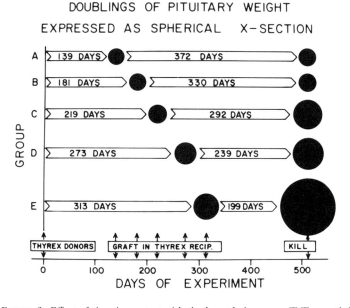

FIGURE 6. Effect of time in contact with the hypothalamus on TtT growth in thyroidectomized mice. See text for experimental details.

Similar primarily physiological alterations may occur during induction of other endocrine-dependent tumors.

Once an initial change has occurred, it may be retained for long periods. Thus inocula of dependent TtT cells in intact euthyroid animals may remain dormant for many months, only to give rise to tumors when the host mice are thyroidectomized (Werner and Grinberg, 1961). Furthermore, a "memory" of previous treatment is retained by mouse testicular interstitial cells during tumor induction by estrogen. Uninterrupted treatment of genetically susceptible male mice with estrogen for a period of 6 months resulted in testicular interstitial cell tumors in 66% of the mice. When the treatment period was divided into segments of 2 months and 4 months separated by 6 months without estrogen, the same final tumor incidence was obtained—i.e., the changes induced during the first 2 months of treatment were not reversed or repaired during the 6-month interval without treatment (Andervont et al., 1957).

As a rule of thumb, but not a universal, those tumor induction procedures involving a nonendocrine carcinogenic agent as well as endocrine factors are more apt to result in initially autonomous neoplasms than those resulting from endocrine imbalance alone. For example, ovarian tumors comprised of the same spectrum of functional cell types can be induced in mice either by irradiation of both ovaries or by transplantation of the ovaries to gonadectomized recipients at sites which drain into the hepatic portal system. Both procedures bring about hypersecretion of gonadotropins—in the first case as the result of destruction of the primary oocytes and consequent prevention of maturing oocyte-dependent ovarian hormone secretion, and in the second as a result of estrogen inactivation in the liver before it reaches the hypothalamic-hypophyseal system (cf. Clifton, 1959). Tumors produced by the two procedures differ, however, in that those induced by radiation, once formed, usually grow on transplantation to intramuscular or subcutaneous sites in intact animals—i.e., do not require elevated gonadotropin titers. Those induced by grafting in the portal system usually grow on transplantation only in sites draining into the portal system in gonadectomized recipients—i.e., retain dependence on elevated gonadotropins.

Similarly, those testicular interstitial cell tumors and anterior pituitary tumors which originate in irradiated mice are most usually autonomous in the first transplant generations, whereas those induced by endocrine imbalance are usually dependent, or at the least highly responsive (Furth et al., 1973). As previously noted, the MTV-related mammary carcinomas of mice are most usually refractory to hormonal manipulation. Although many chemical-carcinogen- or radiation-induced rat mammary carcinomas are highly responsive to hormonal manipulation, only a few are dependent on hormone imbalance.

The electrophilic nature of most ultimate chemical carcinogens and their consequent reactivity with macromolecules (Miller and Miller, 1974), the well-known action of radiation on nucleic acids and chromosomes (Elkind and Whitmore, 1967), the integration of oncogenic viral nucleic acid or viral-directed nucleic acid into the genome of the infected cell (Temin, 1971), and the autonomous nature of most of the tumors they induce all are consistent with the hypothesis that the primary event in oncogenesis by these agents is genetic in nature. The expression of the genetic change thereby induced may depend, of course, on the hormonal milieu. In contrast, the relationship of the oncogenic action of hormones to their normal physiological effects and the dependent nature of the majority of tumors induced by hormone imbalance alone suggest that the initial alterations are phenotypic in nature—i.e., at the level of gene expression, and perhaps comparable to differentiation. With continued hormonal stimulation, and the consequent elevated proliferation rate, dependent tumor cells are probably rendered more susceptible to genetic variation due to chance and/or to low levels of carcinogenic agents, and thus progression proceeds.

3.3. Latency and Susceptibility

As a general but not universal rule, the induction periods of tumors which result from endocrine imbalance alone, and of many of those resulting from exposure to carcinogenic agents, occupy a significant percentage of the organism's life span. In the simplest cases, this may be the result of the time required for a slight excess in cell division above that necessary to replace dying cells to become apparent. For example, in one rat strain, if one cell of every 100 cells initially present in the anterior pituitary gland were to divide, and all of its progeny were to survive and divide every 30 days, the resultant changes in weight of the entire gland would approximate those seen during the 9–14 months required for MtT induction by chronic estrogen administration (Clifton and Meyer, 1956).

Alternatively, the long induction period may result from the time required for one or more intracellular alterations to occur, as during TtT induction noted above.

Finally, a prolonged induction period may result from the requirement for a specific age-dependent change in the internal milieu before a previously acquired intracellular alteration can be expressed in tumor formation. For example, X-ray treatment of the clavicular area of infants was employed as therapy or prophylaxis for thymic enlargement (status thymicolymphaticus, now known not to be a disease entity), which was believed responsible for crib deaths, and for some other benign conditions. Many such children developed thyroid adenomas or carcinomas years later, at puberty or thereafter (Hemplemann, 1969)—i.e., the radiation-induced cellular change was not expressed until the hormonal alterations of puberty produced additional stimulation of thyroid cell function and growth.

The synthetic estrogen diethylstilbestrol (DES) was used to prevent threatened abortions. A rare "clear-cell" or endometrial carcinoma of the vaginal mucosa has recently been found in high incidence in young women born of pregnancies during which such treatment was employed (Herbst *et al.*, 1971; Greenwald *et al.*, 1971). Such women also displayed patchy vaginal benign adenosis. Similar vaginal adenosis was found in 91% of 63 young women whose mothers had received DES during pregnancy, and the remaining 9% had extensive eversion of the columnar epithelium on the ectocervix (Stafl *et al.*, 1974). This is an example of abnormal differentiation resulting from exposure to the synthetic estrogen at a critical time in differentiation, which progresses to malignancy under the ovarian hormonal stimulation of adolescence.

Among the many unsolved problems in endocrine-induced neoplasms are the bases for differences in susceptibility to tumor formation between species, among inbred strains within species, and even between different functional cell types within the same organ. At the last level, despite the fact that the hypophyseal gonadotropic cells hypertrophy, proliferate, and hypersecrete in response to elevated L·RH after gonadectomy, primary gonadotropic pituitary tumors rarely if ever appear in long-term gonadal hormone-deficient rats or mice (Furth *et al.*, 1973). Similarly, AtT do not develop in adrenalectomized or even adrenogonadectomized animals, although they have been isolated from irradiated mice and have been observed in man (Furth *et al.*, 1973). No experimental procedure for the induction of primary StT has yet been devised, despite the fact that tumors of this type were the first functional hypophyseal neoplasm to be recognized in humans (Turner and Bagnara, 1971). MtT are the most common spontaneous pituitary tumors in rats (Furth *et al.*, 1973) and Friesen *et al.* (1973) found that 25–30% of pituitary tumor patients had elevated MtH levels.

4. Prospects and Conclusions

The evolution of cellular specialization in metazoan organisms required concomitant evolution of intercellular communication and integration systems for control of cell number, function, differentiation, and response to changes in the environment. As illustrated above, much recent endocrine research has been devoted to elucidating the major interface between the two principal integration systems of adult vertebrates, the hypothalamic-hypophyseal system, and to defining the mechanism of hormone action on the responding cell. As noted in our introduction, studies in cancer biology have contributed to, as well as gained from, endocrinology. The neoplastic response to endocrine imbalance most usually represents an extreme which may yield insight into normal hormone action. The dependence of the action of both individual hormones and carcinogens on the previous and concurrent exposure of the responding cells to other hormones has been illustrated in several neoplasia induction systems in endocrine-responsive tissues. And transplantable masses of hormone-responsive and hormone-secreting cells have been made available for study by endocrinologists. By combining the new techniques and findings of basic endocrinology and cancer biology, it seems likely that the near future will bring new prognostic tools to guide endocrine therapy, the substitution of specific endocrine-active drugs or hormone antagonists for endocrine-ablative procedures, and hormone-based measurements by which those with high risk of specific endocrine-related cancers may be identified.

Over the long range, it seems likely that the more subtle chemical systems which mediate intercellular communication will become amenable to similar and specific manipulation, and that cancers of tissue not so obviously endocrine related will become subject to analogous risk prediction and therapy.

The dependence of human life on the integrity of regulatory systems will always bear with it the risk of systematic malfunction, one result of which is neoplasia. The questions of cancer research are the fundamental questions of metazoan life. In view of the complexity of the processes of replication, differentiation, and homeostasis, the wonder is that they usually work so well—not that they occasionally go awry.

5. References

ADAMS, J. B., AND WONG, M., 1972, Paraendocrine behavior of human breast cancer, in: *Estrogen Target Tissues and Neoplasia* (T. L. Dao, ed.), pp. 125–150, University of Chicago Press, Chicago.

ANDERVONT, H. B., SHIMKIN, M. B., AND CANTER, H. Y., 1957, Effect of discontinued estrogenic stimulation upon the development and growth of testicular tumors in mice, *J. Natl. Cancer Inst.* **18**:1.

Annual Clinical Conference on Cancer, Thirteenth, 1968, (University of Texas M. D. Anderson Hospital and Tumor Institute, Houston), Yearbook Medical Book Publishers, Chicago.

BABA, Y., MATSUO, H., AND SCHALLY, A. V., 1971, Structure of the porcine LH- and FSH-releasing hormone. II. Confirmation of the proposed structure by conventional sequential analysis, *Biochem. Biophys. Res. Commun.* **44**:459.

BACKWINKEL, K., AND JACKSON, A. S., 1964, Some features of breast cancer and thyroid deficiency, *Cancer* **17**:1174.

BARKER, K. L., 1971, Estrogen-induced synthesis of histones and a specific non-histone protein in the uterus, *Biochemistry* **10**:284.

BAULIEU, E. E., RAYNAUD, J. P., AND MILGROM, E., 1970, Measurement of steroid binding proteins, in: *Steroid Assay by Protein Binding* (E. Diczfalusy, ed.), Karolinska Symposia on Research Methods in Reproductive Endocrinology, Stockholm.

BEATSON, G. T., 1896, On treatment of inoperable cases of carcinoma of the mamma: Suggestions for a new method of treatment, with illustrative cases, *Lancet* **2**:104.

BERENBLUM, I., AND SHUBIK, P., 1947, The role of croton oil applications, associated with a single painting of a carcinogen, in tumor induction of the mouse's skin, *Br. J. Cancer* **1**:379.

BERNARD, C., 1949, *An Introduction to the Study of Experimental Medicine* (translated from the original text), Henry Schuman, New York.

BEUVING, L. J., AND BERN, H. A., 1972, Hormonal influence upon normal, preneoplastic, and neoplastic mammary gland, in: *Estrogen Target Tissues and Neoplasia* (T. L. Dao, ed.), pp. 257–273, University of Chicago Press, Chicago.

BIRKINSHAW, M., AND FALCONER, I. R., 1972, The localization of prolactin labelled with radioactive iodine in rabbit mammary tissue, *J. Endocrinol.* **55**:323.

BITTNER, J. J., 1942, Possible relationship of the estrogenic hormones, genetic susceptibility, and milk influence in the production of mammary cancer in mice, *Cancer Res.* **2**:710.

BITTNER, J. J., 1946, The cause and control of mammary cancer in mice, *Harvey Lect.* **42**:221.

BLACKWELL, R. E., and GUILLEMIN, R., 1973, Hypothalamic control of adenohypophysial secretions, *Ann. Rev. Physiol.* **35**:357.

BOGARDUS, G. M., AND FINLEY, J. W., 1961, Breast cancer and thyroid disease, *Survery* **49**:461.

BOOT, L. M., KWA, H. G., AND ROPCKE, G., 1973, Radioimmunoassay of mouse prolactin: Prolactin levels in isograft-bearing orchidectomized mice, *Eur. J. Cancer* **9**:185.

BOWERS, C. Y., FRIESEN, H. G., HWANG, P., GUYDA, H. J., AND FOLKERS, K., 1971, Prolactin and thyrotropin release in man by synthetic pyroglutamyl-histidyl-prolinamide, *Biochem. Biophys. Res. Commun.* **45**:1033.

BOYNS, A. R., COLE, E. N., GRIFFITHS, K., ROBERTS, M. M., BUCHAN, R., WILSON, R. G., AND FORREST, A. P. M., 1973, Plasma prolactin in breast cancer, *Eur. J. Cancer* **9**:99.

BRITTEN, R. J., AND DAVIDSON, E. H., 1969, Gene regulation for higher cells: A theory, *Science* **165**:349.

BRUNI, J. E., AND MONTEMURRO, D. G., 1971, Effect of hypothalamic lesions on the genesis of spontaneous mammary gland tumors in the mouse, *Cancer Res.* **31**:854.

BULBROOK, R. D., HAYWARD, J. L., AND SPICER, C. C., 1971, Relation between urinary androgen and corticoid excretion and subsequent breast cancer, *Lancet* **2**:395.

BURGUS, R., DUNN, T., DESIDERIO, D., WARD, D., VALE, W., AND GUILLEMIN, R., 1970, Characterization of the hypothalamic hypophysiotropic TSH-releasing factor (TRF) of ovine origin, *Nature (London)* **226**:321.

BURROWS, H., 1949, *Biological Action of Sex Hormones*, Cambridge University Press, London.

BUTLER, T. P., AND PEARSON, O. H., 1971, Regression of prolactin-dependent rat mammary carcinoma in response to antihormone treatment, *Cancer Res.* **31**:817.

CHEW, E. C., AND HOSHINO, K., 1970, Early histogenesis of transplanted mouse mammary glands. II. Within 96 hours following isografting, *Z. Anat. Entwicklungsgesch.* **132**:318.

CLIFTON, K. H., 1959, Problems in experimental tumorigenesis of the pituitary gland, gonads, adrenal cortices and mammary glands: A review, *Cancer Res.* **19**:2.

CLIFTON, K. H., 1961, Hormones and experimental oncogenesis: Mammary and mammotropic tumors, in: *Proceedings of the Fourth National Cancer Conference*, pp. 41–50, Lippincott, Philadelphia.

CLIFTON, K. H., 1963, Tumor induction in hypophyseal grafts in radiothyroidectomized mice; hypothalamica-hyphpyseal relationships, *Proc. Soc. Exp. Biol. Med.* **114**:559.

CLIFTON, K. H., 1966, Cell population kinetics during the induction of thyrotropic pituitary tumors, *Cancer Res.* **26**:374.

CLIFTON, K. H., AND FURTH, J., 1960, Ducto-alveolar growth in mammary glands of adreno-gonadectomized male rats bearing mammotropic pituitary tumors, *Endocrinology* **66**:893.

CLIFTON, K. H., AND FURTH, J., 1961, Changes in hormone sensitivity of pituitary mammotropes during progression from normal to autonomous, *Cancer Res.* **21**:913.

CLIFTON, K. H., AND MEYER, R. K., 1956, Mechanism of anterior pituitary tumor induction by estrogen, *Anat. Rec.* **125**:65.

CLIFTON, K. H., AND YATVIN, M. B., 1974, Hypothalamic-hypophyseal relationships in induction of thyrotropic pituitary tumors: Further studies, in: *Fifth Perugia Quadrennial International Conference on Cancer*, University of Perugia Publications, Perugia, Italy.

CLIFTON, K. H., DOUPLE, E. B., AND SRIDHARAN, B. N., 1974, unpublished observations.

COHN, N. K., AND CLIFTON, K. H., 1971, Aspects of the biology and radiation response of cloned C3H mouse mammary carcinoma cells *in vitro* and *in vivo*, *Eur. J. Cancer* **7**:505.

CUATRECASAS, P., 1973, Insulin receptor of liver and fat cell membranes, *Fed. Proc.* **32**:1838.

CUATRECASAS, P., 1974, Membrane receptors, *Ann. Rev. Biochem.* **43**:169.

CURRIE, A. R., 1958, *Endocrine Aspects of Breast Cancer* (proceedings of a conference held at the University of Glasgow), Livingstone, Edinburgh.

DANIEL, C. W., AND DEOME, K. B., 1965, Growth of mouse mammary glands *in vivo* after monolayer culture, *Science* **149**:634.

DANIEL, C. W., YOUNG, L. J. T., MEDINA, D., AND DEOME, K. B., 1971, The influence of mammogenic hormones on serially transplanted mouse mammary gland, *Exp. Gerontol.* **6**:95.

DAO, T. L., 1972, *Estrogen Target Tissues and Neoplasia* (workshop at Rosewell Park Memorial Institute, Buffalo), University of Chicago Press, Chicago.

DAO, T. L., 1973, Advances in breast cancer research, in: *Perspectives in Cancer Research and Treatment* (G. P. Murphy, ed.), pp. 31–49, A. R. Liss, New York.

DAO, T. L., AND LIBBY, P. R., 1972, Steroid sulfate formation in human breast tumors and hormone dependency, in: *Estrogen Target Tissues and Neoplasia* (T. L. Dao, ed.), pp. 181–200, University of Chicago Press, Chicago.

DAO, T. L., AND SUNDERLAND, J., 1959, Mammary carcinogenesis by 3-methylcholanthrene. I. Hormonal aspects in tumor incidence and growth, *J. Natl. Cancer Inst.* **23**:567.

DAO, T. L., VARELA, R., AND MORREAL, C., 1972, Metabolic transformation of steroids by human breast cancer, in: *Estrogen Target Tissues and Neoplasia* (T. L. Dao, ed.), pp. 163–179, University of Chicago Press, Chicago.

DEANGELO, A. B., AND GORSKI, J., 1970, Role of RNA synthesis in the estrogen induction of a specific uterine protein, *Proc. Natl. Acad. Sci. U.S.A.* **66**:693.

DEOME, K. B., FAULKIN, L. J., JR., BERN, H. A., AND BLAIR, P. B., 1959, Development of mammary tumors from hyperplastic alveolar nodules transplanted into gland-free mammary fat pads of female C3H mice, *Cancer Res.* **19**:515.

DeOme, K. B., Medina, D., and Young, L., 1970, Interference between the nodule inducing virus and the mammary tumor virus at the level of the neoplastic transformation, in: *Immunity and Tolerance in Oncogenesis* (L. Severi, ed.), pp. 541–549, Division of Cancer Research, Perugia, Italy.

Elkind, M. M., and Whitmore, G. F., 1967, *The Radiology of Cultured Mammalian Cells*, Gordon and Breach, New York.

Erhlich, P., 1906, Über ein transplantables Chondron der Maus, *Arb. Konigl. Inst. Exp. Ther. (Frankfurt am Main)* **1**:65.

Eskin, B. A., 1970, Iodine metabolism and breast cancer, *Trans. N.Y. Acad. Sci.* **32**:911.

Forrest, A. P. M., and Kunkler, P. N., 1968, Prognostic factors in breast cancer, in: *Proceedings of First Tenavous Symposium, Cardiff*, Williams and Wilkins, Baltimore.

Foulds, L., 1954, The experimental study of tumor progression: A review, *Cancer Res.* **14**:327.

Foulds, L., 1956, The histological analysis of mammary tumors of mice. I. Scope of investigations and general principles of analysis. II. The histology of responsiveness and progress. The origin of tumors. III. Organoid tumors. IV. Secretion, *J. Natl. Cancer Inst.* **17**:701.

Fracchia, A. A., Randall, H. T., and Farrow, J. H., 1970, The results of adrenalectomy for advanced breast cancer in 500 consecutive patients, in: *Breast Cancer: Early and Late* (University of Texas M. D. Anderson Hospital and Tumor Institute at Houston), pp. 369–376, Year Book Medical Publishers, Chicago.

Friesen, H. G., 1973, Prolactin, its control and clinical significance, *Clin. Sci.* **44(2)**:2p.

Friesen, H., Tolis, G., Shiu, R., and Huang, P., 1973, Studies on human prolactin: Chemistry, radioreceptor assay and clinical significance, in: *Human Prolactin: Proceedings of the International Symposium on Human Prolactin* (J. L. Pasteels and C. Robyn, eds.), pp. 11–23, American Elsevier, New York.

Furth, J., 1953, Conditioned and autonomous neoplasms: A review, *Cancer Res.* **13**:477.

Furth, J., 1959, A meeting of ways in cancer research: Thoughts on the evolution and nature of neoplasms, *Cancer Res.* **19**:241.

Furth, J., 1973, The role of prolactin in mammary carcinogenesis, in: *Human Prolactin: Proceedings of the International Symposium on Human Prolactin* (J. L. Pasteels and C. Robyn, eds.), pp. 233–248, American Elsevier, New York.

Furth, J., and Clifton, K. H., 1958, Experimental observations on mammotropes and the mammary gland, in: *Endocrine Aspects of Breast Cancer* (A. R., Currie, ed.), pp. 276–282, Livingstone, Edinburgh.

Furth, J., and Clifton, K. H., 1966, Experimental pituitary tumors, in: *The Pituitary Gland*, Vol. 2 (G. W. Harris and B. T. Donovan, eds.), pp. 460–498, Butterworths, London.

Furth, J., Kim, U., and Clifton, K. H., 1960, On evolution of the neoplastic state: Progression from dependence to autonomy, *Natl. Cancer Inst. Monogr.* **2**:148.

Furth, J., Ueda, G., and Clifton, K. H., 1973, The pathophysiology of pituitaries and their tumors: Methodological advances, in: *Methods in Cancer Research*, Vol. 10 (H. Busch, ed.), pp. 201–277, Academic Press, New York.

Gardner, W. U., 1953, Hormonal aspects of experimental tumorigenesis, *Adv. Cancer Res.* **1**:173.

Gardner, W. U., Pfeiffer, C. A., Trentin, J. J., and Wolstenholme, J. T., 1953, Hormonal factors in experimental carcinogenesis, in: *The Physiopathology of Cancer* (F. Homburger and W. H. Fishman, eds.), pp. 225–297, Hoeber-Harper, New York.

Gould, M. N., and Clifton, K. H., 1974, unpublished observations.

Gräf, K. J., Newmann, F., Nishino, Y., Mehring, M., and Hasan, S. H., 1973, The effect of different progestogens on prolactin secretion in rats, in: *Human Prolactin: Proceedings of the International Symposium on Human Prolactin* (J. L. Pasteels and C. Robyn, eds.), pp. 160–162, American Elsevier, New York.

Green, J. D., and Harris, G. W., 1949, Observation of the hypophysio-portal vessels of the living rat, *J. Physiol. (London)* **108**:359.

Greenwald, P., Barlow, J. J., Nasca, P. C., and Burnett, W. S., 1971, Vaginal cancer after maternal treatment with synthetic estrogens, *New Engl. J. Med.* **285**:390.

Griffiths, K., Jones, D., Cameron, E. H. D., Gleave, E. N., and Forrest, A. P. M., 1972, Transformation of steroids by mammary cancer tissue, in: *Estrogen Target Tissues and Neoplasia* (T. L. Dao, ed.), pp. 151–162, University of Chicago Press, Chicago.

Gual, C., and Rosemberg, 1973, *Hypothalamic Hypophysiotropic Hormones* (proceedings of the conference held at Acapulco, Mexico, June 1972), Excerpta Medica, Amsterdam, American Elsevier, New York.

GUILLEMIN, R., 1971, Hypothalamic control of the secretion of adenohypophysical hormones, *Adv. Metab. Disord.* **5**:1.

HARRIS, G. W., 1948, Neural control of the pituitary gland, *Physiol. Rev.* **28**:139.

HAYWARD, J. L., AND BULBROOK, R. D., 1968, Urinary steroids and prognosis in breast cancer, in: *Prognostic Factors in Breast Cancer* (A. P. M. Forrest and P. B. Kunkler, eds.), pp. 383–392, Williams and Wilkins, Baltimore.

HELLSTROM, K. E., 1961, Chromosomal studies on diethylstilbestrol-induced testicular tumors in mice, *J. Natl. Cancer Inst.* **26**:707.

HEMPLEMANN, L. H., 1969, Risk of thyroid neoplasms after irradiation in childhood, *Science* **160**:159.

HERBST, A. I., ULFELDER, U., AND POSKANZER, D. C., 1971, Adenocarcinoma of the vagina, *New Engl. J. Med.* **284**:878.

HERTZ, R., 1957, An appraisal of the concepts of endocrine influence on the etiology, pathogenesis and control of abnormal and neoplastic growth, *Cancer Res.* **17**:423.

HESTON, W. E., 1949, Development of inbred strains in the mouse and their use in cancer research, in: *Lectures on Genetics, Cancer, Growth and Social Behavior*, pp. 9–31, Roscoe B. Jackson Memorial Laboratory, Bar Harbor, Me.

HOBBS, J. R., SALIH, H., FLAX, H., AND BRANDER, W., 1973, Prolactin dependence among human breast cancers, in: *Human Prolactin* (J. L. Pasteels and C. Robyns, eds.), pp. 249–258, Excerpta Medica, Amsterdam, American Elsevier, New York.

HUGGINS, C., 1957, Control of cancers of man by endocrinologic methods, *Cancer Res.* **17**:467.

HUGGINS, C., AND MAINZER, K., 1958, Hormonal promotion and restraint of growth of experimental mammary tumours, in: *Endocrine Aspects of Breast Cancer* (A. R. Currie, ed.), pp. 297–304, Livingstone, Edinburgh.

HUGGINS, C., BRIZIARELLI, G., AND SUTTON, H., 1959, Rapid induction of mammary carcinoma in the rat and the influence of hormones on the tumors, *J. Exp. Med.* **109**:25.

ITO, A., MARTIN, J. M., GRINDELAND, R. E., TAKIZAWA, S., AND FURTH, J., 1971, Mammotropic and somatotropic hormones in sera of normal rats and in rats bearing primary and grafted pituitary tumors, *Int. J. Cancer* **7**:416.

ITO, A., FURTH, J., AND MOY, P., 1972, Growth hormone-secreting variants of a mammotropic tumor, *Cancer Res.* **32**:48.

JABARA, A. G., TOYNE, P. H., AND HARCOURT, A. G., 1973, Effects of time and duration of progesterone administration on mammary tumours induced by 7,12-dimethylbenz(*a*)anthracene in Sprague-Dawley rats, *Br. J. Cancer* **27**:63.

JENSEN, E. V., BLOCK, G. E., SMITH, S., KYSER, K., AND DESOMBRE, E. R., 1972, Estrogen receptors and hormone dependency, in: *Estrogen Target Tissues and Neoplasia* (T. L. Dao, ed.), pp. 23–57, University of Chicago Press, Chicago.

JICK, H., and other members of the Boston Colloborative Drug Surveillance Program, 1974, Reserpine and breast cancer, *Lancet* **2**:695.

KASTIN, A. J., SCHALLY, A. V., GUAL, C., GLICK, S., AND ARIMURA, A., 1972, Clinical evolution in men of a substance with growth hormone-releasing activity in rats, *J. Clin. Endocrinol. Matab.* **35**:326.

KENNEDY, B. J., 1970, Hormonal therapies in breast cancer: Andorgens versus estrogens, in: *Breast Cancer: Early and Late* (University of Texas M. D. Anderson Hospital and Tumor Institute, Houston), pp. 381–386, Year Book Medical Publishers, Chicago.

KIM, U., FURTH, J., AND CLIFTON, K. H., 1960, Relation of mammary tumors to mammotropes. III. Hormone responsiveness of transplanted mammary tumors, *Proc. Soc. Exp. Biol. Med.* **103**:646.

KING, R. J. B., AND MAINWARING, W. I. P., 1974, *Steroid–Cell Interactions*, Butterworths, London.

KIRSCHBAUM, A., 1957, The role of hormones in cancer: Laboratory animals, *Cancer Res.* **17**:432.

KORENMAN, S. G., 1972, Human breast cancer as a steroid hormone target, in: *Estrogen Target Tissues and Neoplasia* (T. L. Dao, ed.), pp. 59–67, University of Chicago Press, Chicago.

KRULICH, L., DHARIWAL, A. P. S., AND MCCANN, S., 1968, Stimulatory and inhibitory effects of purified hypothalamic extracts on growth hormone release from rat pituitary *in vitro*, Endocrinology **83**:783.

KWA, H. G., DEJONG-BAKKER, M., ENGELSMAN, E., AND CLETON, F. J., 1974, Plasma-prolactin in human breast cancer, *Lancet* **1**:433.

LACASAGNE, A., 1939, Relationship of hormones and mammary adenocarcinoma in the mouse, *Am. J. Cancer* **37**:414.

LATHROP, A. E. C., AND LOEB, L., 1913, The influence of pregnancies on the incidence of cancer in mice, *Proc. Soc. Exp. Biol. Med.* **11**:38.

LEMON, H. M., 1969, Endocrine influences on human mammary cancer formation: A critique, *Cancer* **23**:781.

LEMON, H. M., WOTIZ, H. H., PARSONS, L., AND MOZDEN, P. J., 1966, Reduced estriol excretion in patients with breast cancer prior to endocrine therapy, *J. Am. Med. Assoc.* **196**:1128.

LEWISON, E. F., 1961, Prophylactic versus therapeutic castration in the total treatment of breast cancer, in: *Proceedings of the Fourth National Cancer Conference*, pp. 263–265, Lippincott, Philadelphia.

LEWISON, E. F., 1970, Prophylactic versus therapeutic castration, in: *Breast Cancer: Early and Late* (University of Texas M. D. Anderson Hospital and Tumor Institute, Houston), pp. 363–367, Year Book Medical Publishers, Chicago.

LOCKWOOD, D. H., STOCKDALE, F. E., AND TOPPER, Y. J., 1967, Hormone-dependent differentiation of mammary gland: Sequence of action of hormones in relation to cell cycle, *Science* **156**:945.

LOEB, L., AND KIRTZ, M. M., 1939, The effects of transplants of anterior lobes of the hypophysis on the growth of the mammary gland and on the development of mammary gland carcinoma in various strains of mice, *Am. J. Cancer* **36**:56.

LONG, J. A., AND EVANS, H. M., 1922, The oestrous cycle in the rat and its associated phenomena, *Mem. Univ. Calif.* **6**:1.

MACMAHON, B., COLE, P., AND BROWN, J., 1973, Etiology of human breast cancer: A review, *J. Natl. Cancer. Inst.* **50**:21.

MATSUO, H., ARIMURA, A., NAIR, R. M. G., AND SCHALLY, A. V., 1971*a*, Synthesis of the porcine LH- and FSH-releasing hormone by the solid-phase method, *Biochem. Biophys. Res. Commun.* **45**:822.

MATSUO, H., BABA, Y., NAIR, R. M. G., ARIMURA, A., AND SCHALLY, A. V., 1971*b*, Structure of the porcine LH- and FSH-releasing hormone. I. The proposed amino acid sequence, *Biochem. Biophys. Res. Commun.* **43**:1334.

McCANN, S., 1970, in: *Hypophysiotropic Hormones of the Hypothalamus: Assay and Chemistry* (J. Meites, ed.), pp. 90–95, Williams and Wilkins, Baltimore.

McCORMICK, G. M., AND MOON, R. C., 1965, Effect of pregnancy and laction on growth of mammary tumors induced by 7,12-dimethylbenz(a)anthracene (DMBA), *Br. J. Cancer* **24**:160.

McGUIRE, W. L., AND JULIAN, J. A., 1971, Comparison of macromolecular binding of estradiol in hormone-dependent and hormone-independent rat mammary carcinoma, *Cancer Res.* **31**:1440.

McGUIRE, W. L., HUFF, K., JENNINGS, A., AND CHAMNESS, G. C., 1972, Mammary carcinoma: A specific biochemical defect in autonomous tumors, *Science* **175**:335.

MEITES, J., 1970, *Hypophysiotropic Hormones of the Hypothalamus: Assay and Chemistry*, Williams and Wilkins, Baltimore.

MEITES, J., 1972*a*, Relation of prolactin and estrogen to mammary tumorigenesis in the rat, *J. Natl. Cancer Inst.* **48**:1217.

MEITES, J., 1972*b*, The relation of estrogen and prolactin to mammary tumorigenesis in the rat, in: *Estrogen Target Tissues and Neoplasia* (T. L. Dao, ed.), pp. 275–286, University of Chicago Press, Chicago.

MEITES, J., 1973, Control of prolactin secretion in animals, in: *Human Prolactin: Proceedings of the International Symposium on Human Prolactin* (J. L. Pasteels and C. Robyn, eds.), pp. 104–118, American Elseveir, New York.

MEITES, J., AND NICOLL, C. S., 1966, Adenohypophysis: Prolactin, *Ann. Rev. Physiol.* **28**:57.

MEITES, J., CASSELL, E., AND CLARK, J., 1971, Estrogen inhibition of mammary tumor growth in rats; counteraction by prolactin, *Proc. Soc. Exp. Biol. Med.* **137**:1225.

MEITES, J., LU, K. H., WUTTKE, W., WELSCH, C. W., NAGASAWA, H., AND QUADRI, S. K., 1972, Recent studies on functions and control of prolactin secretion in rats, *Recent Prog. Horm. Res.* **28**:471.

MILLER, E. C., AND MILLER, J. A., 1974, Biochemical mechanisms of chemical carcinogenesis, in: *The Molecular Biology of Cancer* (H. Busch, ed.), pp. 377–402, Academic Press, New York.

MILLER, T. R., 1970, Hypophysectomy, in: *Breast Cancer: Early and Late* (The University of Texas M. D. Anderson Hospital and Tumor Institute at Houston), pp. 377–380, Year Book Medical Publishers, Chicago.

MITTRA, I., 1974, Mammotropic effect of prolactin enhanced by thyroidectomy, *Nature (London)* **248**:525.

MITTRA, I., AND HAYWARD, J., 1974, Hypothalamic-pituitary-thyroid axis in breast cancer, *Lancet* **1**:885.

MITTRA, I., HAYWARD, J. L., AND McNEILLY, A. S., 1974, Hypothalamic-pituitary-prolactin axis in breast cancer, *Lancet* **1**:889.

MOON, R. C., 1969, Relationship between previous reproductive history and chemically induced mammary cancer in rats, *Int. J. Cancer* **4**:312.

MOOSSA, A. R., PRICE EVANS, D. A., AND BREWER, A. C., 1973, Thyroid status and breast cancer, *Ann. R. Coll. Surg. Engl.* **53:**178.

MUELLER, G. C., 1971, Estrogen action: A study of the influence of steroid hormones on genetic expression, *Biochem. Soc. Symp.* **32:**1–29.

MÜHLBOCK, O., AND BOOT, L. M., 1959, Induction of mammary cancer in mice without the mammary tumor agent by isografts of hypophyses, *Cancer Res.* **19:**402.

MUKHERJEE, A. S., WASHBURN, L. L., AND BANERJEE, M. R., 1973, Role of insulin as a "permissive" hormone in mammary gland development, *Nature (London)* **246:**159.

MURPHY, G. P., 1973, *Perspectives in Cancer Research and Treatment* (contributions in honor of the seventy-fifth anniversary of the Roswell Park Memorial Institute), A. R. Liss, New York.

NAGASAWA, H., AND YANAI, R., 1970, Effects of prolaction or growth hormone on growth of carcinogen-induced mammary tumors of adreno-overiectomized rats, *Int. J. Cancer* **6:**488.

NAGASAWA, H., AND YANAI, R., 1971*a*, Increased mammary gland response to pituitary mammotropic hormones by estrogen in rats, *Endocrinol. Jpn.* **18:**53.

NAGASAWA, H., AND YANAI, R., 1971*b*, Reduction by pituitary isograft of inhibitory effect of large dose of estrogen on incidence of mammary tumors induced by carcinogen in ovariectomized rats, *Int. J. Cancer* **8:**463.

NAGASAWA, H., CHEN, C., AND MEITES, J., 1973, Relation between growth of carcinogen-induced mammary cancers and serum prolactin values in rats, *Proc. Soc. Exp. Biol. Med.* **142:**625.

NAIR, R. M. G., BARRETT, J. F., BOWERS, C. Y., AND SCHALLY, A. V., 1970, Structure of porcine thyrotropin releasing hormone, *Biochemistry* **9:**1103.

NANDI, S., 1958, Endocrine control of mammary-gland development and function in the C3H/He Crgl mouse, *J. Natl. Cancer Inst.* **21:**1039.

NANDI, S., AND BERN, H. A., 1960, Relation between mammary-gland responses to lactogenic hormone combinations and tumor susceptibility in various strains of mice, *J. Natl. Cancer Inst.* **24:**907

NANDI, S., BERN, H. A., AND DEOME, K. B., 1960, Effect of hormones on growth and neoplastic development of transplanted hyperplastic alveolar nodules of the mammary gland C3H/Crgl mice, *J. Natl. Cancer Inst.* **24:**883.

NIALL, H. D., 1972, The chemistry of the human lactogenic hormones, in: *Prolactin and Carcinogenesis* (A. R. Boyns and K. Griffiths, eds.), pp. 13–20, Alpha Omega Alpha, Cardiff, Wales.

NICOLL, C. S., FIORINDO, R. P., MCKENNEE, C. T., AND PARSONS, J. A., 1970, Assay of hypothalamic factors which regulate prolactin secretion, in: *Hypophysiotropic Hormones of the Hypothalamus* (J. Meites, ed.), pp. 115–150, Williams and Wilkins, Baltimore.

NIKITOVITCH-WINER, M., AND EVERETT, J. W., 1958*a*, Comparative study of luteotropin secretion by hypophysial autotransplants in the rat: Effects of site and stages of the estrous cycle, *Endocrinology* **62:**522.

NIKITOVITCH-WINER, M., AND EVERETT, J. W., 1958*b*, Functional restitution of pituitary grafts re-transplanted from kidney to median eminence, *Endocrinology* **63:**916.

NOBLE, R. L., 1957, Hormonal regulation of tumor growth, *Pharmacol. Rev.* **9:**367.

OKA, T., 1974, Spermidine in hormone-dependent differentiation of mammary gland *in vitro*, *Science* **184:**78.

OKA, T., AND TOPPER, Y. J., 1972, Is prolactin mitogenic for mammary epithelium? *Proc. Natl. Acad. Sci. U.S.A.* **69:**1693.

O'MALLEY, B. W., AND MEANS, A. ., 1972, Molecular biology and estrogen regulation of target tisue growth and differentiation, in: *Estrogen Target Tissues and Neoplasia* (T. L. Dao, ed.), pp. 3–22, University of Chicago Press, Chicago.

PARKE, L., 1973, Detection of prolactin activity by bioassay in human amniotic fluid, *J. Endorinol.* **58:**137.

PASTEELS, J. L., AND ROBYN, C., 1973, *Human Prolactin: Proceedings of the International Symposium on Human Prolactin*, Excerpta Medica, Amsterdam, American Elsevier, New York.

PEARSON, O. H., MOLINA, A., BUTLER, T. P., LLERENA, L., AND NASR, H., 1972, Estrogens and prolactin in mammary cancer, in: *Estrogen Target Tissues and Neoplasia* (T. L. Dao, ed.), pp. 287–305, University of Chicago Press, Chicago.

PITOT, H. C., AND YATVIN, M. B., 1973, Interrelationships of mammalian hormones and enzyme levels *in vivo*, *Physiol. Rev.* **53:**228.

QUADRI, S. K., KLEDZIK, G. S., AND MEITES, J., 1973, Effects of L-dopa and methyldopa on growth of mammary cancers in rats, *Proc. Soc. Exp. Biol. Med.* **142:**759.

ROBISON, G. A., BUTCHER, R. W., AND SUTHERLAND, E. W., 1968, Cyclic AMP, *Ann. Rev. Biochem.* **37:**149.

ROBYN, C. C., DELVOYE, P., NOKIN, J., VEKEMANS, M., BADAWI, M., PEREZ-LOPEZ, F. R., AND L'HERMITE, M., 1973, Prolactin and human reproduction, in: *Human Prolactin: Proceedings of the International Symposium on Human Prolactin* (J. L. Pasteels and C. Robyn, eds.), pp. 167–188, American Elsevier, New York.

RUSSFIELD, A., 1966, *Tumors of Endocrine Glands and Secondary Sex Organs*, Public Health Service Publication No. 1332, Government Printing Office, Washington, D.C.

SCHALLY, A. V., AND BOWERS, C. Y., 1964, Corticotropin-releasing factor and other hypothalamic peptides, *Metabolism* 13:1190.

SCHALLY, A. V., BABA, Y., NAIR, R. M. G., AND BENNETT, C. D., 1971, The amino acid sequence of a peptide with growth hormone-releasing activity isolated from porcine hypothalamus, *J. Biol. Chem.* 246:6647.

SCHALLY, A. V., ARIMURA, A., AND KASTIN, A. J., 1973, Hypothalamic regulatory hormones, *Science* 179:341.

SEGALOFF, A., 1973, Inhibition by progesterone of radiation-estrogen-induced mammary cancer in the rat, *Cancer Res.* 33:1136.

SEGALOFF, A., AND MAXFIELD, W., 1971, The synergism between radiation and estrogen in the production of mammary cancer in the rat, *Cancer Res.* 31:166.

SEIDMAN, H., 1969, *Cancer of the Breast, Statistical and Epidemiological Data*, American Cancer Society, New York.

SHELLABARGER, C. J., AND SOO, V. A., 1973, Effects of neonatally administered sex steroids on 7,12,dimethylbenz(a)anthracene-induced mammary neoplasia in rats, *Cancer Res.* 33:1567.

SHELLABARGER, C. L., CRONKITE, E. P., BOND, V. P., AND LIPPINCOTT, S. W., 1957, The occurence of mammary tumors in the rat after sublethal whole-body irradiation, *Radiat. Res.* 6:501.

SHIU, R. P. C., KELLY, P. A., AND FRIESEN, H. G., 1973, Radioreceptor assay for prolactin and other lactogenic hormones, *Science* 180:968.

SINHA, D., AND MEITES, J., 1965, Effects of thyroidectomy and thyroxine on hypothalamic concentration of "thyrotropin releasing factor" and pituitary content of thyrotropin in rats, *Neuroendocrinology* 1:4.

SINHA, D., COOPER, D., AND DAO, T. L., 1973, The nature of estrogen and prolactin effect on mammary tumorigenesis, *Cancer Res.* 33:411.

SLEMMER, G., 1972, Host response to premalignant mammary tissues, *Natl. Cancer Inst. Monogr.* 35:57.

SNEDDON, A., STEEL, J. M., AND STRONG, J. A., 1968, Effect of thyroid function and of obesity on discriminant function for mammary carcinoma, *Lancet* 2:892.

SOMMERS, S. C., 1955, Endocrine abnormalities in women with breast cancer, *Lab. Invest.* 4:160.

SPENCER, J. G. C., 1954, The influence of the thyroid in malignant disease, *Br. J. Cancer* 8:393.

STAFL, A., MATTINGLY, R. F., FOLEY, D. V., AND FETHERSTON, W. C., 1974, Clinical diagnosis of vaginal adenosis, *Obstet. Gynecol.* 43:118.

STERENTAL, A., DOMINGUEZ, J. M., WEISSMAN, C., AND PEARSON, O. H., 1963, Pituitary role in the estrogen dependency of experimental mammary cancer, *Cancer Res.* 23:481.

STERLING, K., BRENNER, M. A., AND SALDANHA, V. F., 1973, Conversion of thyroxine to triiodothyronine by cultured human cells, *Science* 179:1000.

STRONG, L. C., 1942, The origin of some inbred mice, *Cancer Res.* 2:531.

TALWALKER, P. K., AND MEITES, J., 1961, Mammary lobule-alveolar growth induced by anterior pituitary hormones in adreno-ovariectomized-hypophysectomized rats, *Proc. Soc. Exp. Biol. Med.* 107:880.

TALWALKER, P. K., AND MEITES, J., 1964, Mammary lobulo-alveolar growth in adreno-ovariectomized rats following transplantation of "mammotropic" pituitary tumor, *Proc. Soc. Exp. Biol. Med.* 117:121.

TALWALKER, P. K., RATNER, A., AND MEITES, J., 1963, In vitro inhibition of pituitary prolactin synthesis and release by hypothalamic extract, *Am. J. Physiol.* 205:213.

TASHJIAN, A. H., BAROWSKY, N. J., AND JENSEN, D. K., 1971, Thyrotropin releasing hormone: Direct evidence for stimulation of prolactin production by pituitary cells in culture, *Biochem. Biophys. Res. Commun.* 43:516.

TEMIN, H. M., 1971, Mechanism of cell transformation by RNA tumor viruses, *Ann. Rev. Microbiol.* 25:609.

TURKINGTON, R. W., 1972a, Molecular aspects of prolactin, in: *Lactogenic Hormones* (G. E. W. Wolstenholme and J. Knight, eds.), pp. 111–127, Churchill Livingstone, Edinburgh.

TURKINGTON, R. W., 1972b, Measurement of prolactin activity in human serum by the induction of specific milk proteins *in vitro*: Results in various clinical disorders, in: *Lactogenic Hormones* (G. E. W. Wolstenholme and J. Knight, eds.), pp. 169–184, Churchill Livingstone, Edinburgh.

TURKINGTON, R. W., 1972c, Secretion of prolactin by patients with pituitary and hypothalamic tumors, *J. Clin. Endocrinol.* **34**:159.

TURKINGTON, R. W., UNDERWOOD, L. W., AND VANWYK, J., 1971, Elevated serum prolactin levels after pituitary-stalk section in man, *New Eng. J. Med.* **285**:707.

TURKINGTON, R. W., FRANTZ, W. L., AND MAJUMDER, G. P., 1973, Effector–receptor relations in the action of prolactin, in: *Human Prolactin: Proceedings of the International Symposium on Human Prolactin* (J. L. Pasteels and C. Robyn, eds.), pp. 24–34, American Elsevier, New York.

TURNER, C. D., AND BAGNARA, J. T., 1971, *General Endocrinology*, Saunders, Philadelphia.

UEDA, G., TAKIZAWA, S., MOY, P., MAROLLA, F., AND FURTH, J., 1968, Characterization of four transplantable mammotropic pituitary tumor variants in the rat. *Cancer Res.* **28**:1963.

UEDA, G., MOY, P., AND FURTH, J., 1973, Multihormonal activities of normal and neoplastic pituitary cells as indicated by immunohistochemical staining, *Int. J. Cancer* **12**:100.

WAELBROECK-VAN GAVER, C., 1969, Tumeurs hypophysaires induites par les oestrogens chez le rat. II. Etude cytogenetique, *Eur. J. Cancer* **5**:119.

WELSCH, C. W., AND GRIBLER, C., 1973, Prophylaxis of spontaneously developing mammary carcinoma in C3H/HeJ female mice by suppression of prolactin, *Cancer Res.* **33**:2939.

WELSCH, C. W., JENKINS, T. W., AND MEITES, J., 1970, Increased incidence of mammary tumors in the female rat grafted with multiple pituitaries, *Cancer Res.* **30**:1024.

WERNER, S. C., AND GRINBERG, P., 1961, Studies with mouse pituitary thyrotropic tumors. I. Survival of implants during prolonged suppression by thyroid hormone, *Cancer Res.* **21**:522.

WOTIZ, H. H., SHANE, J. A., VIGERSKY, R., AND BRECHER, P. I., 1968, The regulatory role of oestriol in the proliferative action of oestradiol, in: *Prognostic Factors in Breast Cancer* (A. P. M. Forrest and P. B. Kunkler, eds.), pp. 368–382, Livingstone, London.

ZONDEK, B., 1941, *Clinical and Experimental Investigations on the Genital Functions and Their Hormonal Regulation*, William and Wilkins, Baltimore.

11

Chalones (Specific and Endogenous Mitotic Inhibitors) and Cancer

J. C. HOUCK AND A. M. ATTALLAH

1. Introduction

During the past decade, considerable attention has been addressed to the possibility of control of cell proliferation by specific and endogenous negative-feedback inhibitors of mitosis (Weiss, 1952; Weiss and Kavanau, 1957). Bullough (1962) and Bullough and Laurence (1960, 1966) have chosen to call these cell-specific, but not species-specific, endogenous inhibitors "chalones"—a word coined by Sir E. A. Shafer in 1916, and derived from the nautical Greek word meaning "to slow down."

A number of attempts have been made by various investigators to demonstrate the existence of a cell-specific and endogenous inhibitor of the mitotic cycle, both *in vivo* and *in vitro* (Iversen, 1961; Chopra *et al.*, 1972; Elgjo and Hennings, 1971; Marks, 1973; Moorhead *et al.*, 1969; Garcia-Giralt *et al.*, 1970; Houck *et al.*, 1971; Florentin *et al.*, 1973; Papageorgiou *et al.*, 1974; Attallah *et al.*, 1975). It has been clearly demonstrated and confirmed that extracts of epidermis, but not of other tissues, will inhibit the proliferation of epidermal cells both *in vitro* and *in vivo* (Bullough and Laurence, 1960, 1966; Bullough, 1962; Iversen, 1961; Chopra *et al.*, 1972; Elgjo and Hennings, 1971; Marks, 1973). Catecholamines must be added to the *in vitro* medium in order to demonstrate this response of epidermal

J. C. HOUCK AND A. M. ATTALLAH • Research Foundation of Children's Hospital National Medical Center, Washington, D.C. Supported in part by grants from the National Institutes of Health, CA12743, CA14484, and AM17167, and a contract from the Office of Naval Research, N00014-71-C-0203.

tissue extracts, however (Bullough and Laurence, 1960; Bullough, 1962). No species specificity has been demonstrated for this epidermal "chalone" effect (Bullough and Laurence, 1966); further, no apparent cytotoxicity of epidermal extracts was demonstrable in the *in vivo* assays (Iversen, 1961). The inhibitory effects *in vitro* were demonstrated to be reversible.

On the basis of this type of information from both *in vivo* and *in vitro* studies, Bullough and Laurence have developed the concept of the control of proliferation of a number of cells by an endogenous cell-specific, but not species-specific, and noncytotoxic negative-feedback inhibitor of mitosis (Bullough and Laurence, 1960, 1966; Bullough, 1962). The theory was that displacement or destruction of the chalone would permit the entrance of the cell into the cell cycle and that this mitotic activity would continue until sufficiently large amounts of inhibitor had been accumulated to arrest the cells in some portion of the cell cycle, presumably G_1 or G_2.

The existence of a cell-specific and endogenous mitotic inhibitor for both epidermal and lymphocytic cells has been confirmed by a number of workers (Moorhead *et al.*, 1969; Garcia-Giralt *et al.*, 1970; Houck *et al.*, 1971; Florentin *et al.*, 1973; Papageorgiou *et al.*, 1974; Attallah *et al.*, 1975) and, to a large extent, it is on the quality of the evidence offered for these two putative chalones that the case for the existence of chalones must rest.

2. Properties of Chalones

The four primary properties of a putative chalone involve (1) cell specificity, (2) endogenous origin of the inhibitor, (3) lack of species specificity, and (4) reversibility or lack of cytotoxicity of the preparation.

2.1. Epidermal Chalone

Bullough and Laurence used a short-term culture system involving pieces of mouse ear and assayed the effectiveness of their epidermal chalone by counting the number of epidermal cells blocked in metaphase by colcemid some 4 h after the addition of putative chalone preparations (Bullough and Laurence, 1960, 1966; Bullough, 1962). Thus they were able to establish mitotic indices in the germinal layer of the epidermis of the mouse ear in short-term culture in the presence of both epinephrine and cortisone. Increased incubation times usually resulted in a decreased efficiency in mitotic inhibition, demonstrated by the various extracts under study, presumably because of the catabolism of epinephrine via monamineoxidases, which are contained in the connective tissue of mouse ear. Reintroduction of epinephrine into the culture system permitted the prolonged incubation system to demonstrate, again quantitatively, similar inhibition of mitotic indices that were found with shorter-term incubation. Extracts of the epidermis from pig skin containing inhibitory activity toward mouse epidermal mitosis had no effect on the mitotic indices of mouse sebaceous glands, lymphoma, or melanoma (Bullough and Laurence, 1966). However, similar extracts of pig epidermis will demonstrate mitotic inhibitory activity on human epidermis, HeLa, and rabbit lens cells (Bullough and Laurence, 1966).

Extracts prepared from pig liver and striated muscle, mouse brain, kidney, liver, lung, rectum, lymphoma, and melanoma, or sheep lymphocytes or bovine granulocytes had no effect on the proliferation of mouse epidermal cells *in vitro*. Contrarily, similar extracts from the skin of man, mouse, rat, guinea pig, rabbit, and codfish, from pig esophagus, lung, and gingiva, from rabbit lens and mouse lens and lung tumors, from epidermal tumors, human gingiva, and human lung tumors, and even the urine from both mouse and man demonstrated significant mitotic inhibitory activities on the proliferation of mouse epidermal cells *in vitro*. The conclusion from these data was that (1) there is no species specificity for the epidermal chalone and (2) although there is a great deal of cell specificity for chalone action it may not be totally specific for epidermal cells but rather be a general epithelial chalone.

2.2. Lymphocyte Chalone

2.2.1. Specificity

The inhibitory activity for the transformation and proliferation of human lymphocytes which can be demonstrated in aqueous extracts of lymphoid tissue (spleen, lymph node, and thymus) has been shown by us to be concentrated in a molecular weight range between 30,000 and 50,000 daltons, using Amicon Diaflo ultrafilters (Houck *et al.*, 1971). These ultrafiltrates, after lyophilization, were reconstituted in the appropriate tissue culture medium (199), supplemented with 10% or 20% calf serum and antibiotics in the usual fashion at a concentration of 100 μg/ml. This medium was used to cultivate 10^6 human peripheral lymphocytes which had been stimulated with PHA for 72 h, and during the last 6 h of incubation a pulse of [^{3}H]thymidine (1 μCi) was added. After these cells had been rinsed three times in cold isotonic saline (4°C), they were precipitated with 5% trichloroacetic acid (TCA). The resulting precipitate was harvested by centrifugation and rinsed three times with cold TCA to remove all but the macromolecular bound [^{3}H]thymidine. After solubilization and mixing with the appropriate liquid scintillator, the amount of [^{3}H]thymidine in the acid-insoluble DNA was determined in the usual fashion in liquid scintillation radioactive counting.

In a similar manner, these lymphoid tissue extracts were also incubated for 24 h with (1) bone marrow cells from the rat, (2) diploid human fibroblasts, (3) HeLa cells, and (4) human choriocarcinoma cells, and the [^{3}H]thymidine uptake into acid-insoluble DNA by these cells was determined. The effect of ultrafiltered extracts from brain, muscle, and lung of calf on the [^{3}H]thymidine uptake of the various target cells was also determined. The percent inhibition of the normal uptake by these five cell types of [^{3}H]thymidine that was demonstrated by these various extracts is summarized in Table 1. These data indicate that lymphoid

TABLE 1

Inhibitory Effects of "Chalone" Extracts Obtained from Various Calf Tissues on the [³H]Thymidine Uptake by Various in Vitro Cell Systems

	Percent inhibition of				
Extract of	PHA	Bone marrow	Fibro-blasts	HeLa	Chorio-carcinoma
Spleen (100 μg/ml)	99	12	0	0	0
Thymus (100 μg/ml)	84	0	0	0	0
Lymph node (100 μg/ml)	99	10	0	0	0
Brain (500 μg/ml)	0	—	0	0	0
Muscle (500 μg/ml)	0	—	0	0	0
Lung (500 μg/ml)	0	—	33	0	0

tissue extracts could almost completely inhibit the incorporation of [³H]thymidine into the acid-insoluble DNA of human lymphocytes stimulated by the lectin phytohemagglutinin (PHA). These same extracts at the same concentrations had a negligible effect on the uptake of a similar pulse of [³H]thymidine into the acid-insoluble DNA of the various kinds of cells found in rat bone marrow cultures. No inhibition of [³H]thymidine uptake by these extracts was demonstrated against human fibroblasts, choriocarcinoma cells, or HeLa cells after 24 h incubation. Extracts of calf brain, muscle, kidney, and lung which had been subjected to the same kind of ultrafiltration demonstrated absolutely no inhibitory effects on the PHA-stimulated transformation of human lymphocytes and, in fact, had no inhibitory effects against the [³H]thymidine uptake by fibroblasts, HeLa cells, or choriocarcinoma cells, with the singular exception of the extracts of lung against diploid human fibroblasts in culture. Presumably this inhibitory activity proceeds from contaminating fibroblast chalone (Houck *et al.*, 1972) in these extracts of the lung.

It would be reasonable to assume that spleen extract would also be contaminated with fibroblast chalone, since the amount of connective tissue in the spleen, like the lung, is considerable. The lack of demonstration of this inhibition by spleen extracts of fibroblast DNA synthesis may very well be because of the smaller concentrations of lymphoid tissue extracts (100 μg/ml) than of lung (500 μg/ml) employed in this study.

Lymphoid tissue extracts from six different species were prepared by aqueous extraction of acetone powders of these tissues in the cold and subsequent ultrafiltration to collect a molecular weight range between 30,000 and 50,000 daltons, as described above, for normal circulating lymphocytes *in vitro*, and the percent of inhibition of these extracts on the uptake after 6 h of a pulse of

[3H]thymidine into acid-insoluble DNA was determined. This data are summarized in Table 2 and indicate that ultrafiltered aqueous extracts prepared from the lymphoid tissue of six different species were similarly inhibitory toward the PHA-stimulated transformation of human lymphocytes in culture.

Thus the inhibitory activity of lymphoid tissue against a lectin-stimulated transformation of human lymphocytes *in vitro* would seem to be reasonably cell specific but not species specific.

A rather subtle display of cell specificity has been proposed for the lymphocyte chalone *vis-à-vis* T, or thymus-derived, cells and B, or bone-marrow-derived cells. Florentin *et al.* (1973) have shown that extracts of thymus which will inhibit PHA-stimulated lymphocyte transformation, a largely T-cell phenomenon, will not inhibit the functions of antigen stimulation specific for B cells in rats *in vivo*. Extracts of spleen which should theoretically contain both T- and B-derived lymphocytes, however, are capable of inhibiting the antigen stimulation of lymphocyte function in terms of IgM synthesis at similar concentrations. We have found that extracts of thymus will not inhibit the uptake of [3H]thymidine into acid-insoluble DNA by NC-37 diploid human lymphoblasts *in vitro* (Attallah and Houck, 1975; Attallah *et al.*, 1975). These cells are known to be B cells in that they synthesize immunoglobulins and bind the C_3 portion of the complement chain (Pattengale *et al.*, 1973). Further, these NC-37 cells are known to contain the genome to express Epstein-Barr virus, an important property of B cells.

TABLE 2

Percent Inhibition of Lymphocyte Transformation in Vitro Demonstrated by Various Concentrations of Chalone Prepared from the Lymphoid Tissue of Various Species

	Percent inhibition of PHA-lymphocyte transformation by		
	100 μg/ml	50 μg/ml	25 μg/ml
Bovine			
Thymus	84	48	25
Spleen	99	60	33
Porcine			
Thymus	89	50	22
Spleen	99	60	30
Lymph node	100	58	—
Canine			
Spleen	95	48	25
Rabbit			
Thymus	80	48	—
Spleen	99	56	—
Guinea pig			
Thymus	90	50	—
Spleen	99	55	—
Rat			
Spleen	94	55	30
Lymph node	99	61	24

An experiment which is not consistent with T- and B-cell specificities is that β-lipopolysaccharide from *Salmonella typhosa*, which is known to stimulate transformation of B cells (Peavy *et al.*, 1970), can be inhibited significantly by relatively small amounts of thymus-derived chalone (Sunshine and Houck, unpublished results). Normally, the endotoxin will cause approximately 8–10 times as much incorporation of [^{3}H]thymidine into acid-insoluble DNA by B lymphocytes which have been collected from mouse spleen via Hypaque–Ficol gradient (Boyum, 1968), but in the presence of as little as 50 μg/ml of the ultrafiltered extract from calf thymus over 90% of this response is completely inhibited. There are two separate assay systems involved in these experiments: that of Florentin *et al.* (1973), using an antigen specific for B cells both *in vitro* and *in vivo*, and ours, using endotoxin which functions as a mitogen for mouse B cells *in vitro*. Further, the precise end point used in the studies of Florentin *et al.* (1973) was the synthesis of IgM by sensitized lymphocytes, whereas our studies concern the uptake of tritiated thymidine into acid-insoluble DNA; these two procedural differences may be of considerable significance. Our data suggest the possibility that the original suggestion of Florentin *et al.* (1973) that there was a specificity of T-derived chalone for T cells as opposed to B cells may well be true in immunologically stimulated systems, whereas it would appear that B-cell-derived chalone can effectively inhibit the lectin-stimulated transformation of T cells *in vitro* as well as the spontaneous mitotic activity of an established B-cell lymphocyte line. These findings suggest an exquisitely fine cell specificity for lymphocyte chalone.

2.2.2. *Endogenous Origin*

An established cell line of human diploid lymphocytes known as NC-37 originated from the peripheral blood leukocytes of a patient with pneumonia and has been shown to have B-cell characteristics (Pattengale *et al.*, 1973). Established cell lines of NC-37 contain only lymphoblastic cells. These cells can be cultivated in very large quantities, and extracts of the cells themselves have been shown to be able to inhibit the transformation of lymphocytes *in vitro* (Houck and Irausquin, 1973). Significant amounts of this inhibitory activity can also be recovered from the "used" medium during the cultivation of these cells for 3–4 days *in vitro*.

This "used" medium was subjected to ultrafiltration procedures, and the 30,000–50,000 dalton fraction obtained will inhibit the uptake of [^{3}H]thymidine into the DNA of PHA-stimulated lymphocytes but not into diploid human fibroblasts or HeLa cells *in vitro*. Some of these data are summarized in Table 3 and indicate that the "used" medium from NC-37 cells after ultrafiltration contains a sufficient amount of inhibitory activity against [^{3}H]thymidine incorporation into the acid-insoluble DNA of NC-37 to give approximately 50% inhibition of the mitotic activity of these established cell lines *in vitro* at about 150 μg/ml. Less than 25 μg/ml of this same ultrafiltration fraction was required to demonstrate over 50% inhibition of DNA synthesis after PHA stimulation of circulating lymphocytes *in vitro*. Thus it would appear that a specific mitotic inhibitor for

lymphocytes can be recovered from pure cell cultures of human lymphoblasts. **293**
Therefore, this mitotic inhibitor would appear to be endogenous to lymphocytes. CHALONES
AND CANCER

2.2.3. Interpretation of Mitotic Inhibition in Vitro

Ultrafiltrates of the aqueous extract of calf spleen demonstrate a significant inhibition of the uptake of [^{3}H]thymidine into the acid-insoluble DNA content of NC-37 cells *in vitro* after as little as 6 h incubation. The inhibitory activity of spleen extracts, then, is not confined to lymphocyte systems which are stimulated by lectins and suggests that lectin binding cannot be the explanation for the mitotic inhibition of the ultrafiltrate from spleen for lymphocytes *in vitro*.

Since extracts of lymphoid tissue are known to contain significantly large amounts of endogenous thymidine, there is a reasonable possibility of "cold" thymidine contaminating the ultrafiltrate from lymphoid tissue extracts, increasing the pool size of the thymidine, and by dilution decreasing the [^{3}H]thymidine of stimulated lymphocytes *in vitro*. Theoretically, ultrafiltration and washing on a 30,000 dalton filter should reduce considerably this possibility. However, because of this remote possibility of endogenous thymidine diluting the pool size of [^{3}H]thymidine, the effects of 50 μg/ml of an ultrafiltrate of the aqueous extract of calf spleen on the percent of lymphoblasts determined morphologically were studied at various hours after stimulation of 10^6 normal human lymphocytes by PHA *in vitro* in parallel with the determination of the inhibition of [^{3}H]thymidine incorporation into acid-insoluble DNA content of these cells. These results are summarized in Table 4 and indicate that not only is the incorporation of [^{3}H]thymidine into acid-insoluble DNA inhibited by incubation of PHA-stimulated human lymphocytes with the appropriate lymphoid tissue ultrafiltrate, but so, in parallel fashion, is the percent of morphologically transformed lymphoblasts in the population of these cells *in vitro*. These data further suggest that pool-size dilution with cold endogenous thymidine of the [^{3}H]thymidine is an unlikely explanation of the inhibitory effects of these lymphoid tissue extracts.

TABLE 3

Inhibitory Effects of Sieved (30,000–50,000) "Used" Medium from NC-37 Cells in vitro *on the Incorporation of [^{3}H]Thymidine into DNA by PHA-Stimulated Human Lymphocytes (T Cells) and by NC-37 Human Lymphoblasts (B Cells) in Vitro*

Concentration (μg/ml)	Percent inhibition of	
	T cell (PHA)	B cell (NC-37)
0		
25	60[a]	11
50	93[a]	8
100	98[a] (Con A)	40[a]
150	99[a]	55[a]
200	100[a]	68[a]

[a] Significantly inhibited ($P < 0.05$).

TABLE 4

Inhibitory Effects of 50 μg/ml Spleen "Chalone" Concentrate (30,000–50,000 Daltons) on the Percent Lymphoblastic Population and [³H]Thymidine Uptake by 10⁶ PHA-Stimulated Human Lymphocytes in Vitro

Hours after PHA	Percent blasts		Percent [³H]thymidine inhibition
	PHA alone	PHA and chalone	
0	0	0	0
24	14	2	—
48	30	15	56
72	60	23	51
133	75	20	98

However, it is also possible that a significant amount of thymidine could inhibit the proliferation of lymphocytes for a number of reasons other than pool-size dilution (see Section 3). Therefore, circulating human lymphocytes were collected from the blood of two donors and partially purified by Ficol–Hypaque gradients (Boyum, 1968). Lymphocytes (2.5×10^5) from each donor were mixed together to give a total of 5×10^5 human lymphocytes per milliliter of culture and incubated for 5 days with various concentrations of the ultrafiltrate from the aqueous extract of calf thymus prepared as described above. After 5 days incubation at 37°C, the number of cells was counted, their viability was determined by the exclusion of trypan blue, and the percent inhibition of a 6 h pulse of 1 μCi of [³H]thymidine into the acid-insoluble DNA content of these cells was measured. These results, summarized in Table 5, indicate that without chalone after 5 days in mixed lymphocyte culture, wherein each donor's lymphocytes act as an immunological stimulant on the other lymphocytes (two-way mixed lymphocyte culture), the cell number went from 5×10^5 to 14×10^5, approximately a 300% increase in cell number, all of which excluded vital dye.

In the presence of 200 μg of the 30,000–50,000 dalton ultrafiltrate from aqueous extracts of calf thymus, the cell number increased from 5.0 to 5.8×10^5, all of which remained capable of excluding vital dye. Even with as little as 50 μg of

TABLE 5

Effects of Thymus Chalone Concentrate on [³H]Thymidine Uptake into the Trichloroacetic Acid Insoluble Fraction and on the Cell Number of 5×10^5 Human Lymphocytes After 5 Days in Mixed Lymphocyte Culture

Chalone concentration (μg/ml)	Percent [³H]thymidine inhibition	Number of cells	Viability (%)
0	0	14×10^5	100
50	98	—	—
100	98	—	—
200	98	5.8×10^5	100

this thymus ultrafiltrate, approximately 98% of the [^{3}H]thymidine incorporation into the acid-insoluble DNA content of these cells was inhibited.

These data, generated by Dr. Geoffrey Sunshine of this laboratory, indicate that the proliferation of immunologically stimulated lymphocytes, which would normally increase their viable cell number some threefold, was completely inhibited by incubation with the chalone concentrate from the ultrafiltration of calf thymus extracts. Similar results have been obtained using ultrafiltrates from cow spleen.

Finally, the efficacy of lymphocyte chalone *in vivo* has been demonstrated in terms of the inhibition of lymphocyte function in the graft-vs.–host reaction by Garcia-Giralt *et al.* (1972) and for skin allograft survival by ourselves (Houck *et al.*, 1973*b*).

2.3. Recent Supporting Studies by Others

These claims of lymphocyte chalone activity in extracts of spleen which have been ultrafiltered have been confirmed by Lord *et al.* (1974), utilizing a novel and extremely sensitive procedure for the determination of changes in the cytoplasmic viscosity of cells prior to their entrance into S phase. Specifically, they have developed a technique for measuring the polarization fluorescence of cells *in vitro* and have been able to show that there is a significant increase in the "structuredness," or a change in the ratio of polarization fluorescence, in those cells which are destined to enter the mitotic cycle. The entrance of the lymphocyte into the mitotic cycle when stimulated by PHA *in vitro*, as measured by this procedure, is inhibited by the 30,000–50,000 dalton range of ultrafiltered spleen extracts, but not inhibited by molecular weight extracts of larger or smaller size. Further, this inhibition by these ultrafiltrates from spleen extracts can be shown to be cell specific, since it will not interfere with the "structuredness" of either granulocytes or erythropoietic cells *in vitro*. Finally, this inhibitory activity appears to be reversible and therefore presumably not cytotoxic.

Another type of confirmation for the existence of a specific and endogenous mitotic inhibitor for lymphocytes has been presented by Papageorgiou *et al.* (1974), who have shown that the used medium from "crowded" cultures of normal lymphocytes contains a factor processing many of the properties described by us for lymphocyte chalone.

These data suggest very strongly that lymphoid tissue, but not other types of tissues, contains a macromolecule of molecular weight someplace between 30,000 and 50,000 daltons which will specifically inhibit the proliferation of lymphocytes *in vitro*. This inhibitory activity is not species specific but is cell specific and is endogenous to lymphocytes. This inhibitory activity of these ultrafiltrates on lymphoid tissue cannot be explained on the basis of (1) lectin binding, since both Tables 3 and 5 indicate the inhibition of lymphocyte proliferating systems which do not involve lectin; (2) thymidine pool-size dilution or alteration by phosphorylation via the activity of extracellular thymidine kinase, since neither the number of lymphoblasts inhibited nor the number of total cells found after mixed lymphocyte culture would be subject to errors in thymidine uptake deter-mination; (3) cytotoxic contamination of these inhibitory tissue extracts, which is rendered unlikely (a) by the viability studies during long-term incubation with the putative lymphocyte chalone as shown in Table 5 and (b) by the demonstration of the reversibility of this mitotic inhibition after rinsing of NC-37 cells *in vitro* after 4 h incubation (Houck *et al.*, 1973*a*). Therefore, the data described above suggest strongly that there exists in the lymphocyte an endogenous, cell-specific but not species-specific, reversible and not cytotoxic mitotic inhibitor which could be called, in accordance with the original suggestion and definitions of Bullough and Laurence, a lymphocyte chalone.

3. Critique

It is difficult to criticize on a theoretical basis the concept of a specific endogenous mitotic inhibitor or chalone. Careful kinetic and theoretical analysis for the existence of a specific negative-feedback inhibitor of mitosis has been conducted by Weiss and Kavanaugh (1957). Indeed, the idea of a chalone is enormously pleasing to most biologists who have had experience with proliferating cell systems *in vivo*. Evidence for the very existence of chalones is still not totally convincing, however, because there are considerable experimental difficulties in establishing unequivocally the validity of a specific chalone for a specific cell system. This critique will therefore address itself to some of the major technical problems involved in establishing the reality of a particular chalone *in vitro*.

The primary experimental problems *in vitro* revolve around two questions, namely, artifacts in assay techniques and cytotoxicity.

3.1. Assay Artifacts in Vitro

There are three primary techniques for demonstrating the entrance of a cell into a mitotic cycle: (1) to actually count the mitotic figures which have been trapped in metaphase by such inhibitors as colcemid or vinblastine, (2) to actually determine the number of viable cells in an attempt to determine their increase after a given incubation time, and (3) to measure the uptake of tritiated thymidine into acid-insoluble DNA by these cells as they enter into the S-phase portion of the cell cycle—this last being a prerequisite for mitosis. Determination of the mitotic index of the numbers of cells in metaphase vs. the total number of cells is extremely slow and tedious but reasonably reliable. Similarly, the actual counting of the number of cells in a proliferating culture is subject largely to arithmetical rather than methodological error, but, again, this technique represents a reliable method for demonstrating proliferation of cells *in vitro*. The most convenient and yet perhaps the most unreliable method for determining cell proliferation *in vitro*, however, is the uptake of [³H]thymidine into the acid-insoluble DNA content of these cells. There are at least two major reasons why this technique is subject to potential errors of interpretation.

First, a number of tissues contain enzymes capable of phosphorylating or degrading the radioactively labeled thymidine so that it can no longer function as a precursor to DNA synthesis, either because it cannot enter the cell or because it is no longer in the metabolic pathway leading to the synthesis of DNA. The possibility exists that extracts of whole tissues could be contaminated by these normally intracellular metabolic enzymes of the thymidine pathway. Thus the exogenous thymidine which has been labeled with tritium could be destroyed or altered by these enzymes so that it is no longer a reliable measure of the ability of these cells to synthesize DNA *in vitro*. For example, both the reticuloendothelial system and the liver contain very large amounts of thymidine kinase, which would be capable of phosphorylating a very high proportion of the [^{3}H]thymidine added to the cultures in the presence of the putative chalone-containing tissue extract. In this fashion, a spurious demonstration of an apparent inhibition of mitosis could result.

This particular objection can be partially overcome by the appropriate controls as well as by the direct determination of the thymidine kinase or hydrolase activities in a given tissue extract. It is interesting to note that, from our experience, extensive dialysis against water of extracts containing these thymidine-phosphorylating enzymes results in the complete disappearance of this activity, either because of their precipitation as a euglobulin or because of the loss of essential cofactors for the activity which are not found in the simplified culture medium MEM or 199.

A second problem relating to thymidine uptake as a measure of the entrance of cell populations into this phase of the cell cycle is particularly prominent when the putative chalone activity has a low molecular weight, i.e., less than 5000 daltons, as suggested for granulocyte, melanocyte, and liver. That is, these tissue extracts could well be—and probably are—contaminated with unlabeled or cold nucleosides and nucleotides, including thymidine. These low molecular weight nucleosides could dilute out the pool size of the labeled thymidine added to the system under study. Thus an apparent inhibition of thymidine uptake, and hence of cell entrance into the S phase, could be a result of a simple decrease in the probability of a cell's incorporating labeled thymidine molecules. This "pool-size dilution" problem can, in part, be obviated by extensive ultrafiltration of the tissue extracts to remove these low molecular weight nucleosides and nucleotides. This technique, however, is inappropriate when the tissue extracts being studied contain low molecular weight chalones. Further, this pool-size dilution problem cannot necessarily be solved by a demonstration of tissue specificity of the putative chalone. If the intracellular normal thymidine pool is significantly different in two different tissues, then the tissue with the larger thymidine pool shows the least effect of further pool-size dilution after the addition of chalone extracts contaminated with cold thymidine, and this might suggest a spurious tissue specificity of the chalone activity of these extracts.

A further complication of thymidine uptake studies is that various tissue proteins can nonspecifically bind thymidine and thus spuriously indicate thymidine incorporation into DNA (Morley and Kingdon, 1972). This absorption of [^{3}H]thymidine onto tissue proteins not only results in a TCA-precipitable complex mimicking the incorporation of [^{3}H]thymidine into macromolecular DNA but may also reduce the concentration of free or unbound labeled thymidine available for incorporation into DNA. Either way, the singular interpretation of [^{3}H]thymidine incorporation rates under these conditions as representing the net entrance of the cell population under study into S phase is obviously unsupportable and misleading.

Radioactive markers of macromolecular assembly of DNA during S phase other than thymidine could be considered. For example, adenine and formate are incorporated into DNA, although both are also incorporated into RNA. However, a chemical isolation of DNA from RNA is not difficult, and this process, which has not been used extensively in the chalone literature to date, could establish the significance of the alteration in the incorporation rates of these precursors into acid-insoluble DNA in terms of the entrance of these cells into the S-phase portion of their cycle.

In summary, the primary difficulties in interpreting decreases in [^{3}H]thymidine incorporation rates into the acid-insoluble DNA for *in vitro* cell populations in the presence of crude tissue extracts presumably containing a putative chalone are (1) changes in thymidine pool size by contamination of the chalone extract with tissue-derived cold thymidine and (2) alteration of the thymidine so as to render it unavailable for incorporation into the macromolecular synthesis of DNA.

Until recently (Attallah *et al.*, 1975), this type of analysis of the possible artifacts leading to interpretation of mitotic inhibition by crude tissue extracts has not been extensively used by investigators attempting to establish the existence of chalones.

3.2. Cytotoxicity

The most fundamental criticism of experimental work attempting to establish chalonelike activity proceeds from the cytotoxicity of a wide number of tissue extracts *in vitro*. Probably the most important cytotoxic contaminant of tissue extracts would be the complement chain of proteins derived from the blood found in that particular tissue. The latter portion of the interdigitated series of hydrolases (which constitute the complement system) contains a phospholipase and other hydrolases which are capable of enzymatically destroying cell membranes. Therefore, if a latter portion of the complement system was contaminating the tissue extract under study and if it could be activated during the various processes of partial purification employed, this might lead to the destruction of the cells and an apparent inhibition of their mitotic activity. This perhaps is most succinctly summed up in Houck's law: "Dead cells do not divide!" and its corollary: "Dying cells divide damn slowly!"

It is almost impossible to prove that a cell is not being cytotoxically rendered incapable of normal mitotic activity. Usually the evidence for cytotoxicity is based on the failure of nonviable cells to exclude a vital dye, often trypan blue. This is, however, a rather terminal manifestation of the effects of cytotoxic materials on cells *in vitro.* That is, ultimately the entrance of a vital dye into a given cell requires the destruction or loss of integrity of the membrane systems of that cell. One could easily imagine that initially toxic events—which would not yet have had sufficient time to be associated with the loss of integrity of the surface membrane—could have taken place in that cell at the time the incorporation of markers for the entrance of these cells into their mitotic cycle was measured. Obviously, measures of normal mitochondrial function or of glycolytic activity are still quite possible in cells whose ability to exclude vital dye is considerably reduced, because these enzymatic systems still maintain their function within what is clearly a dying cell. So it is possible that a marginally cytotoxic agent could be applied to a given type of cells and, by virtue of making the cells sufficiently "sick," inhibit thereby the enormous energetic expenditures required to enter the S phase. Yet, theoretically, during this period of time the cells may not be sufficiently injured to alter the permeability of their membranes to a highly charged "vital dye." The reversibility of this phenomenon would simply mean that the cytotoxic agent is not sufficiently powerful or is not in sufficient concentration to effect, as yet, irreversible changes, although it is very slowly killing the cells and thereby inhibiting their entrance into the mitotic cell cycle.

The specificity of chalone activity for a particular cell type would not necessarily overcome the argument of cytotoxicity. Certain kinds of cells such as lymphocytes have a very different chemistry about their surface membranes than, say, fibroblasts, which grow attached to glass. It is possible that the fibroblasts attached to glass would not be affected by a mildly cytotoxic agent, whereas lymphocytes in suspension culture would be. This could occur either because part of the fibroblast is masked, being adsorbed to the glass on which it is growing, whereas all the lymphocyte is equally exposed to attack, or because there are intrinsic differences in the susceptibility or the numbers of binding sites on the appropriate cell for a mildly cytotoxic agent. Therefore, it is enormously difficult, if not impossible, to rigorously exclude the possibility that cytotoxicity is complicating the interpretation of *in vitro* data that appear to demonstrate inhibition of mitosis in the presence of tissue extracts. Perhaps the best that could currently be done to exclude cytotoxicity as an explanation for the mitotic inhibition of putative chalone concentrates would be to demonstrate that this inhibitory action was not associated with vital dye staining of the target cells over a long period of incubation and that it was still reversible over this period.

Originally we felt that the inhibition of [³H]thymidine incorporation into cells under the influence of the putative chalone might not be associated with inhibition of the usual rate of uptake of, say, an amino acid or uridine. However, this is not a definitive solution to the question of the cytotoxicity of chalone-containing tissue extracts, for, as will be discussed later, it appears that the chalones which we have studied biochemically are also associated eventually with an inhibition of both protein and RNA synthesis *in vitro.*

In the authors' opinion, it would be unfair to minimize the intellectual difficulty of the question of cytotoxicity as an alternative explanation for the apparent effects of putative chalones *in vitro.* The longest experience we have had with incubating the chalone-containing ultrafiltrates of lymphoid tissue extracts with lymphocytes has been for a total of 7 days in mixed lymphocyte culture. All of the cells in these cultures remained viable, as judged by the exclusion of vital dye. It would have to be believed that by 1 wk, if the chalone content of these extracts were cytotoxic, it should have manifested this cytotoxicity in terms of the exclusion of vital dyes. It is also possible, of course, that responsiveness of these cells in culture to the cytotoxic properties of chalone is distributed on a statistical basis and that during this period of incubation those cells which could be cytotoxically grossly injured have been and hence have disintegrated and been lost morphologically from the culture. Even under these conditions, however, one would expect to find other statistical portions of the population which are now dying and failing to exclude vital dye. Admittedly, this is argumentation rather than definitive experimentation, but we suggest that this is the most powerful single criticism of the chalone and it cannot easily be resolved experimentally. Finally, blood contains a number of macromolecules which can nonspecifically inhibit the uptake of [^{3}H]thymidine by cells *in vitro*. These nonspecific inhibitors considerably complicate the search for real chalones.

3.3. Criticisms of in Vivo Studies of Chalones

The major criticisms *in vivo* relate largely to the immunological complications involved in injecting a variety of foreign materials into an animal and thereby greatly stimulating its immunological rejection mechanisms. In studies of the ability of chalone extracts to inhibit *in vivo* tumor growth, usually a test system involves the use of transplanted tumors within an inbred mouse or rat strain. Under these conditions, however, it is still possible that the added exogenous material contained in the chalone extract could stimulate the animal's immunological defense systems so as to inhibit the tumor growth, not via inhibition of mitotic activity by chalones, but rather via rejection phenomena.

This possibility may be particularly important in the studies described below in terms of granulocyte chalone activity against transplanted Shay chloroleukemia cells in rats. Here low molecular weight materials collected from the granulocytes of rodents (and presumably lymphocytes as well) are injected into an animal. This material is very similar to the "transfer factor" described by Lawrence (1969). The consequence of "transfer factor" in immunologically incompetent patients is to increase enormously the activity of their reticuloendothelial system, permitting them to control previously intractable fungus infections. It is possible that this "transfer factor," when injected into normal rodents, could activate their reticuloendothelial system in a similar fashion and thereby immunologically inhibit the growth of transplanted tumors and even destroy them *in vivo*. Since the experimental tumors transplanted even within a given inbred strain are not homografts, there is the real possibility that—because these tumors have membranes altered chemically and probably immunologically—an immunological rejection of the allograft tumor transplant could gratuitously be stimulated by administration of the crude chalone concentrate. Whether such an immunological stimulation could be accomplished by a "transfer factor" contaminant of leukocyte chalone extracts in a host bearing a transplanted tumor remains unknown. It seems only fair, however, that this particular criticism be included in an objective critique of chalone studies.

Another difficulty in terms of long-term *in vivo* studies, of course, is the possibility that the host animal under study will develop antibodies against the injected chalone-containing tissue extract. One possible exception to this question of antichalone antibody might be the lymphocyte chalone itself, since inhibition of lymphocyte transformation should preclude the release of either cytophilic or circulating antibody from T- and B-cell-type lymphocytes, respectively. In this particular system, long-term exposure to lymphocyte chalone would probably not involve antibody formation to it. Further, since most chalones currently known seem to be of a relatively low molecular weight, their immunogenicity may be relatively low.

4. Chalones and Cancer

4.1. Epidermal Chalone

Bullough and Laurence (1968) originally extracted the rabbit V × 2 epidermal tumor (derived from the Shope papilloma as a poorly differentiated, fast-growing, metastatic squamous cell carcinoma) and were able to demonstrate epidermal chalone activity in these extracts, using the mouse ear *in vitro* assay system. These workers also claimed that this tumor responded to the addition of pig-skin-derived epidermal chalone extracts by demonstrating a decreased mitotic index *in vivo*. Further, the presence of a large V × 2 tumor in a given animal was found to result in a significant depression of the general mitotic rate in the host animal. This result suggested the possibility of the systemic release into the circulation of epidermal chalone activity by the tumor.

The Hewitt epidermal keratinizing squamous carcinoma is maintained by subcutaneous incubation into WHT/Ht albino mice. It is fast growing and typically shows central keratinization and peripheral mitosis. Bullough and Deol (1971) also later reported that these tumor cells synthesize a tissue-specific epidermal chalone that can be easily released into the blood. They based this conclusion on their finding that the animal's normal epidermal mitotic rate was depressed by about 50% while the sebaceous gland's mitotic rate was unaffected in mice carrying this Hewitt carcinoma. This effect was not due to a general metabolic deterioration or to stress because the fall in mitotic rate was epidermal specific.

Aqueous extracts of the Hewitt epidermal carcinoma have been tested *in vitro* on the mitotic index of epidermis and the sebaceous glands. These authors concluded that the Hewitt epidermal carcinoma contained appreciable quantities of the tissue-specific epidermal chalone and that it was active in the first 4 h but not in the second 4 h of incubation *in vitro*, unless the epidermis was washed briefly in a dilute epinephrine solution. These workers also found that there was no significant mitotic depression in the tumor cell with added chalone concentrate and therefore concluded that this was due either to some intrinsic inadequacy in the chalone control mechanism of the tumor cell itself or to an abnormally low chalone concentration preexisting within the tumor cell.

Elgjo and Hennings (1971) chose another assay system, a transplantable keratinizing hamster epithelioma first described by Chernozemski (1967). The aim of their study was to see if the rates of mitosis and DNA synthesis of this tumor were influenced by addition of exogenous epidermal chalone. A preliminary attempt was also made to treat the tumor-bearing animals with repeated injections of epidermal chalone to see if it was possible to induce a regression of the tumors. Their results *in vivo* showed that after injection of epidermal chalone the DNA synthesis and the mitotic rate in the tumors in the ear, epidermis, and cheek pouch epithelium were depressed and the cells were sensitive to the chalone action in both G_1 and G_2 phases but not in S phase. However, in the groups of hamsters treated with repeated injections of chalone they observed no regression of the tumor size during and after treatment. The histological picture of the tumors was similar to that found in untreated tumors. Repeated intraperitoneal injections of the pig skin extract containing epidermal chalone activity killed the animals if given too frequently. Laurence and Elgjo (1971) in an *in vitro* study of the same tumor used by Elgjo and Hennings *in vivo* found that the tumor tissue contained a mitotic inhibitor biologically identical to the epidermal chalone. However, epidermal chalone had no effect on the mitotic rate of the tumor cells *in vitro* even in the presence of the stress hormones. Their explanation for these results was that there was a difference in the dose of colcemid needed for different tissues.

4.2. Melanocyte Chalone

Bullough and Laurence (1968) and Mohr *et al.* (1968) suggested that since skin is known to contain a large population of dispersed melanocytes it is possible that these, too, have their own mitotic control systems and that extracts of skin may contain a melanocyte chalone. Both groups of investigators chose to study Harding–Passey melanomas transplanted into NMRI mice and amelanotic melanomas transplanted into Syrian hamsters. In most of their work, partially purified extracts of pig skin were injected subcutaneously at a site opposite to the tumor. Bullough and Laurence (1968) found that in the fourth hour following the injections of the pig skin extracts into the mouse tumor system *in vivo* the mitotic activity of the outermost growing zone of the melanomas decreased by about 50%. They also cut pieces from the outermost mitotically active zone of hamster tumor and incubated them *in vitro* with chalone extract. The results showed that melanocyte chalone activity also required epinephrine and hydrocortisone. Mohr *et al.* (1968) found that after daily injections into tumor-bearing mice and hamsters for 5 days the tumors in both species responded in the same way; i.e., they became soft and necrotic, the amelanotic melanomas darkened, and then they regressed and ulcerated, and the wounds finally healed. Both Bullough and Laurence (1968) and Mohr *et al.* (1968) found, by using skin extracts obtained via electrophoresis which had been purified for epidermal chalone which was highly active against epidermal mitosis, that no inhibition of melanomas could be demonstrated either *in vivo* or *in vitro*. Both groups suggested that crude skin extracts were contaminated by a melanocyte chalone. These results were apparently not caused by the stressful action of the treatment; for example, the necrosis at the site of injection was stimulated by burning without any effect on the tumors in the absence of melanocyte chalone containing skin extracts. Both groups also showed that extracts of Harding–Passey melanomas prepared in the usual way contained melanoma chalone activity.

Mohr *et al.* (1968) said, "spores of anaerobic bacteria, which might lead to tumor regression as reported by Mose in 1960, were excluded as causative agents morphologically and microbiologically." However, Mohr *et al.* (1972) later reported that the striking melanocyte oncolytic activity found in some of their pig skin fractions was caused by contaminating clostridial spores and not by possible chalone components.

Dewey (1973) found that the growth-inhibiting action of the melanoma extract was specific to melanocytes since his extracts had no effect on the proliferation of Chinese hamster lung cells, transformed human embryo liver cells, and normal human fibroblasts *in vitro*. This chalone activity was demonstrable on melanocytes *in vitro* and was concentrated, using Amicon Diaflo ultrafiltration between 1000 and 10,000 daltons.

Seiji *et al.* (1974) established an *in vitro* assay method using B-16 mouse melanoma melanocytes in tissue culture. They prepared extracts from Harding–Passey mouse melanomas and found that these extracts inhibited DNA and protein synthesis and seemed more inhibitory when epinephrine and hydrocortisone had been added to the tissue culture medium. A single injection of this extract intraperitoneally into mice bearing Harding–Passey mouse melanomas caused a significant reduction of DNA synthesis in this tumor. Seiji *et al.* (1974) also attempted to purify the melanoma melanocyte specific mitotic inhibitor by using ethanol fractionation, gel filtration, and column chromatography. They obtained two fractions containing inhibitory activity, and the inhibitory activities of both these fractions on DNA and protein biosynthesis by melanocytes were well correlated. Tissue specificities were examined, using L cells and HeLa cells, with one of the fractions (weighing less than 5000 daltons) having tissue specificity and the other, higher molecular weight fraction inhibiting DNA and protein synthesis in both L cells and HeLa cells. Both types of inhibitors are still heterogeneous.

The similarity of these results described separately by Dewey (1973) and Seiji *et al.* (1974) suggests that the original observations by Bullough and Laurence (1968) and by Mohr *et al.* (1968) were correct.

J. C. HOUCK
AND
A. M. ATTALLAH

4.3. Fibroblast Chalone and Antichalone

Fibroblasts normally are not mitotically active *in vivo*—except as a consequence of injury and destruction to the connective tissue. The initial events of wound repair involve, subsequent to the vascular response to injury, the proliferation of epithelium, capillaries, and fibroblasts until these last cells reach a high population density within the interstices of the wounded space. These cells usually then cease to be mitotically active, but become active biochemically in terms of the synthesis of collagen and mucopolysaccharides. Fibroblasts which have been cultured from explants of skin, lung, and other organs rich in connective tissue can be cultivated *in vitro*, during which time they logarithmically increase their population number until they come into contact one with the other. At this time in the kinetics of the culture, the cells will reduce their mitotic rate, cease to proliferate, and eventually reach a confluent and stationary phase of culture life when they are said to be "contact inhibited" (Levine *et al.*, 1965; Todaro *et al.*, 1965). This phenomenon of contact inhibition of diploid human fibroblasts in culture is an important characteristic of these cells and can be overcome (1) by creating a mechanical wound in the confluent monolayer by scraping a hole therein (Todaro *et al.*, 1967; Raff and Houck, 1969) or (2) by increasing the concentration of serum in the culture medium from 10% to 20% (Holley and Kiernan, 1968). It is logical to suspect that the control of fibroblast proliferation demonstrated by contact inhibition *in vitro* and wound repair *in vivo* might be mediated through the mechanism of a putative chalone.

Diploid human fibroblasts derived from either cutaneous biopsy explants or WI-38 (Flow Laboratories, Maryland) were cultivated in MEM containing 10% calf serum and supplemented with glutamine and penicillin-streptomycin in the usual fashion. Approximately 2×10^5 of these cells were introduced into small Falcon flasks (25 cm^2) and 24 h later the supernatant medium was decanted and the cells which had adhered to the surface of the plastic were rinsed with serum-free medium and new medium containing 10% calf serum was supplied to the cells at 2 ml per culture. The cells were then allowed to incubate for 24 h with 1 μCi of [^{3}H]thymidine. After this period, the medium was removed, and the cells were rinsed with serum-free medium twice, trypsinized, harvested, and rerinsed in cold (4°C) isotonic saline, aliquots of which were counted in a hemocytometer, and then mixed with 5% cold TCA. The resulting precipitate was rinsed once again with TCA in the cold and allowed to stand in suspension overnight with 5 ml of TCA. The following morning, the suspension was centrifuged and the supernatant removed, and three more rinsings with 5% TCA were performed in order to remove all of the nonspecifically absorbed [^{3}H]thymidine from the precipitated RNA, DNA, and protein. After the final rinsing, the precipitate was solubilized in NCS solubilizer at 80°C (0.5 ml). This solubilized material was then mixed with the liquid scintillation cocktail and counted in the usual fashion. The results are expressed as counts per minute per 10^6 cells.

As a source for a specific and endogenous mitotic inhibitor for fibroblast proliferation, diploid human fibroblasts were grown to a confluent monolayer in

TABLE 6

Inhibitory Effects of Fibroblast Extract Concentration on the Incorporation of [³H]Thymidine by Diploid Human Fibroblasts

	Control	Extract concentration			
		250 μg/ml	500 μg/ml	1 mg/ml	2 mg/ml
Cpm/10⁶ cells	3118	2253	833	889	785
Percent inhibition		28	73	71	75

roller bottles. These cells were rinsed thoroughly with isotonic saline three times to remove adhering serum and other materials, and then were collected by trypsinization and sonically disrupted. After centrifugation of these disrupted cells in the cold, the clear supernatant was removed and dialyzed against 200 vol of water in the cold. After dialysis, the contents of the dialysis bag were centrifuged and the clear supernatant was lyophilized. The inhibitory effects of various concentrations of this fibroblast extract on the incorporation of [³H]thymidine by diploid human fibroblasts in culture are demonstrated in Table 6. At a concentration as low as 500 μg/ml, fibroblast extract prepared in this fashion will inhibit up to 73% of the control uptake of [³H]thymidine by these fibroblasts after 24 h incubation *in vitro*. At a concentration of 1 mg/ml of this fibroblast extract, no similar inhibitory effect on the thymidine uptake by PHA-stimulated lymphocytes *in vitro* or HeLa cells in culture could be demonstrated. The kinetics of the inhibitory effect of this dialyzed and lyophilized extract from diploid human fibroblasts on the uptake of [³H]thymidine by these cells in culture during log phase growth was explored. Within 3 h, there was a significant decrease in the synthesis of DNA by these cells after exposure to 330 μg of extract per milliliter of culture medium, as shown in Table 7. Two doses of extract (0.5 and 2.0 mg/ml) were added to the incubation medium of diploid human fibroblasts in culture. Half of these cultures were then rinsed twice with MEM containing 10% serum, and new medium with 10% serum was added along with [³H]thymidine. Most of the inhibitory activity of the fibroblast extract at 0.5 mg/ml was removed by this

TABLE 7

Kinetics of [³H]Thymidine Uptake by Diploid Human Fibroblasts in the Presence and Absence of 330 μg/ml of Fibroblast Extract

Hours	Control (cpm/10⁶ cells)	Inhibitor (330 μg/ml)	Percent inhibition
2	227	227	18
3	460	267	42
4	807	407	50
24	4266	2026	53

TABLE 8

Results of Rinsing Inhibitor-Treated Fibroblasts with 10% Serum in MEM on the Subsequent Incorporation of [³H]Thymidine

		Cpm/10⁶ cells			
		0.5 mg/ml inhibitor		2 mg/ml inhibitor	
	Control	Non-rinse	Post-rinse	Non-rinse	Post-rinse
	4995	1135	4475	1205	3614
	4868	1240	4727	1234	3834
Mean	4931	1187	4601	1219	3724
Percent inhibition		76	7	75	24

rinsing, as shown in Table 8. Using 2 mg/ml of this extract, only two-thirds of the inhibitory activity could be rinsed from these cells by washing the medium. These results indicate that the bulk of the mitotic inhibition effected by fibroblast extract was reversible when these fibroblasts were rinsed with MEM containing 10% serum, but at higher concentrations of inhibitor not all of this inhibition was reversible. Morphologically, these cells which were inhibited by chalone appeared grossly similar to untreated cells, with no evidence of either rounding up or detachment from the glass surface, both of which are usually characteristic of cytotoxicity.

The extract of diploid human fibroblasts was then subjected to molecular sieving, using Amicon Diaflo ultrafilters. Almost all of the mitotic inhibitory activity on the DNA synthesis rates of these diploid human fibroblasts in culture demonstrated by the extracts during log phase growth was found in the fraction between 30,000 and 50,000 daltons. The molecular weight fraction between 50,000 and 100,000 daltons had absolutely no effect on [³H]thymidine uptake by these cells and very little effect was demonstrable using fractions between 10,000 and 30,000 daltons.

Diploid human fibroblasts in culture were maintained in confluency for 3–4 days in MEM with 10% serum. At the end of this time, the medium was removed, dialyzed exhaustively against water, and centrifuged. The clear supernatant resulting from this centrifugation was lyophilized and the effect of various concentrations of this portion of the "used" medium from the cultivation of these cells on the [³H]thymidine uptake by fresh diploid human fibroblasts was determined. This series of experiments demonstrated that the quantitative uptake of [³H]thymidine was approximately 3200 cpm per 10⁶ cells, and up to 77% of this uptake into acid-insoluble DNA could be inhibited by the addition of 0.5–2.0 mg/ml of the nondialyzable portion of the used medium. There was no nondialyzable mitotic inhibitor in either normal MEM supplemented with 10% serum (unused medium) or similar medium which had been exposed to the cells for only a few hours. Essentially equivalent amounts of inhibitory activity could be demonstrated in the used medium after 3 or 4 days of incubation with diploid human fibroblasts in confluency.

Again, this mitotic inhibitory activity of the nondialyzable portion of used medium from the cultivation of diploid human fibroblasts was not associated with any apparent cytotoxicity, as judged by either morphology or cell detachment of the treated fibroblasts.

The dialyzed and lyophilized used medium from the cultivation of these diploid human fibroblasts *in vitro* was subjected to isoelectric focusing, as described by Vesterberg and Svensson (1966). There were three major isoelectric peaks found in the used medium which had been subjected to isoelectric focusing between pH 3.5 and 4.3, 4.4 and 4.9, and 5.0 to 5.7. At 330 μg/ml, only the most acid peak contained significant amounts of inhibitory activity against fibroblasts' DNA synthesis *in vitro* (see Table 9). The apparent inhibition of 16% of the DNA synthesis of these cells when cultivated with the most alkaline-isoelectric-point material was not statistically significant. When the acid-isoelectric-point material was pooled and subjected to molecular ultrafiltration, essentially all of the inhibitory activity toward DNA synthesis by diploid human fibroblasts in culture was found in the molecular weight range between 30,000 and 50,000 daltons. As little as 50 μg/ml of this fraction which had been subjected to isoelectric focusing and molecular ultrafiltration could inhibit 50% of the [^{3}H]thymidine uptake by diploid human fibroblasts in log phase growth *in vitro*.

These data suggest that extracts of fibroblasts in culture and of a similar molecular weight portion of their used medium after cultivation *in vitro* contain a mitotic inhibitor which is not cytotoxic to fibroblasts and which apparently is specific for these cells *in vitro*. The molecular weight of this material is between 30,000 and 50,000 daltons and its isoelectric point is between 3.5 and 4.3.

This inhibitory activity toward DNA synthesis by diploid human fibroblasts in culture was destroyed by trypsin and was thermolabile after incubation at 55°C for 30 min.

This cell-specific inhibitory activity for the S-phase activity of diploid human fibroblasts could also be found in the same molecular weight range in extracts of such fibroblast-rich tissues as porcine lung. Extracts of skin were found by us to

TABLE 9

Inhibitory Effects of Three Fractions from the Isoelectric Focusing of the Nondialyzable Portion of "Used" Medium on Fibroblast Uptake of [^{3}H]Thymidine

| | Cpm/10^6 cells | | | |
	Control	Peak 1 (pH 3.5–4.3)	Peak 2 (pH 4.4–4.9)	Peak 3 (pH 5.0–5.7)
	4152	2332	5012	3892
	4292	2020	5046	3186
Mean	4222	2176	5029	3539
Percent inhibition		49.5	0	16

contain enormous amounts of cytotoxic materials which were nonspecific in their inhibitory activity for a number of human cells in culture.

Diploid human fibroblasts, after counting in a hemocytometer, were seeded into Leighton tubes at a concentration of 4×10^4 cells per 1.5 ml of medium per tube. After 24 h, these fibroblast cultures were rinsed with balanced salt solution and the medium was changed, reintroducing fresh MEM supplemented with 10% serum. At this point, the number of cells was counted, using a Whipple eyepiece and an inverted microscope, as has been described previously by Raff and Houck (1969). After various periods of incubation, these cultures were counted in triplicate, and the log of the number of cells per square millimeter was plotted against time. The slope of the initial straight-line portion of this plot during the period of log phase growth permitted the population doubling time to be calculated. The effects of various concentrations of crude chalone ultrafiltrate between 30,000 and 50,000 daltons prepared from used medium of diploid human fibroblasts *in vitro* were determined. At 10–20% serum, the population generation time was increased from a normal control of about 35 h to close to 100 h at a concentration of 500 μg/ml. As little as 100 μg of the chalone concentrate from molecular ultrafiltration of used medium from the cultivation of human fibroblasts *in vitro* would prolong the population doubling time of these same cells significantly to about 45 h. The effects of similar concentrations of chalone concentrate from the used medium on the population generation time of a number of cultures cultivated in medium supplemented with only 2.5% or 5.0% serum were determined. In the presence of 5% serum, the doubling time of the population of cells was approximately 60 h; the addition of as little as 50 μg of the chalone concentrate from the ultrafiltration procedure described above increased this to close to 90 h. As has been published elsewhere (Houck *et al.*, 1973c), the amount of chalone concentrate required to effect a 100% increase in the time required for population doubling increased linearly as the concentration of serum in the culture was increased. These data suggest strongly that there is a competition between some element of serum and the putative fibroblast chalone.

We have isolated and purified completely a sialoprotein of approximate molecular weight 120,000 from mammalian serum which is stringently required for diploid human fibroblasts' *in vitro* proliferation (Houck and Cheng, 1973). All the mitogenic activity of mammalian serum from four different species for diploid human fibroblasts in culture is an expression of the concentration of this purified sialoprotein in the medium. Solutions of purified mitogenic sialoprotein from calf serum were prepared at a concentration of 50 μg/ml of MEM supplemented only with glutamine and penicillin-streptomycin. This medium would support the growth of diploid human fibroblasts at a population doubling time of approximately 28 h. When 500 μg of chalone concentrate from the ultrafiltration of used medium was added to this solution of serum mitogen, the medium supported a population doubling time of approximately 110 h. When mixtures of fresh purified serum mitogen (at 50 μg/ml) and 500 μg/ml of chalone concentrate were subjected to molecular sieving through an Amicon Diaflo ultrafilter XM50 (passing materials of molecular weight below 50,000), as has been described elsewhere (Houck *et al.*, 1972, 1973c), the population doubling time supported by this medium was restored essentially to normal (32 h) for that portion of the material which did not pass through a 50,000 molecular weight filter; thus essentially all of the putative chalone had been easily removed from the solution containing purified serum mitogen, suggesting that there was little direct interaction between the fibroblast mitogen from serum and the chalone concentrate.

Therefore, we propose that the purified serum mitogen or sialoprotein most probably acts competitively at the same sites on the cells as does fibroblast chalone. We propose that the control mechanism of fibroblast proliferation *in vitro* and probably *in vivo* resides in the relationship of the concentration of fibroblast chalone to fibroblast mitogen or "antichalone." Contact inhibition *in vitro* would then involve a sharing of a critical chalone concentration between cells which are essentially contiguous through crowding into confluency. The chalone could be displaced from the surface of these cells by the addition of serum containing the appropriate fibroblast mitogen or antichalone. Because of the decreased concentration of chalone through displacement from the cell surface, these cells would continue to proliferate *in vitro*. Similarly, during wound repair *in vivo*, the normally mitotically arrested fibroblasts begin to proliferate at a considerable rate in that portion of the tissue adjacent to the injury. Extravasation of serum into the wounded tissue is, of course, one of the major characteristics of the initial events of the acute inflammatory response. Thus it is probable that the fibroblast mitogen derived from the serum flooding into the injured tissue area around the site of the wound would displace chalone from the fibroblast contained within this marginal area and therefore permit the entrance of these cells into the mitotic cycle. Proliferation of these fibroblasts into the injured tissue would continue until such time as the biological continuity of the microcirculation was restored and the fibroblast mitogen from serum would no longer be flooding the environment around the area of injury. Thus the proliferation of fibroblasts into the wound would cease, and the repair of the lesion by collagenization could begin.

When diploid human fibroblasts are cultivated in the presence of SV40 virus, a certain percentage of these cells are eventually transformed into heteroploid fibrosarcoma cells (Houck and Cheng, 1973). These cells do not require serum for mitotic activity, albeit they are helped by the addition of serum to their medium in terms of proliferation rates. Such transformed WI-38 fibroblasts have been cultivated in our laboratory and they, too, will respond to the addition of the chalone concentrate from the ultrafiltered fraction of either used medium or diploid human fibroblasts themselves. That is, their population generation time as judged from cell counting in Leighton tubes is considerably prolonged by the addition of 500 g/ml of the chalone concentrate. This demonstration of the ability of fibroblast chalone concentrate to inhibit the proliferation of transformed fibroblasts is analogous to the demonstration of chalone inhibition of the proliferation of fibrosarcoma cells *in vitro*.

Osteosarcoma cells have been cultivated *in vitro* from a patient from Los Angeles Children's Hospital (McAllister *et al.*, 1971), and these cells, which adhere to glass, will proliferate unremittingly in the absence of serum, are not contact inhibited, and adhere to each other even more effectively than they do to glass. Their karyology has been determined and is essentially heteroploid. The effect of fibroblast chalone concentrate from used medium on the proliferation rates, determined from cell counting *in vitro*, of human osteosarcoma cells was quite profound—namely, 1 mg/ml completely inhibited the proliferation of these cells *in vitro*. The rinsing of these osteosarcoma cells *in vitro* with serum containing MEM, as described above, restored the proliferative activity of these cells. The readdition of 1 mg/ml of fibroblast chalone concentrate from used medium again essentially arrested the mitotic activity of these cells over a period of 5 days *in vitro*.

On the basis of these experiments involving (1) WI-38 fibroblasts transformed into fibrosarcoma cells and (2) human osteosarcoma cells, we have been able to demonstrate that fibroblast chalone concentrate can effectively inhibit the proliferation of these tumor varieties of fibroblasts *in vitro*. We believe that this constitutes another example of the ability of chalone of a given cell type to control the proliferation of the cancer variety of this cell *in vitro*. Thus tumor cells, despite their unremitting mitotic activity both *in vitro* and *in vivo*, will respond to the addition of chalone from the normal cell by a significant reduction in their rate of proliferation *in vitro*.

4.4. Granulocyte Chalone

The granulocyte chalone is claimed to be specific for granulocytes or polymorphonuclear leukocytes. These cells are found in normal bone marrow and peripheral blood, as well as in certain types of tumors such as chronic myeloid leukemia in man and Shay myelocytic chloroleukemia in rats. Chloroleukemia is a malignant derivative of the granulocytic cell system which when transplanted subcutaneously causes a local tumor with a relatively slow growth rate and when injected intraperitoneally causes a typical generalized leukemia. The tumor cells appear to be immature myelocytes and are characterized by a green color under ordinary light and a bright red under ultraviolet due to the presence of protoporphyrin IX, a component of the enzyme myeloperoxidase, which is specific to granulocytic cells (Rytömaa and Kiviniemi, 1968a).

The primary assay for chalone effect is via the uptake of labeled DNA precursors into DNA in bone marrow preparations *in vitro* (Rytömaa and Kiviniemi, 1968a,b, 1970). Determinations of labeling indices (to show the amount of incorporation per cell) were done by autoradiography, using the stripping film technique (Rytömaa and Kiviniemi, 1968a,b).

Some *in vivo* studies were also performed, using chloroleukemic rats as the experimental animals. Regression of local tumors and survival were used as criteria for chalone activity subsequent to the intraperitoneal injection of chalone extract (Rytömaa and Kiviniemi, 1970; Rytömaa, 1973).

Several factors (Rytömaa and Kiviniemi, 1968a, 1970; Rytömaa, 1973) related to this granulocyte chalone have been studied: (1) the chalone content of various types of normal and leukemic cells, (2) the response of various types of cells to the

chalone extract, (3) the effects of the chalone *in vivo*, and (4) the presence of an
antichalone:

1. It has been claimed that granulocytic chalone is present in normal blood, bone marrow, and serum of rats; in normal blood of humans and cows; in blood, serum, and tumor cells of chloroleukemic rats; and in blood and serum of humans with chronic myeloid leukemia. The amount of chalone in tumor cells, however, is only one-fortieth to one-tenth that found in normal cells, while the amount in the serum of leukemic animals is in great excess of that found in normal serum. This indicates the possibility that in tumors the cells are producing a normal amount of chalone but, for some reason, it is escaping into the serum.

2. While both normal cells and tumor cells respond to the addition of chalone into the culture medium, normal cells are significantly more sensitive to the chalone. To Rytömaa and Kiviniemi (1968b), this would seem to suggest that there are at least two possible reasons for the rapid proliferation of tumor cells: (a) escape of chalone from the cells and (b) decreased sensitivity of the cells to chalone.

3. The *in vivo* assays consisted of treating rats with either implanted subcutaneous tumors or generalized leukemia with subcutaneous injections of chalone extract. In the case of the subcutaneous tumors, 10–30% regressed spontaneously, while the remainder regressed with chalone treatment. In the case of the generalized leukemia, no spontaneous remissions were observed and all control animals died within 24 days of infection; a significant number of the treated animals showed permanent regression of their chloroleukemia (Rytömaa and Kiviniemi, 1970; Rytömaa, 1973).

4. It has been demonstrated that the entry of large numbers of mature granulocytes into the blood from the bone marrow is followed by a reduction in the amount of granulocytic chalone and the concomitant appearance of a specific stimulator, the granulocyte "antichalone," in the serum (Rytömaa and Kiviniemi, 1968b). The antichalone behaves quite differently from chalone on Sephadex gel filtration, since elution parameters of "antichalone" on G75 and G200 indicate a molecular weight of 30,000–35,000. It appears as if a balance between chalone and antichalone is required for granulocytopoiesis. Chalone prevents and "antichalone" promotes the entry of granulocytic precursor cells into the DNA synthesis phase of their cell cycle. Under normal conditions, the chalone prevents the excessive proliferation of granulocytic precursors, while under conditions of acute functional demand, "antichalone," a tissue-specific stimulator, replaces chalone in the serum.

A means must be devised for determining that the chalone is completely tissue specific, however, for while comparative autoradiography of bone marrow suggests that the granulocyte chalone concentrate does not inhibit hematopoiesis markedly, these studies are not quantitatively convincing and other types of cells have not been employed as target cells for this chalone.

The effect of long-term chalone treatment on the growth rate of baby rats was followed in several experiments (Rytömaa and Kiviniemi, 1970). Because these results demonstrated that the treatment did not retard whole body growth, Rytömaa and Kiviniemi (1970) felt that granulocytic chalone had no generalized inhibitory effect on the proliferation of the cells primarily involved in whole body growth. When a crude preparation, effective in Rytömaa's standard *in vitro* assay, was tested on the mitotic activity of the epidermal cells *in vitro*, no effect could be seen (Rytömaa, 1973). Therefore, it appears probable that granulocyte chalone concentrate may well be reasonably cell specific.

A problem relating particularly to the low molecular weight (less than 10,000 daltons) granulocytic chalone is that extracts of lymphoid tissue are known to contain a large amount of cold thymidine. To avoid the possibility of diluting the pool size of labeled thymidine, Rytömaa and Kiviniemi (1968b) showed that inhibition by chalone of DNA synthesis in normal rat bone marrow cells and in chloroleukemic cells *in vitro* is readily demonstrable by means of ^{14}C-labeled formate.

Another approach to this problem has been taken recently by Lord *et al.* (1974), who used the new technique of fluorescence polarization. This technique is based on the excitation of fluorescein molecules released intracellularly by enzymatic hydrolysis of the nonfluorescing fluorescein diacetate (FDA) in the cytoplasm of the emitted fluorescence. Lord *et al.* (1974) have found that the fractions between 10,000 and 500,000 daltons from granulocytes have a significant effect on the "structuredness" of the cytoplasmic matrix (SCM), i.e., inhibit the physicochemical sol–gel alteration precedent to the entrance of these cells into S phase. The high molecular weight fractions from granulocytes or lymph nodes or red blood cells were without effect on the SCM of these cells, further evidence suggesting tissue specificity of granulocytic chalone.

Finally, studies by Benestad *et al.* (1973), using a diffusion chamber implanted intraperitoneally, indicated that only the proliferation of the granulocytic portion of the bone marrow cells contained in the chambers was inhibited by the administration of granulocyte chalone concentrates *in vivo*. These studies using this *in vivo* technique provide the strongest evidence as to the cell specificity of the granulocyte chalone and go a long way toward rebutting the criticism of gratuitous pool-size dilution of labeled DNA precursor uptake.

Paukovits (1973) obtained a granulopoiesis-inhibiting factor (GIF) from medium containing bone marrow. He used ultrafiltration, gel chromatography, and paper electrophoresis techniques to isolate this polypeptide. Paukovits found that the action of GIF was strongly cell type specific and was not species specific. Paukovits thinks that GIF may be identical to granulocytic chalone (Paukovits, 1973). This preparation was highly purified and could not have contained any significant amounts of contaminating "cold" thymidine.

All this evidence suggests strongly that granulocytic chalone exists and will specifically inhibit the proliferation both *in vitro* and *in vivo* of granulocyte tumor cells.

Leukemia is characterized by the uncontrolled proliferation and accumulation of leukemic cells. These cells are incapable of normal maturation and are relatively unresponsive to growth regulation. When the leukemic mass reaches a critical size, the growth rate of the normal and the leukemic cells is decreased. If the number of leukemic cells is reduced sufficiently by therapy, the normal cells are released from this inhibition (Clarkson, 1974). Bichel (1972) has found that recurrent growth of the aspirated JB-1 ascites tumor in one mouse was, at most, completely prevented when the parabiotic partner had a JB-1 ascites tumor at the plateau, suggesting to Bichel the transfer of growth inhibitors via the blood from the full-growing tumor in the parabiotic partner.

The effects of relatively large concentrations of the ultrafiltered spleen extract containing the putative lymphocyte chalone on the proliferation of leukemic lymphocytes *in vitro* was studied using four different established cell lines: (1) L-1210, a mouse leukemic lymphocyte which has been well characterized both *in vivo* and *in vitro*; (2) EL-4, a mouse leukemic lymphocyte (Gorer, 1960); (3) Molt, established from the peripheral blood of a patient during relapses of acute lymphoblastic leukemia with T-cell characteristics (Minowada *et al.*, 1973); and (4) NC-37, a permanent lymphoblastic line with B-cell characteristics (Pattengale *et al.*, 1973) which originated from the peripheral leukocytes of a patient with pneumonia.

The leukemic lymphocyte cell lines were grown in RPMI 1640 medium containing 20% fetal calf serum, glutamine, and 100 units/ml each of penicillin and streptomycin. The NC-37 human lymphoblastic cells were cultured in McCoy's medium with 20% fetal calf serum and 100 units/ml each of penicillin and streptomycin. The ultrafiltered spleen extracts were reconstituted in the appropriate medium before addition to the cultures. DNA synthesis was measured by the amount of [³H]thymidine incorporation into the acid-insoluble DNA fraction. Triplicate cultures were incubated at 37°C for 18 h with the spleen extracts followed by a 6-h pulse of [³H]thymidine. The number of viable cells remaining in similar cultures was determined in triplicate by trypan blue dye exclusion, using a hemocytometer.

The effects of various concentrations of ultrafiltered spleen extracts on the lymphoblastic cell lines are shown in Table 10. It can be seen that (1) the spleen extracts inhibited [³H]thymidine incorporation in all four established lymphocyte cell lines and (2) many of the human and mouse lymphoblasts in these cultures were apparently killed during this incubation period.

Essentially similar cytotoxicity toward leukemic lymphocytes (Molt, L-1210) *in vitro* was also demonstrated by ultrafiltered preparations from other desiccated, defatted calf, cow, and pig spleen powders obtained from the Viobin Corporation. Similar ultrafiltered extracts were prepared from fresh calf spleen and 200 μg/ml of this ultrafiltered material was also found to be capable of killing 45% of the Molt cells *in vitro* after 24 h incubation.

J. C. HOUCK
AND
A. M. ATTALLAH

TABLE 10

Effects of 24-h Incubation at 37°C of Ultrafiltered Spleen Extracts (in Triplicate) on the Mean Number of Viable Cells (Capable of Excluding Trypan Blue Vital Dye) Remaining and Incorporation of [³H]Thymidine (6-h Pulse) into the Acid-Insoluble DNA of Four Established Lymphoblastic Cell Lines

Cell type	Concentration (μg/ml)	Number of viable cells ($\times 10^5$/ml)	Percent dead cells	Cpm/10^6 viable cells	Percent inhibition of DNA
Mouse					
1. L-1210	0	8.1	10	37,500	—
$(5.5 \times 10^5$/ml)[a]	125	4.5	44	15,500	59
	250	2.8	65	14,200	63
2. EL-4	0	8.0	10	13,800	—
$(10.2 \times 10^5$/ml)[a]	125	3.3	59	14,400	0
	250	1.4	83	8,900	33
Human					
1. Molt	0	7.0	10	110,000	—
$(6.8 \times 10^5$/ml)[a]	125	3.3	53	12,000	89
	250	2.0	72	8,000	93
2. NC-37	0	7.2	10	13,600	—
$(6.2 \times 10^5$/ml)[a]	125	4.0	44	1,140	92
	250	3.5	51	250	98

[a] Initial seed number.

These same spleen extracts were incubated with normal human lymphocytes and normal mouse spleen cells. Triplicate cultures of 5×10^5 human lymphocytes with or without PHA were incubated with or without 200 μg/ml of ultrafiltered spleen, as described previously (Houck *et al.*, 1971; Houck and Irausquin, 1973). There was no reduction in the number of viable cells after 72 h, as judged by vital dye exclusion. Despite this lack of extract cytotoxicity, 50 μg/ml inhibited over 50% of the PHA-stimulated transformation of these cells, as measured both morphologically and by [³H]thymidine incorporation into acid-insoluble DNA. Similarly, incubation of mouse spleen cells for 48 h with or without 200 μg/ml of spleen extract showed no apparent cytotoxicity.

Ultrafiltered extracts of cow and pig kidney were prepared as described above. Neither of these extracts, at concentrations similar to that of the spleen preparations, demonstrated any inhibition of [³H]thymidine incorporation or cytotoxicity toward L-1210 or Molt cells after 48 h incubation *in vitro*. Finally, similar ultrafiltered extracts of fresh calf thymus were prepared and were demonstrated to be extremely cytotoxic to Molt cells but not to normal human lymphocytes *in vitro*.

Thus it would appear that 30,000–50,000 dalton extracts of lymphoid tissue, but not of nonlymphoid tissues, from cow and pig are capable of specifically inhibiting the mitotic activity of both mouse and human lymphoblastic cell lines and, more importantly, are uniquely cytotoxic to these cells *in vitro*.

The cytotoxicity of these extracts was also determined on primary cultures of EL-4 lymphoblasts. The EL-4 lymphoid tumor, originally induced in C57 mice by

TABLE 11

315
CHALONES
AND CANCER

TABLE 11

Cytotoxicity and DNA Inhibition Produced by Incubating Various Concentrations of Spleen Ultrafiltered Extracts with Primary Cultures of 5×10^5/ml EL-4 Mouse Lymphocytes in Triplicate for 48 h in Vitro

Concentration (μg/ml)	Number of cells ($\times 10^5$/ml)	Percent viable cells	Percent inhibition of DNA
0	6.5	66	0
75	7.2	45[a]	54[a]
125	5.7	24[a]	81[a]
250	6.9	17[a]	98[a]
500	5.9	5[a]	99[a]

[a] Means found to be significantly different from 0 concentration control ($P < 0.05$).

the carcinogen 9,10-dimethyl-1,2-benzanthracene (Gorer, 1960), has been carried in several laboratories as a transplantable ascites tumor (kindly provided by Dr. John R. Wunderlick of the National Cancer Institute, National Institutes of Health). These animals were killed, and the EL-4 cells were removed from their *in vivo* peritoneal incubation medium, were counted by hemocytometry in the usual fashion, and on the basis of the exclusion of vital dye were found to be well over 95% viable. These primary cultures were incubated in triplicate, as described above, for 48 h with various concentrations of the desiccated, defatted ultrafiltered spleen extract. The effects of these extracts on the incorporation of a 6-h pulse of [^{3}H]thymidine into acid-insoluble DNA and on the viability of these cells as determined by vital dye exclusion are presented in Table 11. It can be seen that while the mean number of cells was not significantly reduced, the percentage of these cells remaining viable was again reduced in direct proportion to the dose of the spleen extract employed.

Finally, we determined the cytotoxic effects of 100 or 200 μg/ml of ultrafiltered spleen extract on cultures of L-1210 lymphoblasts, which have been shown by Garcia-Giralt and Macieira-Coelho (1974) to be inhibited in terms of DNA synthesis but not in terms of cell proliferation or cytotoxicity when cultured at 100,000 cells/ml. Therefore, we studied cultures which had been seeded initially with varying numbers of cells and incubated for 48 h at 37°C. These results are presented in Table 12. Concentrations of L-1210 from 5 to 10×10^5 cells/ml (cell concentrations used routinely in most laboratories) incubated with both 100 μg and 200 μg of the spleen ultrafiltered extract had a significant number of dead cells, as judged by their inability to exclude vital dye. With 2.3×10^5 or fewer cells per milliliter, 100 μg/ml of ultrafiltered spleen extract no longer demonstrated cytotoxic effects, while 200 μg/ml of ultrafiltered spleen extract still demonstrated a 40% cytotoxicity. However, this dose was without cytotoxic effect on cultures initially seeded with 0.8×10^5 lymphoblasts per milliliter and did not inhibit their proliferation. In contrast to our results, Hryniuk *et al.* (1969) have shown that as cells approach their saturation density, thereby slowing their growth rate, longer periods of exposure to the same concentration of S-phase poisons are required to effect cell death.

TABLE 12

Effects of Inoculum Size on the Cytotoxicity of 100 or 200 µg/ml of Ultrafiltered Spleen Extracts on L-1210 Mouse Leukemic Lymphocytes After 48 h Incubation in Triplicate at 37°C

Number of cells seeded ($\times 10^5$/ml)	Number of viable cells ($\times 10^5$/ml) after incubation with spleen extract		
	0 µg/ml	100 µg/ml	200 µg/ml
9.5	14.0	5.3[a]	5.4[a]
5.3	6.5	3.6[a]	3.6[a]
2.3	6.4	6.3	3.7[a]
0.8	2.3	2.4	2.2

[a] Means found to be significantly different from 0 concentration control ($P < 0.05$).

The significance and mechanism of this cell-concentration-dependent specific cytotoxicity against established cell lines of mouse and human lymphoblasts is unclear, as is the relevance of proliferating lymphocytes *in vitro* to the *in vivo* human condition. However, this finding (Attallah and Houck, 1975a) that normally noncytotoxic concentrations of ultrafiltered spleen extracts containing lymphocyte chalone activity appear to be specifically cytotoxic for crowded cultures of leukemic lymphocytes *in vitro* seems to be deserving of attention.

4.6. Evidence for a Putative Colon Chalone

An established cell line of human colon carcinoma cells (SW-48) was obtained from Dr. Albert Liebovitz (Scott and White Clinic, Temple, Texas). These cells proliferate in L-15 medium containing 10% serum and make very considerable amounts of mucus *in vitro*. Morphologically, these heteroploid cells resemble very closely those found in human colon carcinoma *in vivo*.

We have obtained from the cultivation of large numbers of these human colon carcinoma cells their "used" medium after approximately 7 days *in vitro*. Pooled samples of this "used" medium were subjected to molecular ultrafiltration, using the Amicon Diaflo ultrafiltration system. The "used" medium was thereby subdivided into fractions in excess of 300,000 daltons, between 50,000 and 300,000 daltons, between 10,000 and 50,000 daltons, and between 1000 and 10,000 daltons. These molecular weight fractions were concentrated and washed extensively with water to remove salt and lyophilized, as described previously.

A number of cultures were established in triplicate which had been seeded with $1.7–6.0 \times 10^5$ colon carcinoma cells into L-15 medium containing 10% fetal calf serum and supplemented with gentamycin and fungizone. The number of cells per flask was determined in triplicate by harvesting these cells via trypsin in EDTA and counting the resulting cell suspension in a hemocytometer in triplicate. The mean cell number per flask was calculated and the standard deviation of these means after up to 5 days of incubation was found to be about ±7%. The population doubling time for these cells was calculated from the slope of a linear plot of the log of the mean cell number per flask after 0, 24, 43, 48, 54, 69, 95, and 120 h of incubation at 37°C to be 24–48 h.

One day after inoculation of colon carcinoma cells into large numbers of 25-cm² Falcon flasks, these cultures were incubated with various concentrations (0, 0.5, 1.0, 2.0, and 3.0 mg/ml) of the four molecular weight fractions of the "used" medium described above. Three days later, these cultures were harvested and suspensions of these cells were prepared and counted in a hemocytometer. Cytotoxicity was indicated by loss of cell numbers via detachment of the cells from the plastic surface. The mean cell number per flask and percentage of inhibition was recorded, as indicated in Table 13. These data indicate that a very considerable amount of noncytotoxic inhibition of the proliferation of human colon carcinoma cells *in vitro* could be demonstrated by 1 mg/ml or more of the molecular weight fraction of the "used" medium between 10,000 and 50,000 daltons. The fraction between 1000 and 10,000 daltons was essentially cytotoxic, as was the fraction in excess of 300,000 daltons. The fraction between 50,000 and 300,000 daltons had no apparent inhibitory or cytotoxic activity on these colon carcinoma cells *in vitro*.

The molecular weight fraction between 10,000 and 50,000 daltons from the "used" medium of the cultivation of human colon carcinoma cells *in vitro* was found to have no inhibitory effect at 1 or 3 mg/ml on the PHA-stimulated transformation of diploid human lymphocytes *in vitro* or on the proliferation of diploid human fibroblasts (WI-38), as judged by cell count studies in Leighton tubes *in vitro*.

TABLE 13

Effects of Concentrations of Various Molecular Weight Fractions of the "Used" Medium from the Cultivation of Human Colon Carcinoma Cells in Vitro on the Number of These Cells per Culture (in Triplicate) After 72 h Incubation

Concentration of mol wt fraction	Mean cell number ($\times 10^5$)		Percent inhibition
	0 time	72 h	
None	1.72	6.32	—
Over 300,000			
(1, 2, or 3 mg/ml)	1.72	Reduced numbers	Cytotoxic
50,000–300,000			
(1, 2, or 3 mg/ml)	4.00	18.6	0
10,000–50,000			
0 mg/ml	2.00	5.8	—
0.5 mg/ml	2.00	5.4	10
1.0 mg/ml	2.00	4.0	47
2.0 mg/ml	2.00	2.8	79
3.0 mg/ml	2.00	2.5	87
1000–10,000			
(1, 2, or 3 mg/ml)	2.00	Reduced numbers	Cytotoxic

318

J. C. HOUCK
AND
A. M. ATTALLAH

The 10,000–50,000 dalton fraction of the "used" medium from the cultivation of human colon carcinoma cells was subdivided into two fractions between 10,000 and 30,000 daltons and between 30,000 and 50,000 daltons via Amicon Diaflo ultrafiltration. One milligram of the fraction between 10,000 and 30,000 daltons inhibited the proliferation of these colon carcinoma cells by 35%, whereas a similar concentration of the 30,000–50,000 dalton fraction inhibited the proliferation of these cells by 100%, as summarized in Table 14.

The mucosal lining of a sample of aganglionic human colon from a patient with Hirschprung's disease was obtained by dissection and approximately 1 g of this sample was extracted in 0.15 M sodium chloride in the cold (10 ml/g) overnight. (10 ml/g) centrifugation, the clear supernatant was passed through a 50,000 dalton Amicon Diaflo ultrafilter and was concentrated on a 10,000 dalton filter. After repeated washing with distilled water and lyophilization, this material was assayed for its ability to inhibit the proliferation of human colon carcinoma cells *in vitro*. This extract demonstrated 95% inhibition of the proliferation of these cells after 72 h incubation, as also shown in Table 14. While "unused" medium containing serum includes a mildly cytotoxic inhibitor for colon cell proliferation which can be concentrated in the 10,000–50,000 dalton range, the 30,000–50,000 dalton concentrate was without any inhibitory activity on the proliferative rate of these cells *in vitro*.

This endogenous mitotic inhibitor of colon carcinoma cell proliferation *in vitro* was destroyed by preincubation with trypsin and yet was still fully active after incubation for 30 min at 55°C.

Thus there appears to be a specific, endogenous, and noncytotoxic mitotic inhibitor for the proliferation of human colon carcinoma cells *in vitro* which can be obtained from either the "used" medium from the cultivation of these cells after 7 days or from aqueous extracts of human colon epithelium with a molecular weight of about 30,000 daltons. This mitotic inhibition thermostable and contained peptide bonds essential to its inhibitory activity. Therefore, we suggest that the proliferation of colon carcinoma cells *in vitro* may well be under the control of a chalone.

TABLE 14

Inhibitory Effects of the 10,000–30,000 and 30,000–50,000 Dalton Concentrations from "Used" Medium and 0.15 M NaCl Extracts of Human Colon Epithelium on the Number of Human Colon Carcinoma Cells per Culture After 72 h Incubation in Vitro

Mol wt fraction (1 mg/ml)	Mean cell number ($\times 10^5$)		Percent inhibition
	0 time	72 h	
None	3.20	14.3	—
"Used" medium			
30,000–50,000	1.72	1.60	103
10,000–30,000	3.2	10.4	35
Colon extract			
10,000–50,000	3.2	3.8	95

Cyclic AMP has a clearly defined role as a "second messenger" in the action of many hormones (Robison *et al.*, 1968). It has been found that the intracellular level of cyclic AMP in transformed and rapidly growing normal cells is lower than in slowly dividing or stationary normal cells (Sheppard, 1971, 1972). Addition of dibutyryl cyclic AMP to the medium of cultured cells changes their morphology and restores controlled growth to transformed cells (Inbar and Sachs, 1969).

It has been shown that a transient reduction of the cellular cyclic AMP level occurs after confluent monolayers of normal 3T3 cells have been exposed to serum, trypsin, and insulin (Sheppard, 1972). Pharmacological agents which raise the endogenous level of cyclic AMP markedly inhibit the transformation of PHA-stimulated lymphocytes (Smith *et al.*, 1971). Several workers have shown that the activity of adenyl cyclase in transformed cells is less than in untransformed cells (Peery *et al.*, 1971). Insulin causes a decrease in the concentration of intracellular cyclic AMP and inhibits membrane-bound adenylate cyclase (Jimenez de Asua *et al.*, 1973). Cyclic AMP inhibits the mitotic activity of mouse epidermis *in vitro* (Voorhees *et al.*, 1972). Cyclic AMP can prevent lymphocytes from differentiating into antibody-producing cells when it is present during a critical period of the immune induction *in vitro* (Schneider and Kolb, 1973). Iversen (1969) had suggested a possible role for cyclic AMP in epidermal differentiation.

Hakomori *et al.* (1968) have found a difference in the chemical nature of the side groups of the plasma membranes of normal and transformed cells. Studies of cell membranes derived from 3T3 and 3T3-transformed cells have revealed lower amounts of sialic acid in the transformed cell membranes and altered glycoprotein composition of the plasma membranes (Wu *et al.*, 1968). Thus this alteration could be the cause of decreased chalone and/or adenylcyclase activities. It has been shown that the activity of adenyl cyclase is lower in transformed cells than in untransformed cells (Peery *et al.*, 1971). Wright *et al.* (1973) have found a decreased response of adenyl cyclase in psoriatic skin to epinephrine.

Hauschka *et al.* (1972) have indicated that cyclic AMP is capable of significantly inhibiting the uptake of [^{3}H]thymidine into the acid-insoluble DNA fraction of Chang hamster ovary (CHO) fibroblastlike cells. They have found that this cyclic AMP inhibition of thymidine uptake by these cells is mediated through the inhibition of nucleoside kinase activity intracellularly. As DNA synthesis requires the continuous recruitment of nucleoside precursors, it is tempting to speculate that the chalone shuts off the supply of precursors for macromolecular synthesis at some stage before the incorporation of deoxynucleoside triphosphates into DNA but allows the completion of DNA synthesis from those triphosphates formed prior to chalone addition. The phosphorylation of nucleosides (particularly thymidine) by specific kinases is diminished by exogenous cyclic AMP in blasts (Hauschka *et al.*, 1972).

If we postulate that chalone is a part of the cell membrane which regulates the cyclic AMP system, we are able to construct a simple model (Fig. 1) of growth regulation which is consistent with these observations (Attallah, 1975; Attallah and Houck, 1975). For example, normal fibroblasts from several different species were found to inhibit the growth of transformed cells. This growth inhibition could be achieved only if the cells were in contact with one another (Stoker, 1964; Stoker and Shearer, 1966). It was shown that strains of normal cells which attain relatively low population densities in culture (contact inhibition of growth) inhibit each other in mixed culture (Eagle and Levine, 1967). This interstrain inhibition is not species specific (Eagle *et al.*, 1968). Chalone is known to be tissue but not species specific. Further, contact inhibition through chalone bridges on the cell membrane has been proposed (Houck *et al.*, 1972, 1973c). "Wound healing" *in vitro* is initiated when a small patch of cells is scraped away from a stationary-phase monolayer (Raff and Houck, 1969). This could lower the amount of chalone that regulates the cyclic AMP system, subsequently lowering cyclic AMP in cells which in turn start dividing, repair the wound, and accumulate enough chalone to eventually become contact-inhibited through chalone bridges (Attallah and Houck, 1975). A report on fibroblasts derived from human skin indicated that these cells gave greater adenyl cyclase activity at the time the cultures become confluent and that rates of cell division decreased (Zacchello *et al.*, 1972).

Houck and Cheng (1973) were able to purify the mitogenic factor from serum which apparently acts as an antichalone, thereby serving to displace preexisting chalone from the surface of the fibroblast and permitting the cell to enter the mitotic phase of its cell cycle (Houck *et al.*, 1973c). Proteolytic enzymes could have the same effect by destroying either the existing chalone on the cell membrane or

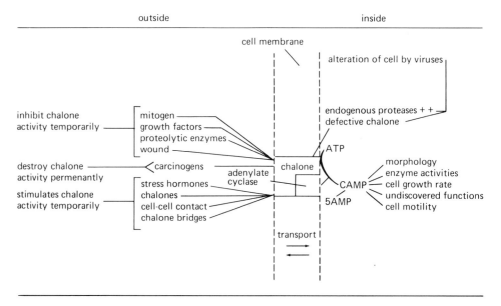

FIGURE 1. A schematic representation of the chalone–cyclic AMP system hypothesis, in which several factors interact with chalone, altering its inhibitory activity either temporarily or permanently and thereby increasing or decreasing cyclic AMP concentration intracellularly via adenyl cyclase activity modulation (see text for details). From Attallah (1975).

the sites to which it is bound, thus allowing the cell to escape from mitotic control until the necessary amount of new chalone was synthesized so that the concentration of chalone shared by these cells would again be sufficient to control mitosis. Other compounds that act on the cell surface also stimulate growth. These include proteases bound to Sepharose beads (Burger, 1971) and neuraminidase (Vaheri *et al.*, 1972). Their effects are transitory and generally permit only one round of cell division after the agent is removed. Several transformed cell lines were found to produce a protease that depends on serum for its activation (Ossowski *et al.*, 1973). Schnebli (1972) reported such an increase in proteaselike activity in DNA-virus-transformed cells. It was found that a number of protease inhibitors selectively inhibited the growth of transformed cells (Schnebli and Burger, 1972).

A cancer cell does not contain as much chalone and will not respond to chalone as effectively as do normal cells, according to Bullough and Laurence (1968*a*) and Rytömaa and Kiviniemi (1968*a*). These authors have claimed that chalones escape from the cancer cells into the bloodstream of tumor-bearing animals. The observed decreased sensitivity of the transformed cell's adenyl cyclase to hormones reported by Peery *et al.* (1971) has suggested an alteration of the cell's hormone receptor site or surface structure with transformation. This difference between neoplastic and normal cells reported by Bullough and Laurence (1968), Rytömaa and Kiviniemi (1968*a*), and Peery *et al.* (1971) might be attributed to the large amount of proteolytic enzymes produced by these cancer cells, consequently altering either the chalone or its binding site. Another possibility would be the modification of all or part of the genome that produces a defective chalone (see Fig. 1). A possible explanation for these results thus might be to suppose that the chalone glycoprotein contains two active sites: one site specific for the cell membrane and the other site nonspecifically stimulating the adenyl cyclase activity on the membrane (Attallah, 1975; Attallah and Houck, 1975*b*).

As a consequence of the action of this cell-specific stimulator of adenyl cyclase activity, the intracellular concentration of cyclic AMP would be maintained at a relatively high level and the cell would then be unable to enter the mitotic cycle because of a decrease in nucleoside kinase activity and hence a lack of DNA and RNA precursors. This possibility that chalone involves the cyclic AMP system clearly deserves further investigation; a necessary proof of this proposed mechanism for chalone activity is the demonstration of an increased adenyl cyclase activity in broken membrane preparations with the addition of the appropriate chalone.

6. Proposed Practical Potential of Chalones

We have attempted to summarize both the available literature and our own most recent data to indicate that for at least six cell systems there are sufficient data to suggest that chalones obtained by extracting the appropriate tissue or cell system are capable of inhibiting the proliferation of the cancerous variety of that cell type

TABLE 15

Summary Chart of Chalones and Cancer

	Epidermis		Melanocyte	Fibroblast	Granulocyte	Lymphocyte	Colon
Cell cycle	G_1	G_2	G_1	G_1	G_1	G_1	G_1
Mol wt	100,000	30,000–40,000	2000	30,000–50,000	4000	30,000–50,000	30,000–50,000
Lability to treatment by							
Proteases	No	Yes	Yes	Yes	Yes	Yes	Yes
RNase	No	—	Yes	—	—	No	—
DNase	—	—	—	—	—	No	—
Heat	No	Yes	Yes	Yes	—	Yes	No
Source	Pig skin, hairless mice, keratinizing cell	Skin of various mammals, basal cell	Harding–Passey melanoma, tumor pig skin	Used media of fibroblasts	Rat bone marrow, granulocyte, spleen	Lymphocytes, lymph node, spleen, thymus of various mammals	Mucosa cells, intestine, used media of carcinoma cells
Assay system							
In vitro	[³H]Thymidine uptake in mouse skin	Colcemid technique	[³H]Thymidine uptake, cell number, average mitotic count	[³H]Thymidine uptake, cell number	[³H]Thymidine autoradiography of short-term culture of rat bone marrow	[³H]Thymidine uptake, cell number, lymphoblast number	Cell number
In vivo	[³H]Thymidine uptake in mouse skin	Colcemid technique	DNA synthesis in Swiss mice with Harding-Passey melanoma	—	[³H]Thymidine uptake by cells in diffusion chamber	GVH, allograft, xenograft survival	—
Tumor inhibition	Hamster carcinoma	Mitotic depressions of V × 2 epidermal tumor of rabbits in vitro, in vivo	Mouse and hamster melanoma melanocytes	Human osteosarcoma proliferation inhibited	Inhibition of DNA synthesis, chloroleukemia (rat), chronic myeloid leukemia (man)	Cytotoxic for leukemic cells in man and mouse	Proliferation inhibited

in vitro and, in some cases, *in vivo* (Table 15). The quality of the data offered to support the contention that chalone-rich concentrates are capable of inhibiting the proliferation of the appropriate tumor cells varies considerably; sufficiently adequate data exist, however, to suggest that the phenomenon of chalone control of mitotic activity of tumor cells is a reasonable possibility.

The potential practical application of these findings may not be directly related to inhibiting tumor growth by increasing the systemic concentration of the appropriate chalone, but rather may reside in the fact that for the most part chalones appear to inhibit the proliferation of cells in the G_1 portion of their cell cycle and that a great deal more chalone is required to inhibit a cancer cell than to inhibit the proliferation of a normal cell. Therefore, perhaps it would be possible to introduce a large amount of the appropriate chalone *in vivo* which would arrest both normal and tumor cell proliferation in G_1. If this inhibition by chalone could be maintained over a period of 24–36 h, which would certainly encompass the normal cell cycle of most proliferative cells, these cells would be trapped in G_1 precedent to the S phase when DNA synthesis occurs. A reduction, then, of the concentration of the appropriate chalone would release these cells from their G_1 inhibition and they would, in a synchronized fashion, march into S phase and at this point they would be enormously vulnerable to the various kinds of DNA inhibitors and S-phase poisons. The reduction of the concentration of the chalone would not be sufficient, however, to release the normal cell from its G_1 inhibition, and so the proliferation of the normal cell would continue to be inhibited. Therefore, these normal cells would be protected from the cytotoxic effects of the appropriate chemotherapeutic agent. On this basis, we believe it is possible that chalones may constitute an important addition to the existing modalities of chemotherapy by (1) synchronization of the target cell and (2) protecting the normal cell from the chemotherapy. If such a critical pharmacological concentration (still inhibiting normal but not tumor cells) could be defined for chalones, then their ability to synchronize tumor cells and protect normal cells would be enormously important in terms of improving the efficacy of the current modalities of chemotherapy *in vivo*. It is this possibility that suggests that it would be well worthwhile for oncologists to pay considerable attention to the development of the chalone concept, that is, the control of mitotic replication via specific and endogenous negative-feedback inhibitors of mitosis.

7. References

ATTALLAH, A. M., 1975, A proposed mechanism of chalone action, *Clin. Proc. CHNMC,* in press.

ATTALLAH, A. M., AND HOUCK, J. C., 1975a, Lymphocyte chalone concentrates and their effects upon leukemic cells *in vitro, Proc. Intr. Symp. Hematology.*

ATTALLAH, A. M., AND HOUCK, J. C., 1975b, *The Lymphocyte Chalone. In Chalones,* Elsevier, Amsterdam, in press.

ATTALLAH, A. M., SUNSHINE, G., HUNT, C. V., AND HOUCK, J. C., 1975, The specific and endogenous mitotic inhibitor of lymphocytes (chalones), *Exp. Cell. Res.,* in press.

BENESTAD, H., RYTÖMAA, T., AND KIVINIEMI, K., 1973, The cell-specific effect of the granulocytic chalone demonstrated with the diffusion chamber technique, *Cell Tissue Kinet.* **6:**147.

BICHEL, P., 1972, Specific growth regulation in three ascitic tumours, *Eur. J. Cancer* **8**:167.

BOYUM, A., 1968, Isolation of mononuclear cells and granulocytes from human blood: Isolation of mononuclear cells by one centrifugation, and of granulocytes by combining centrifugation and sedimentation at 1 G, *Scand. J. Clin. Lab. Invest.* **21**:77 (Suppl. 97).

BULLOUGH, W. S., 1962, The control of mitotic activity in adult mammalian tissues, *Biol. Rev.* **37**:307.

BULLOUGH, W. S., AND DEOL, J. U., 1971, Chalone induced mitotic inhibition in the Hewitt keratinising epidermal carcinoma of the mouse, *Eur. J. Cancer* **7**:425.

BULLOUGH, W. S., AND LAURENCE, E. B., 1960, The control of epidermal mitotic activity in the mouse, *Proc. R. Soc. London Sci. B* **151**:517.

BULLOUGH, W. S., AND LAURENCE, E. B., 1966, Tissue homeostasis in adult mammals in: *Advances in Biology of Skin*, Vol. VII: *Carcinogenesis* (W. Montagna and R. Dobson, eds.), pp. 135–164, Pergamon Press, New York.

BULLOUGH, W. S., AND LAURENCE, E. B., 1968a, Control of mitosis in rabbit V × 2 epidermal tumours by means of the epidermal chalone, *Eur. J. Cancer* **4**:587.

BULLOUGH, W. S., AND LAURENCE, E. B., 1968b, Melanocyte chalone and mitotic control in melanomata, *Nature (London)* **270**:137.

BURGER, M. M., 1971, *Current Topics in Cellular Regulation*, New York, Academic Press, Vol. 3, p. 135.

CHERNOZEMSKI, I. N., 1967, New transplantable hamster tumor: A squamous cell carcinoma of the skin, *J. Natl. Cancer Inst.* **39**:1081.

CHOPRA, D. P., RUERY, J. Y., AND FLAXMAN, B. A., 1972, Demonstration of a tissue-specific inhibitor of mitosis of human epidermal cells *in vitro*, *J. Invest. Dermatol.* **59**:207.

CLARKSON, B. D., 1974, The survival value of the dormant state in neoplastic and normal cell populations, in: *Control of Proliferation in Animal Cells* (B. Clarkson and R. Baserga, eds.), pp. 945–973, Cold Spring Harbor Laboratory, Cold Spring Harbor, N.Y.

DEWEY, D. L., 1973, The melanocyte chalone, *Natl. Cancer Inst. Monogr.* **38**:213.

EAGLE, H., AND LEVINE, E., 1967, Growth regulatory effects of cellular interaction, *Nature (London)* **213**:1102.

EAGLE, H., LEVINE, E., AND KOPROWSKI, H., 1968, Species specificity in growth regulatory effects of cellular interaction, *Nature (London)* **220**:266.

ELGJO, K., AND HENNINGS, H., 1971, Epidermal chalone and cell proliferation in a transplantable squamous cell carinoma in hamsters. I. *In vivo* results, *Virchows Arch. Zellpathol.* **7**:1.

FLORENTIN, I., KIGER, N., AND MATHE, G., 1973, T lymphocyte specificity of a lymphocyte inhibiting factor (chalone) extracted from the thymus, *Eur. J. Immunol.* **3**:135.

GARCIA-GIRALT, E., AND MACIEIRA-COELHO, A., 1974, Differential effect of a lymphoid chalone on the target and non-target cells *in vitro*, in: *Lymphocyte Recognition and Effector Mechanisms* (K. Lindahl-Kiessling and D. Osobu, eds.), pp. 457–474, Academic Press, New York.

GARCIA-GIRALT, E., LASALVIA, E., FLORENTIN, I., AND MATHE, G., 1970, Evidence for a lymphocyte chalone, *Eur. J. Clin. Biol. Res.* **15**:1012.

GARCIA-GIRALT, E., MORALES, H., LASALVIA, E., AND MATHE, G., 1972, Suppression of graft-versus-host reaction by spleen extract, *J. Immunol.* **109**:878.

GORER, P. A., 1960, The isoantigens of malignant cells, in: *Biological Approaches to Cancer Chemotherapy* (R. J. C. Harris, ed.), pp. 219–230, Academic Press, London.

HAKOMORI, S., TEATHER, C., AND ANDREWS, H., 1968, Organizational difference of cell surface "hematoside" in normal and virally transformed cells, *Biochem. Biophys. Res. Commun.* **33**:563.

HAUSCHKA, P. V., EVERHART, L. P., AND RUBIN, R. W., 1972, Alteraction of nucleoside transport of Chinese hamster cells by dibutyryl adenosine 3′-5′-cyclic monphosphate, *Proc. Natl. Acad. Sci. U.S.A.* **69**:3542.

HOLLEY, R. W., AND KIERNAN, J. A., 1968, "Contact-inhibition" of cell division in 3T3 cells, *Proc. Natl. Acad. Sci. U.S.A.* **60**:300.

HOUCK, J. C., AND CHENG, R. F., 1973, Isolation, purification, and chemical characterization of the serum mitogen for diploid human fibroblasts, *J. Cell. Physiol.* **81**:257.

HOUCK, J. C., AND IRASUQUIN, H., 1973, Some properties of the lymphocyte chalone, *Natl. Cancer Inst. Monogr.* **38**:117.

HOUCK, J., IRAUSQUIN, H., AND LEIKIN, S., 1971, Lymphocyte DNA synthesis inhibition, *Science* **173**:1139.

HOUCK, J. C., WEIL, R. L., AND SHARMA, V. K., 1972, Evidence for a fibroblast chalone, *Nature New Biol.* **240**:210.

HOUCK, J. C., CHENG, R. F., AND SHARMA, V. K., 1973a, Control of fibroblast proliferation, *Natl. Cancer Inst. Monogr.* **38**:161.

HOUCK, J. C., ATTALLAH, A. M., AND LILLY, J. R., 1973b, Some immunosuppressive properties of lymphocyte chalone, *Nature (London)* **245:**148.

HOUCK, J. C., SHARMA, V. K., AND CHENG, R. F., 1973c, Fibroblast chalone and serum mitogen (anti-chalone), *Nature New Biol.* **246:**111.

HRYNIUK, W. M., FISCHER, G. A., AND BERTINO, J. R., 1969, S-phase cells of rapidly growing and resting populations: Differences in response to methotrexate, *Mol. Pharmacol.* **5:**557.

INBAR, M., AND SACHS, L., 1969, Structural differences in sites on the surface membrane of normal and transformed cells, *Nature (London)* **223:**710.

IVERSEN, O. H., 1961, The regulation of cell numbers in epidermis, *Acta Pathol. Microbiol. Scand. Suppl.* **148:**91.

IVERSEN, O. H., 1969, Chalones of the skin, in: *Homeostatic Regulators* (E. Wolstenholme and J. Knight,. eds.), pp. 29–56, Churchill, London.

JIMENEZ, A. L., SURIAN, E. S., FLAWIA, N. M., AND TORRES, H. N., 1973, Effect of insulin on the growth pattern and adenylate cyclase activity of BHK Fibroblasts, *PNAS. USA.* **70:**1388.

LAURENCE, E. B., AND ELGJO, K., 1971, Epidermal chalone and cell proliferation in a transplantable squamous cell carcinoma in hamsters. II. *In vitro* results, *Virchows Arch. Zellpathol.* **7:**8.

LAWRENCE, H. S., 1969, Transfer factor, *Adv. Immunol.* **11:**195.

LEVINE, E. M., BECKER, Y., BOONE, C. W., AND EAGLE, H., 1965, Contact inhibition, macromolecular synthesis, and polyribosomes in cultured human diploid fibroblasts, *Proc. Natl. Acad. Sci. U.S A.* **53:**350.

LORD, B., CERCEK, L., CERCEK, B., SHAH, G., DEXTER, T., AND LAJTHA, L., 1974, Inhibitors of hemopoietic cell proliferation? Specificity of action in the hemopoietic system, *Br. J. Cancer* **29:**168.

MARKS, F., 1973, A tissue-specific factor inhibiting DNA synthesis in mouse epidermis, *Natl. Cancer Inst. Monogr.* **38:**79.

MCALLISTER, R. M., GARDNER, M. B., GREENE, A. E., BRADT, C., NICHOLS, W. W., AND LANDING, B. H., 1971, Cultivation *in vitro* of cells derived from a human osteosarcoma, *Cancer* **27:**397.

MINOWADA, J., OHNUMA, Y., AND MOORE, G. E., 1973, Rosette-forming human lymphoid cell lines. I. Establishment and evidence for origin of thymus-derived lymphocytes, *J. Natl. Cancer Inst.* **49:**891.

MOHR, U., ALTHOFF, J., KINZEL, V., SUSS, R., AND VOLM, M., 1968, Melanoma regression induced by chalone: A new tumor-inhibiting principle acting *in vivo, Nature (London)* **220:**138.

MOHR, U., HONDIUS-BOLDINGH, W., AND ALTHOFF, J., 1972, Identification of contaminating clostridium spores as the oncolytic agent in some chalone preparations, *Cancer Res.* **32:**1117.

MOORHEAD, J. F., PARASKOVA-TCHERNOZENSKA, E., PIRRIE, A. J., AND HAYES, C., 1969, Lymphoid inhibitor of human lymphocyte DNA synthesis and mitosis *in vitro, Nature (London)* **224:**1207.

MORLEY, C. G. D., AND KINGDON, H. S., 1972, Use of ^{3}H-thymidine for measurement of DNA synthesis in rat liver—A warning, *Anal. Biochem.* **45:**298.

OSSOWSKI, L., UNKELESS, J., TOBIA, A., QUIGLEY, J. R., RIFKIN, D., AND REICH, E., 1973, An enzymatic function associated with transformation of fibroblasts by oncogenic viruses, *J. Exp. Med.* **137:**112.

PAPAGEORGIOU, P. S., TIBBETS, L., SOROKIN, C. F., AND GLADE, P. R., 1974, Presence of a reversible inhibitor(s) for human lymphoid cell RNA, protein, and DNA synthesis in the extracts of established human cell lines, *Cell. Immunol.* **11:**354.

PATTENGALE, P. K., SMITH, R. W., AND GERBER, P., 1973, Selective transformation of B lymphocytes by EB virus, *Lancet,* July 14, p. 53.

PAUKOVITS, W. R., 1973, Granulopoiesis-inhibiting factor: Demonstration and preliminary chemical and biological characterization of a specific polypeptide (chalone), *Natl. Cancer Inst. Monogr.* **38:**147.

PEAVY, D. L., ADLER, W. H., AND SMITH, R. T., 1970, The mitogenic effects of endotoxin and staphylococcal enterotoxin B on mouse spleen cells and human peripheral lymphocytes, *J. Immunol.* **105:**1453.

PEERY, C. V., JOHNSON, G. S., AND PASTAN, I., 1971, Adenyl cyclase in normal and transformed fibroblasts in tissue culture, *J. Biol. Chem.* **246:**5785.

RAFF, E. C., AND HOUCK, J. C., 1969, Migration and proliferation of diploid human fibroblasts following "wounding" of confluent monolayers, *J. Cell. Physiol.* **74:**235.

ROBISON, G. A., BUTCHER, R. W., AND SUTHERLAND, E. W., 1968, Cyclic AMP, *Ann. Rev. Biochem.* **37:**149.

RYTÖMAA, T., 1973, Chalone of the granulocyte system, *Natl. Cancer Inst. Monogr.* **38:**143.

RYTÖMAA, T., AND KIVINIEMI, K., 1968a, Control of DNA duplication in rat chloroleukemia by means of the granulocytic chalone, *Eur. J. Cancer* **4:**595.

RYTÖMAA, T., AND KIVINIEMI, K., 1968b, Control of granulocyte production. I. Chalone and antichalone, two specific humoral regulators, *Cell Tissue Kinet.* **1:**329.

RYTÖMAA, T., AND KIVINIEMI, K., 1968c, Control of granulocyte production. II. Mode of action of chalone and antichalone, *Cell Tissue Kinet.* **1**:341.

RYTÖMAA, T., AND KIVINIEMI, K., 1969, Chloroma regression induced by the granulocytic chalone, *Nature (London)* **222**:996.

RYTÖMAA, T., AND KIVINIEMI, K., 1970, Regression of generalized leukemia in rat induced by the granulocytic chalone, *Eur. J. Cancer* **6**:401.

SCHAFER, E. A., 1916, *The Endocrine Organs*, Longmans Green, London.

SCHNEBLI, H. P., 1972, A protease-like activity associated with malignant cells, *Schweiz. Med. Wochenschr.* **102**:1194.

SCHNFBLI, H. P., AND BURGER, M. M., 1972, Selective inhibition of growth of transformed cells by protease inhibitors, *Proc. Natl. Acad. Sci. U.S.A.* **69**:3825.

SCHNEIDER, R., AND KOLB, H., 1973, Influence of cyclic AMP on early events of immune induction, *Nature*, **244**:224.

SEIJI, M., NAKANO, H., AKIBA, H., AND KATO, T., 1974, Inhibition of DNA and protein synthesis in melanocytes by a melanoma extract, *J. Invest. Dermatol.* **62**:11.

SHEPPARD, J. R., 1971, Restoration of contact-inhibited growth to transformed cells by dibutyryl adenasine 3′,5′-cyclic monophosphate, *PNAS. USA.* **68**:1316.

SHEPPARD, J. R., 1972, Difference in the cyclic adenosine 3′,5′-monophosphate levels in normal and transformed cells, *Nature New Biol.* **236**:14.

SMITH, J. W., STEINER, A. L., AND PARKER, C. W., 1971, Human lymphocyte metabolism: Effects of cyclic and noncyclic nucleotides on stimulation by phytohemagglutinin, *J. Clin. Invest.* **50**:442.

STOKER, M., 1964, Regulation of growth and orientation in hamster cells transformed by polyoma virus, *Virology* **24**:164.

STOKER, M., AND SHEARER, O. C., 1966, Growth inhibition of polyoma-transformed cells by contact with static normal fibroblasts, *J. Cell Sci.* **1**:297.

TODARO, G. J., LAZAR, G. K., AND GREEN, H., 1965, The initiation of cell division in a contact-inhibited mammalian cell line, *J. Cell. Comp. Physiol.* **66**:325.

TODARO, G. J., MATSUYA, Y., BLOOM, S., ROBBINS, A., AND GREEN, H., 1967, Stimulation of RNA synthesis and cell division in resting cells by a factor present in serum, in: *Growth Regulating Substances for Animal Cells in Culture* (V. Defendi and M. Stoker, eds.), Wistar Institute Symposium, Monograph 7, Wistar Institute Press, Philadelphia.

VAHERI, A., RUOSLAHTI, E., NORDLING, S., 1972, Neurominidase stimulates division and sugar uptake in density-inhibited cell cultures, *Nature New Biol.*, **238**:24.

VESTERBERG, O., AND SVENSSON, H., 1966, Isoelectric fractionation analysis and characterization of ampholytes in natural pH gradients. IV. Further studies on the resolving power in connection with separation of myoglobins, *Acta Chem. Scand.* **20**:820.

VOORHEES, J. J., DUELL, E. A., AND KELSEY, W. H., 1972, Dibutyryl cyclic AMP inhibition of epidermal cell division, *Arch. Dermatol.* **105**:384.

WEISS, P., 1952, Self regulation of organ growth by its own products, *Science* **115**:487.

WEISS, P., AND KAVANAU, J. L., 1957, A model of growth and growth control in mathematical terms, *J. Gen. Physiol.* **41**:1.

WRIGHT, R. K., MANDY, S. H., HALPRIN, K. M., AND HSIA, S. L., 1973, Defects and deficiency of adenyl cyclase in psoriatic skin, *Arch. Dermatol.* **107**:47.

WU, H., MEEZAN, E., BLACK, P. H., AND ROBBINS, P. W., 1968, Comparative studies on the carbohydrate containing membrane components of normal and transformed fibroblasts, *Biochemistry* **8**:2509.

ZACCHELLA, F., BENSON, P. F., AND GIANNELLI, F., *et al.*, 1972, Induction of adenylate cyclase activity in culture human fibroblasts during increasing cell population density, *Biochem. J.* **126**:27.

Extracellular Compartments of Solid Tumors

PIETRO M. GULLINO

1. Introduction

Neoplastic cells can multiply to constitute a solid tumor only when new formation of stroma and vessels occurs and a pericellular environment suitable for cell survival and growth is maintained. Conventionally, the extracellular space of solid tumors is divided into two major compartments, vascular and interstitial. This chapter discusses some physiopathological parameters which characterize both compartments.

2. Tumor Vascular Compartment

2.1. Absence of Vascularization

Greene (1941a,b) was the first to observe that fragments of neoplastic tissues could survive for months in the anterior chamber of the rabbit eye "as a parasitic tissue culture" without visible vascularization. Folkman *et al.* (1962, 1963) repeated Greene's observation in perfused canine thyroids. Mouse melanoma cells implanted in the gland grew rapidly to form nodules, but their size never exceeded a few millimeters in diameter. Folkman hypothesized that absence of

PIETRO M. GULLINO • Laboratory of Pathophysiology, National Cancer Institute, National Institutes of Health, Bethesda, Maryland.

extensive growth was related to a lack of vascularization, since endothelial cells damaged by perfusion were unable to initiate neovascularization. In pursuing this hypothesis, Folkman *et al.* (1971) partially isolated a tumor factor capable of eliciting angiogenesis from the host vascular system. Moreover, Gimbrone *et al.* (1972) developed the concept of tumor dormancy due to a lack of neovascularization. They observed that fragments of Brown–Pearce carcinoma implanted on the iris of susceptible rabbits were rapidly vascularized and grew to destroy the eye within days. In contrast, implants placed in the anterior chamber of the eye, at a maximal distance from the iris, grew into spheroids of a few millimeters in diameter but remained arrested (dormant) for weeks. When, however, these spheroids were transferred onto the iris, vascularization occurred and growth was rapidly resumed. A new concept for solid tumor therapy was based on these observations: specific blockade of tumor-induced angiogenesis may effectively control neoplastic growth (Folkman, 1972).

2.2. Angiogenesis Induced by Preneoplastic Lesions

The hypothesis that neovascularization is a necessary condition for malignant growth of a solid tumor was extended to the study of preneoplastic lesions of the mammary gland by Gimbrone and Gullino (1974). DeOme *et al.* (1959) showed that the aging mammary gland of several strains of mice contained foci of hyperplastic parenchyma. They classified the foci as hyperplastic alveolar nodules (HAN) and showed that they were a tissue with a very high risk of becoming neoplastic (preneoplastic lesions). This risk has been quantitated by Medina (1973), who succeeded in propagating by transplantation into the fat pad two lines of HAN: D-1, with a rate of neoplastic transformation of less than 10%, and D-2, which produced carcinomas in more than 70% of the transplants. When these were tested in the rabbit eye, Gimbrone and Gullino (1974) observed that vascularization of the iris grafts occurred consistently in mammary tumor grafts, rarely in implants of resting mammary gland, and in about 30% of HAN transplants taken at random in aging C3H" females. Specifically, iris grafts on the D-2 line stimulated neovascularization in 80% of the cases, grafts of the D-1 line in only 30%. Thus ability to elicit angiogenesis could be used as a criterion to differentiate the biological characteristics of some mammary tissue before morphological or clinical signs of neoplasia occurred.

2.3. Morphogenesis of the Vascular Network

2.3.1. Vessel Growth

Slit-lamp stereomicroscopy permits the observation of new-formed vessels which originate from the limbal plexus and migrate toward a tumor fragment grafted in the cornea. In this model, one can follow *in vivo*, without manipulations, the morphogenesis of the tumor vascular network. In a Brown–Pearce transplant, new vessels appear within 3–4 days, and the overall growth pattern can be described as a network of sprouts and loops originating from the host vessels closest to the implant. The endothelium proliferates actively and gives rise to buds which grow in length and width; their tips are thought to be solid cords of cells which are secondarily canalized. Where growing sprouts meet, they fuse, giving rise to loops or cross-connections and, ultimately, to intricate networks. The morphogenesis of vessels colonizing the tumor isograft is quite similar to that of the regenerating capillaries as described in the cornea damaged by silver nitrate (Schoefl, 1963). The ultrastructure of capillary sprouts induced by melanomas in the hamster cheek pouch has been described by Warren (1966; Warren *et al.,* 1972). Also, he found a close correlation, at the ultrastructural level, between capillaries elicited by neoplastic tissue and those elicited by inflammatory stimulation. As the original nucleus of neoplastic cells becomes colonized by the new-formed vessels, growth of both cells and vessles proceeds very rapidly.

True capillaries are defined as having a diameter close to that of an erythrocyte (7–10 μm) and have walls constituted by three layers: (1) the endothelium, (2) the basement membrane and pericytes, and (3) the adventitia (Bruns and Palade, 1968). The endothelium may have a "continuous" or a "fenestrated" cytoplasm; the endocytoplasmic vesicles as well as the intercellular junctions play a basic role in attaining physiological permeability (Karnovsky, 1968). Tumor capillaries have not been studied as extensively as normal ones. It is generally accepted that tumor capillaries differ from normal ones in two major features: (1) the diameter of most of them is larger, and (2) the endothelial lining as well as the basement membrane may be irregular, discontinuous, and so markedly attenuated as to make it appear that plasmalemma of adjacent neoplastic cells constitutes the vessel wall. In a transplantable mammary carcinoma, Vogel (1965) classified the tumor vessels which had walls constituted only of endothelial cells as capillaries (less than 12 μm diameter) and sinusoids (greater than 12 μm diameter). The first constituted 12% of vascular volume, the second 32%. The average surface area of capillaries was calculated in 45 mm^2/mm^3 of tissue, the average vessel length in 1700 mm/mm^3. For the sinusoids, the values were 11 mm^2/mm^3 and 50 mm/mm^3, respectively. When surface area, length, and vascular volume were studied per unit weight, Vogel (1965) found that small and large tumors constituted a vascular volume about 16% of tumor size, and this total volume remained rather constant over a tenfold change in tumor weight. However, for tumor weight of 18 mg, vessel length was 820 mm/mm^3 and surface area was 34 mm^2/mm^3; whereas for mean tumor weight of 1853 mg the values were 47 mm/mm^3 and 7 mm^2/mm^3, respectively. Thus morphogenesis of the tumor vascular net comprises not only new formation of capillaries, which occurs mostly along the pattern of physiological angiogenesis, but also modulation of the length, width, and surface area of the new-formed network, which, in turn, depends on at least two other parameters: density and growth of cell population, and thrombosis followed by occlusion of vessels.

329

EXTRA-
CELLULAR
COMPARTMENTS
OF SOLID
TUMORS

2.3.2. Relationship Between Vessels of Host and Tumor

Using a modification of the transparent chamber technique (Sandison, 1924), Merwin and Algire (1956) observed in mice that the original vessels of thyroid tissue isografts survived and provided most of the implant vessels, but that, in mammary carcinoma isografts, only very few of the original vessels survived and that they produced no new sprouts. Thus the survival of the preexisting vascular network is a common event in isografts of normal tissues (Davis and Traut, 1925) but a rare exception in tumor transplants, where neovascularization prevails. The vascular network of the tumor is constituted not only by the new-formed vessels but also by the vessels of the organ in which the tumor is located, because they are incorporated into the growing mass. For instance, if a tumor is transplanted into a rat kidney and a cast of the vascular system is prepared, one can still identify major branches of the renal artery and vein when the tumor has reached 10–15 g in size. The vessels incorporated by the tumor are stretched to supply a mass of tissue ten- to fifteenfold larger than the original kidney (Gullino and Grantham, 1962). To understand the physiological behavior of the tumor network, it is indispensable to remember that this network is constituted by both new-formed and preexisting vessels and that host vessels surviving in the tumor mass usually retain, at least in part, the contractile and nervous apparatuses which make them responsive to physiological stimuli.

2.3.3. Cell Population as Organizer of the Vascular Network

The possibility that the cell of origin of a tumor acts as "organizer" in the morphogenesis of the tumor vascular network was put forward by Wright (1937, 1938). He observed that liver carcinomas, considered to derive from cells of the bile ducts, were vascularized by the hepatic artery, not by the portal system, and that bronchial carcinomas were vascularized by the bronchial and not by the pulmonary artery. Breedis and Young (1954) observed, however, that liver metastases of several types of tumors, naturally occurring or produced by inoculation of cell suspensions, were also prevalently vascularized by the hepatic artery. Moreover, by infusing [46]Sc-tagged ceramic or plastic microspheres, Blanchard et al. (1965) showed that the hepatic artery brought tenfold more radioactivity to liver implants of V × 2 carcinoma than the mesenteric vein. The reasons for a prevalent vascularization by the hepatic artery of liver metastases are not clear at this time. Vessels which can survive the pressure of a growing cell population may be the only ones capable of generating this new network.

Evidence for a regulatory influence of the neoplastic cell population over the volume of vessels formed by the host is only indirect. Carcinomas and sarcomas within a 2–10 g range had a rather constant vascular space over many transplant generations, regardless of the host tissue receiving the transplant. Moreover, when two cell populations with different biological properties were isolated from the same hepatoma, tumors with a different vascular volume were obtained and the difference persisted over subsequent transplant generations (Gullino and Grantham, 1964).

The role of neoplastic cell populations in shaping the architecture of the neoplastic network was studied by Goodall *et al.* (1965). They observed that the cell populations of two melanomas, one breast carcinoma, and a hemangiopericytoma were indeed able to influence density, orientation, and the geometric relationship of new-formed vessels. The study was done using the transparent chamber method as modified by Sanders and Shubik (1964) for the hamster cheek pouch. It may be that the special conditions under which the tumor develops within the chamber have an influence on the final results.

331
EXTRA-
CELLULAR
COMPARTMENTS
OF SOLID
TUMORS

In our experience with the rabbit eye, Brown-Pearce carcinoma has recognizable characteristics in the formation of vascular loops, but not V × 2 carcinoma or heterografts of mouse mammary carcinomas. Moreover, Eddy and Casarett (1973) found in a hamster neurilemmoma studied in the transparent chamber that anastomosing of vascular sprouts occurs randomly, although ultimately a characteristic vascular pattern appears which, at least in part, is shaped by the histological features of the tissue.

Present knowledge suggests that the uniqueness of the tumor vascular pattern in relation to tumor type and architecture is sometimes recognizable, but no generalization can be made. The same forces which shape the histological structure are probably modulating the angiographic pattern (Lewis, 1927; Margulis *et al.*, 1961; Milne *et al.*, 1967).

A change in the standard architecture of the vascular network of an organ invaded by a tumor occurs either by distortion, due to the new-formed mass, or by the overlapping of a new pattern of distribution, or by both. For years, radiologists have exploited this observation for diagnostic purposes, using contrast media to visualize the neoplastic network. Patterns have been described as pathognomonic of certain tumors, but details of those findings are beyond the scope of this chapter.

2.4. Vascular Volume

2.4.1. Measurements

Two methods have been utilized to measure the vascular space of tumors. One is based on a marker mixed in the circulating blood and recovered from the tumor; the second is based on morphometric analyses of tumor serial sections. With the first method, one determines the percentage of tumor weight occupied by the blood present in the vascular system at the time of measurement. Two sources of errors of this procedure are the diffusion of the marker outside the vessels and/or the uneven distribution of the marker because of intermittent function of some section of the network. With the second method, the vascular surface area of fixed tissues is measured and referred to either the total area or the viable portion of the tumor. The inability to detect fully the microvasculature and/or the distortion of vessels due to tissue fixation are the two most serious limitations of this method.

2.4.2. Vascular Space and Surface Area

The vascular space of five transplanted rat hepatocarcinomas was found to be 4.5–12.4% of tumor weight, as compared with 18.6% of the host liver. A

375×10^3 mol wt dextran was used as the marker, and the tumors were measured in a weight range of 1–13 g (Gullino and Grantham, 1964). In mice, the vascular space of transplanted carcinomas of the ovary and mammae was found to be 1.5–4.7% of the tumor weight; ^{32}P-tagged erythrocytes were used as the marker (Storey *et al.*, 1951). The vascular space of Walker 256 carcinoma, a transplantable mammary carcinoma of the rat, was found to be 10.6% of the tumor weight when measured with dextran as the marker (Gullino and Grantham, 1964) and 4.0% of the tumor weight by ^{51}Cr-tagged erythrocytes (Song and Levitt, 1971); we confirmed this finding in our laboratory.

The difference in values may be due, in part, to inherent errors in both methods, as mentioned earlier, in part, to a lower hematocrit in capillaries as contrasted to large vessels, but also to the size of the tumors measured (3.5–13 g in the first, 1.0–4.0 g in the second). Hilmas and Gillette (1974) showed by morphometric analysis that in the microvasculature of a mouse mammary carcinoma vessel diameter widened as the tumor grew. Vogel (1965) made the same observation in another mouse mammary carcinoma; he calculated that the ratio between sinusoidal (greater than 12 μm) and capillary (4–12 μm) vessels was about 0.5 in tumors weighing 0.1 g, but 3.0 for tumors of 2.4 g. DS carcinosarcomas growing from 3.5–11.0 g reduced the size of their vascular bed from 3.3–0.3% of tumor mass (Vaupel, 1974).

The total vascular volume was reported by Vogel (1965) and Hilmas and Gillette (1974) to remain rather steady at 15–18% of viable-tumor volume for carcinomas in a 0.1–2.4 g range. In general, as the tumor increases in size the vascular surface area decreases (Vaupel *et al.*, 1971). This decrease, however, varies extensively from one tumor to another and also within a single tumor, depending on size. Vogel (1965), for instance, observed a fivefold reduction in capillary surface area when mammary carcinomas of 18 mg average weight were compared with 1853-mg tumors. However, the same tumor, in an average weight range of 100–770 mg, had a capillary surface area reduced by only 26%. This reduction in surface area depends mainly on the fact that less of the total vascular volume is constituted by capillaries (less than 12 μm) and more by sinusoidal vessels (greater than 12 μm). The ratio between these two components must be considered when assessing the physiological meaning of tumor vascular space measurements, and, in general, one must remember that the entire vasculature of a growing tumor is subject to continuous change in shape, length, and diameter of each component vessel.

The reduction of vascular surface area as tumor size increases has been attributed by Tannock (1970) to a difference in turnover times between endothelial and neoplastic cells. In a mammary carcinoma of the C3H mouse, he calculated a turnover time for neoplastic cells of about 22 h, but 50–60 h for endothelial cells. Since the mean labeling index of capillary endothelial cells remained constant between 10 and 40 h after a single injection of tritiated thymidine, Tannock concluded that the capillary endothelial cells in the tumor were not derived from a faster-proliferating precursor population and therefore that they lagged behind the increase in the number of neoplastic cells. This interpretation seems to be reinforced by the observation that the turnover time of endothelial cells in new-formed bone capillaries is also 50 h 3 days after a fracture, when the labeling index is high (Tannock and Hayashi, 1972).

333

EXTRA-
CELLULAR
COMPARTMENTS
OF SOLID
TUMORS

2.5. Blood Supply

The expression "blood supply" has mistakenly been applied to describe tumor vascularity. Here it is used to indicate blood flow through the vascular network and the conditions that can modify this flow.

2.5.1. Blood Flow Measurements

If all the blood flowing through the network of an organ is collected in an efferent vein, the simplest way to measure the flow is by cannulating the vein and measuring the efferent blood volume under controlled arterial pressure. A tumor preparation which allows this experimental approach was developed (Gullino and Grantham, 1961a), and the blood flow of five rat hepatomas was found to be 8.2 ml/h/g, on the average, or about one-twentieth that of normal liver (Gullino and Grantham, 1961b).

By direct determination of blood flow using anesthetized, operated-on animals, one cannot distinguish between blood circulating through the vascular network and blood crossing arteriovenous shunts. However, control of direct determinations can be obtained by an indirect method based on the fractional distribution of a labeled compound. A foreign substance, after a single, rapid, intravenous injection, will initially be distributed to the organs in proportion to their blood flow and will then be carried away by the venous discharge. Sapirstein (1958) observed that, for a short period, the amount of substance lost by venous drainage is negligible as compared to that delivered by the artery. Moreover, this period is longest for substances such as ^{42}KCl or ^{86}RbCl, which have a large volume of distribution within the tissue and which diffuse out of the vascular system with little hindrance. Gullino and Grantham (1961b) demonstrated that the observations of Sapirstein (1958) also hold for neoplastic tissue.

An intravenous injection of ^{86}RbCl in the rat foot produced an inflow of radioactivity into the tumor which started about 14 s after the injection, then increased for 20 s, reaching a plateau during the next 20 s. If the animals were killed 40 s after the injection, the label present in the tumor could be considered as representing the fraction of cardiac output reaching the tumor; blood flow could be calculated in unanesthetized animals. Results, with direct and indirect methods, generally indicated that transplanted tumors had a blood supply smaller than that of their tissues of origin (Gullino and Grantham, 1961b; Urbach, 1961; Cataland et al., 1962).

A preparation has been obtained in which the whole efferent blood of a primary mammary tumor was collected by a single vein (Grantham et al., 1973). The blood flow of primary, 7,12-dimethylbenz[α]anthracene-induced mammary carcinomas of rats was measured by the direct method in tumors weighing 2.0–3.5 g and found to be 2–8 ml/h/g (Butler and Gullino, 1974a). Thus primary mammary tumors were shown to have a blood flow of the same order of magnitude as transplanted ones.

In some reports, tumor blood flow was interpreted to be equal to or higher than in the tissue of origin. Bierman *et al.* (1952*a*) observed that in metastatic lesions of 12 patients the oxygen content and saturation level of the venous blood draining the neoplasm were higher than in the host venous blood. They suggested that considerable arteriovenous shunting or lack of oxygen extraction could explain the results, but they concluded that an increased and more rapid blood flow through the tumors was probable. This conclusion was supported by skin calorimetry measurements of melanomas and skin metastases of a variety of human tumors. Persistent increased temperature was found over the neoplastic lesions and interpreted to indicate an elevated blood supply (Bierman *et al.*, 1952*b*). Wollman and Reed (1963) reported a radioiodide clearance from rat thyroid tumors corresponding to a blood flow from 0.08–0.5 ml/g/min. The first value is close to the ones reported (Gullino and Grantham, 1961*b*; Cataland *et al.*, 1962), but the last value is much larger. Before accepting this value, it should be made certain that the vascular network of the host tissue, surviving among the islands of growing tumor, was not the major carrier of the labeled material.

The possible importance of a persistent vascular network from the organ in which the tumor grows is emphasized in studies comparing tumor size and blood flow per unit weight. For instance, Cataland *et al.* (1962) observed a threefold reduction in blood flow (per gram) when a mouse mammary carcinoma increased in size from 0.1–1.0 g, but no significant decrease of flow in tumors growing from 1.0–5.0 g and a small reduction from 5.0–10.0 g. It seems reasonable to consider that the blood flow of 1.0–5.0 g tumors is the actual supply to the tumor and that the sharp initial drop in flow is the consequence of a gradual demolition of the host-tissue network by the spreading tumor. Necrosis is not likely to be a major factor in the initial drop of blood flow; otherwise, one would expect a comparable change between tumors of 1.0 and 10.0 g.

In primary canine lymphosarcomas, regional blood flow determined by the thermal dilution technique (Tuttle and Sadler, 1964) was estimated at about 18 ml/g/min on the outer margin of the tumor mass and 1.2 ml/g/min in the central portions (Straw *et al.*, 1974). This shows a very good irroration of tumor masses where persistence of the primative vascular network of the lymph node is hardly probable. Lymphomas and melanomas may well have a much better supply of blood than carcinomas and fibrosarcomas.

2.5.2. Efficiency of Blood Supply

As a tumor grows larger, the supply of blood per unit weight decreases (Gullino and Grantham, 1961*b*; Cataland *et al.*, 1962; Vogel and Haynes, 1966). Injections of bloodborne substances have shown that some regions of the tumor cannot be reached. This old observation was quantitated by Tannock and Steel (1969), using ^{51}Cr-tagged erythrocytes and transplanted rat mammary carcinoma. In well-perfused areas, only 2% of tumor vessels did not contain labeled cells; in poorly

335

EXTRA-
CELLULAR
COMPARTMENTS
OF SOLID
TUMORS

perfused areas, the opposite was found. An assessment of the perviousness of the network has been made, using intravenous injections of lissamine green. Goldacre and Sylven (1962) described in subcutaneously transplanted tumors of rats and mice an outermost zone uniformly green, followed by a zone, about 150 μm thick, in which only traces of color were visible. Inside this zone was a line of intense green, and, more centrally, there was only unstained or lightly stained tissue which was microscopically necrotic. Goldacre and Sylven (1962) established that the intensely colored line was due to necrobiotic cells accumulating color. With intravenous injections of various colors given at appropriate intervals, they were able to mark the necrobiotic lines as the tumor grew and to follow the progression of necrosis in the center of the tumor. In mammary carcinomas of ABL mice, the necrotic center progressed 1·0–1·5 mm per day.

Many years ago, pathologists described vascular thrombosis in tumors and attributed necrosis to vascular occlusion. It is a fact, however, that in histological sections one can find surprisingly well-preserved capillaries, full of well-preserved erythrocytes, surrounded by necrotic-looking tumor cells. It is difficult to imagine that such vessels had been occluded and that necrosis of surrounding cells occurred by nutrient starvation while both the endothelial lining and the trapped erythrocytes remained intact. This impression has been corroborated by Rubin and Casarett (1966). Tannock and Steel (1969) estimated the relative proportions of viable and necrotic tissue by Chalkley's method (1943) and compared these with the distribution through the tumor of ^{51}Cr-labeled erythrocytes injected intravenously into the host. The ratio of the labeling index of blood in tumor imprints to that in the general circulation plotted against the proportion of viable tissue in corresponding sections gave a series of points close to the 45° line, indicating a similar red cell concentration in viable and necrotic areas. Thus the assessment of blood supply efficiency by morphological determination of the extent of necrosis may be misleading, and the findings of Goldacre and Sylven (1962) support it. They transplanted necrotic areas of mammary carcinomas and sarcoma 37, and they found that in about 50% of the transplants a tumor grew. Evidently a large number of viable cells were present in necrotic-looking regions.

Regurgitation and intermittent circulation (i.e., periods of stasis) followed by resumption of blood flow, sometimes in a direction opposite to the previous one, are probably the "normal" features of the vascular transport system of tumors. The observations with the transparent chamber confirm this hypothesis (Goodall et al., 1965). "Tissue pressure" due to continuous cell proliferation may be of particular importance in producing an intermittent circulation and possibly an overall dampening of the transport efficiency. This problem will be discussed later.

Evidence that arrest of cell division or cell destruction improves vascular transport in tumors was obtained by Reinhold (1971). Microangiograms of tumors grown in a sheetlike fashion with a thickness of about 50 μm were obtained during a course of fractionated radiotherapy with daily fractions of 576 rad. An improvement of the tumor microcirculation was found, most marked at the seventh day of treatment when the tumors had just regressed beyond their initial size. Improved circulation was obtained also with chemotherapy. Vogel and Haynes (1966) observed that 100-mg mammary carcinomas of mice were perfused 700 times their own weight in blood per day, but that thiotepa-treated (6 days) tumors which were 100 mg at the time of measurements were perfused with blood equivalent to 1200 times their weight per day. Butler and Gullino (1974a) observed also that MTW-9 mammary carcinomas of rats increased their blood flow per gram by 25–30% when they regressed to about half their initial size following a sharp reduction of the mammotropin level in the blood.

2.5.3. Regulation of Circulation

Control of tumor flow concerns vessels of the host tissue incorporated and distorted by the invading tumor, as well as newly formed vessels derived from the host network under the effect of an angiogenesis factor(s) produced by the neoplastic cell population. In preparations where all of the tumor blood was collected by a single vein, the vessel was cannulated and blood outflow was measured before and after vasoactive drugs were injected into the host. In four hepatomas, one lymphosarcoma, and a mammary carcinoma of the rat, the flow of tumor efferent blood was decreased by epinephrine, by a reduction in tumor temperature, and by removal of the celiac ganglion; in contrast, acetyl-β-methylcholine increased the outflow. These data were interpreted as showing that the network of the tumors responded to vasoactive drugs, just as did the ovarian vessels which supplied the tumor preparation (Gullino and Grantham, 1961a, 1962). With the transparent chamber technique, Algire and Legallais (1951) also observed in mouse sarcomas and mammary carcinomas a decrease of capillary circulation when hypotension was produced in the host. Moreover, they used several hypotensive preparations in an effort to produce irreversible ischemic damage to the tumor vasculature (Algire et al., 1952, 1954).

Several reports, however, suggest that regulation of blood supply to neoplastic tissues may be different from that of the host tissue invaded by the tumor. Using skin calorimetry, Natadze (1959) observed that, in mouse mammary carcinomas, local application of epinephrine, histamine, or acetylcholine did not change the calorimetric readings of the tumor, but that epinephrine decreased, and the other drugs increased, the temperature of the adjacent normal skin. Natadze (1959) concluded that tumor vasculature did not respond to the vasoactive drugs, and he suggested that persistent, marked dilation of tumor efferent vessels probably caused the abnormal behavior. Another explanation is possible—for calorimetric measurements, the tumor is a system with large capacitance since blood is mostly contained in dilated, capillarylike vessels which empty slowly.

Edlich et al. (1966) reported a very large blood flow (0·68 ml/min/g) in an amelanotic melanoma of the hamster, corresponding to about tenfold the flow of underlying muscle and fivefold that of the surrounding skin. Tissue blood flow was estimated by [^{131}I]antipyrine distribution. Infusion of small doses of epinephrine increased the muscle flow by 186% but decreased tumor flow by 87%. Infusion with low doses of catecholamine, which did not produce significant effects in muscle or skin, reduced the mean tumor flow by 84%.

Altered drug response of tumor vessels has been described in a variety of
neoplasms studied with angiographic techniques (Abrams, 1964; Kahn, 1965;
Rockoff *et al.*, 1966). Results varied, depending on the tumor, from a lack of
response to partial or physiological response to excessive response. Control of
circulation in tumors is an open question, at present.

337

EXTRA-
CELLULAR
COMPARTMENTS
OF SOLID
TUMORS

3. Tumor Interstitial Compartment

3.1. Collagen Content

Collagen is usually measured by tissue content of hydroxyproline, since it is
generally accepted that this amino acid occurs almost exclusively in the scleropro-
teins of the connective tissue (Tristram, 1953). In a series of rat and mouse
hepatomas produced with a variety of carcinogens, Gullino *et al.* (1962) observed
that the production of collagen was greater in tumors than in the liver of origin
(Table 1) and that the greatest difference was about sixfold when expressed per
milligram of nitrogen or about tenfold per microgram of DNA. For each tumor,
collagen production remained constant over many transplant generations,
regardless of the transplant site. In eight of nine rat hepatomas, collagen content
increased proportionally with tumor growth from about 2–10 g size. Only in
hepatoma 5123 was the increase of neoplastic tissue faster than that of collagen.
Hepatoma 5123 reflects the conditions of the regenerating liver. At 14 days after
hepatectomy, the wet weight of the liver is almost equal to the original weight, but
the collagen content is only about two-thirds (Table 1).

In subcutaneous implants of Guerin rat carcinoma, Grabowska (1959)
described a rapid reduction of collagen content as the tumor grew to 1.5 g in size,
but a constant content for tumors between 1.5 and 30 g. Since the collagen of the
subcutaneous area in very small tumors becomes incorporated among the islands
of growing cells, the initial reduction can be explained by a destruction of the
host-tissue collagen by the growing neoplastic cells. Therefore, Grabowska's data
also indicate that collagen content of Guerin carcinoma was constant within a
2–30 g range of tumor sizes as found in hepatomas. The collagen content of
sarcomas followed the same general pattern as found in carcinomas. No appreciable "accumulation" of collagen was observed during tumor growth (Grabowska,
1959; Gullino and Grantham, 1963).

3.2. Influence of Host and Neoplastic Cell Population on Collagen Production

Tumor collagen is produced by the host, but the rate of synthesis is regulated by
the neoplastic cell population (Gullino and Grantham, 1963). A demonstration
that the host was the source of tumor collagen was obtained by separating
neoplastic cells of Novikoff hepatoma from fibroblasts. First, a partial separation
was obtained by spinning dissociated tissue in solutions of polyvinylpyrrolidone-
sucrose (Greenfield and Whitaker, 1961). The fraction enriched with epithelial

TABLE 1

Collagen Content of Hepatocarcinomas and Liver[a]

Strain/sex	Tissue denomination	Weight (g)	Hydroxyproline (μg/mg N)	Collagen (mg/100 mg protein)
Hepatocarcinomas[b]				
Rat lines				
Sprague-Dawley ♂	Novikoff	4.1 ± 14.6	10.9 ± 0.8[c]	1.30
Fisher 344 ♀	LC 18	2.9 ± 6.2	10.9 ± 0.5	1.30
A × C ♀	3683	3.3 ± 9.0	17.4 ± 0.6	2.06
A × C ♀	3924A	2.2 ± 7.4	30.5 ± 1.8	3.69
Buffalo ♂	T3-2	4.2 ± 11.1	32.4 ± 1.2	3.82
OM ♂	HC	4.0 ± 7.8	42.6 ± 2.0	5.04
OM ♀	LC	3.9 ± 6.6	20.9 ± 1.3	2.46
OM ♀	3	3.5 ± 7.8	28.1 ± 2.0	4.34
Buffalo ♂	5123	3.4 ± 9.6	36.6 ± 2.0	4.34
Mouse lines				
C3H ♂	129 solid	0.75 ± 3.6	8.9 ± 0.5	1.06
C3H ♂	129 ascites	0.40 ± 1.4	19.7 ± 1.3	2.30
C3H ♀	134 solid	0.60 ± 2.1	18.2 ± 1.1	2.16
C3H ♀	134 ascites	0.60 ± 1.5	17.3 ± 0.8	2.05
Normal Liver				
Rat lines				
Sprague-Dawley ♂	Normal	190–210[d]	8.6 ± 0.4	1.02
Fisher 344 ♀	Normal	130–145	9.0 ± 0.2	1.06
A × C ♀	Normal	180–200	8.5 ± 0.1	1.01
Buffalo ♂	Normal	190–210	5.9 ± 0.2	0.68
Sprague-Dawley ♂	14 days regenerating	190–210	5.3 ± 0.3	0.63
Buffalo ♂	14 days regenerating	190–210	3.4 ± 0.2	0.39

[a] From Gullino and Grantham (1962).
[b] Additional information in *J. Natl. Cancer Inst.* 27:679, 1961.
[c] ± SD.
[d] Host weight.

cells was then transferred into a Millipore chamber placed in the abdominal cavity of Sprague-Dawley rats (Shelton and Rice, 1958). After about 20 days, the chamber was filled, in part by a fluid rich in floating neoplastic cells and in part by a jelly tissue adherent to the filter and containing mainly fibroblasts and collagen fibers. When only the fluid was transferred into a new chamber, a neoplastic cell population grew with a hydroxyproline content smaller than that of the previous generation. After six to ten passages, hydroxyproline became undetectable in some chambers and no collagen was visible on the filter; but the chamber's fluid was rich in neoplastic epithelial cells. These cells, free of fibroblasts, were transplanted in syngeneic rats and solid tumors were produced, either subcutaneously or in tissue-isolated preparations. The collagen content of these tumors was about 10 μg of hydroxyproline per milligram of nitrogen, just as for the standard transplants of Novikoff hepatoma (Table 1) in which neoplastic cells and fibroblasts were mixed. Thus the fibroblasts carried with the transplant could be eliminated without changing the collagen content of the grown tumor. Results obtained with Novikoff hepatoma transplanted into Sprague-Dawley rats were reproduced in hepatomas 129 and 134 transplanted into C3H mice (Gullino and Grantham, 1963), suggesting that collagen production by the host is a general event in solid tumors.

339
EXTRA-
CELLULAR
COMPARTMENTS
OF SOLID
TUMORS

The ability of the neoplastic cell population to control the collagen content of the tumor was studied in hepatoma 129 of C3H mice (Gullino and Grantham, 1963). This tumor had been carried for several years in two forms, solid and ascites. The two sublines have a different cell population, as shown by the DNA content per nucleus, which in the solid line is about twice that of the ascites line. Solid tumors obtained by transplanting ascites cells were found to contain 20 μg of hydroxyproline per milligram of nitrogen. However, within six subsequent transplant generations as solid tumors the hydroxyproline content gradually dropped to 9 μg per milligram of nitrogen, which is the content consistently found in the tumors carried as solid lines. Fragments of the solid tumors obtained from the ascites cells after six transplant generations were retransplanted intraperitoneally, and the ascites form of hepatoma 129 was again obtained after ten transplant generations. The ascites cells of this generation were then able to produce solid tumors with about 20 μg of hydroxyproline per milligram of nitrogen. Thus, as the relative composition of the hepatoma 129 cell population was modulated by the influence of transplantation sites, the collagen production evoked from the host by the changing population also changed. The same conclusion was reached using a rat tumor. Rechcigl and Sidransky (1962) isolated from an ethionine-induced hepatoma two cell populations characterized by catalase activities of 183 units (HC) and 21 units (LC), respectively. Tumors of the HC line invariably contained about twice as much collagen as the LC line (Table 1), and the difference persisted in subsequent transplant generations—another example of modulation of collagen content by a changing cell population.

Indirect proof that the neoplastic cell population, and not the host, controls the rate of collagen production by solid tumors was obtained in transplants of Novikoff hepatomas and osteogenic sarcomas in various strains of cortisonized rats. In all transplants which grew to 2 g or more in size, the collagen content of the Novikoff hepatoma was similar to that of the strain of origin. Thus, despite the change of host, collagen production evoked by a stable cell population remained constant (Gullino and Grantham, 1963).

3.3. Collagen During Oncogenesis

The hydroxyproline content of mouse skin treated for more than 20 wk with 20-methylcholanthrene in acetone was studied by Van den Hooff (1962). There was a steep rise from 0 to 2 wk, followed by a decrease to subnormal values from 2 to 10 wk, and a second rise from 10 to 15 wk; at that time, the carcinoma appeared. A most complete histological study of dermal changes in the course of skin carcinogenesis by 20-methylcholanthrene dissolved in acetone was conducted by Orr (1938). Only during the third week of treatment did he observe the first changes: collagen fibers became finer and lost their refractility. The alterations became progressively more marked, but the thickness of the involved dermis was variable. After warts appeared (10–16 wk), an increase in the dermis thickness was sometimes observed, which coincides with the rise of hydroxyproline content found by Van den Hooff (1962). Vasiliev (1959) listed four characteristic alterations of the connective tissue during skin carcinogenesis produced by a paraffin pellet containing the carcinogen: (1) long-lasting lymphoid infiltration, (2) inhibition of fibroblast differentiation, (3) accumulation of lipids in the cytoplasm of connective tissue cells, and (4) altered fibrogenesis around the pellet. Studies on collagen behavior during carcinogenesis have been primarily descriptive (Orr, 1940; Maltoni and Prodi, 1960) and are only indirectly related to the objectives of this chapter.

3.4. Tumor Interstitial Fluid

3.4.1. TIF Sampling

In the tissue space limited by the endothelial wall of capillaries and the plasma membrane of neoplastic cells, there is a fluid phase which is usually designated as tumor interstitial fluid (TIF). Two procedures for sampling TIF are available. One is based on visualization by dissection of the exterior tumor surface, the production of small pouches on it by blunt instruments, and sampling by capillaries of fluid accumulating in these pouches (Sylven and Bois, 1960). The second procedure is based on a 13-mm chamber with walls constituted by Millipore filters of 0.45 μm pore diameter. The chamber is placed in a pouch of the subcutaneous tissue with a few fragments of a transplantable tumor, and within a few days a neoplasm grows to incorporate the chamber. Neoplastic cells grow against the filters but do not pass through the pores. In contrast, the fluid surrounding the neoplastic cells does enter the chamber cavity and can be sampled (Gullino et al., 1964).

The major objection to the first procedure is the damage produced by the dissection and formation of pouches. Cells are, no doubt, destroyed by the procedure; and the fluid collected in the pouches is a mixture of cellular sap and pericellular fluid. The major objection to the second procedure is the lack of knowledge of the possible influence of the chamber on the tumor cell population and on the "selective" effect of the filter. Three arguments sustain the supposition that the objections do not invalidate the latter method: (1) The pore size of the filters is huge as compared with the molecules present in TIF. (2) Samples collected inside and outside a chamber immersed in plasma have identical compositions. (3) When two chambers are placed close to each other in a subcutaneous pouch or a tumor, proteins with enzymatic activity placed in one chamber are retrieved in the adjacent one. Thus enzymes when present in TIF can be sampled by the chamber (Gullino and Lanzerotti, 1972).

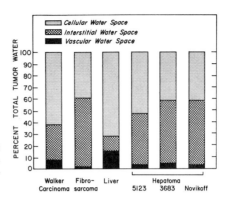

341

EXTRA-
CELLULAR
COMPARTMENTS
OF SOLID
TUMORS

FIGURE 1. Relative proportion of water spaces in neoplastic tissues. Note the sharp difference in vascular and interstitial water spaces between normal liver and hepatocarcinomas.

3.4.2. TIF Volume

The volume of the interstitial space relative to that occupied by the vascular and cell compartments was estimated by subtracting the vascular from the extracellular water space (Gullino *et al.*, 1965*a*). ^{24}NaCl, Na^{36}Cl, and D-[1-^{14}C]mannitol were used as markers of the extracellular space, and dextran 500 as a marker of the vascular space. Figure 1 reports the relative proportions of cellular, interstitial, and vascular spaces referred to total tumor water, since this is the common solvent in which the markers distribute themselves. The interstitial water space of all tumors studied was very large, between 30 and 60% of the tumor water, depending on tumor type. Hepatomas, in particular, had an interstitial water space 3–4 times larger than that in the liver of the host. Using an *in vitro* approach, Humphrey (1961) also reported that hepatomas had serum albumin and inulin spaces larger than those in the liver. The implications of these structural characteristics are not fully understood and have thus far been little studied.

3.4.3. TIF Composition

Cell necrosis is a common event in any solid tumor, and it is generally accepted that dead cells are digested in the interstitial spaces where macrophages and lytic enzymes operate. This concept is based primarily on morphological evidence. Cell dissolution suggests a "spilling over" of cell components into the pericellular environment, despite the fact that survival and growth of a cell population require a physiological stability of the interstitial compartment. Investigators have reported data both in favour of and against these propositions.

A relative "isolation" of necrotic areas from the surrounding tissue has been shown by Goldacre and Sylven (1962), using dye diffusion tests. In mammary tumors regressing after hormonal deprivation of the host, Kerr *et al.* (1972) observed that cell fragments had well-preserved outer membranes. Sylven and Niemi (1972) have described autolytic vacuoles, as revealed by a naphthylamidase reaction at pH 5.5, in neoplastic cells undergoing destruction but with their plasma membrane still unbroken. Increased activity of six lysosomal enzymes during mammary tumor regression has been reported by Lanzerotti and Gullino (1972). The increase was localized in the cells, however; and no activity was found in the pericellular fluid, either before or during regression (Gullino and Lanzerotti, 1972).

Contrary to these observations, which indicate that cell destruction is a rather "localized" process, other studies suggest that profound changes are produced in the pericellular fluid by necrosis of neoplastic cells. Sylven and Bois-Svensson (1965) and Sylven (1968), using their capillary-sampling procedure, described high levels of proteolytic and lysosomal enzyme activities in TIF, particularly in necrotic areas. "Leakage" of enzymes from neoplastic cells has been described on several occasions (Poole and Williams, 1967; Bosmann, 1969); and tumor invasion has been attributed to the ability to "digest" the stroma (Simpson, 1954). The validity of results in this area is still very much dependent on the sampling procedure, in particular on the ability to sample TIF without damaging cells.

From data obtained with tumor-isolated preparations (Gullino and Grantham, 1961a) and the micropore chamber sampling procedure (Gullino et al., 1964), a diagram emphasizing differences between vascular and interstitial compartments of Walker 256 mammary carcinoma is presented in Fig. 2.

A micropore chamber incorporated within a tumor (Gullino et al., 1964) drains a yellow serumlike fluid which becomes hemorrhagic as the tumor size increases. The density of this fluid was 1014 vs. 1019 for aortic serum of the same animal, or 1017 for ascites fluid, or 1014 for fluid draining from a subcutaneously implanted chamber free of tumor.

The gross composition of TIF (not hemorrhagic) was found to be rather constant. The major differences between TIF and aortic plasma were evident in

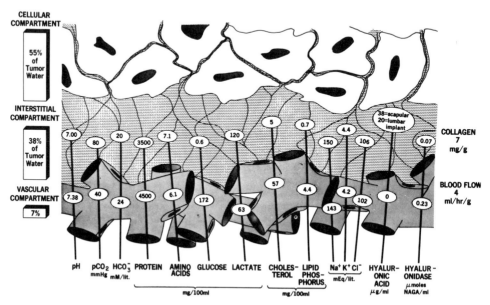

FIGURE 2. Schematic presentation of vascular, interstitial, and cellular compartments of Walker 256 mammary carcinoma. The three blocks on the left represent the total size of each compartment. Constituents of serum and interstitial fluid are listed at the bottom. Each vertical line connects two numbers, one superimposed on the vascular compartment and the other on the interstitial compartment to represent the quantities of these constituents. On the right, collagen content of the interstitial compartment and average blood flow of the vascular compartment are given.

glucose, lactate, cholesterol, and lipid phosphorus content. Also, protein concentration was lower; and free amino acid levels were higher in TIF than in aortic plasma (Fig. 2).

343

EXTRA-
CELLULAR
COMPARTMENTS
OF SOLID
TUMORS

Of particular importance is the relationship between hyaluronic acid and hyaluronidase in TIF, since glucosaminoglycans have a fundamental role in the diffusion of molecules between vascular and interstitial compartments. Using the micropore sampling technique, Fiszer-Szafarz and Gullino (1970a) observed that hyaluronic acid content of subcutaneous interstitial fluid was 53.5 μg/ml in the scapular region, but only 37.2 μg/ml in the lumbar region. When Walker carcinoma was implanted, hyaluronic acid concentration of the interstitial fluid reached the level characteristic for this tumor (20 μg/ml), and remained constant regardless of the implant site. Moreover, the presence of the tumor was sufficient to induce a decrease of about 25% in the hyaluronic acid concentration of subcutaneous areas distant from the tumor. One reason for the low concentration of hyaluronic acid in the tumor may have been the increase of TIF hyaluronidase activity, which was 57% higher than that of subcutaneous interstitial fluid (Fiszer-Szafarz and Gullino, 1970b). The possibility that high hyaluronidase activity in TIF makes the tumor a source of polysaccharide fragments, which continuously drain into the general circulation, should be studied, especially in relation to the immunological status of the host.

3.4.4. Acid–Base Status

Regardless of necrosis, the metabolic characteristics of neoplastic tissue, i.e., glycolysis, have peculiar effects on interstitial fluid physiology. The acidosis of TIF compared with plasma was on the order of 0.3 pH unit (Gullino $et\ al.$, 1965b): H$^+$ concentration of the fluid surrounding the neoplastic cells of a solid tumor $in\ vivo$ was about twice that of arterial plasma, the CO_2 tension of TIF doubled that of arterial plasma, while the level of bicarbonate ions was about 20% lower (Table 2). The relatively large concentration of lactic acid in TIF suggested to Gullino $et\ al.$ (1965b) an effective way of augmenting further the difference in H$^+$ concentration between tumor and host tissues. Addition of sodium bicarbonate (0·1%) to the drinking water of tumor-bearing rats increased, within 3–4 days, the difference in pH between TIF and afferent blood to about 0.6 pH unit, while the pCO$_2$ tension in TIF reached the enormous value of 120–130 mm Hg, close to threefold that of tumor blood. Exploitation of this observation for chemotherapeutic purposes could be rewarding.

4. Efficiency of Exchange Between Cellular and Extracellular Compartments of Tumors

4.1. Lymphatic Drainage

In normal organs, the physiological behavior of the microvascular system is based on two properties of the vessel wall, permeability and resistance. Permeability involves transcellular passage of respiratory gases and lipid-soluble molecules by

TABLE 2

pH and CO$_2$ Partition in Tumor Interstitial Fluid (TIF) and Plasma of Tumor Afferent Blood (PAB)[a]

Tumor[b]	pH		pCO$_2$ (mm Hg)		Dissolved CO$_2$ (mM)		Bicarbonate ion (mM)	
	TIF	PAB	TIF	PAB	TIF	PAB	TIF	PAB
Novikoff	6.95 ± 0.17[c]	7.38 ± 0.09	80 ± 10	43 ± 3	2.5 ± 0.2	1.4 ± 0.1	18.6 ± 4.1	24.7 ± 2.0
Hepatoma 3683	7.00 ± 2.14	7.36 ± 0.05	84 ± 7	48 ± 2	2.6 ± 0.3	1.4 ± 0.2	20.8 ± 3.4	24.7 ± 2.1
Hepatoma 5123	7.19 ± 0.08	7.42 ± 0.06	59 ± 3	43 ± 2	2.0 ± 0.2	1.6 ± 0.2	24.3 ± 3.6	26.2 ± 1.0
Walker 256 carcinoma	7.00 ± 0.14	7.39 ± 0.09	79 ± 6	40 ± 4	2.4 ± 0.4	1.2 ± 0.2	19.3 ± 4.3	23.3 ± 3.0
Fibrosarcoma 4956	7.09 ± 0.12	7.41 ± 0.03	71 ± 5	45 ± 3	2.1 ± 0.31	1.3 ± 0.1	20.9 ± 3.4	25.4 ± 2.2

[a] From Gullino *et al.* (1965b).
[b] Weight range of 10–20 g.
[c] ± SD.

diffusion, active permeation of large molecules by pinocytosis, or intercellular transfer along pores or slits of the endothelial layer. Resistance of the capillary wall is guaranteed by the basement membrane and the "compactness" of the endothelial layer (cell junctions) (Bruns and Palade, 1968). Maintenance of the fluid balance in the tissue spaces is based on hydrostatic and colloido-osmotic pressures operating on a vascular network with uneven permeability and with asymmetry of the exchange area, since the venous site of the capillary bed is usually larger than the arterial counterpart (Hammersen, 1970). In such a system, lymph drainage is a factor of primary importance in maintaining fluid balance (Hauck, 1971).

345
EXTRA-
CELLULAR
COMPARTMENTS
OF SOLID
TUMORS

Microcirculation of the solid tumor occurs in new-formed vessels, often with a "stretched" endothelial lining and a rudimentary or absent basement membrane. Consequently, diapedesis of erythrocytes and deposition of fibrin on and around the vessels are frequently observed in a variety of tumors (Day *et al.*, 1959*a,b*). A lymphatic system as an anatomical entity is not demonstrable in tumors, and Evans' (1908) description of lymphatic vessels in an intestinal tumor remains an exceptional finding. However, convective currents within the tumor mass have been predicted by Swabb *et al.* (1974) in a study on the relationship between solute diffusive and convective fluxes in the extravascular spaces of hepatomas. Reinhold (1971) also measured the speed of extravascular transfer of pyranin in a C3HBA mammary carcinoma. Values up to 25 μ/s were determined, higher than expected for simple diffusion. Moreover, Butler and Gullino (1974*a*) were able to measure, in mammary carcinomas, a reduction of efferent vs. afferent fluid of 0.2 ml/h/g, corresponding to about 5% of the blood supply. This fluid, which failed to leave the tumor via the efferent vein, was probably oozing out at the tumor surface. Suggestive of this possibility is the common finding of accumulation of dye and intense edema of the subcutaneous tissue surrounding large tumors (Underwood and Carr, 1972).

The existence of convective currents within the tumor could be favored by the relatively low hyaluronic acid content of tumor interstitial fluid. Tissue glucosaminoglycans concentration and solute molecular weight are known to be the two most important parameters which determine whether extravascular transport of solutes occurs predominantly by diffusion or convection.

Hyaluronic acid content of Walker carcinoma interstitial fluid has been found to be 20.1 μg/ml, as compared with 36.6 μg/ml for the subcutaneous tissue where the tumor grew (Fiszer-Szafarz and Gullino, 1970*a*). Hexosamine content of Ehrlich and Krebs carcinomas was about 0.27 mg/g (Brada, 1965) as compared with 1.44 mg/g of subcutaneous tissue in which they were transplanted (Pearce, 1965).

The interstitial fluid "tension" within the solid tumor is another parameter to be considered in assessing the existence of convective currents which may be equated with lymphatic drainage. If a micropore chamber is embedded in the subcutaneous tissue, interstitial fluid starts draining out within 24 h and can be stopped with a pressure of 7–9 mm Hg. If the micropore chamber drains tumor interstitial fluid, pressures up to 16 mm Hg may be necessary to stop drainage (Gullino *et al.*,

1964). The volume of interstitial fluid draining out of identical micropore chambers is about threefold larger in tumors than in the subcutaneous-embedded chamber (Butler and Gullino, 1974a). Thus indications of an increased hydraulic pressure within the tumor are available, but its role in the exchange between vascular and cellular compartments is still obscure.

4.2. Oxygen Supply and Utilization

After Warburg described the high aerobic glycolysis of tumors (formation of lactic acid from glucose in the presence of oxygen), attention was mainly focused on the relationship between neoplastic transformation and the biochemical conditions responsible for the reduced capacity of neoplastic cells to utilize oxygen *in vitro* (review in Aisenberg, 1961). Later, biochemists became convinced that aerobic glycolysis did not necessarily mean "damaged respiration" but could depend on a peculiar glucose metabolism of the cell as it became neoplastic (Weinhouse, 1956). Only later was the utilization of oxygen *in vivo* measured in tumors which were studied *in toto* as isolated organs (Gullino *et al.*, 1967a).

Rat carcinomas and sarcomas were able to remove about 50% of the oxygen carried by the afferent blood. When more oxygen was supplied, the oxygen removal ratio remained about 50%, and total oxygen consumption increased. Walker 256 mammary carcinoma, 5123 hepatoma, and 4956 fibrosarcoma consumed 3.3, 5.3, and 1.0 μl O_2/h/mg dry weight. These Q_{O_2} values are similar to those found *in vitro* with slices of the same tumors (Dickens, 1936; Aisenberg and Morris, 1963), although the comparison has probably little meaning, since Q_{O_2} *in vitro* is very dependent on the medium in which the tissues are assayed. The respiratory quotients (CO_2 of venous blood minus CO_2 of arterial blood divided by O_2 consumed per hour) for the three tumors were 1.25, 1.0, and 0.76, respectively. This difference suggests that the relative proportions of various metabolic fuels utilized differed for each tumor type.

Experiments probing the relationship between oxygen supply and utilization by the tumor *in vivo* revealed that reduction of available oxygen, obtained by either anemia or hypooxygenation, induced a parallel reduction in consumption. The oxygen removal capacity of the tumor increased in most cases, but the blood supply did not; therefore, net utilization decreased (Gullino *et al.*, 1967a; Vaupel, 1974).

Lack of oxygen has been considered a major cause of neoplastic cell necrosis. Thomlinson and Gray (1955) first called attention to the pattern of necrosis in squamous carcinomas of the lung, especially of bronchial origin. They observed that, in general, there was no central necrosis in tumor cords less than 160 μm in radius and that there was no tumor cord more than 200 μm in radius without central necrosis. Moreover, regardless of the radius of the necrotic center, the thickness of the surrounding sheath of tumor cells never exceeded 180 μm; i.e., no apparently intact tumor cell was seen more than 180 μm from the stroma. A value of 145 μm was calculated as an approximate estimate of the oxygen gradients to be expected within the tumor cords when the partial pressure of oxygen at the surface is 40 mm Hg. Thomlinson and Gray (1955) concluded that necrosis within a cord was consistent with a limitation of oxygen diffusion. Goldacre and Sylven (1962) estimated a similar value for the oxygen diffusion length (150 μm) by assessing diffusion of a dye into the necrotic centers of a variety of tumors. A third and similar estimate was made by Rajewsky (1965), who demonstrated that the depth of the *in vitro* labeling of tumors with [³H]thymidine depended on the oxygen tension of the medium. Similarity of estimates, however, does not demonstrate that a lack of oxygen is the cause of necrosis. Lack of other metabolites or accumulation of catabolites may, for instance, be more pertinent. Tannock (1968) utilized the techniques of thymidine autoradiography to study cell proliferation in a mouse mammary tumor in which viable tissue was arranged cylindrically around tumor blood vessels. He concluded that the growth fraction was reduced as cells moved away from the central vessel. Moreover, estimates of oxygen and glucose diffusion lengths, as well as concentrations of lactate and carbon dioxide in tumor cords, convinced him that necrosis in this tumor could also be explained by limited oxygen diffusion. Tannock (1968) substantiated his hypothesis by observing that tumor growth was reduced in hypoxic animals. One must, however, remember that animals kept under hypoxia reduce their growth rate and are generally in poor health. Since Warburg *et al.* (1927) observed tumor damage in hypoxic animals, the experiment on tumor growth control by oxygen deprivation of the host has been repeated often. The results have been variable and sometimes difficult to interpret (Campbell and Cramer, 1928; Pollock *et al.*, 1942; Barach and Bickerman, 1954).

The data available on catabolite concentration distribution within neoplastic tissues do not permit, at this time, a quantitative evaluation of the role which such an event may have in tumor necrosis.

Availability of oxygen to neoplastic tissue has another important aspect. Radiosensitivity of clonogenic cells depends on the concentration of oxygen around these cells at the time of irradiation (Thomlinson, 1973). Radiologists have long been concerned about the "anoxic" cells which are able to resist the damaging effects of radiation. However, an assessment of the length of time neoplastic cells can survive with a deficiency or absence of oxygen, regardless of radiation damages, is impossible to make. Two observations point to an exceptional "resistance." Goldacre and Sylven (1962) obtained 56% "takes" when transplanting necrotic areas of carcinomas and sarcomas. Gullino (1968) perfused Walker 256 mammary carcinomas for more than 50 h with perfusates carrying only 10% of the oxygen normally consumed by the tumor *in vivo*. When fragments of the perfused tumor were transplanted subcutaneously, they grew as well as normal transplants.

4.3. Glucose Consumption and Lactate Production

Glucose utilization by tumors *in vivo* may be a useful method for assessing one aspect of metabolite exchange between cellular and extracellular compartments

347

EXTRA-
CELLULAR
COMPARTMENTS
OF SOLID
TUMORS

of tumors. Walker 256 mammary carcinoma, 5123 hepatoma, and 4956 fibrosarcoma, transplanted into rats, utilized 0.95, 0.55, and 0.45 g of glucose/h/100 g wet tumor weight, respectively (Gullino *et al.*, 1967*b*). These results corresponded to 28%, 23%, and 32% of the glucose supplied by blood and represent a large consumption. By comparison, the brain, one of the organs with the highest glucose utilization, consumes 0.2–0.6 g/h/100 g (Scheinberg and Stead, 1949). Glucose consumption in tumors is directly dependent on the blood concentration. Neoplastic tissue is unable to increase the glucose removal rate and maintain during hypoglycemia the same consumption as in normoglycemia. Support for these statements derives from experiments in which blood flow and arterial–venous difference in glucose content of tumor blood were measured in Walker 256 mammary carcinomas, 5123 hepatomas, and 4956 fibrosarcomas (Gullino *et al.*, 1967*b*). Hyperglycemia of 300 mg/100 ml serum produced a burst of glucose consumption by the neoplastic cell population. A threefold increment over normal uptake was observed within the first hour; then a "saturation level" was reached within the next few hours. At this level, carcinomas utilized about 30% more glucose than under normoglycemic conditions, but sarcomas reduced utilization by about 30%. Hypoglycemia of 50 g/100 ml serum reduced glucose consumption to about one-half that of normoglycemia in carcinomas and sarcomas. Thus, under hypoglycemic conditions, the tumor adapts itself to a lower utilization of glucose which can last for days, but, under hyperglycemia, glucose consumption increases to a plateau which depends on the type of neoplastic cell population.

Unexpected findings were obtained when the relationship between vascular and extravascular concentration of glucose was studied. Under normoglycemic conditions, the interstitial fluid of tumors, sampled by the micropore chamber procedure, had a negligible amount of glucose. In contrast, the subcutaneous interstitial fluid, sampled from the same host and in the same manner, had a glucose level only 10–15% lower than that of plasma. During hyperglycemia (300 mg %), the interstitial fluid content of glucose remained negligible for a few hours, then started to rise, and equilibrated with the plasma level within 24 h. Passage from hyper- to normoglycemia reconstituted the sharp concentration gradient for glucose as normally found in tumors (Gullino *et al.*, 1967*b*). Thus glucose concentration in the pericellular fluid of solid tumors is normally very low, as low as in ascites fluid (Kemp and Mendel, 1957); but glucose consumption is very high. The sharp concentration gradient maintained by the vascular walls appears to result from the fact that consumption by the cell population is higher than the diffusion capability across the vascular wall. Glucose consumption by the tumor can be saturated only when diffusion across the vascular wall is increased by elevation of glucose concentration in the plasma.

The physiological effect of increased glucose consumption on the biological properties of the neoplastic cell population is poorly understood. Tumor growth rate was not related to glucose utilization, nor was tumor growth improved under continuous hyperglycemia; in fact, it was slower in alloxan-diabetic rats (Shapot,

1972). In our experience, 4956 fibrosarcomas, for example, grew three times faster than 5123 hepatomas, but they consumed about 20% less glucose, which was delivered by a blood flow about 30% smaller in a vascular space only one-fourth as large (Gullino *et al.*, 1967*c*).

349
EXTRA-
CELLULAR
COMPARTMENTS
OF SOLID
TUMORS

One particular aspect of glucose utilization by tumors concerns lactate production. Aerobic glycolysis is such a remarkable event in the life of neoplastic tissues that production of lactate has traditionally been bound to the nature of neoplasia. However, one can obtain, *in vivo*, a high production of lactate in nonneoplastic tissues. For instance, the lactate content of the interstitial fluid increased in all rats bearing a micropore chamber implanted in the subcutaneous area (Gullino *et al.*, 1967*c*). In the majority of these animals, a sarcoma is produced around the chamber within 10–18 months, but lactate production and decreased pH are observed within 2 wk after chamber implantation. Libenson and Jena (1974) believe that persistent low pH may be a determining factor in oncogenesis; yet the causes for the large lactate production, long before any neoplastic transformation is demonstrable, remain unknown.

Carcinomas and sarcomas *in vivo* converted into lactate about 35% of the glucose utilized. This estimate was based on the assumption that for each mole of lactate eliminated into the tumor efferent blood $\frac{1}{2}$ mole of glucose was consumed (Gullino *et al.*, 1967*b*). Glycolytic efficiency of tumors can be changed *in vivo*. For example, when the glucose supply was reduced to one-half or less of the physiological level, the relative proportion of glucose transformed into lactate increased. In fact, during severe and prolonged hypoglycemia, almost all glucose utilized by a tumor was accounted for by the lactate of the efferent blood. However, when a large supply of glucose followed a period of glucose starvation, the tumor increased its glucose consumption tremendously; but practically no lactate was eliminated during the first 30 min of hyperglycemia. The role of glucose starvation in producing the dissociation between glucose consumption and lactate production *in vivo* remains unclear.

The amount of glucose utilized *in vivo* was larger than the quantity of glucose that most tumors could oxidize. With both glycolytic and oxidative energy pathways available, the neoplastic cell has often been considered to be in an advantageous position for survival, in the sense that it could shift from respiration to fermentation, or *vice versa*, depending on oxygen availability. We were unable to find any indication that this indeed does happen *in vivo*. Tumors with low oxygen consumption utilized proportionally smaller amounts of glucose. When glycolysis was measured in the same tumor before and after an acute shortage of oxygen, there was no clear indication that glucose utilization or lactate production was enhanced during hypoxemia. Actually, any increase of glucose consumption required an increase in oxygen utilization. Moreover, when an abrupt deprivation of oxygen was inflicted on the tumor during active glucose consumption, both utilization of glucose and production of lactate ceased (Gullino *et al.*, 1967*c*). The role of glycolysis in the broad picture of neoplastic transformation remains largely unknown.

PIETRO M.
GULLINO

4.4. Passage of Neoplastic Cells Through Capillary Walls

Penetration of neoplastic cells into the vascular network of the tumor and host is a frequent event. Displacement due to continuous growth of the neoplastic cell population and irregularity of the new-formed vascular wall are conditions which indicate that shedding of cells into the bloodstream may occur. Manipulation of the tumor is a common way to increase cell shedding into the general circulation. For instance, Gazet (1966) observed a fivefold increase in the number of circulating cells when a $V \times 2$ carcinoma implanted in a thigh was massaged. Presence of neoplastic cells in the blood of tumor-bearing hosts has been reported frequently; however, quantitation of cell shedding and an estimation of the circulating cell load for a given size of tumor are difficult to obtain. Butler and Gullino (1974b) measured a shedding of about 4×10^6 neoplastic cells/24 h/g tumor in MTW-9 mammary carcinoma of the rat. These neoplastic cells were rapidly cleared from the circulation, so that their number in the aortic blood of the host was one-tenth the number present in the efferent tumor blood. A 2-g tumor produced, every 24 h, a circulating cell load similar to the inoculum necessary for the transplant. Nonetheless, MTW-9 did not metastasize. The conditions necessary for development of metastasis from circulating neoplastic cells are described elsewhere in this volume.

ACKNOWLEDGMENTS

I am grateful to my collaborators for their help over the years and to Miss Rosemary Connelly and Miss Ursula Walz for their valuable contribution to the preparation of the manuscript.

5. References

ABRAMS, H. L., 1964, Altered drug response of tumour vessels in man, *Nature (London)* **201**:167.

AISENBERG, A. C., 1961, *The Glycolysis and Respiration of Tumors*, Academic Press, New York.

AISENBERG, A. C., AND MORRIS, H. P., 1963, Energy pathways of hepatomas H-35 and 7800, *Cancer Res.* **23**:566.

ALGIRE, G. H., AND LEGALLAIS, F. Y., 1951, Vascular reactions of normal and malignant tissues *in vivo.* IV. The effect of peripheral hypotension on transplanted tumors, *J. Natl. Cancer Inst.* **12**:399.

ALGIRE, G. H., LEGALLAIS, F. Y., AND ANDERSON, B. F., 1952, Vascular reactions of normal and malignant tissues *in vivo.* V. The role of hypotension in the action of a bacterial polysaccharide on tumors, *J. Natl. Cancer Inst.* **12**:1279.

ALGIRE, G. H., LEGALLAIS, F. Y., AND ANDERSON, B. F., 1954, Vascular reactions of normal and malignant tissues *in vivo.* VI. The role of hypotension in the action of components of podophyllin on transplanted sarcomas, *J. Natl. Cancer Inst.* **14**:879.

BARACH, A. L., AND BICKERMAN, H. A., 1954, The effect of anoxia on tumor growth with special reference to sarcoma 180 implanted in C57 mice, *Cancer Res.* **14**:672.

BIERMAN, H. R., KELLY, K. H., AND SINGER, G., 1952a, Studies on the blood supply of tumors in man. IV. The increased oxygen content of venous blood draining neoplasms, *J. Natl. Cancer Inst.* **12**:701.

BIERMAN, H. R., GILFILLAN, R. S., KELLY, K. H., KUZMA, O. T., AND NOBLE, M., 1952b, Studies on the blood supply of tumors in man. V. Skin temperatures of superficial neoplastic lesions, *J. Natl. Cancer Inst.* **13**:1.

351

EXTRA-
CELLULAR
COMPARTMENTS
OF SOLID
TUMORS

BLANCHARD, R. J. W., GROTENHUIS, L., LAFAVE, J. W., AND PERRY, J. F., JR., 1965, Blood supply to hepatic V2 carcinoma implants as measured by radioactive microspheres, *Proc. Soc. Exp. Biol. Med.* **118:**465.

BOSMANN, H. B., 1969, Glycoprotein degradation: Glycosidases in fibroblasts transformed by oncogenic viruses, *Exp. Cell Res.* **54:**217.

BRADA, Z., 1965, Host–tumor relationship. XX. The hexosamine content of the tumour as a marker of relations between the tumour stroma and tumour cells, *Neoplasma* **12:**373.

BREEDIS, C., AND YOUNG, G., 1954, The blood supply of neoplasms in the liver, *Am. J. Pathol.* **30:**969.

BRUNS, R. R., AND PALADE, G. E., 1968, Studies on blood capillaries. I. General organization of blood capillaries in muscle, *J. Cell Biol.* **37:**244.

BUTLER, T. P., AND GULLINO, P. M., 1975*a*, in preparation.

BUTLER, T. P., AND GULLINO, P. M., 1975*b*, Quantitation of cell shedding into efferent blood of mammary adenocarcinoma, *Cancer Res.* in press.

CAMPBELL, J. A., AND CRAMER, W., 1928, Some effects of oxygen pressure in the inspired air upon cancer growth and body-weight of rats and mice, *Lancet* **1:**828.

CATALAND, S., COHEN, C., AND SAPIRSTEIN, L. A., 1962, Relationship between size and perfusion rate of transplanted tumors, *J. Natl. Cancer Inst.* **29:**389.

CHALKLEY, H. W., 1943, Method for the quantitative morphologic analysis of tissues, *J. Natl. Cancer Inst.* **4:**47.

DAVIS, J. S., AND TRAUT, H. F., 1925, Origin and development of blood supply of whole thickness skin grafts, *Ann. Surg.* **82:**871.

DAY, E. D., PLANINSEK, J. A., AND PRESSMAN, D., 1959*a*, Localization *in vivo* of radioiodinated anti-rat-fibrin antibodies and radioiodinated rat fibrinogen in the Murphy rat lymphosarcoma and other transplantable rat tumors, *J. Natl. Cancer Inst.* **22:**413.

DAY, E. D., PLANINSEK, J. A., AND PRESSMAN, D., 1959*b*, Localization of radioiodinated rat fibrinogen in transplanted rat tumors, *J. Natl. Cancer Inst.* **23:**799.

DeOME, K. B., FAULKIN, L. J., JR., BERN, H. A., AND BLAIR, P. B., 1959, Development of mammary tumors from hyperplastic alveolar nodules transplanted into gland-free mammary fat pads of female C3H mice, *Cancer Res.* **19:**515.

DICKENS, F., 1936, The metabolism of normal and tumour tissue. XVII. The action of some derivatives of phenazine, quinoline and pyridine on the Pasteur reaction, *Biochem. J.* **30:**1233.

EDDY, H. A., AND CASARETT, G. W., 1973, Development of the vascular system in the hamster malignant neurilemmoma, *Microvasc. Res.* **6:**63.

EDLICH, R. F., ROGERS, W., DeSHAZO, C. V., JR., AND AUST, J. B., 1966, Effect of vasoactive drugs on tissue blood flow in the hamster melanoma, *Cancer Res.* **26:**1420.

EVANS, H. M., 1908, On the occurrence of newly-formed lymphatic vessels in malignant growths, *Johns Hopkins Hosp. Bull.* **19:**232.

FISZER-SZARFARZ, B., AND GULLINO, P. M., 1970*a*, Hyaluronic acid content of the interstitial fluid of Walker carcinoma 256, *Proc. Soc. Exp. Biol. Med.* **133:**597.

FISZER-SZAFARZ, B., AND GULLINO, P. M., 1970*b*, Hyaluronidase activity of normal and neoplastic interstitial fluid, *Proc. Soc. Exp. Biol. Med.* **133:**805.

FOLKMAN, J., 1972, Anti-angiogenesis: New concept for therapy of solid tumors, *Ann. Surg.* **175:**409.

FOLKMAN, M. J., LONG, D. M., JR., AND BECKER, F. F., 1962, Tumor growth in organ culture, *Surg. Forum* **13:**81.

FOLKMAN, J., LONG, D. M., JR., AND BECKER, F. F., 1963, Growth and metastasis of tumor in organ culture, *Cancer* **16:**453.

FOLKMAN, J., MERLER, E., ABERNATHY, C., AND WILLIAMS, G., 1971, Isolation of a tumor factor responsible for angiogenesis, *J. Exp. Med.* **133:**275.

GAZET, J. C., 1966, The detection of viable circulating cancer cells, *Acta Cytol.* **10:**119.

GIMBRONE, M. A., JR., AND GULLINO, P. M., 1975, Neovascularization induced by intraocular xenografts of normal, prenoplastic and neoplastic mouse mammary tissues, *J. Natl. Cancer Institute*, in press.

GIMBRONE, M. A., JR., LEAPMAN, S. B., COTRAN, R. S., AND FOLKMAN, J., 1972, Tumor dormancy *in vivo* by prevention of neovascularization, *J. Exp. Med.* **136:**261.

GOLDACRE, R. J., AND SYLVEN, B., 1962, On the access of blood-borne dyes to various tumour regions, *Br. J. Cancer* **16:**306.

GOODALL, C. M., SANDERS, A. G., AND SHUBIK, P., 1965, Studies ot vascular patterns in living tumors with a transparent chamber inserted in hamster cheek pouch, *J. Natl. Cancer Inst.* **35:**497.

GRABOWSKA, M., 1959, Collagen content of normal connective tissue, of tissue surrounding a tumour and of growing rat sarcoma, *Nature (London)* **183**:1186.

GRANTHAM, F. H., HILL, D. M., AND GULLINO, P. M., 1973, Primary mammary tumors connected to the host by a single artery and vein, *J. Natl. Cancer Inst.* **50**:1381.

GREENE, H. S. N., 1941*a*, Heterologous transplantation of mammalian tumors. I. The transfer of rabbit tumors to alien species, *J. Exp. Med.* **73**:461.

GREENE, H. S. N., 1941*b*, Heterologous transplantation of mammalian tumors. II. The transfer of human tumors to alien species, *J. Exp. Med.* **73**:475.

GREENFIELD, R. E., AND WHITAKER, B. M., 1961, The use of intravenous-trypsin and solutions of polyvinylpyrrolidone (PVP) for the isolation of cells from tissues of the rat, *Proc. Am. Assoc. Cancer Res.* **3**:230.

GULLINO, P. M., 1968, *In-vitro* perfusion of tumors, in: *Organ Perfusion and Preservation* (J. C. Norman, J. Folkman, W. G. Hardison, L. E. Rudolf, and F. J. Veith, eds.), pp. 877–898, Appleton-Century-Crofts, New York.

GULLINO, P. M., AND GRANTHAM, F. H., 1961*a*, Studies on the exchange of fluids between host and tumor. I. A method for growing "tissue-isolated" tumors in laboratory animals, *J. Natl. Cancer Inst.* **27**:679.

GULLINO, P. M., AND GRANTHAM, F. H., 1961*b*, Studies on the exchange of fluids between host and tumor. II. The blood flow of hepatomas and other tumors in rats and mice, *J. Natl. Cancer Inst.* **27**:1465.

GULLINO, P. M., AND GRANTHAM, F. H., 1962, Studies on the exchange of fluids between host and tumor. III. Regulation of blood flow in hepatomas and other rat tumors, *J. Natl. Cancer Inst.* **28**:211.

GULLINO, P. M., AND GRANTHAM, F. H., 1963, The influence of the host and the neoplastic cell population on the collagen content of a tumor mass, *Cancer Res.* **23**:648.

GULLINO, P. M., AND GRANTHAM, F. H., 1964, The vascular space of growing tumors, *Cancer Res.* **24**:1727.

GULLINO, P. M., AND LANZEROTTI, R. H., 1972, Mammary tumor regression. II. Autophagy of neoplastic cells, *J. Natl. Cancer Inst.* **49**:1349.

GULLINO, P. M., GRANTHAM, F. H., AND CLARK, S. H., 1962, The collagen content of transplanted tumors, *Cancer Res.* **22**:1031.

GULLINO, P. M., CLARK, S. H., AND GRANTHAM, F. H., 1964, The interstitial fluid of solid tumors, *Cancer Res.* **24**:780.

GULLINO, P. M., GRANTHAM, F. H., AND SMITH, S. H., 1965*a*, The interstitial water space of tumors, *Cancer Res.* **25**:727.

GULLINO, P. M., GRANTHAM, F. H., SMITH, S. H., AND HAGGERTY, A. C., 1965*b*, Modification of the acid–base status of the internal milieu of tumors, *J. Natl. Cancer Inst.* **34**:857.

GULLINO, P. M., GRANTHAM, F. H., AND COURTNEY, A. H., 1967*a*, Utilization of oxygen by transplanted tumors *in vivo*, *Cancer Res.* **27**:1020.

GULLINO, P. M., GRANTHAM, F. H., AND COURTNEY, A. H., 1967*b*, Glucose consumption by transplanted tumors *in vivo*, *Cancer Res.* **27**:1031.

GULLINO, P. M., GRANTHAM, F. H., COURTNEY, A., AND LOSONCZY, I., 1967*c*, Relationship between oxygen and glucose consumption by transplanted tumors *in vivo*, *Cancer Res.* **27**:1041.

HAMMERSEN, F., 1970, The terminal vascular bed in skeletal muscle with special regard to the problem of shunts, in: *Capillary Permeability* (C. Crone and N. A. Lassen, eds.), pp. 351–365, Academic Press, New York.

HAUCK, G., 1971, Physiology of the microvascular system, *Angiologica* **8**:236.

HILMAS, D. E., AND GILLETTE, E. L., 1974, Morphometric analyses of the microvasculature of tumors during growth and after X-irradiation, *Cancer* **33**:103.

HUMPHREY, E. W., 1961, A comparison of the permeability of normal liver and of hepatoma to sucrose and inulin, *Cancer Res.* **21**:1573.

KHAN, P. C., 1965, The epinephrine effect in selective renal angiography, *Radiology* **85**:301.

KARNOVSKY, M. J., 1968, The ultrastructural basis of transcapillary exchanges, *J. Gen. Physiol.* **52**:64s.

KEMP, A., AND MENDEL, B., 1957, How does the Ehrlich ascites tumour obtain its energy for growth? *Nature (London)* **180**:131.

KERR, J. F. R., WYLLIE, A. H., AND CURRIE, A. R., 1972, Apoptosis: A basic biological phenomenon with wide-ranging implications in tissue kinetics, *Br. J. Cancer* **26**:239.

LANZEROTTI, R. H., AND GULLINO, P. M., 1972, Activities and quantities of lysosomal enzymes during mammary tumor regression, *Cancer Res.* **32**:2679.

LEWIS, W. H., 1927, The vascular patterns of tumors, *Bull. Johns Hopkins Hosp.* **41**:156.

LIBENSON, L., AND JENA, M., 1974, Extracellular pH and neoplastic transformations, *Cancer Res.* **34**:953.

MALTONI, C., AND PRODI, G., 1960, The behaviour of connective tissue in the genesis and development of tumours, in: *Recent Contributions to Cancer Research in Italy*, Vol. 1, (P. Bucalossi and U. Veronesi, eds.), pp. 49–155, Casa Ed. Ambrosiane, Milan, Italy.

MARGULIS, A. R., CARLSSON, E., AND McALISTER, W. H., 1961, Angiography of malignant tumors in mice, *Acta Radiol.* **56**:179.

MEDINA, D., 1973, Preneoplastic lesions in mouse mammary tumorigenesis, in: *Methods in Cancer Research* (H. Busch, ed.), pp. 3–53, Academic Press, New York.

MERWIN, R. M., AND ALGIRE, G. H., 1956, The role of graft and host vessels in the vascularization of grafts of normal and neoplastic tissue, *J. Natl. Cancer Inst.* **17**:23.

MILNE, E. N. C., MARGULIS, A. R., NOONAN, C. D., AND STOUGHTON, J. I., 1967, Histologic type-specific vascular patterns in rat tumors, *Cancer* **10**:1635.

NATADZE, T. D., 1959, Regulation of blood circulation in malignant tumours, *Vopr. Onkol.* **5**:654.

ORR, J. W., 1938, The changes antecedent to tumour formation during the treatment of mouse skin with carcinogenic hydrocarbons, *J. Pathol. Bacteriol.* **46**:495.

ORR, J. W., 1940, The histology of the rat's liver during the course of carcinogenesis by butter-yellow (*p*-dimethylaminoazobenzene), *J. Pathol. Bacteriol.* **50**:393.

PEARCE, R. H., 1965, Glycosaminoglycans and glycoproteins in skin, in: *The Amino Sugars*, Vol. 2A, (E. A. Balazs and R. W. Jeanloz, eds.), pp. 149–195, Academic Press, New York.

POLLACK, M. A., TAYLOR, A., AND SORTOMME, C. L., 1942, The effect of variations in oxygen pressure upon tumor transplants, *Cancer Res.* **2**:828.

POOLE, A. R., AND WILLIAMS, D. C., 1967, *In vivo* effect of an invasive malignant rat tumour on cartilage, *Nature (London)* **214**:1342.

RAJEWSKY, M. F., 1965, *In vitro* studies of cell proliferation in tumours. II. Characteristics of a standardised *in vitro* system for the measurement of ³H-thymidine incorporation into tissue explants, *Eur. J. Cancer* **1**:281.

RECHCIGL, M., JR., AND SIDRANSKY, H., 1962, Isolation of two lines of transplantable, ethionine-induced rat hepatomas of high and low catalase activity from a primary tumor, *J. Natl. Cancer Inst.* **28**:1411.

REINHOLD, H. S., 1971, Improved microcirculation in irradiated tumours, *Eur. J. Cancer* **7**:273.

ROCKOFF, S. D., DOPPMAN, J., BLOCK, J. B., AND KETCHAM, A., 1966, Variable response of tumor vessels to intra-arterial epinephrine, *Invest. Radiol.* **1**:205.

RUBIN, P., AND CASARETT, G., 1966, Microcirculation of tumors. I. Anatomy, function, and necrosis, *Clin. Radiol.* **17**:220.

SANDERS, A. G., AND SHUBIK, P., 1964, A transparent window for use in the Syrian hamster, *Israel J. Exp. Med.* **11**:118.

SANDISON, J. C., 1924, A new method for the microscopic study of living growing tissues by the introduction of a transparent chamber in the rabbit's ear, *Anat. Rec.* **28**:281.

SAPIRSTEIN, L. A., 1958, Regional blood flow by fractional distribution of indicators, *Am. J. Physiol.* **193**:161.

SCHEINBERG, P., AND STEAD, E. A., JR., 1949, The cerebral blood flow in male subjects as measured by the nitrous oxide technique: Normal values for blood flow, oxygen utilization, glucose utilization, and peripheral resistance, with observations on the effect of tilting and anxiety, *J. Clin. Invest.* **28**:1163.

SCHOEFL, G. I., 1963, Studies on inflammation. III. Growing capillaries: Their structure and permeability, *Virchows Arch. Pathol. Anat.* **337**:141.

SHAPOT, V. S., 1972, Some biochemical aspects of the relationship between the tumor and the host, *Adv. Cancer Res.* **15**:253.

SHELTON, E., AND RICE, M. E., 1958, Studies on mouse lymphomas. II. Behavior of three lymphomas in diffusion chambers in relation to their invasive capacity in the host, *J. Natl. Cancer Inst.* **21**:137.

SIMPSON, W. L., 1954, Connective tissue and cancer, in: *Connective Tissue in Health and Disease* (G. Asboe-Hansen, ed.), pp. 225–238, Munksgaard, Copenhagen.

SONG, C. W., AND LEVITT, S. H., 1971, Quantitative study of vascularity in Walker carcinoma 256, *Cancer Res.* **31**:587.

STOREY, R. H., WISH, L., AND FURTH, J., 1951, Organ erythrocyte and plasma volumes of tumor-bearing mice, *Cancer Res.* **11**:943.

353

EXTRA-
CELLULAR
COMPARTMENTS
OF SOLID
TUMORS

STRAW, J. A., HART, M. M., KLUBES, P., ZAHARKO, D. S., AND DEDRICK, R. L., 1974, Distribution of anticancer agents in spontaneous animal tumors. I. Regional blood flow and methotrexate distribution in canine lymphosarcoma, *J. Natl. Cancer Inst.* **52**:1327.

SWABB, E. A., WEI, J., AND GULLINO, P. M., 1974, Diffusion and convection in normal and neoplastic tissues, *Cancer Res.*, **34**:2814.

SYLVEN, B., 1968, Lysosomal enzyme activity in the interstitial fluid of solid mouse tumour transplants, *Eur. J. Cancer* **4**:463.

SYLVEN, B., AND BOIS, I., 1960, Protein content and enzymatic assays of interstitial fluid from some normal tissues and transplanted mouse tumors, *Cancer Res.* **20**:831.

SYLVEN, B., AND BOIS-SVENSSON, I., 1965, On the chemical pathology of interstitial fluid. I. Proteolytic activities in transplanted mouse tumors, *Cancer Res.* **25**:458.

SYLVEN, B., AND NIEMI, M., 1972, Histochemical evidence of cell death in transplanted tumours, *Virchows Arch. Abt. B Zellpathol.* **10**:127.

TANNOCK, I. F., 1968, The relation between cell proliferation and the vascular system in a transplanted mouse mammary tumour, *Br. J. Cancer* **22**:258.

TANNOCK, I. F., 1970, Population kinetics of carcinoma cells, capillary endothelial cells, and fibroblasts in a transplanted mouse mammary tumor, *Cancer Res.* **30**:2470.

TANNOCK, I. F., AND HAYASHI, S., 1972, The proliferation of capillary endothelial cells, *Cancer Res.* **32**:77.

TANNOCK, I. F., AND STEEL, G. G., 1969, Quantitative techniques for study of the anatomy and function of small blood vessels in tumors, *J. Natl. Cancer Inst.* **42**:771.

THOMLINSON, R. H., 1973, Radiation and the vascularity of tumours, *Br. Med. Bull.* **29**:29.

THOMLINSON, R. H., AND GRAY, L. H., 1955, The histological structure of some human lung cancers and the possible implications for radiotherapy, *Br. J. Cancer* **9**:539.

TRISTRAM, G. R., 1953, The amino acid composition of proteins, in: *The Proteins*, Vol. 1A, (H. Neurath and K. Bailey, eds.), p. 221, Academic Press, New York.

TUTTLE, E. P., JR., AND SADLER, J. H., 1964, Measurement of renal tissue fluid turnover rates by thermal washout technique, in: *Hypertension: Proceedings of the Council for High Blood Pressure Research*, Vol. 13, pp. 3–16, American Heart Association, New York.

UNDERWOOD, J. C. E., AND CARR, I., 1972, The ultrastructure and permeability characteristics of the blood vessels of a transplantable rat sarcoma, *J. Pathol.* **107**:157.

URBACH, F., 1961, The blood supply of tumors, in: *Advances in Biology of Skin*, Vol. 2: *Blood Vessels and Circulation* (W. Montagna and R. A. Ellis, eds.), pp. 123–149, Pergamon Press, New York.

VAN DEN HOOFF, A., 1962, Chemical and morphological collagen changes in the course of 20-methylcholanthrene-induced carcinogenesis in mouse skin, *Oncologia* **15**:161.

VASILIEV, J. M., 1959, Early changes in the subcutaneous connective tissue of rats after implantation of pellets containing carcinogenic polycyclic hydrocarbons, *J. Natl. Cancer Inst.* **23**:441.

VAUPEL, P., 1974, *Atemgaswechsel und Glucosestoffwechsel von Tumoren (DS-Carcinosarkom) in vivo*, Akademie der Wissenschaften und der Literatur, Mainz, in Kommission bei F. Steiner Verlag, Wiesbaden.

VAUPEL, P., GUNTHER, H., AND GROTE, J., 1971, Atemgaswechsel und Glucosestoffwechsel von Tumoren (DS-Carcinosarkom) *in vivo*. I. Experimentelle Untersuchungen der versorgungsbestimmenden Parameter, *Z. Gesamte Exp. Med.* **156**:283.

VOGEL, A. W., 1965, Intratumoral vascular changes with increased size of a mammary adenocarcinoma: New method and results, *J. Natl. Cancer Inst.* **34**:571.

VOGEL, A. W., AND HAYNES, J., 1966, Mammary adenocarcinoma (72j) blood flow in mice treated with thioTEPA, *J. Natl. Cancer Inst.* **37**:293.

WARBURG, O., WIND, F., AND NEGELEIN, E., 1927, The metabolism of tumors in the body, *J. Gen. Physiol.* **8**:519.

WARREN, B. A., 1966, The ultrastructure of capillary sprouts induced by melanoma transplants in the golden hamster, *J. R. Microsc. Soc.* **86**:177.

WARREN, B. A., GREENBLATT, M., AND KOMMINENI, V. R. C., 1972, Tumour angiogenesis: Ultrastructure of endothelial cells in mitosis, *Br. J. Exp. Pathol.* **53**:216.

WEINHOUSE, S., 1956, On respiratory impairment in cancer cells, *Science* **124**:267.

WOLLMAN, S. H., AND REED, F. E., 1963, Clearance of blood radioiodide by transplantable tumors of the thyroid gland in the unanesthetized rat, *J. Natl. Cancer Inst.* **31**:1479.

WRIGHT, R. D., 1937, The blood supply of newly developed epithelial tissue in the liver, *J. Pathol. Bacteriol.* **45**:405.

WRIGHT, R. D., 1938, The blood supply of abnormal tissue in the lung, *J. Pathol. Bacteriol.* **47**:489.

13

Tumor Angiogenesis

JUDAH FOLKMAN

1. Introduction

Two central issues preoccupy many investigators in cancer biology. (1) How is the normal cell transformed to a malignant cell? (2) How is the transformed state maintained? From studies addressed to these questions has come the realization that malignant transformation, while necessary for the development of a tumor, may not be sufficient! Not all cells transformed to malignancy *in vitro* will produce a tumor. To become a successful tumor, transformed cells must express additional characteristics. Thus a third issue can be introduced. How is the tumorigenic state attained?

No doubt, it will be found that numerous properties are essential before a malignant tumor can "succeed" in its host. These properties may include the release of specific proteases (Reich, 1974) or the synthesis of tumor-specific antigens (Currie, 1973). However, tumor angiogenesis, the capacity of a tumor to continuously elicit neovascularization in host vessels, may be one of the characteristics fundamental to the tumorigenic state. In this chapter, we will examine the proposal that the ability of a young malignant tumor to stimulate capillary proliferation in the host may be essential for progressive tumor growth and for the expression of malignant potential. A first consideration is the early phase of tumor growth *before* connection to the host's vascular system.

2. The Avascular Phase of Tumor Growth

Most if not all solid tumors arising spontaneously, or from metastasized cells, or by transplantation in experimental animals begin as avascular aggregates of malignant cells. The tumor population exchanges nutrients and catabolites with the

JUDAH FOLKMAN • Department of Surgery, Children's Hospital Medical Center and Harvard Medical School, Boston, Massachusetts

surrounding interstitial tissue by a process of simple diffusion. This phase of tumor growth is usually microscopic and visible only in a few clinical and experimental situations. Carcinoma *in situ* can be diagnosed in the skin, in the eye, in the bladder, and most commonly in the uterine cervix. In the cervix (Süss *et al.*, 1973), neoplastic cell masses sit superficial to the basement membrane and may remain for years without penetrating it. At some point, this membrane is penetrated and almost simultaneously the tumor becomes vascularized. In fact, carcinoma *in situ* of the cervix may be thought of as a general model for the avascular phase of the majority of carcinomas. This is because carcinomas generally originate in the avascular epithelial compartment (Fig. 1). There is a common histological pattern in the skin, pharynx, gastrointestinal tract, respiratory tract, and genitourinary tract in which the epithelial compartment is separated from blood vessels by a basement membrane (Eisenstein *et al.*, 1973). Most carcinomas begin in this compartment and remain small nodules, often less than 2 mm in diameter. This small size is generally determined by the growth constraints placed on a three-dimensional aggregate of cells forced to survive by simple diffusion. Growth of an avascular three-dimensional aggregate of tumor cells is self-inhibiting. This can be better understood by examining tumor growth *in vitro*.

If any group of cells is to continue growing, the surface area of the aggregate population must be sufficient to allow adequate absorption of nutrients (oxygen included) and escape of waste catabolites (Folkman *et al.*, 1974). Tumor cells in flat tissue culture grow in only two dimensions. The third dimension reaches equilibrium as a thin layer of cells pile up, but rarely exceeds a thickness of six to eight cell layers. The cell population will expand indefinitely in two dimensions as

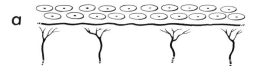

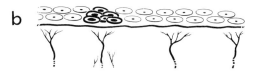

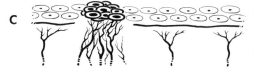

FIGURE 1. (a) Epithelium of the skin, gut, respiratory tract, and genitourinary tract shown as an avascular compartment. A basement membrane separates blood vessels from the epithelial compartment. (b) Carcinomas arising in this epithelium also are avascular until the basement membrane is violated and new vessels penetrate the tumor, as shown in (c). Although this diagram is drawn to suggest that the vessels might invade the basement membrane before the tumor does, there is no proof of which is the first to invade the membrane.

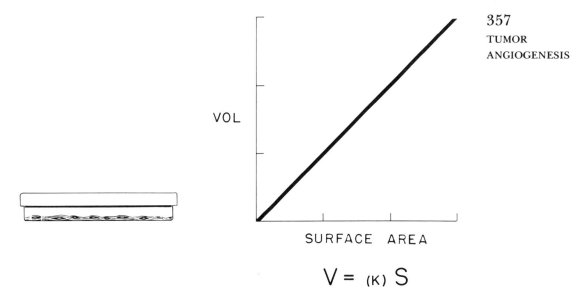

VOL

SURFACE AREA

$$V = (K) \, S$$

FIGURE 2. Relation of surface area to volume when growth occurs in two dimensions *in vitro*. From Folkman *et al.* (1974) with permission of Cold Spring Harbor Laboratory.

long as (1) the medium is changed frequently and (2) enough open space is provided (i.e., the dish is enlarged or cells are repeatedly transferred to a new dish). Under these conditions, two-dimensional growth is *not* self-limiting, because the surface area of a flat population increases in direct proportion to the volume of the population (Folkman and Hochberg, 1973) (Fig. 2).

By contrast, when tumor cells are cultured in suspension (spinner or soft agar), growth occurs in *three* dimensions. In this configuration, growth is self-limiting despite frequent changes of media and provision for abundant open space. As the three-dimensional aggregate enlarges, its volume increases by the third power, while surface area increases only by the second power (Fig. 3). Eventually the cell population approaches a volume at which surface area is insufficient for adequate diffusion of nutrients and catabolites. Further growth is impossible. Such a cell population is not dead, but dormant. The outer cells are proliferating while the cells in the center are dying. A steady state is reached when the peripheral proliferating cells balance those dying in the center. For a number of tumors grown in soft agar, the maximum number of viable cells in one study was less than 10^6, and the mean diameter ranged from 3 to 4 mm (Folkman and Hochberg, 1973). This is a form of population dormancy. The tumor spheroid grown in suspension culture or soft agar is an analogue of the avascular tumor *in vivo*. The vast majority of solid tumors in mouse or man grow from their earliest inception as three-dimensional aggregates. Tumors appear as spheroids or ellipsoids in the kidney, liver, lung, intestine, breast, brain, and lymph nodes (Willis, 1973). It is rare that a tumor expands in a flat plane. Later during tumor progression, one

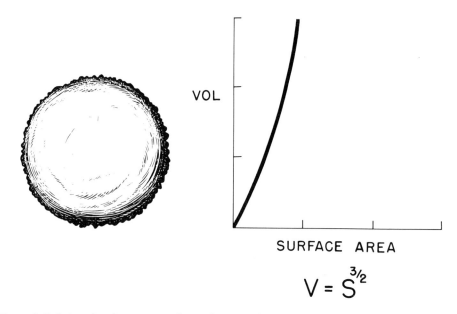

$$V = S^{3/2}$$

FIGURE 3. Relation of surface area to volume when growth is spheroidal or three-dimensional as in soft agar, or in the avascular phase of tumor growth *in vivo*. From Folkman *et al.* (1974) with permission of Cold Spring Harbor Laboratory.

may see laminar growth in nerve sheaths or along peritoneal or pleural linings. Because the avascular phase is usually imperceptible, it is not readily appreciated that a three-dimensional aggregate of tumor cells in the avascular state will limit its own growth to a population of less than 10^6 cells. However, in certain experimental situations the avascular phase is easily observed. Tumors implanted into the chorioallantoic membrane of the chick embryo remain avascular for about 72 h (Knighton *et al.*, 1975). The avascular phase is also visible in the transparent chamber implanted in the rabbit ear (Algire and Chalkley, 1945), the hamster cheek pouch (Warren and Shubik, 1966), or the subcutaneous tissue of the rat (Yamaura and Sato, 1973). Also, tumors implanted in the anterior chamber or the corneal stroma will remain in the avascular phase for much longer periods, depending on the distance of the tumor implant from the iris or limbal vessels. In fact, the self-limiting effect of three-dimensional avascular growth can be illustrated by lengthening the duration of the avascular phase in the anterior chamber to weeks or months. During this time, avascular tumors cannot grow beyond 1 mm³ (Gimbrone *et al.*, 1972). They remain viable, however, and growth is reinstituted once vascularization takes place. In summary, the hallmark of the avascular phase is limited growth, and, if the onset of vascularization is delayed, population dormancy.

The avascular phase of human cancer is witnessed by dermatologists, ophthalmologists, and gynecologists. For example, retinoblastoma metastasizes into the vitreous. These vitreous seedings are small spherical tumors less than 1 mm in diameter with a necrotic center (Folkman, 1974b) (Fig. 4). Vessels from the retina do not reach them. Carcinoma of the cervix *in situ* is another example. Petersen (1956) followed 127 patients with this tumor, untreated for 10 years. In 33%, the avascular lesion progressed to stage I carcinoma or beyond. In the other patients, the *in situ* lesion remained stationary or regressed completely.

3. The Vascular Phase of Tumor Growth

Rapid growth and in some tumors exponential growth starts with vascularization. Gimbrone *et al.* (1972) showed that a Brown–Pearce tumor implanted in the anterior chamber near the iris vessels will be vascularized in 5–6 days (Fig. 5). During the next 2 wk the tumor may enlarge to 16,000 times its original avascular volume. Chick embryo tumor implants maintained a dormant diameter of 0.93 ± 0.29 mm during the avascular phase and reached a mean diameter of 8.0 ± 2.5 mm 7 days after vascularization (Knighton *et al.*, 1975). The avascular tumor has an area of central necrosis; this disappears 48 h after vascularization (Ausprunk *et al.*, 1975). Open capillaries course throughout the tumor while it is between 1 mm^3 and 1 cm^3 in size and most cells are viable (Goldacre and Sylven, 1962). Central necrosis may reappear as the tumor exceeds 1 cm^3. Tissue pressure rises in the center of the expanding tumor, compressing the deeper capillaries (Young *et al.*, 1950). Blood flow stops in the depths of the large tumor, leaving only a thin rind supplied by proliferating capillaries.

Vascularization may be responsible for other malignant characteristics of neoplasms in addition to rapid growth. Immunological enhancement may require vascularization. Herberman (1974) has pointed out that serum blocking factors are generally present only when there is detectable tumor. Detectable tumors in man or in experimental animals are almost always vascularized. Currie (1973) has suggested that circulating tumor antigen may inhibit tumor immunity in man. It is possible that this antigen pours into the bloodstream only after vascularization and rapid growth. Direct proof is lacking at this writing. However, indirect evidence is provided by an analogous experiment. India ink particles will not diffuse through the rabbit cornea because of their size, 250 Å (Cotran and Remensynder, 1968). Smolin and Hyndiuk (1971) observed that India ink will diffuse out of a cornea which has been neovascularized by inflammatory vessels. We modified their experiment by mixing particles of India ink with a tumor implanted in a corneal pocket. These particles remain with the tumor in its corneal pocket, and the tumor appears as a black disc with sharply defined edges. When the tumor is penetrated by proliferating capillaries, the India ink particles quickly leave the tumor bed and enter the circulation and the regional lymph nodes. This implies that large macromolecules or pieces of tumor membrane may enter the circulation after tumor vascularization. It is also possible that metastatic cells may be shed into the circulation only after the onset of vascularization. The avascular tumor may be unable to shed metastases. Finally, vascularization may be responsible for malignant progression or "malignant drift." Klein and Klein (1955)

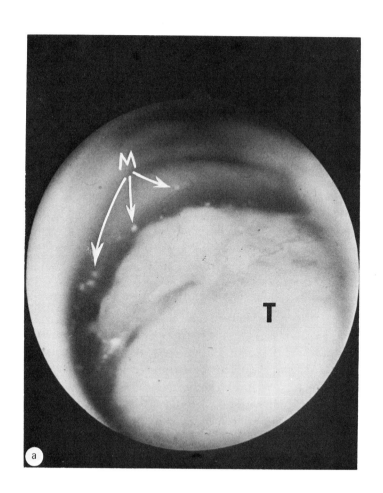

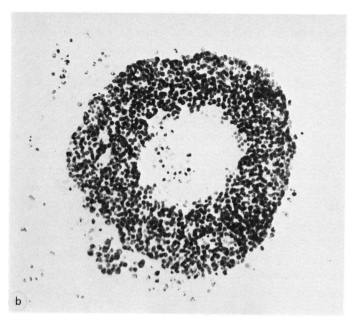

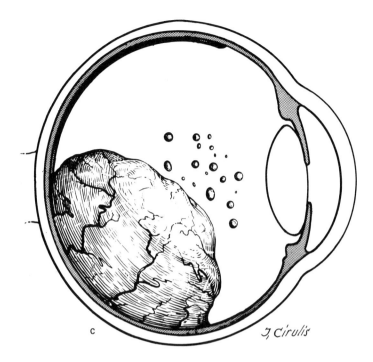

FIGURE 4. (a) A retinal tumor (T) as viewed through an opthalmosscope in a child. The tumor fills the vitreous space. Above this tumor are small vitreous metastases (M) suspended throughout the vitreous. (b) Microsection of one of the spheroids of retinoblastoma. Hematoxylin and eosin; ×240 reduced 20% for reproduction. (c) Vascularized tumor and avascular metastases. From Folkman (1974*b*) with permission of the publisher.

described how tumors increase their malignant characteristics during repeated propagation. With continued cell proliferation, daughter cells gradually increase their growth rate, lose signs of differentiation, become independent of certain growth-regulating factors, become heterotransplantable, and eventually grow in suspension culture. Malignant drift seems to be a function of the number of cell divisions, and occurs in steps. Because the number of mitosing cells is so much higher in the vascular tumor than in the avascular phase, it would be expected that vascularization might expedite malignant progression. For this reason, a tumor kept in the avascular phase for a long period might not progress or drift. This hypothesis has not yet been tested experimentally.

The sudden shift to rapid growth after vascularization raises the question of mechanism. Why is it that a new capillary precipitates such rapid tumor growth on penetrating the tumor? One explanation is that tumor cells tend to grow in the configuration of a capillary unit. Tannock and Steel (1969) have shown that tumor cells are found a mean distance of approximately $100\,\mu m$ from the nearest open capillary. Thomlinson and Gray (1955) have pointed out that the oxygen diffusion distance for most tissues is about $150\,\mu m$. From our own studies (Brem and Folkman, 1975), we know that a tumor-induced capillary may grow as fast as 0.8 mm/day. A cylinder of tumor with a $150\,\mu m$ radius surrounding a capillary of

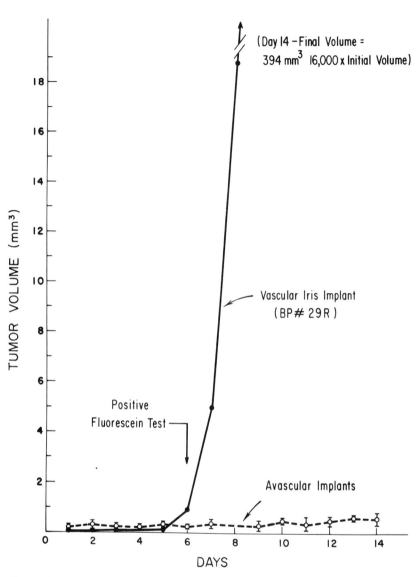

FIGURE 5. A Brown–Pearce tumor implanted on the iris suddenly grows exponentially after it is vascularized. By comparison, the mean daily volumes of ten avascular tumors in the anterior chamber remain small. The onset of vascularization is indicated by the positive fluorescein test on day 6. From Gimbrone *et al.* (1972) with permission of the publisher.

1.0 mm may contain up to 10^4 tumor cells (Fig. 6). From a series of histological sections of experimental and human tumors, we have estimated that a capillary of 1 mm length contains approximately 20–100 endothelial cells. Therefore, if the capillary elongates by the length of one endothelial cell, approximately 100 new tumor cells can be supported. Thus vascularization is an amplification step by which each new capillary permits a burst of new tumor growth. Knasek (1974) has

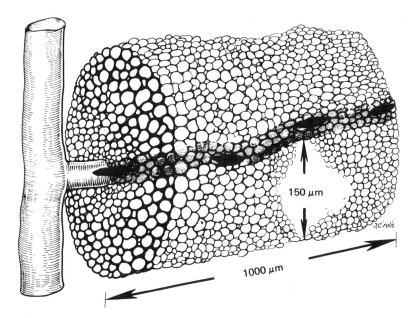

FIGURE 6. Depiction of tumor cells growing in a capillary unit. Since a relatively small number of endothelial cells are required to make a capillary which supports a much larger population of tumor cells, an amplification step exists. Because of this amplification step, the inhibition of a few endothelial cells would bring about growth cessation in a larger tumor population.

demonstrated an *in vitro* model of this principle. Cells were cultured on semipermeable membranes in the shape of capillaries 200 μm in diameter. Cell densities attained within the capillary culture units were similar to those of solid tissue *in vivo*, i.e., approximately 10^8 cells/cm³ of tissue. This amplification step can, however, be viewed as a potential control point, as will be described below. For every endothelial cell inhibited, a hundredfold reduction in tumor cell population may occur.

4. Humoral Mediation of Tumor Angiogenesis

If in fact tumor growth is so dependent on neovascularization, then it is essential to understand the mechanism by which neovascularization is induced. For more than 100 years, pathologists have noted that increased numbers of blood vessels are associated with solid tumors (Virchow, 1863; Goldman, 1907; Lewis, 1927; Hasegawe, 1934; Ide *et al.*, 1939; Urbach, 1961; Day, 1964). In 1945, Algire and Chalkley emphasized that malignant tumors could continuously elicit new capillaries from the host, and that this in some way might underlie the autonomous growth of these tumors. However, until the 1960s the literature on tumor angiogenesis was mainly descriptive and not mechanistic. In 1968, Greenblatt and Shubik first suggested that a diffusible material might be responsible for induction of neovascularization. Tumors separated from the vascular bed of the hamster cheek pouch by a Millipore filter induced new vessels. This was confirmed by Ehrmann and Knoth (1968) and also demonstrated in the CAM by Gitterman and Luell (1969). We have observed the phenomenon in subcutaneous air sacs of the rat back. These studies implied that a diffusible material from the tumor crossed the filter. But there were two other possible explanations. The filter was only 25 μm thick, and it could be argued that cytoplasmic processes of tumor cells could contact endothelial cells through the pores. Second, it was possible that the vascular response beneath the filter represented only vasodilation, not true capillary proliferation. In a series of papers, we demonstrated that the vascular response was true capillary proliferation and that endothelial DNA synthesis and mitosis preceded the sprouting of new capillaries (Cavallo et al., 1972, 1973). We also showed that tumor stimulation of capillary proliferation can operate over distances greater than the thickness of a Millipore filter (Gimbrone et al., 1972, 1973d, 1974b).

The maximum distance between the edge of a tumor and the vessels it stimulated was found to be 2.5 mm in the rabbit cornea, 3 mm in the subcutaneous air sac of the rat, and 5 mm in the anterior chamber of the rabbit eye.

4.1. Tumor Angiogenesis Factor

We have isolated a diffusible factor secreted by tumor cells which is mitogenic to vascular endothelium and stimulates capillary proliferation. Tumor angiogenesis factor (TAF) has been found in the nuclei and cytoplasm of solid and ascites experimental tumors, and also in human tumors (Folkman et al., 1971; Folkman, 1974a). The cytoplasmic form was originally obtained by cell disruption followed by Sephadex chromatography. The nucleus was found to contain angiogenesis activity in the nonhistone pool of chromatin proteins (Tuan et al., 1973). The histone proteins and DNA were free of TAF activity. More recently, we have found cell disruption to be unnecessary. TAF can be obtained from tumor cells in culture by replacing the medium with Ringer's solution for 3 h (Folkman, 1974c). The Ringer's solution is then dialyzed against distilled water and lyophilized. The resultant protein pool contains angiogenesis activity and is used as the crude starting material for purification. At this writing, purification is still in progress and characterization has not been completed. However, a variety of mouse, rat, and human tumor lines have been shown to secrete TAF (Folkman and Klagsbrun, 1975) (Table 1). A long-established "normal" cell line, the WI-38, produced TAF in culture. However, primary mouse embryo or human neonatal fibroblasts in culture did not produce TAF (Table 2). It is possible that long-established cell lines may make biochemical transformations in culture to produce TAF without other malignant changes. A variety of normal tissues including mouse placenta, liver, skeletal muscle, and myocardium do not stimulate

TABLE 1

365

TUMOR
ANGIOGENESIS

Species	Cells giving positive TAF response[a]	Minimum number of cells to obtain positive assay
Mouse	BALB/c 3T3 embryo[b]	3×10^6
	BALB/c SVT-2 (SV40 virus transformed 3T3)	3×10^6
	B-16 melanoma	5×10^6
Rat	Walker 256	6×10^6
Human	WI-38 embryonic lung (passage 24)	4×10^6
	SVWI-26 (SV40 virus transformed WI-26)	4×10^6
	Glioblastoma	10^6
	Meningioma	10^5
	HeLa[c]	N.D.[d]

[a] As measured by bioassay on chick embryo chorioallantoic membrane. Cells are exponentially growing in T-75 tissue culture flasks.
[b] Contact-inhibited cell line but grows as tumor on CAM.
[c] Positive for cells grown in suspension but negative for cells grown as monolayer.
[d] No data.

angiogenesis in the cornea or the CAM. Allogeneic lymph node grafts may produce delayed hypersensitivity in the cornea followed by weak neovascularization (Auerbach, 1974b). Syngeneic nodes from the same rabbit do not stimulate angiogenesis.

4.2. Bioassay for Tumor Angiogenesis Factor

The chorioallantoic membrane of the 9- to 10-day chick embryo is used to assay fractions for TAF activity. Fertile eggs are washed with formalin (1 : 4000), allowed to air dry, and wiped with povidone-iodine (Betadine). One milliliter of albumin is aspirated on day 3. A window is made in the shell on day 5 or 6 as described by Leighton (1967), so that the chorioallantoic membrane drops away from the shell. The window is covered with cellophane tape. On day 9 or 10, a $\frac{1}{2}$-mm sliver of Millipore filter ($25 \mu m$ thick) is placed on the CAM, where it adheres. Fractions to be tested are sterilized by Millipore filtration and

TABLE 2

Species	Cells giving negative TAF response	Maximum number of cells tested which still gave negative response[a]
Mouse	BALB/c primary embryo	$>6 \times 10^6$
Human	Skin fibroblast (passage 11)	$>10^7$

[a] Might be higher but not tested.

366

T.A.F. ASSAY on C.A.M.

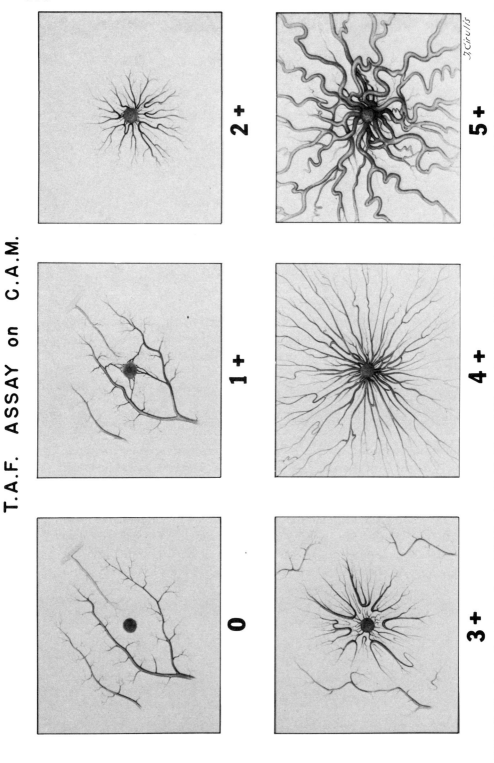

0

1 +

2 +

3 +

4 +

5 +

FIGURE 7. The chorioallantoic membrane (CAM) at days 13–15. A 1-mm Millipore disc soaked in TAF fraction is placed over a tiny hole in the CAM made with a No. 30 needle. New vascular loops, mostly capillaries and small venules, converge on the disc if the fraction is active. The density of these new vessels is assigned a grade of 0 to 5+. From Knighton et al. (unpublished data).

lyophilized. A tiny crystal is placed on the CAM at the edge of the Millipore filter, and a hole is punched in the membrane with a No. 30 hypodermic needle. After 48–72 h, new vessels begin to converge toward the implant site. Their density is graded on a scale of 0 to 5+ (Fig. 7). Alternatively, concentrated solutions of the test fraction can be soaked into the Millipore filter. Up to 50–100 eggs can be used per day. In a study of tumor vascularization in the chick embryo, Knighton *et al.* (1975) found that tumors implanted from day 3 (yolk sac vessels) up to day 12 (CAM vessels 5–12) induced capillary proliferation and were generally vascularized by 72 h. However, when TAF fractions were implanted at various days, the converging network of vessels was not discernible until these fractions were implanted on day 9 or 10. Ausprunk *et al.* (1974) have shown that the vessels in the yolk are growing at ceiling rates (labeling index 23%) until day 11, when normal growth suddenly slows and the labeling index decreases to 2.8%. It is possible that the rapidly growing young CAM cannot display the effect of an additional stimulus to capillary proliferation until its own normal growth has slowed.

The rabbit cornea can also be used. A 1-mm pocket is made in the cornea in anesthetized rabbits as previously described (Gimbrone *et al.*, 1974b) (Fig. 8). The

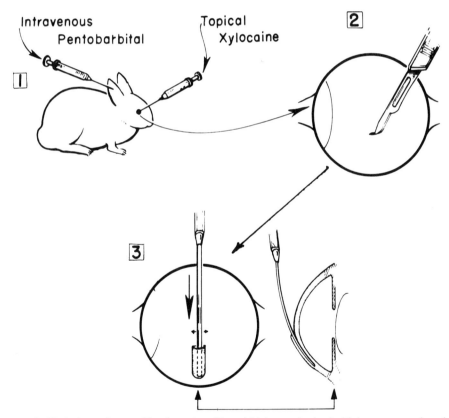

FIGURE 8. Technique of corneal implantation. The rabbit is anesthetized with intravenous phenobarbital and xylocaine applied topically to the cornea. An incision is made halfway through the thickness of the cornea. An intrastromal pocket is made with a malleable iris spatula. The pocket ends approximately 1–2 mm from the limbus. Tumor fragments are inserted into the pocket. From Gimbrone *et al.* (1974b) with permission of the publisher.

test fraction is inserted in the pocket. This method is more quantitative than the CAM because vessel growth rates can be measured daily. But it has the disadvantage of expense and also that test fractions can diffuse out of the pocket and thus may have to be absorbed in slow-release polymers before implantation. However, the corneal pocket is excellent for testing angiogenesis capacity of tissues from many species.

5. Biology of Tumor Angiogenesis Factor

5.1. Relation to Mitotic Index (Effect of X-Irradiation)

The capacity of a tumor to induce angiogenesis or to secrete TAF in culture is not inhibited by X-ray irradiation sufficient to stop mitosis but not to kill the tumor cell. Auerbach *et al.* (1975) irradiated free grafts of tumor tissue before implantation into either the chorioallantoic membrane or the rabbit cornea. Tumor grafts which received 2000 or 4000 r did not grow, but did induce capillary proliferation at the same rate elicited by nonirradiated tumors. Normal tissues, whether irradiated or not, did not initiate capillary proliferation (Tables 3 and 4). Reduction in angiogenesis activity was not observed until tumor grafts were irradiated with 16,000 r. When the tumor grafts were killed by freezing or heating, no angiogenesis activity was present. These studies imply that TAF synthesis may continue in the absence of mitosis. Until recently, many investigators believed that tumor neovascularization was a nonspecific effect of higher metabolism and increased release of metabolic products, because fast-growing tumors seem to induce more capillary proliferation. This is shown not to be the case because mitotic activity can be dissociated from angiogenesis capacity by irradiation of the graft. It is important to note that the *vascular bed* was not irradiated in these experiments. In conventional radiotherapy of solid tumors, the vascular endothelium and the tumor cell population are both exposed to irradiation. Theoretically, the radiosensitivity of the endothelium should be maximized during stimulation by TAF, and also because the endothelium is well oxygenated at least in peripheral vessels. The continued stimulation and proliferation of endothelial cells throughout the course of radiotherapy may account in

TABLE 3
Irradiated Tumor Graft: Ability to Induce Angiogenesis in Cornea[a]

| Tissue | Number positive/total | |
	No irradiation	4000 r
V2 carcinoma	10/10	14/16
Muscle (rabbit)	0/4	0/4
Placenta (13-day mouse)	0/3	0/4

[a] From Auerbach *et al.* (1975) with permission of the publisher.

TABLE 4

369

TUMOR

ANGIOGENESIS

TABLE 4
Irradiated Tumor Graft: Ability to Induce Angiogenesis on CAM[a]

Tissue	Number positive/total		
	No irradiation	2000 r	4000 r
Walker sarcoma	9/10	14/19	7/8
Mouse teratoma	8/11	5/6	6/6
Mouse melanoma	5/6	4/5	5/5
V2 carcinoma	7/7	7/8	
Mouse placenta	0/7	0/7	
Mouse muscle	0/4	0/2	

[a] From Auerbach *et al.* (1975) with permission of the publisher.

part for its success. As endothelial cells are killed by radiation, the tumor should shrink just as it would if vascular proliferation were stopped by any other means. However, unless every tumor cell is killed, a tumor reduced to the avascular state may be able to revascularize itself after a prolonged time. Revascularization may occur even though every cell is not in the cell cycle. Escape from radiotherapy would depend (1) on the time required to regenerate new vascular endothelium and (2) on the distance of competent endothelial cells from surviving avascular tumor cells.

5.2. Correlation with Malignant Progression

Gimbrone and Gullino (1974) have demonstrated that certain preneoplastic tissues can induce vasoproliferation in a manner similar to that of tumors (see Chapter 12, this volume). This capacity for neovascularization occurred before malignant transformation as measured by morphological and biochemical criteria. They demonstrated a correlation between this neovascular capacity and the predicted tumorigenic potential of a given preneoplastic tissue. They studied a strain of C3H mice with a high incidence of spontaneous mammary cancer; angiogenesis capacity of the mammary tissues was tested by implanting them on the iris of the rabbit eye. Normal mammary tissues did not induce capillary proliferation. Two types of hyperplastic nodules developed: the D-1 line, with a 2–9% incidence of transforming into a tumor, and the D-2 line, with a 45–60% incidence of transforming into a tumor. Both lines were similar morphologically and cytochemically. Yet 32% of the D-1 implants exhibited neovascular capacity while 76% of the D-2 implants exhibited neovascular capacity. When mammary carcinomas appeared, virtually all of them induced vasoproliferation, regardless of their histological classification. The neovascular response was not inhibited by corticosteroid treatment. Fragments of grossly necrotic mammary carcinomas produced no detectable changes in iris vessels. If carcinogenesis is a multistage process, then the production of TAF or the capacity to induce neovascularization may be an early step in the progression to malignancy. These studies imply that

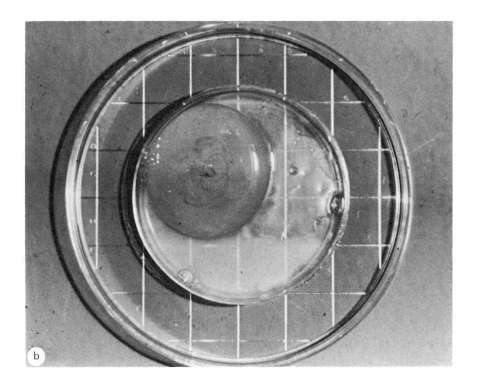

TUMOR

9 cm

74.6 cm

a

J. Cirulis

b

FIGURE 9. (a) Petri dish technique for long-term cultivation of chick embryo. Contents of 3-day embryo are placed in the bottom of a 20- by 100-mm plastic petri dish by cracking the shell against the dish. The dish is placed inside a larger petri dish (25 by 150 mm) containing a thin layer of water for humidification. The larger dish is covered and placed in a humidified incubator at 37°C. Rapid fresh air circulation is essential. (b) Initial culture, 3.5 days of prior incubation. (c) A 7.5-day embryo; developing chorioallantoic membrane is in the center. (d) An 11.5-day embryo; chorioallantoic membrane now covers entire petri dish surface. From Auerbach *et al.* (1974) with permission of the publisher.

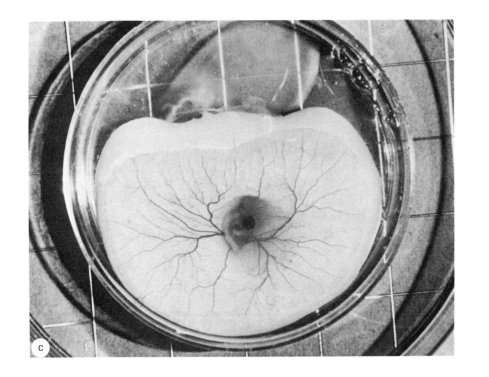

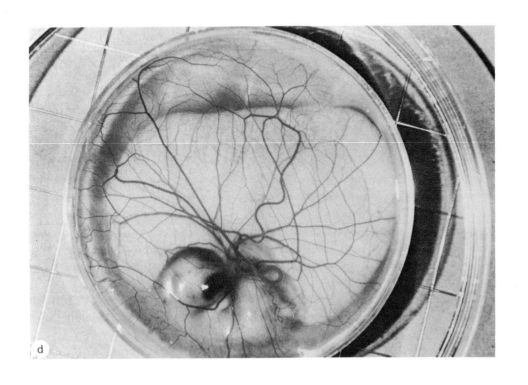

TAF begins to be secreted by a cell destined to become malignant prior to any morphological indication of malignancy. This is additional evidence that TAF release and mitotic rate operate independently. A similar mechanism may be functioning in tissue culture. Established lines of so-called normal cells may begin to produce TAF in culture before they have expressed other characteristics of spontaneous transformation.

5.3. Relation to Host Immunity

From recent studies, we know that expression of tumor angiogenesis is also independent of the state of host immunocompetence. Chick embryos were cultured in petri dishes by a new technique that permits accurate observation, from day 3 to days 17–18, of the vascularization of tumor implants (Auerbach *et al.*, 1974). Tumors implanted on yolk sac vessels on day 3 stimulated new capillaries at the same rate and were vascularized at the same time as tumors later implanted to day 15 on the CAM. Similar results were obtained with embryos which remained in their shells (Knighton *et al.*, 1975). The immune system does not develop until after days 12–14 of embryonation (Auerbach, 1974*a*). This study implies that tumor angiogenesis operates independently of delayed hypersensitivity. It also suggests that the vascular component of delayed hypersensitivity may be mediated by another mechanism (Fig. 9).

6. Biology of Proliferating Capillaries

6.1. Formation of New Capillaries

Capillary proliferation occurs infrequently during adult life of an animal. The vascular endothelium is a relatively quiescent tissue compared to the bone marrow or other high-speed renewal systems. The [^{3}H]thymidine labeling index of endothelium in adult rats is 0.5% or less (Spaet and Lejnieks, 1967). Engerman *et al.* (1967) found the labeling index in the myocardium to be 0.13%, while it was only 0.01% in the retina. Zones of increased endothelial turnover are known to occur in large vessels near areas of turbulence such as aortic coarctation. Bursts of capillary proliferation occur only infrequently: when wounds heal, during some forms of chronic inflammation, and occasionally during delayed hypersensitivity.

When capillary proliferation begins, the morphological events are similar no matter what the stimulus. The major difference between tumor-induced new capillaries and embryonic capillaries or those proliferating in response to a wound or inflammation is that tumor-induced vessels grow faster and continuously. The most rapidly growing vessels in the CAM of the chick embryo may reach a peak labeling index of 23% (Ausprunk *et al.*, 1974). In the neighbourhood of a tumor implant, whether among developing vessels or mature vessels, the labeling index may be 37% or more.

The major event in the formation of a new capillary is budding of the side wall of a small venule or other capillary. Prior to this, arterioles dilate, capillaries become engorged (Schoefl, 1963; Yamaura and Sato, 1973), and endothelial cells synthesize new DNA in preparation for mitosis (Cavallo *et al.*, 1973). At about this time, the basement membrane of the blood vessel becomes fragmented as though lysed. The budlike processes become blind sprouts. These sprouts anastomose with each other to form loops through which blood begins to circulate in one direction. The tips of the newly formed sprouts invade the avascular area, often arranging themselves parallel to each other. This is especially well illustrated where capillaries advance toward a tumor like railway tracks. There may be a hemorrhagic band at the tip of each sprout, but most sprouts are sealed at their end. The growth of a new vessel depends not only on endothelial mitosis but also on the ability of endothelial cells to migrate. Yamagami (1970) did an electron microscopic study of new vessels in the cornea induced by inflammatory agents. Endothelial cells at the very tip of an advancing capillary were migrating forward. Endothelial mitosis was occurring several cells distant from the tip. Ryan (1973) also has emphasized the importance of endothelial migration in capillary proliferation. This may explain why relatively few endothelial cells are required to produce a capillary 1 mm long.

When a wound heals or its edges contract together, capillary proliferation ceases. By contrast, tumor vessels are continuously elicited unless the tumor is completely killed. Also, capillary proliferation induced by tumor is not accompanied by inflammation (Cavallo *et al.*, 1972; Fauve *et al.*, 1974). In fact, a cornea with tumor-induced new vessels is almost always free of edema and cellular infiltrate.

The mean rate of capillary growth in the cornea containing tumor is 0.3 mm/day (Folkman, 1974c). However, as the vessels approach the tumor, they may increase their growth rate to 0.61 ± 0.14 mm/day (Brem and Folkman, 1975). Newly formed vessels regress when TAF or tumor or other stimulus is removed. We have observed this in the cornea. Capillaries 2 mm or longer will fade away completely over a period of 1–2 wk. While new capillaries seem to have a short half-life, little is known about the mechanism of this regression, nor has it been quantitated. It is not known what determines whether new vessels will mature or acquire smooth muscle and remain in the area they have entered.

Little is known about the mediation of capillary proliferation in chronic inflammation or in delayed hypersensitivity. However, sensitized lymphoid cells may play a role in the neovascular component of delayed hypersensitivity. Sidky and Auerbach (1975) showed that syngeneic lymph node grafts to the subcutaneous space of mice and to the cornea (Auerbach, 1974b) of rabbits did not induce neovascularization. However, allogeneic grafts induced a weak neovascular response. Allogeneic lymph node grafts from athymic nude mice did not induce neovascularization. Graham and Shannon (1972) showed that endothelial cells incorporated [³H]thymidine on exposure to lymphoid cells passing through the vascular wall in experimental immune arthritis.

Although both embryonic tissues and tumors become vascularized after transplantation as free grafts, there are some major differences in how this happens. Ausprunk *et al.* (1975) have recently clarified this issue with a study of adult and embryonic rat tissues which were grafted to the CAM of the chick embryo. A comparison was made with grafts of the rat tumor Walker carcinosarcoma 256. All grafts were 1 mm or less and were observed daily by stereomicroscopy, *in vivo* by colloidal carbon injections to determine the precise onset of graft circulation, and by histological sections of [^{3}H]thymidine-labeled autoradiographs. Adult tissues were skeletal muscle, heart, liver, and kidney from 5-wk-old rats. Embryonic tissues were limb bud, heart, liver, and kidney obtained from 15- to 17-day rat embryos and chorioallantoic membrane and heart from 7- and 11-day chick embryos.

The results are summarized in Fig. 10. In tumor tissue, preexisting blood vessels within the tumor graft disintegrated by 24 h after implantation. Revascularization did not occur until at least day 3 and only by penetration of proliferating *host* vessels in the neighborhood of the tumor graft. By contrast, in the embryonic graft, preexisting vessels did *not* disintegrate. They anastomosed to host vessels within 24–48 h. There was minimal or no neovascularization on the part of the host vessels. No embryonic tissue was able to stimulate neovasculariza-

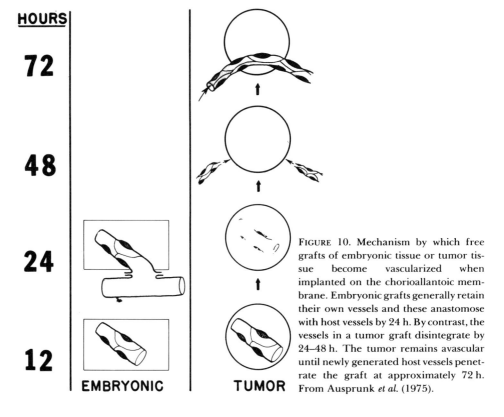

HOURS

72

48

24

12

EMBRYONIC　**TUMOR**

FIGURE 10. Mechanism by which free grafts of embryonic tissue or tumor tissue become vascularized when implanted on the chorioallantoic membrane. Embryonic grafts generally retain their own vessels and these anastomose with host vessels by 24 h. By contrast, the vessels in a tumor graft disintegrate by 24–48 h. The tumor remains avascular until newly generated host vessels penetrate the graft at approximately 72 h. From Ausprunk *et al.* (1975).

tion in the host! In adult tissues, the preexisting graft vessels disintegrated, although this took longer than tumor vessels, i.e., 9 days. Also, adult tissues did not stimulate capillary proliferation in the host. There was *no* reattachment of their circulation with the host.

When adult tissues were compared to tumor grafts, both developed central necrosis, and in both the preexisting vessels disintegrated. New vessels grew only into the tumor, at which time the necrotic center was replaced with viable tumor. The adult graft was unable to stimulate new vessels, and the necrotic center persisted, leaving only a thin rim of viable tissue.

This study indicates that only tumor grafts acquire their blood supply solely by stimulating formation of new blood vessels from the host. By contrast, revascularization of normal tissue grafts, when it does occur, is predominantly the result of fusion of preexisting vessels with the host circulation.

6.3. Vascular Endothelium in Vitro

We have cultured vascular endothelium in this laboratory for the past 3 years (Sade *et al.*, 1972). If endothelium could be stimulated by TAF to proliferate in culture, an *in vitro* assay for TAF might be feasible. Human endothelial cells from the umbilical vein have been carried in culture (Gimbrone *et al.*, 1973*a,b,c*, 1974*a*) by modification of a method first described by Jaffe *et al.* (1972).

Primary endothelial cells form a monolayer of uniform polygonal cells within 1 wk. They are characterized as endothelial cells by the presence of Weibel–Palade bodies (Weibel and Palade, 1964), pinocytotic vesicles, small amounts of 60 Å fibrils located at the periphery of the cells, 100 Å fibrils located close to the nuclei, rod-shaped nuclei which only rarely show branching, and ellipsoid nuclei having a fine granular pattern of chromatin. One to three distinct nucleoli are present in each nucleus (Haudenschild *et al.*, 1975*a,b*). These cells exhibit a unique pattern of growth in that they synthesize DNA only when subconfluent. The percentage of [^{3}H]thymidine-labeled cells in sparse cultures may be as high as 40%. However, in confluent cultures the percent of labeled nuclei is less than 3%. This cannot be increased by any concentration of calf or human serum. By contrast, confluent cultures of Balb/c-3T3 cells and primary human foreskin fibroblasts will increase their labeling index to 80% after stimulation with fresh serum. Thus endothelial cells *in vitro* are under a particularly stringent form of growth control. So far, we have not been able to directly stimulate endothelial cells *in vitro* with purified preparations of TAF or with tumor cell supernates, although these are active in *in vivo* assays. This suggests that TAF may stimulate endothelial proliferation *in vivo* by an indirect route. For example, TAF might stimulate some other cell to release a specific protease which induces endothelial proliferation. On the other hand, it is possible that these cultured endothelial cells from umbilical vein may be different than those at the level of capillaries and venules. We do not know if endothelium of large veins can be stimulated by tumor *in vivo*. At this writing, endothelial cultures are not useful as an *in vitro* assay for TAF.

7.1. Potential Approaches to Antiangiogenesis

It is apparent from Fig. 11 that vascularization acts like a switch, permitting a solid tumor to display its full potential for growth. Once vascularization takes place, a tumor will tend to grow rapidly. Its maximum rate is probably determined genetically and modified, if at all, by host factors, such as immune status and nutrition. From a conventional therapeutic standpoint, after vascularization has occurred most tumors are beyond the point of no return.

By contrast, the avascular phase is restrictive to growth. Dormancy is the rule; full growth potential cannot be expressed. When the avascular state is prolonged, the tiny dormant tumor may be extremely vulnerable to host defenses which would be inadequate for the vascularized tumor. Experimental tumors main-

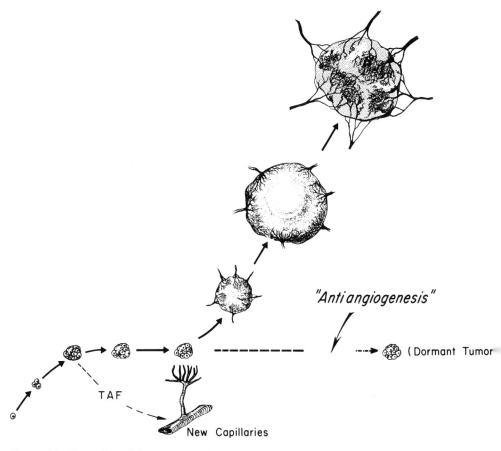

FIGURE 11. Illustration of three concepts basic to tumor growth: (1) Solid tumors pass through an avascular and a vascular stage. (2) New host capillaries are stimulated by a humoral factor (TAF) released by the tumor. Rapid growth follows. (3) If this humoral signal is inhibited, or if capillaries are prevented from penetrating the tumor, further growth is blocked and the tumor enters a dormant phase. Antiangiogenesis implies a possible therapeutic approach. From Folkman (1974c) with permission of the publisher.

tained in the avascular state for months were eventually rejected immunologically
when vascularization did occur (Brem and Folkman, 1975). Yet, under usual
conditions, when the avascular period was only a few days, carcinoma used in this
system has never spontaneously regressed. In Petersen's (1956) study of women
with untreated carcinoma of the cervix *in situ*, more than 60% of the *in situ* lesions
remained stationary for up to 10 years or regressed without ever vascularizing.
Therefore, any means of preventing capillary proliferation induced by tumor
might prolong the avascular state indefinitely. The already vascularized tumor
might be forced to return to the avascular, *in situ* state. We have proposed the term
"antiangiogenesis" for a therapeutic approach based on this principle (Folkman,
1971, 1972, 1975).

Therefore, it would seem prudent to examine the ways in which tumor-induced
capillary proliferation might be inhibited.

At this writing, we can envision at least four points in the interaction between
tumor and vascular endothelium, at which angiogenesis might be interrupted
(Fig. 12). There may well be others.

7.1.1. Interruption of TAF Synthesis

Interruption of TAF synthesis represents an unknown area. The site of synthesis
and the structure of TAF are as yet unknown. At present, there are no compounds
which will inhibit synthesis of TAF. Eventually this may be feasible.

7.1.2. Inhibition of TAF Directly While It Is in Transit

Inhibition of TAF directly while it is in transit might be accomplished with a
specific anti-TAF antibody. Such an antibody would diffuse from the bloodstream

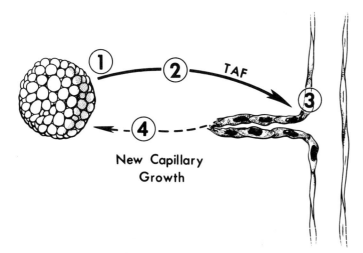

FIGURE 12. Four points at which tumor angiogenesis might theoretically be
interrupted: (1) Interruption of TAF synthesis. (2) Neutralization of TAF
after its release from a tumor. (3) Prevention of endothelial cell proliferation and migration. (4) Prevention of vessels from penetrating a tumor.
From Folkman (1974c) with permission of the publisher.

and theoretically neutralize TAF before it reached the endothelium. It is also possible that TAF requires some intermediate cell for its activity, or that TAF has to be activated in some way before it reaches vessels. This is still conjecture, but it is a potential point of inhibition.

7.1.3. Prevention of Endothelial Mitosis

TAF is mitogenic to endothelial cells only. If they possess a unique receptor for TAF, an inactive analogue of TAF might be used as an inhibitor. Alternatively, a general inhibitor for capillary proliferation would accomplish the same effect, without necessarily blocking TAF. We have recently extracted such an inhibitor from cartilage (Brem and Folkman, 1975). This is described below. Endothelial cells can be injured by circulating endotoxin (McGrath and Stewart, 1969). Some cases of tumor regressions following gram-negative infection may be explained on the basis of circulating endotoxin (Parr *et al.*, 1973).

7.1.4. Prevention of Tumor Penetration by Vessels

After new capillaries have formed, they might possibly be prevented from reaching the tumor. For example, iris vessels proliferate in response to a tumor suspended in the anterior chamber of the eye. Vessels never reach the tumor because they cannot grow through the aqueous humor. Alternatively, a specific inhibitor of endothelial cell migration might prevent tumor vascularization, because cell migration is such an important component of capillary advance.

Once a tumor is vascularized and has grown, it is still possible that inhibition of endothelial proliferation at that point might lead to capillary regression followed by tumor regression. The short half-life of proliferating capillaries may be the reason.

Furthermore, it is possible that agents which cause endothelial cells within tumor vessels to differentiate or mature might slow tumor growth or prevent metastases (LeServe and Hellmann, 1972).

By whatever mechanism antiangiogenesis can be achieved, our experimental studies of tumor growth in the isolated perfused organ (Folkman *et al.*, 1963, 1966; Folkman, 1970; Folkman and Gimbrone, 1971), the anterior eye chamber, the chick embryo, and soft agar indicate that tumors held in the avascular state should remain dormant. An example of our recent experimental application of antiangiogenesis is described below.

7.2. Inhibition of Angiogenesis by a Diffusible Factor from Cartilage

Human embryonic cartilage is known to be vascularized, but vessels disappear in the early neonatal period (Haraldsson, 1962; Blackwood, 1965). A possible explanation is that a factor inhibitory for capillary proliferation might be turned on during the maturation of neonatal cartilage. Eisenstein *et al.* (1973) have reported that cartilage placed on the chorioallantoic membrane did not become vascularized. Recently, we have shown that tumor-induced vessels are inhibited by a diffusible factor from neonatal rabbit cartilage (Brem and Folkman, 1975; Brem *et al.*, 1975). Keuttner *et al.* (1975) have demonstrated that endothelial cells in culture are inhibited by a factor isolated from cartilage.

In our studies (Brem and Folkman, 1975), Walker carcinosarcoma or TAF obtained from the Walker tumor was implanted on the chorioallantoic membrane as a source of neovascularization. A 1-mm piece of neonatal cartilage from rabbit scapula was implanted 1–2 mm from the neovascularizing source. An avascular zone of 1–2 mm width developed around the cartilage (Fig. 13). A similar experiment was repeated in the rabbit cornea, in order to quantitate the inhibitory effect of cartilage on vessel growth. Pieces of neonatal rabbit cartilage (1.0 by 1.5 mm) were implanted in a pocket made in the corneal stroma. V2 carcinoma (1.5 by 1.5 mm) was also implanted in the pocket according to the configuration in Fig. 14. Controls for the active cartilage included cartilage which was boiled, pieces of neonatal cornea of the same size as the cartilage implant, and fragments of neonatal bone. Each cornea was examined every other day with a slit-lamp stereomicroscope. One hundred and forty-four corneas were studied. Measurements of the growth rate of new vessels were made with an accuracy of ±0.1 mm. The results are summarized in Figs. 15 and 16. In every case, tumor grew slowly as a thin intracorneal plate. It remained avascular until one edge grew within

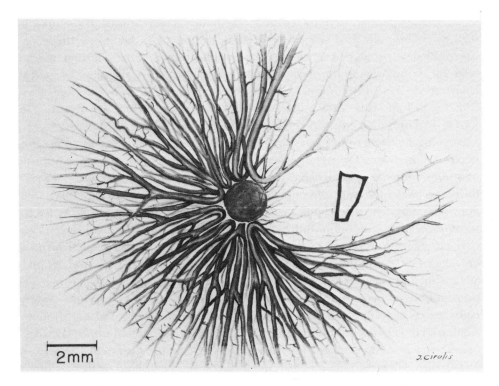

FIGURE 13. Diagram of chorioallantoic membrane. Neovascularization induced by TAF granules (circle in center) is inhibited in the zone which surrounds a fragment of cartilage implanted on the CAM. From Brem and Folkman (1975) with permission of the publisher.

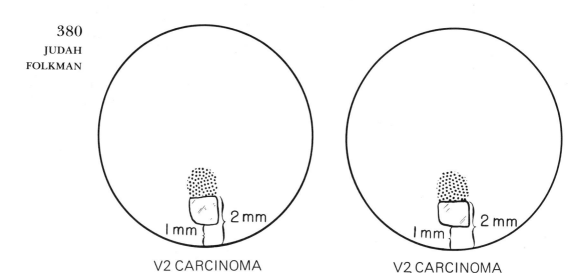

V2 CARCINOMA
+ CARTILAGE

V2 CARCINOMA
+ CONTROL

FIGURE 14. Diagram of rabbit cornea. V2 carcinoma and neonatal rabbit cartilage are implanted together in a corneal pocket. As a control for neonatal cartilage, boiled cartilage, or pieces of neonatal cornea are used. V2 carcinoma is implanted alone as another control.

2.5 ± 0.5 mm of the limbus. At that point, preexisting vessels in the limbus began to proliferate. New capillaries grew toward the tumor. When tumor was alone or with cartilage inactivated by boiling, capillaries grew toward the tumor at 0.22 ± 0.12 mm/day during the first week. By the end of the first week, there were up to 30 new capillaries advancing toward the tumor. The rate increased to 0.48 ± 0.16 mm/day by the second week. Within 3 wk after the onset of neovascularization, all of the tumors were large, exophytic masses enveloping the eye (Fig. 15F). At this time, the capillaries were growing at the rate of 0.61 ± 0.14 mm/day. None of these tumors regressed.

By contrast, when tumor was implanted with active neonatal cartilage, the time of onset of neovascularization was similar to that in corneas containing only tumor or tumor with inactive cartilage control. By the end of the first week, a major difference was observed; the density of vessel growth was less (Fig. 15A). Only approximately five new capillaries were advancing toward the tumor. By the second week, another major difference was observed: as the vessel tips grew close to the cartilage, the rate of vessel growth slowed. The average vessel growth was only 0.12 ± 0.16 mm/day (Figs. 15B and 16). In some corneas, the vessels stopped advancing and regressed. In other corneas, vessels appeared to oscillate between brief periods of growth and regression, but without forward progress. Twenty-eight percent of these tumors had not vascularized by the end of 3 months compared to vascularization times of 3 wk for tumors implanted without cartilage or with inactivated cartilage. The unvascularized tumors eventually underwent immunological rejection. No rejections have ever been seen with this tumor during the 4 years it has been carried in the cornea and intramuscularly in our laboratory.

The remaining tumors implanted intracorneally with cartilage eventually became vascularized. This vascularization resulted from the steady growth of the

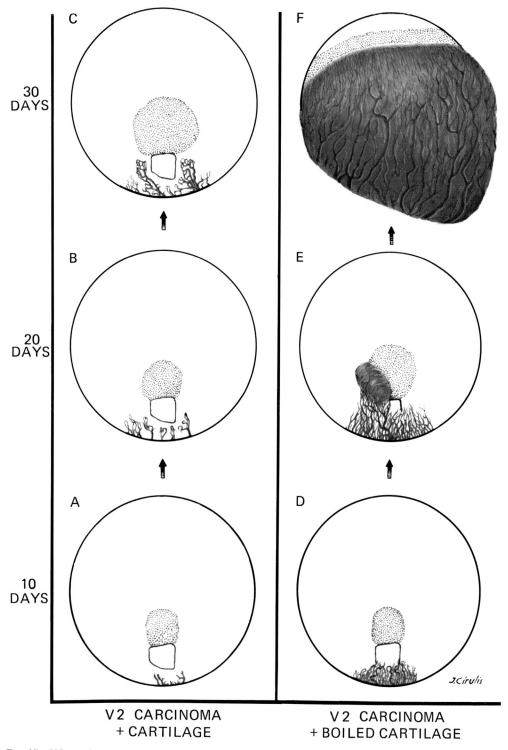

FIG. 15. V2 carcinoma implanted in rabbit corneas with active neonatal cartilage or with boiled cartilage. Scale drawings made by tracing color photographs of the actual specimens. Vessels are inhibited from reaching the tumor when active cartilage is implanted with it (A,B,C). Cartilage inactivated by boiling is implanted with tumor in D. Vessels enter this tumor by day 15 and rapid tumor growth follows (E), leading to a large exophytic mass (F). A similar result (D,E,F) is obtained when the boiled cartilage is replaced by neonatal cornea or when the tumor is implanted alone. The diameter of the cornea is 12 mm. From Brem and Folkman (1975) with permission of the publisher.

tumor plate in two dimensions within the corneal lamellae. Vessels were then elicited at sites of the limbus remote from the cartilage. Once the tumor was vascularized, rapid exponential growth ensued and the cartilage was completely covered by tumor.

In all corneas, the cartilage implant appeared healthy throughout, by histological section. It was not associated with any inflammatory reaction (Fig. 17).

A soluble extract of cartilage has been isolated with the same inhibitory effect in the CAM. Recently, we have shown that newborn calf scapular cartilage has a similar inhibitory effect in the rabbit cornea.

These studies show that a diffusible material released from neonatal cartilage inhibits capillary proliferation induced by tumor. The inhibitory effect operates over short distances of up to 2.0 mm, and displays a gradient from cartilage source to limbal edge of the cornea. The highest concentration of the inhibitor seems to be closest to the cartilage, because capillary tips slow their growth as they approach the cartilage. The inhibitor is effective even in the face of a rising concentration of TAF stimulator which meets the advancing vessels, because the tumor is implanted just beyond the cartilage. The cartilage inhibitor does not appear to neutralize TAF. If this were the case, lesser amounts of TAF should arrive at the limbus. The *onset* of capiillary proliferation in the presence of active cartilage should be delayed. In fact, there was no significant difference between the first appearance of vessels in the corneas containing active cartilage and those containing no cartilage or boiled cartilage. Cartilage appears to continuously produce inhibitor, because the inhibitory effect on capillary growth lasted through the longest observation period of 4 months. At that time, the cartilage appeared viable by histology.

This is the first time to our knowledge that a diffusible material from normal tissue has been shown to inhibit capillary proliferation induced by tumors. The

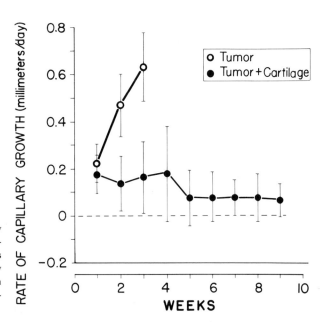

FIGURE 16. Rates of capillary growth with and without cartilage. Note that some vessels exposed to cartilage actually regressed at 4–10 wk. From Brem and Folkman (1975) with permission of the publisher.

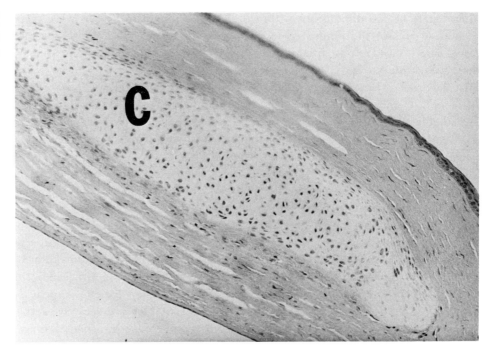

FIGURE 17. Cartilage (C) implant in the rabbit cornea. Hematoxylin and eosin; ×90 reduced 13% for reproduction.

material is not inflammatory in the cornea. When this inhibitory factor is further purified and characterized, it may prove useful as a therapeutic means of maintaining tumor dormancy by "antiangiogenesis" (Folkman, 1971, 1972).

Of further interest is the eventual immunological rejection of V × 2 carcinoma when it is held in the avascular state, especially since this tumor has never been rejected spontaneously in our experience. Immunological rejection was demonstrated by histology. Rechallenge of each animal with fresh tumor implanted in muscle or cornea was followed by tumor rejection.

Two conditions seem necessary for this rejection to proceed: (1) The avascular state must be prolonged beyond the time usually required to vascularize the tumor, in this case more than 3 wk. (2) Vessel tips must be near enough to the edge of the tumor so that immune effector cells can traverse the cornea and reach the tumor. This distance seems to be 0.5 mm or less. Although the normal cornea has no lymphatics, it is known that lymphatics will grow into cornea after vessels have proliferated into it (Collin, 1971). It is possible that lymphatics accompanied the vessels and played a major role in immunization. We did not study lymphatics in these corneas.

The usual avascular period is so short and tumor growth after vascularization so rapid that there may be insufficient time for the host to mount a rejection against a weakly immunogenic tumor. By hurrying through the avascular period into the vascular period of growth, a tumor may escape immune attack.

By contrast, when the avascular period is prolonged in such a way that capillaries are contiguous to the tumor but have not penetrated it, immunization can proceed while tumor growth is restricted! Given time, the immune system may be able to deliver into the avascular tumor enough immune cells, from "offshore capillaries," to kill the tumor (Folkman and Klagsbrun, 1975). The ensuing rejection would be a conventional first-set response. Compare this to an already immunized animal. A fresh tumor implanted in the cornea is rejected at the onset of vascularization, i.e., a second-set response.

It is probable that in tissues other than cornea spontaneously arising tumors or metastases would be surrounded at the start by *contiguous capillaries.* If the capillaries could be prevented from proliferating and penetrating the tumor, then the same conditions might pertain as in the cornea, allowing the immune system sufficient time and providing it with a small enough tumor target for effective rejection.

8. *Theoretical Considerations and Conclusions*

This new information about the mechanism of tumor angiogenesis has also enlarged our understanding of the biology of solid tumor growth. We can now perceive more clearly that fleeting period in the life of a solid tumor when a tiny spheroid of neoplastic cells has yet to be vascularized and is exquisitely vulnerable.

When vascularization proceeds on schedule, a permissive switch is activated, allowing a given tumor to reach its own maximum growth rate. Release of antigens, shedding of metastases, and tumor progression follow, leading to the death of the host.

If vascularization is inhibited and the tumor held in the avascular state, the switch is restrictive. Growth is not permitted beyond a tiny population of cells. It is a population which barely survives, is unable to display its malignant potential, and may be vulnerable to immune rejection by the host.

Tumor angiogenesis is not a side effect. It is not the result of inflammation from necrotic tumor, nor is it a host defense mechanism. Tumor angiogenesis operates independently of mitotic rate and of oxygen tension in tumor cells. It is an essential component of tumor survival. Tumors which induce angiogenesis can be lethal to the host; those incapable of it may be vulnerable to the host.

Tumor angiogenesis is a control point because of a peculiarity of solid tumors themselves. At the onset of neoplasia, the cells of a solid tumor tend to stick together. They crowd each other in a packed population as they grow. Thus they become subject to all the laws of diffusion governing nutrient absorption and waste release which affect the lives of normal cells. It is true that tumor cells may survive lower oxygen tensions and may live in slightly more garbage than normal cells, but these are not the conditions sufficient for massive growth. They are the conditions of the avascular phase, of bare survival, of population dormancy!

Tumor angiogenesis would not be a control point if solid tumor cells proliferated in the circulation as do leukemia cells. But solid tumor cells rarely survive a long trip in the circulation. Tumor angiogenesis would not be a control point if solid tumors all progressed immediately to the ascites state. Few of all known tumors in man ever reach the ascites stage. Hundreds of cell generations are required for tumor progression to the ascites stage. If the first clone of a solid tumor could march through tissues in a straight line, like a needle only a few cells in diameter, tumor angiogenesis would not be a control point. But solid tumors don't behave this way. They tend to grow as spheroids, or ellipsoids, or little balls in most organs. This growth configuration of early solid tumors is their Achilles' heel. Because they form packed aggregates, they are vulnerable through their supply line.

Holley (1972) has proposed that normal cells may maintain their state of growth cessation by keeping certain nutrients (growth factors) out of their cytoplasm. The many genetic and epigenetic regulators of cell growth may act through a final common path: a simple principle, no nutrient...no growth. An avascular population of malignant cells may behave in a similar fashion. Their growth is limited by the availability of nutrients, controlled in the absence of vascularization by ratio of surface area to volume.

In neoplasia new vessels must be induced from the host. Because this induction is humoral and occurs over distances of millimeters, it represents a form of information transfer between malignant tumor and nonmalignant vascular endothelium. Under usual conditions, the vascular endothelium can be viewed as a differentiated, resting population with a low labeling index. This population is turned on and caused to proliferate in response to even a tiny tumor population. The response of capillary endothelium seems to be twofold: (1) *Migration.* Endothelial cells which are at the leading edge of an advancing new capillary migrate toward the tumor implant. In the cornea studies, the rate of migration increases as the capillary tip nears the tumor. This implies that some component of the capillary, perhaps its endothelium, has gradient-sensing ability. (2) *Mitosis.* Tumor also has a mitogenic effect on capillary endothelium. However, it is not yet clear whether TAF induces mitosis directly or whether it must be processed by some other cell. It is also possible that TAF may act solely as a chemotatic stimulus of endothelium at the tip of the capillary. This could lead secondarily to mitosis of other endothelial cells as they became separated from their neighbors. Furthermore, it is not yet clear whether large vessel endothelium will respond to tumor in the same way as capillary endothelium. If there is a difference, it may explain why umbilical vein endothelium in culture does not seem to be turned on with TAF or tumor.

Some pieces of the puzzle are becoming clear, however. For example, the evidence is fairly strong that the majority of normal (nonmalignant tissues) transferred as free grafts *do not* have the capacity to stimulate new capillary growth in the host. Furthermore, the work of Gimbrone and Gullino indicates that the appearance of this capacity for angiogenesis in tumor cells, may be an early event in the stepwise transformation of normal cells to the fully malignant state. Finally, the evidence from Auerbach's work implies that tumor angiogenesis capacity does not seem to be coupled to mitotic rate of the tumor cell. Tumor angiogenesis did not diminish when mitosis was stopped completely. This fact makes a stronger case for the specificity of neovascularization induced by tumor.

Because tumor angiogenesis can be viewed as a control point in tumor growth, there are some obvious therapeutic implications. If it should ever become possible to inhibit or delay tumor angiogenesis on a larger scale than in the cornea model, then it may be feasible that *in-situ* carcinomas could be contained in the avascular stage. From what we know of the rapid turnover of new capillaries, it is possible that an already vascularized tumor may be forced to return to the *in-situ* stage.

An even more fundamental question is whether the growth of normal tissue or embryonic tissue might in fact be controlled by the timing of vascularization or by its density. For example, on a purely theoretical basis, bone length might be regulated by inhibitors of vascularization located in the cartilage. As another example, the epithelial component of epidermis, intestinal mucosa, bladder mucosa, cervix, and other tissues can be viewed as an avascular compartment. Possibly it is this avascular condition which prevents these epithelial populations from proliferating excessively. Suppose that a capillary inhibitor (like the one in cartilage) also exists in the basement membrane which separates avascular epithelial compartments from their blood vessels. If this were the case, then failure of this inhibitor or its loss might be one explanation for neovascularization of the dermis in psoriasis. A similar hypothesis might be applied to other situations of pathologic neovascularization. If articular cartilage or vitreous contain an inhibitor of capillary proliferation, then some forms of neovascularization in arthritis, and vascularization of the vitreous in diabetes, may represent a failure of this inhibitor.

In conclusion, tumor angiogenesis is a powerful control point in the growth of a solid tumor. What has been learned about tumor angiogenesis may also be applicable in other disease states where neovascularization is prominent. A thorough understanding of the mechanism by which tumors induce capillary proliferation may reveal the basis of normal capillary behavior.

ACKNOWLEDGMENTS

This work was supported by Grants CA-14019 from the National Cancer Institute and DT-2A from the American Cancer Society, and also by a gift from the Alza Corporation. We thank Mr. Carl Cobb and Ms. Jane Dittrich for editorial assistance and Mrs. Polly Breen for preparation of the manuscript. The color plate was drawn by Mr. Janis Cirulis.

9. References

ALGIRE, G. H., AND CHALKEY, H. W., 1945, Vascular reactions of normal and malignant tissues *in vivo*. I. Vascular reactions of mice to wounds and to normal and neoplastic transplants, *J. Natl. Cancer Inst.* **6:**73–85.

AUERBACH, R., 1974*a*, Development of immunity, in: *Concepts of Development* (J. Lash and J. R. Whittaker, eds.), pp. 261–271, Sinauer Associates, Stamford, Conn.

AUERBACH, R., 1974*b*, unpublished data.

AUERBACH, R., KUBAI, L., KNIGHTON, D. R., AND FOLKMAN, J., 1974, A simple procedure for the long-term cultivation of chicken embryos, *Dev. Biol.* **41:**391–394.

AUERBACH, R., ARENSMAN, R., KUBAI, L., AND FOLKMAN, J., 1975, Tumor angiogenesis: Lack of inhibition by irradiation, *Int. J. Cancer* **15:**241–245.

AUSPRUNK, D. H., KNIGHTON, D. R., AND FOLKMAN, J., 1974, Differentiation of vascular endothelium in the chick chorioallantois: A structural and autoradiographic study, *Dev. Biol.* **38:**237–248.

AUSPRUNK, D. H., KNIGHTON, D. R., AND FOLKMAN, J., 1975, Vascularization of normal and neoplastic tissues grafted to the chick chorioallantois: Role of host and pre-existing graft blood vessels, *Am. J. Porhol.* **79:**597–610.

BLACKWOOD, H. J. J., 1965, Vascularization of the condylar cartilage of the human mandible, *J. Anat.* **99:**551–563.

BREM, H., AND FOLKMAN, J., 1975, Inhibition of tumor angiogenesis mediated by cartilage, *J. Exp. Med.* **141:**427–439.

BREM, H., ARENSMAN, R., AND FOLKMAN, J., 1975, Inhibition of tumor angiogenesis by a diffusible factor from cartilage in: *Extracellular Matrix Influences on Gene Expression* (H. Slavkin, ed.), pp. 767–772, Academic Press, New York.

CAVALLO, T., SADE, R., FOLKMAN, J., AND COTRAN, R. S., 1972, Tumor angiogenesis: Rapid induction of endothelial mitoses demonstrated by autoradiography, *J. Cell Biol.* **54:**408–420.

CAVALLO, T., SADE, R. M., FOLKMAN, J., AND COTRAN, R. S., 1973, Endothelial regeneration: Ultrastructural and autoradiographic studies of the early proliferative response in tumor angiogenesis, *Am. J. Pathol.* **70:**345–362.

COLLIN, H. B., 1971, The fine structure of growing corneal lymphatics, *J. Pathol.* **104:**99–113.

COTRAN, R. S., AND REMENSYNDER, J. P., 1968, The structural basis of increased vascular permeability after graded thermal injury—Light and electron microscopic studies, *Ann. N.Y. Acad. Sci.* **150:**495–509.

CURRIE, G., 1973, The role of circulating antigen as an inhibitor of tumor immunity in man, *Br. J. Cancer* **28:**153–161 (Suppl. I).

DAY, E. D., 1964, Vascular relationships of tumor and host, in: *Progress in Experimental Tumor Research*, Vol. 4 (F. Homburger, ed.), pp. 58–84, Hafner, New York.

EHRMANN, R. L., AND KNOTH, M., 1968, Choriocarcinoma: Transfilter stimulation of vasoproliferation in the hamster cheek pouch—Studied by light and electron microscopy, *J. Natl. Cancer Inst.* **41:**1329–1341.

EISENSTEIN, R., SORGENTE, N., SOBLE, L. W., MILLER, A., AND KUETTNER, K. E., 1973, The resistance of certain tissues to invasion, *Am. J. Pathol.* **73:**765–774.

ENGERMAN, R. L., PFAFFENBACH, D., AND DAVIES, M. D., 1967, Cell turnover of capillaries, *Lab. Invest.* **17:**738.

FAUVE, R. M., HEVIN, B., JACOB, H., GAILLARD, J. A., AND JACOB, F., 1974, Anti-inflammatory effects of murine malignant cells, *Proc. Natl. Acad. Sci. U.S.A.* **71:**4052–4056.

FOLKMAN, 1970, The intestine as an organ culture, in: *Carcinoma of the Colon and Antecedent Epithelium* (W. J. Burdette, ed.), Chapter 6, Thomas, Springfield, Ill.

FOLKMAN, J., 1971, Tumor angiogenesis: Therapeutic implications, *New Engl. J. Med.* **285:**1182–1186.

FOLKMAN, J., 1972, Anti-angiogenesis: New concept for therapy of solid tumors, *Ann. Surg.* **175:**409–416.

FOLKMAN, J., 1974a, Tumor angiogenesis: Role in regulation of tumor growth, in: *Thirtieth Symposium of the Society for Developmental Biology: Macromolecules Regulating Growth and Development* (E. Hay, ed.), pp. 43–52, Academic Press, New York.

FOLKMAN, J., 1974b, Tumor angiogenesis factor, *Cancer Res.* **34:**2109–2113.

FOLKMAN, J., 1974c, Tumor angiogenesis, in: *Advances in Cancer Research*, Vol. 19 (G. Klein and S. Weinhouse, eds.), pp. 331–358, Academic Press, New York.

FOLKMAN, J., 1975, Tumor angiogenesis: A possible control point in tumor growth, *Ann. Intern. Med.* **82:**96–100.

FOLKMAN, J., AND GIMBRONE, M., 1971, Perfusion of the thyroid, in: *Karolinska Symposia on Research Methods in Reproductive Endocrinology, 4th Symposium: Perfusion Techniques* (E. Diczfalusy, ed.), Karolinska Institutet, Stockholm.

FOLKMAN, J., AND HOCHBERG, M., 1973, Self-regulation of growth in three dimensions, *J. Exp. Med.* **138:**745–753.

FOLKMAN, J., AND KLAGSBRUN, M., 1975, Tumor angiogenesis: Effect on tumor growth and immunity, in: *Symposium on Fundamental Aspects of Neoplasia* (A. Gottlieb, ed.), Rutgers University, New Brunswick, N.J., Springer, New York.

FOLKMAN, J., LONG, D. M., AND BECKER, F. F., 1963, Growth and metastasis of tumor in organ culture, *Cancer* **16:**453–467.

FOLKMAN, J., COLE, P., AND ZIMMERMAN, S., 1966, Tumor behavior in isolated perfused organs: *In vitro* growth and metastases of biopsy material in rabbit thyroid and canine intestinal segment, *Ann. Surg.* **164:**491–502.

FOLKMAN, J., MERLER, E., ABERNATHY, C., AND WILLIAMS, G., 1970, Isolation of a tumor factor responsible for neovascularization, *J. Clin. Invest.* **49:**30a (abst. no. 95, June).

FOLKMAN, J., MERLER, E., ABERNATHY, C., AND WILLIAMS, G., 1971, Isolation of a tumor factor responsible for angiogenesis, *J. Exp. Med.* **133**:275–288.

FOLKMAN, J., HOCHBERG, M., AND KNIGHTON, D., 1974, Self-regulation of growth in three dimensions: The role of surface area limitation, in: *Cold Spring Harbor Symposium: Control of Animal Cell Proliferation* (B. Clarkson and R. Baserga, eds), pp. 833–842, Cold Spring Harbor Laboratory, Cold Spring Harbor, N.Y.

GIMBRONE, M. A., JR., AND GULLINO, P. M., 1975, Neovascularization induced by intraocular xenografts of normal, pre-neoplastic and neoplastic mouse mammary tissues, *J. Nat. Cancer Inst.* in press.

GIMBRONE, M. A., JR., LEAPMAN, S., COTRAN, R. S., AND FOLKMAN, J., 1972, Tumor dormancy *in vivo* by prevention of neovascularization, *J. Exp. Med.* **136**:261–276.

GIMBRONE, M. A., JR., COTRAN, R. S., AND FOLKMAN, J., 1973a, Endothelial regeneration and turnover: Studies with human endothelial cell cultures, *Microvasc. Res.* **6**:249.

GIMBRONE, M. A., JR., COTRAN, R. S., AND FOLKMAN, J., 1973b, Endothelial regeneration: Studies with human endothelium cells in culture, *Ser. Haematol.* **4**:453–459.

GIMBRONE, M. A., JR., COTRAN, R. S., HAUDENSCHILD, C., AND FOLKMAN, J., 1973c, Growth and ultrastructure of human vascular endothelium and smooth muscle cells in culture, *J. Cell Biol.* **59**:109a.

GIMBRONE, M. A., JR., LEAPMAN, S., COTRAN, R. S., AND FOLKMAN, J., 1973d, Tumor angiogenesis: Iris neovascularization at a distance from experimental intraocular tumors, *J. Natl. Cancer Inst.* **50**:219–228.

GIMBRONE, M. A., JR., COTRAN, R. S., AND FOLKMAN, J., 1974a, Human vascular endothelial cells in culture: Growth and DNA synthesis, *J. Cell Biol.* **60**:673–685.

GIMBRONE, M. A., JR., COTRAN, R. S., AND FOLKMAN, J., 1974b, Tumor growth and neovascularization: An experimental model using rabbit cornea, *J. Natl. Cancer Inst.* **52**:413–427.

GITTERMAN, C. A., AND LUELL, S., 1969, Transfilter induction of vascular proliferation on the chorioallantoic membranes of embryonated eggs, *Proc. Am. Assoc. Cancer Res.* **10**:29.

GOLDACRE, R. J., AND SYLVEN, B., 1962, On the access of bloodborne dyes to various tumor regions, *Br. J. Cancer* **16**:306–322.

GOLDMAN, E., 1907, The growth of malignant disease in man and the lower animals with special reference to the vascular system, *Lancet* **2**:1236.

GRAHAM, R. C., AND SHANNON, S. L., 1972, Peroxidase arthritis. II. Lymphoid cell–endothelial interactions during a developing immunologic inflammatory response, *Am. J. Pathol.* **69**:7–24.

GREENBLATT, M., AND SHUBIK, P., 1968, Tumor angiogenesis: Transfilter diffusion studies in the hamster by the transparent chamber technique, *J. Natl. Cancer Inst.* **41**:111–124.

HARALDSSON, S., 1962, The vascular pattern of growing and full-grown human epiphysis, *Acta Anat.* **48**:156–167.

HASEGAWE, K., 1934, Experimental study of the nutritious blood vessels of sarcoma in rabbits, *Gann* **28**:32.

HAUDENSCHILD, C. C., ZAHNISER, D., AND KLAGSBRUN, M., 1975a, Human vascular endothelial cells in culture. No response to serum growth factors. *Exper. Cell Res.* in press.

HAUDENSCHILD, C. C., COTRAN, R. S., GIMBRONE, M. A., AND FOLKMAN, J., 1975b, Fine structure of vascular endothelium in culture, *J. Ultrastruct. Res.* **50**:22–32.

HERBERMAN, R., 1974, Cell-mediated immunity to tumor cells, in: *Advances in Cancer Research*, Vol. 19 (G. Klein and S. Weinhouse, eds.), pp. 207–293, Academic Press, New York.

HOLLEY, R. W., 1972, A unifying hypothesis concerning the nature of malignant growth, *Proc. Natl. Acad. Sci.* **69**:2840.

IDE, A. G., BAKER, N. H., AND WARREN, S. L., 1939, Vascularization of the Brown–Pearce rabbit epithelioma transplant as seen in the transparent ear chambers, *Am. J. Roentgenol. Radium Ther.* **42**:891–899.

JAFFE, E. A., NACHMAN, R. L., BECKER, C. G., AND MINICK, R. C., 1972, Culture of human endothelial cells derived from human umbilical cord veins, *Circulation* **46(2)**:252 (abst.).

KLEIN, G., AND KLEIN, E., 1955, Variation in cell populations of transplanted tumors as indicated by studies on the ascites transformation, *Exp. Cell Res. Suppl.* **3**:218–229.

KNASEK, R. A., 1974, Solid tumor masses formed *in vitro* from cells cultured on artificial capillaries, *Fed. Proc.* **33**:1978–1981.

KNIGHTON, D., AUSPRUNK, D., TAPPER, D., AND FOLKMAN, J., 1975, Study of the avascular and vascular phases of tumor growth in the chick embryo, unpublished data.

388

JUDAH
FOLKMAN

KUETTNER, K. E., PITA, J. C., HOWELL, D. S., SORGENTE, N., AND EISENSTEIN, R., 1975, Regulation of epiphyseal cartilage maturation, in: *Extracellular Matrix Influences on Gene Expression* (H. Slavkin, ed.), pp. 435–440, Academic Press, New York.

LEIGHTON, J., 1967, The spread of cancer explored in the embryonated egg, in: *The Spread of Cancer*, pp. 115–192, Academic Press, New York.

LESERVE, A. W., AND HELLMANN, K., 1972, Metastases and the normalization of tumor blood vessels by ICRF 159: A new type of drug action, *Br. Med. J.* **1**:597–601.

LEWIS, W. H., 1927, The vascular pattern of tumors, *Johns Hopkins Hosp. Bull.* **41**:156.

MCGRATH, J. M., AND STEWART, G. J., 1969, The effects of endotoxin on vascular endothelium, *J. Exp. Med.* **129**:833–848.

PARR, I., WHEELER, E., AND ALEXANDER, P., 1973, Similarities of the anti-tumour actions of endotoxin, Lipid A and double stranded RNA, *Br. J. Cancer* **27**:370–389.

PETERSEN, O., 1956, Spontaneous course of cervical precancerous conditions, *Am. J. Obstet. Gynecol.* **72**:1063–1071.

REICH, E., 1974, Tumor associated fibrinolysis, in: *Control of Proliferation in Animal Cells* (B. Clarkson and R. Baserga, eds.), Cold Spring Harbor Laboratory, Cold Spring Harbor, N.Y.

RYAN, T. J., 1973, Factors influencing growth of vascular endothelium in the skin, in: *The Physiology and Pathophysiology of the Skin* (A. Jarret, ed.), pp. 779–805, Academic Press, New York.

SADE, R. M., AND FOLKMAN, J., 1972, En face stripping of vascular endothelium, *Microvasc. Res.* **4**:77–80.

SADE, R. M., FOLKMAN, J., AND COTRAN, R. S., 1972, DNA synthesis in endothelium of aortic segments *in vitro*, *Exp. Cell Res.* **74**:297–306.

SCHOEFL, G. I., 1963, Studies on inflammation. III. Growing capillaries: Their structure and permeability, *Virchows Arch. Pathol. Physiol.* **337**:97–141.

SIDKY, Y. A., AND AUERBACH, R., 1975, Lymphocyte induced angiogenesis: A quantitative and sensitive assay of graft-versus-host reaction, *J. Exp. Med.* **141**:1084–1100.

SMOLIN, G., AND HYNDIUK, R., 1971, Lymphatic drainage from vascularized rabbit cornea, *Am. J. Opthalmol.* **72**:147–151.

SPAET, T. H., AND LEJNIEKS, I., 1967, Mitotic activity of rabbit blood vessels, *Proc. Soc. Exp. Biol. Med.* **125**:1197–1201.

SÜSS, R., KINZEL, V., AND SCRIBNER, J. D., 1973, *Cancer Experiments and Concepts*, p. 70, Springer, New York.

TANNOCK, I. F., AND STEEL, G. G., 1969, Quantitative techniques for study of the anatomy and function of small blood vessels in tumors, *J. Natl. Cancer Inst.* **42**:771–782.

THOMLINSON, R. H., AND GRAY, L. H., 1955, The histological structure of some human lung cancers and the possible implications for radiotherapy, *Br. J. Cancer* **9**:539–549.

TUAN, D., SMITH, S., FOLKMAN, J., AND MERLER, E., 1973, Isolation of the non-histone proteins of rat Walker carcinoma 256: Their association with tumor angiogenesis, *Biochemistry* **12**:3159–3165.

URBACH, F., 1961, The blood supply of tumors, in: *Advances in Biology of the Skin* (W. Montagna and R. A. Ellis, eds.), pp. 123–149, Pergamon Press, New York.

VIRCHOW, R., 1863, *Die Krankhaften Geschwulste*, August Hirschwald, Berlin.

WARREN, B. A., AND SHUBIK, P., 1966, The growth of the blood supply to melanoma transplants in the hamster cheek pouch, *Lab. Invest.* **15**:464–478.

WEIBEL, E. R., AND PALADE, G. E., 1964, New cytoplasmic components in arterial endothelia, *J. Cell Biol.* **23**:101–112.

WILLIS, R. A., 1973, *Pathology of Tumors*, Butterworths, London.

YAMAGAMI, I., 1970, Electronmicroscopic study on the cornea. I. Mechanism of experimental new vessel formation, *Jpn. J. Opthalmol.* **14**:41–58.

YAMAURA, H., AND SATO, H., 1973, Experimental studies of angiogenesis in AH109A ascites tumor transplanted to a transparent chamber in rats, in: *Chemotherapy of Cancer Dissemination and Metastasis* (S. Garattini and G. Franchi, eds.), pp. 149–175, Raven Press, New York.

YOUNG, J. S., LUMSDEN, C. E., AND STALKER, A. L., 1950, The significance of the "tissue pressure" of normal testicular and of neoplastic (Brown–Pearce carcinoma) tissue in the rabbit, *J. Pathol. Bacteriol.* **62**:313.

14

Regulation of Energy Metabolism in Normal and Tumor Tissues

Charles E. Wenner

1. Aerobic Glycolysis of Neoplastic Cells: The Warburg Effect

A metabolic imbalance exists in progressively malignant tumor cells. The observation that rapidly growing tumor cells have a high aerobic glycolysis was first reported by Warburg (1931), who considered that elevated glycolysis was a consequence of an impairment in the respiratory mechanism of cells caused by carcinogens. Warburg noted that in all of the tumors he examined respiration was low and glycolysis was high. In Warburg's proposal, the carcinogenic agent is presumed to interfere with cell respiration and the cell either dies or adopts a fermentative mechanism to derive energy necessary for survival. The carcinogenic agent, whether it be a virus, anaerobiosis, X-ray, or chemical carcinogen, is presumed to damage respiration either by interfering with the extent of respiration (i.e., quantitatively) or by impairing the effect of respiration, rendering it incapable of suppressing glycolysis. Warburg's theory implied that damage to respiration should be irreversible, but as yet there has not been an unequivocal demonstration that the respiration of tumors is disturbed. Following Warburg's initial observation of a low rate of respiration in tumors, it was demonstrated that in some tumors the rate of respiration is normal and that several noncancer tissues have appreciable rates of aerobic glycolysis, such as the retina, leukocytes, kidney, medulla, and intestinal mucosa. Mitochondria from

Charles E. Wenner • Department of Experimental Biology, Roswell Park Memorial Institute, Buffalo, New York neoplastic tissues have a full complement of the enzymes of the citric acid cycle and also functional respiratory pigments which serve as the components of the electron transport chain (*cf.* Wenner, 1967). Further, as emphasized by Weinhouse (1965), neoplasms exhibit a normal Pasteur effect when measured in terms of the Meyerhof oxidation quotient. That is, the oxygen which is consumed by malignant cells is just as effective in quantitatively inhibiting the formation of glycolysis end products as that consumed by normal tissues. One of the most potent arguments against the Warburg hypothesis is the demonstration that the series of minimal-deviation hepatomas exhibit low rates of aerobic glycolysis and respire at rates which do not appear to differ from that of their normal counterpart, the liver. Thus aerobic glycolysis is not necessarily an essential feature of malignancy.

Despite the failure to observe a unique biochemical pattern of energy metabolism in all tumor cells, a correlation of growth rate with increasing glycolysis is observed in the hepatoma series (Burk *et al.*, 1967). However, the question as to whether this is related to the primary event in oncogenesis is unanswered.

Racker (1972) has proposed a new hypothesis which focuses on "the findings of Warburg as a significant feature of cancer pathogenesis." He proposes that "tumors can be caused by a number of different primary lesions," all of which "have in common the ability to cause a persistent alteration in the intracellular pH thereby upsetting the normal regulatory mechanism that prevents uncontrolled growth."

Thus the so-called Warburg effect remains, and, in this author's opinion, is deserving of further study in view of the reported correlation between growth rate and glycolysis (Burk *et al.*, 1967). The increased aerobic glycolysis may reflect cellular alterations which favor growing cells.

1.1. Relationship Between Respiration and Glycolysis

Before discussing possible explanations for an elevated aerobic glycolysis, it is perhaps useful to discuss the regulation of carbohydrate metabolism, particularly the interrelationships of respiration and glycolysis. The fundamental controls which operate on these processes at the cellular level are part of the basic system on which the action of external controls, such as hormones and growth factors, is superimposed.

Inhibition of glycolysis by oxidative phosphorylation is known as the Pasteur effect. The uncouplers of oxidative phosphorylation reverse the inhibition of glycolysis, indicating that phosphorylation of ADP and inorganic phosphate (P_i) and not respiration is important to the control mechanism. As pointed out by Racker, the Pasteur effect is explained as follows: "The enzymes of glycolysis can metabolize glucose only when (a) inorganic phosphate and ADP are available for the oxidation of glyceraldehyde-3-phosphate, and (b) the ATP : ADP ratio and the concentration of P_i and other allosteric effects of glycolytic enzymes are suitable for catalytic action."

Some key enzymes of glycolysis are regulated allosterically by the ATP : ADP ratios as well as by P_i levels. As first demonstrated by Bücher and Rüssman (1964), the key enzymes subject to regulation are those whose substrates and products are displaced from equilibrium in the cell. As an example, the phosphofructokinase reaction is inhibited by high concentrations of ATP but stimulated by P_i. Further, inorganic phosphate reverses product inhibition of hexokinase by glucose-6-phosphate; also, inorganic phosphate as well as the NAD : NADH ratio regulates the oxidation of glyceraldehyde-3-phosphate. The NAD : NADH ratio is dependent on the availability of an electron acceptor such as pyruvate, and pyruvate formation from phosphoenolpyruvate is dependent on ADP availability. It is thus apparent that the levels of ATP, ADP, and P_i determine the rate of glycolysis by their interaction at several key steps in the fermentation scheme.

The rate of respiration is also markedly dependent on the availability of ADP and P_i, and this dependence is known as respiratory control. Thus the cofactors of the phosphorylation system are common to both glycolysis and respiration. Further, there is competition between these two systems for ADP and P_i, which are in limited supply. As chemical work (e.g., biosynthesis) or osmotic work such as ion transport is performed, energy is utilized and ADP and P_i become available for further generation of energy. The inhibition of glucose utilization by oxygen then is attributed in part to the lesser availability of cofactors of the phosphorylation system under aerobic conditions.

1.2. Control of Aerobic Glycolysis by Ion Transport

There are several factors which can contribute to the availability of these cofactors of the phosphorylating system and to low-energy states in the cell. For example, apart from ATP breakdown resulting from biosynthetic needs, the energy-dependent uptake of K^+ or active extrusion of Ca^{2+} contributes to the availability of cofactors of phosphorylation. The former process is catalyzed by the ouabain-sensitive enzyme $(Na^+ + K^+)$-ATPase and is important for maintenance of cell volume and maintenance of the membrane potential, as well as for protein and DNA synthesis. The latter process is catalyzed by the enzyme Ca^{2+}-ATPase, and current thought is that this ATP-dependent enzyme plays a role in intracellular Ca^{2+} homeostasis, although to a somewhat lesser extent than the mitochondrial energy-linked uptake of Ca^{2+} (cf. Borle, 1973). Another factor important to the breakdown of ATP is the mitochondrial ATPase. In addition, other ATPases not yet identified have been reported as contributing to the phosphate pool (Suolinna et al., 1974).

Is there then a common factor which contributes to the high aerobic glycolysis of tumors? Recent evidence has indicated that the high aerobic glycolysis can be attributed to different factors depending on the type of tumor. This is perhaps not unexpected in view of the diversity of tissues from which tumors are derived. For example, Racker, whose earlier studies on glucose utilization by Ehrlich ascites tumor cells suggested that P_i is the rate-limiting step, has shown that in this tissue

TABLE 1

Control of Lactate Formation in Various Cell Lines[a]

Additions	Ascites	3T3	Py-3T3	Neuro-blastoma	BHK	Py-BHK
None	0.35	0.41	0.86	0.98	0.6	0.7
Oubain (10^{-3} M)	0.12	0.60	0.70	0.57	0.5	0.7
DNP (10^{-4} M)	1.28	0.69	1.40	1.63	1.5	2.0
Rutamycin (8 μg/ml)	0.45	0.18	0.27	0.60	1.2	1.7

[a] Ehrlich ascites cells were maintained in mice, harvested, washed, and analyzed as described previously (Scholnick *et al.*, 1973). The other cell lines were grown *in vitro* in 75-cm². Falcon plastic flasks in Dulbecco's modified Eagle's medium with 5% calf serum, 5% fetal calf serum, 20 mM Hepes buffer, 20 units/ml of penicillin, and 200 μg/ml of streptomycin. The cells were suspended in the buffer used for the measurement of glycolysis, but with 0.1% EDTA and without $MgCl_2$, and then washed twice with the assay buffer. The latter was the same as used for the ascites cells but also contained 0.1 M sucrose. All values are expressed as μmoles of lactate/30 min/mg protein. From Suolinna *et al.* (1974).

the high aerobic glycolysis rate is dependent on active K^+ pumping since ouabain produced marked lowering of aerobic glycolysis (Scholnick *et al.*, 1973). In contrast, aerobic glycolysis in virus-transformed mouse embryonic fibroblasts Py-3T3 (as well as in 3T3 cells) appears to be supported by mitochondrial ATPase (Table 1). In other tumor cells, there is yet another ATPase which is susceptible to inhibition by flavones such as quercetin. Thus in each tumor examined the increased glycolysis is attributed to a different factor, but in each case there appears to be acceleration of ATP breakdown.

There are few studies in which the effects of different ATPase inhibitors on respiration and glycolysis can be compared between normal tissues and their neoplastic counterparts. Van Rossum *et al.* (1971) have studied the effect of the $(Na^+ + K^+)$-ATPase inhibitor ouabain on respiration and glycolysis in rat liver and the rapidly growing Morris hepatoma 3924A. In each tissue, ouabain (0.75–1.0 mM) inhibited endogenous respiration by about 30%. Similarly, ouabain inhibited the rate of anaerobic glycolysis by one-third in slices of rat hepatoma. It thus appears that the utilization of energy for transport mediated by $(Na^+ + K^+)$-ATPase is approximately the same in these tissues. Further study is necessary, however, with shorter incubation periods to confirm these findings.

Comparisons of $(Na^+ + K^+)$-activated ATPase activity have been made with normal and transformed cells in culture. Kasarov and Friedman (1974) have shown that $(Na^+ + K^+)$-ATPase activity is increased four- to fivefold when mouse and rat fibroblasts are transformed spontaneously or transformed by SV40, murine sarcoma, and murine leukemia viruses. Also, an increase was observed in XC cells, a line established from a Wistar rat tumor induced with Rous sarcoma virus. A concern is that the expression of $(Na^+ + K^+)$-ATPase is variable; for example, Skou (1965) has shown that detergents markedly increase $(Na^+ + K^+)$-ATPase activity. Thus one is not certain that total activity is being measured. Kimelberg and Mayhew (1974) have also reported that cells transformed by SV40 and Rous sarcoma virus show an enhanced $(Na^+ + K^+)$-ATPase. Further, their studies are supported by the demonstration of an increased uptake of the K^+ analogue ^{86}Rb in transformed cells. These results are of particular interest when considered with the observations of Hatanaka and Hanafusa (1970) to be discussed in more detail later. These workers showed that chick embryonic fibroblasts transformed by Rous sarcoma virus show increased glycolysis in culture. It is not certain whether the increased glycolysis reflected by these differences is due to malignant transformation or due to increase in cell growth, but the possibility that an enhanced $(Na^+ + K^+)$-ATPase contributes to an increase in aerobic glycolysis of the transformed cultured mouse embryonic fibroblasts is suggested by these separate experiments.

1.3. Are Differences in Membrane Fluidity in Transformed Cells Responsible for Observed Differences in Transport Enzymes?

The question arises as to what is responsible for increased sugar, amino acid, and cation transport as well as $(Na^+ + K^+)$-ATPase activity in transformed cells. One explanation is that an enhanced membrane fluidity in transformed cells is responsible for both the reported differences in membrane transport and the activity of membrane transport enzymes. Indirect evidence for altered membrane fluidity comes from lectin binding studies (cf. Robbins and Nicolson, Chap. 1, Vol. 4), but it is not yet established whether the increased clustering seen in transformed cells reflects a decrease in viscosity of membrane lipids, or whether subcellular elements as microtubules control protein mobility and activity.

Although the use of probes to detect membrane fluidity has not provided consistently uniform results, some workers have provided evidence that membrane lipid fluidity is enhanced when cells are transformed. Barnett et al. (1974) have reported, from studies with the use of a spin label which is presumed to localize in the plasma cell membrane, that membranes of chemically transformed (MC-3T3) and spontaneously transformed 3T3 cells are significantly more fluid than normal 3T3 embryonic fibroblasts. This is in contrast to the failure of other workers to observe changes with a similar probe in which fatty acids were spin labeled (cf. Gaffney, 1975; Robbins et al., 1975). However, subsequent studies have indicated that the probe used by Barnett was incorrectly identified (R. Barnett, personal communication). A dissimilar partitioning of probes might account for these differences, but further study is necessary to establish the significance of these observations. In any case, failure to demonstrate changes does not rule out the possibility that changes in lipid fluidity are primary to changes in $(Na^+ + K^+)$-ATPase since conventional spectroscopic techniques report average values and may not detect changes of fluidity in lipids adjacent to membrane enzymes.

Shinitzky and Inbar (1974) have reported with the use of fluorescent polarization techniques that transformed lymphocytes have greater fluidity than normal lymphocytes. These studies as well as experiments described by Robbins and Nicolson (Chap. 1, Vol. 4) of the binding of plant lectins to cell surfaces further suggest that membrane fluidity is enhanced in transformed cells. Maximal activation of $(Na^+ + K^+)$-ATPase activity has been shown in reconstituted enzyme phospholipid systems to be dependent on the state of fluidity of the phospholipids (Kimelberg and Papahadjopoulos, 1972; Kimelberg and Mayhew, 1975), and Arrhenius plots of the $(Na^+ + K^+)$-ATPase activity of SV40 3T3 cells have been interpreted as being consistent with the concept that enhanced membrane fluidity is responsible for the observed increase in $(Na^+ + K^+)$-ATPase (Kimelberg and Mayhew, 1975).

Inbar and Shinitzky (1974) reported that the plasma cell membranes derived from transformed cells have a decreased cholesterol content; this condition would be expected on the basis of model membrane studies to lead to greater fluidity of the phospholipid components of plasma cell membranes (Engelman and Rothman, 1973). However, factors other than the properties of the phospholipids of the plasma membrane may be involved; for example, changes in fluidity could result from interaction of peripheral membrane proteins with intrinsic membrane proteins, as discussed by Robbins and Nicolson in Volume 4.

Another factor which would be expected to influence membrane fluidity is the interaction of divalent cations at the cell surface. Studies on the interaction of Ca^{2+} with phospholipid bilayers have shown that asymmetry of Ca^{2+} distribution across negatively charged phosphatidylserine bilayers leads to instability of the model membrane (Ohki and Papahadjopoulos, 1972). Also, Ca^{2+} (0.5 mM) induces an altered phase transition of both phosphatidylglycerol and phosphatidylserine bilayers (Jacobson and Papahadjopoulos, 1975).

Alternatively, Ca^{2+} might interact with a submembranous assembly of components, e.g., actin-containing fibers as microfilaments, and myosin-like proteins, and/or possibly microtubules. The structural arrangements of chick fibroblast actin have been compared in normal and transformed cells, and actin appears to be less polymerized in cells transformed by Rous sarcoma virus (Robbins *et al.*, 1974). Further, Pollack *et al.* (1975) have shown by immunofluorescent visualization with the use of antibodies directed specifically against actin that SV 40 transformation of 3T3 cells leads to a decrease in the presence of actin-containing sheaths, and that reversion of the SV 101 line is accompanied by an increase in these structures. In view of the inhibition of microtubule polymerization by Ca^{2+} (*cf.* Borisey *et al.*, 1974), it is of interest to learn whether transformation results in changes in its organization. Clarification of the role of these subcellular elements in the mobility of membrane proteins appears necessary in order to advance our understanding of the mechanism by which Ca^{2+} contributes to changes in structural and functional properties of membranes.

1.4. Ca^{2+} Interactions with Plasma Cell Membranes

A Ca^{2+} interaction with the plasma cell surface is indicated by experiments which show that Ca^{2+} modifies the permeability of cells to monovalent cations. In our

experience, introduction of extracellular Ca^{2+} (0.1–5.0 mM) to Ehrlich Lettré
ascites tumor cells in Krebs–Ringer buffer permits higher levels of ouabain-
sensitive entrapment of $^{42}K^+$ by ascites tumor cells (Wenner and Hackney, in
preparation). Further, Ca^{2+} prevents the rapid efflux of $^{42}K^+$ from $^{42}K^+$-preloaded
cells. The ability of Ca^{2+} to stimulate net K^+ uptake and to maintain $^{42}K^+$
contents of preloaded ascites tumor cells is superior to that of Mg^{2+}. No
stimulation of $^{42}K^+$ uptake or prevention of leakage of $^{42}K^+$ from preloaded cells is
observed with the introduction of La^{3+} (0.05–1.0 mM) (*cf.* Levinson *et al.*, 1972)[1].
In fact, La^{3+} promotes $^{42}K^+$ leakage of preloaded Ehrlich ascites cells. While
increased retention of K^+ might arise from Ca^{2+} interaction with phospholipid
bilayers, this action would involve more than charge neutralization in view of the
ion selectivity. However, it is also possible that Ca^{2+} maintains intracellular K^+
contents by affecting lipid–protein interactions, or by altering the activity of
membrane proteins directly.

Studies of Gilbert (1971) indicate that Ca^{2+} requirements for maintenance of
membrane K^+ contents differ in some normal and neoplastic cells. The absence of
Ca^{2+} or low concentrations of Ca^{2+} (10^{-5}–10^{-4} M) lead to leakage of cellular K^+
content of normal cells, but the ability of three transplanted rat tumors to
maintain cellular potassium contents in incubation media containing low Ca^{2+} was
much better than that of normal tissues. The concentration of Ca^{2+} necessary for
normal tissues to maintain K^+ levels was an order of magnitude higher. These
studies suggest that Ca^{2+} interaction with the plasma membrane is responsible for
the observed differences in K^+ levels. The authors attribute the differences in
normal and tumor cells as due to a higher apparent affinity of the sites for Ca^{2+} in
tumor cells. In their studies, Ca^{2+} and Mg^{2+} were equally effective in maintaining
K^+ contents in tumor slices but Ca^{2+} was superior to Mg^{2+} in liver slices. As pointed
out by the authors, an increased density of surface negative charges could increase
the apparent affinity for the "receptor" sites but would not be expected to alter the
relative affinities for Ca^{2+} and Mg^{2+}. It should be pointed out, however, that
comparisons were not made between normal and neoplastic cells of homologous
tissues, and it should not be construed from these experiments that tumors in
general have physicochemically different receptor sites from their normal counterpart. Nevertheless, in view of the reported differences between normal and
tumor tissues in the ability of Ca^{2+} and Mg^{2+} to protect leakage of K^+ contents, the
question arises as to whether the binding of Ca^{2+} differs in normal and neoplastic
cells. If so, do these differences contribute to the presumed alterations in
membrane fluidity of transformed cells?

395
REGULATION
OF ENERGY
METABOLISM
IN NORMAL
AND TUMOR
TISSUES

---

[1] Although La^{3+} behaves like Ca^{2+} in some biological systems, our studies as well as studies by Levinson
et al. (1972) indicate that Ca^{2+} (to 5.0 mM) exhibits properties different from those of La^{3+}. (However,
at concentrations of Ca^{2+} greater than 10.0 mM, Ca^{2+} also promotes release of K^+ or Rb^+ from
preloaded cells.) We observed, in agreement with Levinson *et al.* (1972), that La^{3+} (0.04−1.0 mM)
decreases the K^+ content of Ehrlich ascites tumor cells. It is also of interest that Levinson *et al.* (1972)
have shown that La^{3+} binding to ascites tumor cells is unaffected by phospholipase treatment or by
lipid extraction with chloroform–methanol. However, the addition of pronase to lipid-extracted cells
did cause the release of La^{3+}.

2. Energy-Linked Functions of Tumor Mitochondria

As mentioned previously, earlier studies focused on possible structural or functional aberrations of mitochondria of neoplastic cells as an explanation of the high aerobic glycolysis of tumors. However, attempts to demonstrate unique differences in mitochondria from tumors have failed. Mitochondria from neoplastic cells have a full complement of the enzymes of the citric acid cycle, and contain all of the functional respiratory pigments of the electron transport chain (*cf.* Wenner, 1967). Tumor mitochondria are also fully capable of carrying out oxidative phosphorylation (Wenner, 1967). Despite these significant similarities, some minor differences in oxidative phosphorylation properties of tumor mitochondria other than those mentioned in Section 1.2 have been reported. For example, Pederson and Morris (1974) reported that isolated mitochondria from minimally deviated Morris hepatoma and Ehrlich ascites tumor cells are deficient in uncoupler-stimulated adenosine triphosphatase activity. This finding is in contrast to what is observed in mitochondria from normal cells, but the generalization that tumor mitochondria have an atypical dinitrophenol-stimulated ATPase is blunted by the observation that azo-dye-induced tumors grown in ascites form and another strain of Ehrlich ascites tumor cells exhibit intermediate responses which resemble those of the tissue of origin (Pedersen and Morris, 1974). Thus a spectrum of responses of uncoupler stimulation is observed depending on the cell type. In other studies concerned with ion transport by tumor mitochondria, some differences in swelling properties of tumors have been reported (Feo *et al.*, 1973); however, only a relatively small number of tumors were examined. Recently, several workers have reported differences which appear to be more significant. These differences arise in the mitochondrial uptake of a key divalent cation, Ca^{2+}. Since mitochondrial uptake of Ca^{2+} is also pertinent to an evaluation of cellular Ca^{2+} homeostasis, these studies require further attention. They are of particular interest in view of its possible role in influencing membrane fluidity as described in Section 1.3.

2.1. Regulation of Intracellular Ca^{2+} by Energy-Linked Mitochondrial Uptake

The concentration of Ca^{2+} is not only involved in the regulation of glycolysis (Bygrave, 1966) and respiration (*cf.* Lehninger *et al.*, 1967) but has also been reported necessary for activation of guanyl cyclase (Schultz *et al.*, 1973), intercellular communication (Lowenstein, 1966), activation of protein phosphokinases (*cf.* Rasmussen *et al.*, 1972), and, as already mentioned, permeability to Na^+ and K^+, and possibly plasma cell membrane fluidity as well. Ca^{2+} also appears to be the most permeant cation to mitochondria, and therefore it would appear to be the principal ion involved in regulating the distribution of anions in the cell. Thus study of the interplay between Ca^{2+} transport by the plasma membrane and by mitochondria of tumor cells appears warranted. The mitochondrial Ca^{2+} pumping system appears to be the principal component in the maintenance of low intracellular Ca^{2+} levels in the tumor cells studied, and it is this system that will be emphasized in this review. The question then arises as to whether tumor mitochondria differ from their normal counterpart in the energy-linked transport of Ca^{2+}.

397
REGULATION
OF ENERGY
METABOLISM
IN NORMAL
AND TUMOR
TISSUES

The Ca^{2+} pumping system has been studied largely in rodent liver mitochondria, and the stoichiometry of Ca^{2+} uptake to oxygen utilization and proton release has been established under different experimental conditions with liver mitochondria. There seems little question that tumor mitochondria can actively support Ca^{2+} uptake. For example, the use of a spectrophotometric technique involving murexide permitted demonstration of energy-linked Ca^{2+} accumulation by intact Ehrlich ascites tumor cells (Cittadini *et al.*, 1971) and later from isolated mitochondria of these cells (Cittadini *et al.*, 1973). Further, the latter report indicated that respiratory jumps were observed on addition of Ca^{2+} (200 μM) to mitochondria of these cells. The latter observation has also been reported by Thorne and Bygrave (1973), and confirmed in our laboratory. Reynafarje and Lehninger (1973) have studied the stoichiometry of Ca^{2+} accumulation by mitochondria derived from L-1210 mouse leukemic cells. From these studies by Dr. Britton Chance and A. L. Lehninger's group, there arise two aspects of calcium uptake by tumor cells which appear unusual (Cittadini *et al.*, 1973; Reynafarje and Lehninger, 1973). The first property in which some differences arise concerns the stoichiometry of Ca^{2+} uptake by isolated tumor mitochondria; the second property to be discussed is the reported failure of glucose to support uptake of Ca^{2+} by intact ascites tumor cells.

2.2. Possible Differences in $Ca^{2+} : O$ and $Ca^{2+} : H^+$ Stoichiometries in Mitochondria of Normal and Neoplastic Cells

The stoichiometry of mitochondrial Ca^{2+} accumulated/oxygen utilized differs in the presence and absence of permeant anions. Thus when inorganic phosphate is present 2.0 Ca^{2+} ions are taken up from the medium by isolated animal tissue mitochondria per pair of electrons passing each energy-conserving site of the respiratory chain. This ratio has been obtained by a number of investigators working with liver mitochondria, and it has been observed by Reynafarje and Lehninger (1973) with L-1210 mitochondria, as well as with mitochondria derived from Ehrlich ascites tumor cells by this author. However, in the absence of phosphate, the ratio is greater than 2 in mitochondria isolated from either source. Reynafarje and Lehninger (1974) were able to show an early burst of H^+ ejection on addition of Ca^{2+} in the absence of a permeant anion. This extremely rapid proton release is presumed to result from an energy-requiring Ca^{2+}–H^+ exchange reaction. When corrected for this initially rapid Ca^{2+}–H^+ ion exchange, tumor mitochondria as well as normal mitochondria showed the characteristic $Ca^{2+} : O$ ratio of 2.0. The superstoichiometry is thus attributed to an initially rapid energy-dependent Ca^{2+} binding, superimposed on the slower, normal uptake of Ca^{2+} and ejection of H^+.

L-1210 mitochondria are more sensitive than liver mitochondria to stimulation of respiration by Ca^{2+} in that the K_m for stimulation by Ca^{2+} is 8 μM in the tumor mitochondria, in contrast to 50 μM for liver mitochondria. These values, however, are uncorrected for complexation of Ca^{2+} by other components of the medium.

The ratio of Ca^{2+} accumulation/H^+ ejection also shows superstoichiometry, and the $Ca^{2+} : H^+$ ratio is greater with L-1210 mitochondria than that derived from normal liver. Possibly the numbers of membrane binding sites differ in the two mitochondrial types. The nature of the possible binding sites is poorly understood, but it does appear that tumor mitochondria have a high affinity for energy-dependent Ca^{2+} binding. Alternatively, the differences in the $Ca^{2+} : H^+$ ratios may reflect some subtle changes in a $Ca^{2+} : H^+$ exchange process. Comparisons of more mitochondrial types are necessary before it can be established whether tumor mitochondria, in general, display greater superstoichiometries in $Ca^{2+} : O$ and $Ca^{2+} : H^+$ ratios than normal mitochondria.

2.3. Ca^{2+} Uptake by Intact Ascites Tumor Cells: Influence of Glycolyzable Substrates

A second property of tumor cells which appears unique was reported by Cittadini et al. (1973). These workers observed that glucose fails to support the uptake of Ca^{2+} by intact Ehrlich ascites tumor cells. This is somewhat surprising since ATP formed from glycolysis should be fully capable of supporting energy-requiring Ca^{2+} uptake by ascites tumor mitochondria. One possible reason for the failure to observe glucose-supported Ca^{2+} uptake is that a compatible anion such as inorganic phosphate becomes less available when glucose is present; however, a more likely explanation is that the initially rapid phosphorylation of glucose by hexokinase leads to a marked lowering of the ATP level. The above-mentioned experiments were carried out at room temperature and the results differ from experiments with ELD ascites tumor cells carried out in our laboratory at 37°C. We have observed that $^{45}Ca^{2+}$ uptake at physiological temperatures is supported by glucose under anaerobic conditions (R. Resch, R. Hines, and C. E. Wenner, unpublished experiments). Although the adenylate charge is maintained fairly well when utilization of ATP is accelerated (presumably by activation of adenylate deaminase), it is nevertheless possible that the transient drop in the ATP level upon glucose addition would not support Ca^{2+} uptake.

As stated in the previous section, direct comparisons of stoichiometric Ca^{2+} uptake by tumor mitochondria with that derived from normal tissues have not been made, and it is not yet possible to establish whether these observations in intact cells represent differences between mitochondria of normal and tumor tissues or differences in tissue source. Studies carried out with normal mammary cells and with other tumor tissues are of interest to determine whether an increased mitochondrial affinity of Ca^{2+} provides an advantage for rapidly growing cells.

3. Early Changes in Metabolism Accompanying Cell Transformation

3.1. Enhanced Glucose Uptake Concomitant with Virus-Induced Morphological Changes

The question arises as to whether the altered carbohydrate metabolism which develops when cells are transformed reflects some change in membrane function. Conceivably a change in membrane properties could result in increased availability of substrate requisite for cell growth. Demonstration then of an altered membrane function associated with transformed cells provides one approach to an understanding of the etiology of malignancy. Hatanaka and Hanafusa (1970) have reported that an early event in cell transformation by Rous sarcoma virus is a marked increase in glucose transport, but it can be questioned whether phosphorylation or transport of hexoses is accelerated under these conditions. These authors carried out sequential studies at hourly intervals during the process of chick embryo cell transformation, and reported an increased rate of sugar transport concomitant with changes in cell morphology. The authors also reported a marked reduction in the K_m of 2-deoxyglucose uptake in these cells following Rous sarcoma virus infection, which was considered to be a result of the expression of specific sarcoma virus genes. This finding has been questioned by Weber (1973), whose studies with the nonphosphorylatable 3-O-methylglucose and nonmetabolizable 2-deoxyglucose indicate that V_{max} but not K_m is significantly altered by cell transformation. The latter results suggest that the type of transport site is not altered.

Evidence that the apparent enhancement of 2-deoxyglucose uptake is not due to an enhancement of the transport process has been brought forth by Romano and Colby (1973). These authors measured the intracellular pools of both the free [2-^{14}C]deoxyglucose and phosphorylated [2-^{14}C]deoxyglucose phosphate in four lines of mouse embryonic fibroblasts—3T3, SV40-3T3 transformed cells, 3T6, and a flat revertant SV-3T3-FL. These measurements showed that both the rate of 2-deoxyglucose uptake and the final steady-state concentration of free 2-deoxyglucose are basically the same in each cell type. The increased total intracellular 2-deoxyglucose is accounted for by the increase in the phosphorylated derivative in the SV40-3T3 cells. An increase in the phosphorylated 2-deoxyglucose is observed as well with the untransformed 3T6 cells, a density-independent cell type, but not the revertant transformed cells, which grow slowly. Thus these studies suggest that enhanced hexose uptake is not specifically attributable to the viral genome but is representative of a "pleiotropic response" which reflects the overall growth rate.

Thus the initial phosphorylation of glucose may represent one of several metabolic steps modulated in accord with the rate of growth. Changes in $(Na^+ + K^+)$-ATPase activity may also be one of these responses. Further work is necessary to resolve whether these processes are interrelated. The use of the virus-transforming system, where a large percentage of cells become transformed, and the availability of cell lines which permit examination of whether changes in a particular activity are specifically mediated by the presence of the viral genome offer considerable promise to resolve the question of whether changes of specific membrane properties play an essential role in cell transformation.

3.2. Cocarcinogen-Induced Changes in Cyclic Nucleotides and Ca^{2+} Movements

Some studies have suggested a role for Ca^{2+} in triggering mechanisms by which cell growth is accelerated (Rasmussen *et al.*, 1972; Whitfield *et al.*, 1973), and the question arises of whether changes in Ca^{2+} movements are important to tumor development. Interest in Ca^{2+} movements also stems from studies with mitogenic plant lectins, which induce a cycle of cell division. There are parallelisms between these studies and experiments with agents which induce cell proliferation such as the cocarcinogenic phorbol esters. In both systems, there has been increasing understanding of the role of regulatory cyclic nucleotides in cell proliferation and to a lesser extent an awareness of the dependence of cyclic nucleotides on Ca^{2+} movements in cell proliferation. This subject has been reviewed by Goldberg *et al.* (1974), and the concept of cyclic AMP as the single primary regulatory component of cells is questioned. The basic discovery of Sutherland of cyclic 3',5'-AMP as a second messenger has been extended by Goldberg *et al.* (1974) in the dualism concept, where cAMP and cGMP serve as the principal determinants in deciding the fate of specific cellular processes. The regulation of cell division in cell cultures had earlier been attributed solely to levels of cAMP (Willingham *et al.*, 1972). Although attempts to find differences in concentration of adenyl cyclase in normal and transformed cells have not been successful, the K_m for ATP of the adenyl cyclase of cells transformed by Rous sarcoma virus is higher than that of chick embryo fibroblasts (Anderson *et al.*, 1973). Some evidence has also been reported that Ca^{2+} regulates cell proliferation by raising cAMP levels in bone marrow and thymic tissue (Whitfield *et al.*, 1973), but the mechanisms involved in the triggering of cellular proliferation have not as yet been established with certainty. Recently, several studies have focused on promoters of carcinogenesis, and of particular interest is the potent cocarcinogen derived from croton oil, tetradecanoyl phorbol acetate (TPA).

In 3T3 cells, TPA induces cell division which is associated with an extremely rapid tenfold increase in cGMP levels (Estensen *et al.*, 1974; Goldberg *et al.*, 1974). Since phorbol esters are surface active (Jacobson *et al.*, in press), it is important to learn whether these transient changes are relevant to tumor promotion. A critical test is to examine whether stereoisomeric phorbol esters which are inactive as promoters produce similar responses.

In many ways, these findings are analogous to results observed with plant lectins which induce cell division. It has been suggested that the intracellular expression of cGMP has an obligatory requirement for increased translocation or transport

401
REGULATION
OF ENERGY
METABOLISM
IN NORMAL
AND TUMOR
TISSUES

of Ca^{2+} into the cell (Goldberg *et al.*, 1974). In this regard, it is of interest that the mitogen phytohemagglutinin, which enhances proliferation in lymphocytes, induces within 15 min a progressive increase in ^{45}Ca accumulation. Furthermore, Zucker *et al.* (1974) have demonstrated that TPA also stimulates Ca^{2+}-dependent platelet aggregation and Ca^{2+}-dependent release of 5-hydroxytryptamine and adenine nucleotides from platelets within 30 s, suggesting that TPA is capable of inducing efflux of these components present in platelet storage organelles. In view of these findings and previous studies of Ca^{2+}-induced release of cell effectors, TPA may possibly alter Ca^{2+} transport as a consequence of interaction with a cell surface receptor. An increased availability of Ca^{2+} may subsequently activate guanyl cyclase, as reported by Schultz *et al.* (1973). Thus TPA-induced increases in cGMP levels may be mediated by increased intracellular Ca^{2+}.

The specificity of TPA (the 4-α-stereoisomer is inactive as a promoter) implies a specific protein interaction, and it should be noted that TPA at fairly low concentrations (10^{-7}–10^{-6} M) induces a decrease in the electrophoretic mobility of Ehrlich ascites tumor cells (Wenner *et al.*, 1974). A failure of TPA to produce specific changes in the electrophoretic mobility of phospholipid model membranes or to increase permeability in synthetic phospholipid bilayers (Jacobson *et al.*, in preparation) is suggestive that a specific membrane protein is the receptor for TPA.

Goldberg *et al.* (1974) have reported that cGMP (10^{-11} M) stimulates RNA synthesis by isolated intact lymphocyte nuclei. Thus, TPA-induced cell proliferation may be mediated by alteration of Ca^{2+} movements which enhance cyclic GMP levels.

The question remains as to how cocarcinogens, which probably interact with the cell surface, send a message to the internal machinery of the cell. Whether this is due to increased transport, or change in cyclic AMP or cyclic GMP levels, has not yet been ascertained. As pointed out by Dulbecco and Elkington (1975) "changes in these parameters might also be coordinate effects not primarily responsible for the mitogenic effect." These workers observed that externally added Ca^{2+} by itself induced DNA replication when added to resting cultures of Balb/c3T3 cells supportive of the idea that Ca^{2+} serves as an intracellular mediator of the regulation of growth. Since other workers have shown that the addition of Ca^{2+} ionophores to lymphocytes induce mitogenesis (*c.f.* Dulbecco and Elkington, 1975), it may well be that an increased concentration of intracellular Ca^{2+}, or an increased interaction of Ca^{2+} with cellular constituents, or a change in ionic distribution, leads to a triggering of the growth process.

4. References

ANDERSON, W. B., JOHNSON, G. S., AND PASTAN, I., 1973, Transformation of chick-embryo fibroblasts by wild-type and temperature-sensitive Rous sarcoma virus alters adenylate cyclase activity, *Proc. Natl. Acad. Sci. U.S.A.* **70**:1055.
BARNETT, R., FURCHT, L., AND SCOTT, R., 1974, Differences in membrane fluidity and structure in contact-inhibited and transformed cells, *Proc. Natl. Acad. Sci. U.S.A.* **71**:1992.

BORISY, G. G., OLMSTED, J. B., MARCUM, J. M., AND ALLEN, C., 1974, Microtubule assembly *in vitro*, *Fed. Proc.* **33**:167.

BORLE, A. B., 1973, Calcium metabolism at the cellular level, *Fed. Proc.* **32**:1944.

BÜCHER, T., AND RÜSSMAN, W., 1964, Equilibrium and nonequilibrium in the glycolysis system, *Angew. Chem. Int. Ed.* **t3**:426.

BURK, D., WOODS, M., AND HUNTER, J., 1967, On the significance of glycolysis for cancer growth, with special reference to Morris rat hepatomas, *J. Natl. Cancer Inst.* **38**:839.

BYGRAVE, F. L., 1966, The effect of Ca ions on the glycolytic activity of Ehrlich ascites cells, *Biochem. J.* **101**:480.

CITTADINI, A., SCARPA, A., AND CHANCE, B., 1971, Kinetic evidence for Ca^{++} uptake by intact Ehrlich ascites tumor cells, *FEBS Letters* **18**:98.

CITTADINI, A., SCARPA, A., AND CHANCE, B., 1973, Calcium transport in intact Ehrlich ascites tumor cells, *Biochim. Biophys. Acta* **291**:246.

DULBECCO, R., AND ELKINGTON, J., 1975, Induction of growth in resting fibroblastic cell cultures by Ca^{2+}, *Proc. Nat. Acad. Sci. U.S.A.* **72**:1584.

ENGELMAN, D., AND ROTHMAN, J., 1973, The planar organization of DPPC–cholesterol bilayers, *J. Biol. Chem.* **247**:3694.

ESTENSEN, R. D., HADDEN, J. W., HADDEN, F., TOURAINE, F., TOURAINE, J., HADDEN, M., AND GOLDBERG, N. D., 1974, in: *Control of Proliferation in Animal Cells* (B. Clarkson and R. Baserga, eds.), pp. 627–634, Cold Spring Harbor Press, Cold Spring Harbor, N.Y.

FEO, F., BONELLI, G., CANUTO, R., AND GARCEA, R., 1973, Further observations on the effect of trypsin on the volume and functions of mitochondria isolated from normal liver and AH-130 Yoshida ascites hepatoma, *Cancer Res.* **33**:1804.

GAFFNEY, B. J., 1975, Fatty acid chain flexibility in the membranes of normal and transformed fibroblasts, *Proc. Natl. Acad. Sci. U.S.A.* **72**:664.

GILBERT, I. G. F., 1971, The effects of divalent cations on the ionic permeability of cell membranes in normal and tumor tissues, *Eur. J. Cancer* **8**:99.

GOLDBERG, N. D., HADDOX, M. D., DUNHAM, E., LOPEZ, C., AND HADDEN, J. W., 1974, The Yin Yang hypothesis of biological control: Opposing influences of cyclic GMP and cyclic AMP in the regulation of cell proliferation and other biological processes, in: *Control of Proliferation in Animal Cells* (B. Clarkson and R. Baserga, eds.), p. 609, Academic Press, New York.

HATANAKA, M., 1974, Transport of sugars in tumor cell membranes, *Biochim. Biophys. Acta* **355**:77.

HATANAKA, M., AND HANAFUSA, H., 1970, Analysis of a functional change in membrane in the process of cell transformation by Rous sarcoma virus; alterations in the characteristics of sugar transport, *Virology* **41**:647.

HICKIE, R. A., AND KALANT, I., 1967, Ca^{++} and Mg^{++} content of rat liver and Morris hepatoma, *Cancer Res.* **27**:1053.

INBAR, M., AND SHINITZKY, M., 1974, Increase of cholesterol level in the surface membrane of lymphoma cells and its inhibitory effect on ascites tumor development, *Proc. Natl. Acad. Sci. U.S.A.* **71**:2128.

JACOBSON, K., AND PAPAHADJOPOULOS, D., 1975, Phase transitions and phase separations in phospholipid vesicles induced by changes in temperature, pH or concentration of bivalent cations, *Biochem.* **14**:152.

JACOBSON, K., WENNER, C. E., KEMP, G., AND PAPAHADJOPOULOS, D., Surface properties of phorbol esters and their interaction with lipid monolayers and bilayers, *Cancer Res.* (in press).

KASAROV, L. B., AND FRIEDMAN, H., 1974, Enhanced Na^+-K^+-activated adenosine triphosphatase activity in transformed fibroblasts, *Cancer Res.* **34**:1862.

KIMELBERG, H. K., AND MAYHEW, E., 1975, Increased ouabain-sensitive $^{86}Rb^+$ uptake and $(Na^+ + K^+)$ stimulated ATPase activity in transformed cell lines, *J. Biol. Chem.* **250**:100–104.

KIMELBERG, H. K., AND PAPAHADJOPOULOS, D., 1972, Phospholipid requirements for $(Na^+ + K^+)$-ATPase activity: Head-group specificity and fatty acid fluidity, *Biochim. Biophys. Acta* **282**:272.

LEHNINGER, A. L., CARAFOLI, E., AND ROSSI, C. S., 1967, Energy-linked ion movements in mitochondrial systems, in: *Advances in Enzymology*, Vol. 29 (F. F. Nord ed.), p. 259, Interscience, New York.

LEVINSON, C., MIKITEN, T. M., AND SMITH, T. C., 1972, Lanthanum-induced alterations in cellular electrolytes and membrane potential in Ehrlich ascites tumor cells, *J. Cell. Physiol.* **79**:299.

LOWENSTEIN, W. R., 1966, Permeability of membrane junctions, in: Biological Membranes: Recent Progress (W. R. Lowenstein, ed.), *Ann. N.Y. Acad. Sci.* **137**:441.

PAPAHADJOPOULOS, A., AND OHKI, S., 1969, Stability of asymmetric phospholipid membranes, *Science* **164**:1075.

403
REGULATION
OF ENERGY
METABOLISM
IN NORMAL
AND TUMOR
TISSUES

PEDERSEN, P., AND MORRIS, H. P., 1974, Uncoupler-stimulated adenosine triphosphatase activity: Deficiency in intact mitochondria from Morris hepatoma and ascites tumor cells, *J. Biol. Chem.* **249**:3327.

POLLACK, R., OSBORN, M., AND WEBER, K., 1975, Patterns of organization of actin and myosin in normal and transformed cultured cells, *Proc. Natl. Acad. Sci. U.S.A.* **72**:994.

RACKER, E., 1972, Bioenergetics and the problem of tumor growth, *Am. Sci.* **60**:56.

RASMUSSEN, H., GOODMAN, D., AND TENENHOUSE, A., 1972, The role of cyclic AMP and calcium in cell activation, *Crit. Rev. Biochem.* **1**:95.

RASMUSSEN, H., BORDIER, P., KUROKAWA, K., NAGATA, N., AND OGATA, E., 1974, Hormonal control of skeletal and mineral homeostasis, *Am. J. Med.* **56**:751.

REYNAFARJE, B., AND LEHNINGER, A. L., 1973, Ca^{2+} transport by mitochondria from L1210 mouse ascites tumor cells, *Proc. Natl. Acad. Sci. U.S.A.* **70**:1744.

REYNAFARJE, B., AND LEHNINGER, A. L., 1974, The cause of superstoichiometric Ca^{2+} uptake and H^+ ejection in L1210 mouse ascites tumor mitochondria, *Biochem. Biophys. Res. Commun.* **57**:286.

ROBBINS, P. W., WICKUS, G. C., BRANTON, P. E., GAFFNEY, B. J., HIRSCHBERG, G. B., FUCHS, P., AND BLUMBERG, P. M., 1974, The chick fibroblast cell surface following transformation by Rous sarcoma virus, *Cold Spring Harbor Symp. Quant. Biol.* **39**:1173.

ROMANO, A. H., AND COLBY, C., 1973, SV 40 virus transformation of mouse 3T3 cells does not specifically enhance sugar transport, *Science* **179**:1240.

SCHOLNICK, P., LANG, D., AND RACKER, E., 1973, Regulatory mechanisms in carbohydrate metabolism. IX. Stimulation of aerobic glycolysis by energy-linked ion transport and inhibition by dextran sulfate, *J. Biol. Chem.* **248**:5175.

SCHULTZ, G., HARDMAN, J. G., HURWITZ, L., AND SUTHERLAND, E. W., 1973, Importance of calcium for the control of cyclic GMP levels, *Fed. Proc.* **32**:773.

SELKIRK, J. K., ELWOOD, J. C., AND MORRIS, H. P., 1971, Study on the proposed role of phospholipid in tumor cell membrane, *Cancer Res.* **31**:27.

SHINITZKY, M., AND INBAR, M., 1974, Difference in microviscosity induced by different cholesterol levels on the surface membrane lipid layer of normal lymphocytes and of malignant lymphoma cells, *J. Mol. Biol.* **85**:603.

SKOU, J. C., 1965, Enzymatic basis for active transport of Na^+ and K^+ across the cell membrane, *Physiol. Rev.* **45**:596.

SUOLINNA, E., LANG, D., AND RACKER, E., 1974, Quercetin, an artificial regulator of the high aerobic glycolysis of tumor cells, *J. Natl. Cancer Inst.* **53**:1515.

THORNE, R. F., AND BYGRAVE, F. L., 1973, Interaction of calcium with mitochondria isolated from Ehrlich ascites tumor cells, *Biochem. Biophys. Res. Commun.* **50**:294.

VAN ROSSUM, G. D. V., GOSALVEZ, M., GALEOTTI, T., AND MORRIS, H. P., 1971, Net movements of monovalent and bivalent cations and their relation to energy metabolism in slices of hepatoma 392 4A and of a mammary tumor, *Biochim. Biophys. Acta* **245**:263.

WARBURG, O., 1931, *The Metabolism of Tumors*, R. R. Smith, New York.

WEBER, M. J., 1973, Hexose transport in normal and in Rous sarcoma virus-transformed cells, *J. Biol. Chem.* **248**:2978.

WEINHOUSE, S., 1955, Oxidative metabolism of neoplastic tissues, *Adv. Cancer Res.* Ed. A. Haddow and J. P. Greenstein, **3**:269, Academic Press, New York.

WENNER, C. E., 1967, Progress in tumor enzymology, in: *Advances in Enzymology*, Vol. 29 (F. F. Nord, ed.), p. 321, Interscience, New York.

WENNER, C. E., HACKNEY, J. H., KIMELBERG, H., AND MAYHEW, E., 1974, Membrane effects of phorbol esters, *Cancer Res.* **34**:1731.

WHITE, J. G., GUNDU, H. R., AND ESTENSEN, R. D., 1974, Investigation of the release reaction in platelets exposed to phorbol myristate acetate, *Am. J. Pathol.* **75**:301.

WHITFIELD, J. F., RIXON, R. H., MacMANUS, J. P., AND BALK, S. D., 1973, Calcium, cyclic adenosine 3′,5′-monophosphate, and the control of cell proliferation: A review, *In Vitro* **8**:257.

WILLINGHAM, M. C., JOHNSON, G. S., AND PASTAN, I., 1972, Control of DNA synthesis and mitosis in 3t3 cells by cyclic AMP, *Biochem. Biophys. Res. Commun.* **48**:743.

WU, R., AND RACKER, E., 1959, Regulatory mechanisms in carbohydrate metabolism. IV. Pasteur effect and Crabtree effect in ascites tumor cells, *J. Biol. Chem.* **234**:1036.

ZUCKER, M. B., TROLL, W., AND BELMAN, S., 1974, The tumor-promoter phorbol ester (12-O-tetradecanoyl-phorbol-12-acetate), a potent aggregating agent for blood platelets, *J. Cell Biol.* **60**:325.

15

DNA-Nucleoproteins

Giovanni Rovera

1. Introduction

The transformed state of a neoplastic cell could be due to and maintained by stable alterations at the level of the genome. The genetic evidence supporting this theory has been reviewed by Comings (1973). Two mechanisms are usually suggested to explain the stability of the changes at the level of the genome: either the lesion affects the genetic code of the cell, or the genetic code is normal and an alteration in the epigenetic mechanisms that control the expression of specific genes is responsible for the transformed phenotype. The two proposed mechanisms are not mutually exclusive and the transformed state could of course be maintained by one or the other or both of these mechanisms.

The former mechanism is suggested by the evidence that carcinogens are also mutagens (for review, see Miller and Miller, 1974) and by the fact that oncogenic viruses are integrated into the host cell DNA in transformed cells (for review and discussion, see Tooze, 1973), the latter by the fact that under particular conditions neoplastic cells and tumors can differentiate and cease to proliferate (Pierce *et al.*, 1960; Pierce and Wallace, 1971; Lehman *et al.*, 1974). The second mechanism has a strong emotional appeal that resides in the hope that transformed cells could be made to redifferentiate and induced to enter permanently into the resting phase of the cell cycle so that tumor growth would be arrested.

The molecular bases of the lesions that are responsible for the transformed state at the level of the genome are practically unknown. We can hypothesize that at least two groups of genes could be affected by the cancer transformation and at least two altered phenotypes must coexist for the full expression of malignancy.

GIOVANNI ROVERA • Department of Pathology, Temple University School of Medicine, Philadelphia, Pennsylvania and a Scholar of the Leukemia Society of America. Present Address: Wistar Institute, Philadelphia, Pennsylvania.

The altered phenotypes are (1) loss of control in the mechanisms regulating cell proliferation and (2) capacity to infiltrate the surrounding tissues and grow in distant organs (for discussion, see Tooze, 1973). These two different phenotypes are not linked and can coexist independently in noncancerous tissues. For example, loss of control of cellular proliferation can be observed in psoriasis (Halprin and Taylor, 1971), and capacity to infiltrate surrounding tissues and to metastasize has been reported for normal trophoblastic cells (Haines, 1955; Attwood and Park, 1961).

2. Gene Regulation in Eukaryotes

The chromosomes of eukaryotic cells contain DNA and several species of proteins and RNAs. They can be isolated from interphase cells using various biochemical methods as "chromatin," i.e., a nucleoprotein complex obtained after the removal of cytoplasmic and soluble nuclear components. The chromatin represents the structure that is responsible for the storing and expression of the various information necessary for the cellular functions. Pardon *et al.* (1967) and Hewish and Burgoyne (1973) have given some evidence that the chromatin is constituted of repeated structures, and Kornberg (1974) has proposed that the backbone chromatin structure is based on repeating subunits of 200 base pairs of DNA and two of each of the histones, with the exception of F_1, which occurs only once per subunit. Further evidence for this model has been given by Noll (1974). To this backbone other proteins (the so-called nonhistone chromosomal proteins) and different RNA species are bound. Most of the data published on structure and function of chromatin can be found in the review written by Simpson (1973).

As discussed by Rutter *et al.* (1973) and by Monahan and Hall (1974), three groups of models are currently proposed by different authors to explain how the expression of a particular gene or set of genes can be controlled in eukaryotes. These models are not mutually exclusive and the relatively small amount of data obtained so far does not permit us to discard any. These three models stress the importance of (1) the proteins of the chromatin as gene repressors or inducers, (2) the repeated sequences of DNA that are characteristic of eukaryotes and absent in prokaryotes, and (3) the physical conformation of the chromatin.

The first group of hypotheses is in several respects very similar to the mechanisms of the positive and negative regulation of gene expression as has been observed in prokaryotes. It has been advanced in one form or another by several authors (Huang and Bonner, 1962; Allfrey *et al.*, 1963; Paul and Gilmour, 1968; Gilmour and Paul, 1969). generally speaking, it has been proposed that histones and nonhistone chromosomal proteins by binding to segments of DNA make different portions of the genome available or unavailable to RNA polymerase molecules. The evidence supporting this hypothesis resides mainly in experiments in which the chromatin constituents were disassembled onto DNA and various classes of proteins and then reassembled *in vitro*, and the control of the synthesis of a specific messenger RNA (e.g., hemoglobin) or of different RNA species was evaluated (Kamiyama and Wang, 1971; Spelsberg *et al.*, 1971; Stein *et al.*, 1972; Gilmour and Paul, 1973).

407

DNA-
NUCLEOPROTEINS

The second group of hypotheses stresses the fact that eukaryotic cells have a large number of sequences of DNA that are repeated hundreds of times (Britten and Davidson, 1969; Georgiev *et al.*, 1973). Some of these repeated sequences of DNA could function as monitors of the cellular environment by binding to specific proteins. They could code for species of RNA that in turn would control the expression of structural genes by regulating the transcript of specific messenger RNAs (Bekhor *et al.*, 1969; Huang and Huang, 1969).

The third hypothesis deals more with the physical state of the segments of chromatin involved in transcription and how changes in the physical state could control changes in gene expression (Crick, 1971). In Crick's model, a large fraction of globular supercoiled DNA would exist in the chromatin and would contain the recognition sites for the control of gene transcription. A small fraction of fibrous extended DNA would represent the part of the chromatin containing the genes coding for specific messenger RNAs. Sobell (1973) has pointed out that studies on protein–nucleic acid interaction suggest the existence of an alternate branched configuration for DNA caused by proteins with a specific structure bound to symmetrically arranged polynucleotide base sequences. In this case, the specific sequence of DNA could be recognized by tetrameric proteins which are similar in structure and function to the same repressors in prokaryotes (Pirrotta *et al.*, 1970). The mechanism that has been proposed could produce rearrangement of hydrogen bonds of the original linear DNA duplex to form a cloverleaf structure. White *et al.* (1972) has also proposed that these cloverleaf structures could represent initiation and termination sites for RNA synthesis.

3. DNA

The DNA of eukaryotes differs from that of the prokaryotes in the fact it is about 1000 times larger and contains a large number of DNA sequences that are repeated hundreds and thousands of times. The most repeated sequences are represented by the so-called satellite DNA (for review, see Walker, 1971). This DNA is associated with the constitutive heterochromatin of the cell (Yunis, 1970) and probably has a structural role associated with the centromeric region of the chromosome. It is common belief that nothing is transcribed *in vivo* from satellite DNA (Flamm *et al.*, 1969) and its sequence of bases suggests that it cannot code for a meaningful polypeptide.

A second group, less frequently repeated than the satellite DNA, is the intermediate DNA (Britten and Kohne, 1968). Davidson *et al.* (1973) have shown that 50% of the mammalian genome consists of repetitive sequences, 300 nucleotides long, interspersed with nonrepetitive sequences 700–900 nucleotides long. Another 25% of the genomes consists of repetitive sequences interspersed with nonrepetitive sequences longer than 4000 nucleotides. Repeated sequences can be found arranged in tandem (Thomas *et al.*, 1970), and it has been estimated (Thomas and Lee, 1973) that as much as half of the DNA in mammalian cells is composed of tandemly repeated sequences clustered in groups called g regions. In the mouse genome g regions there are approximately 40,000. The types of RNA transcribed from intermediate DNA change during tissue development (Denis, 1966; Davidson, 1969). This RNA is confined to the cell nucleus, where it turns over rapidly (Shearer and McCarthy, 1967) and does not code for polypeptides. It has been suggested that this RNA itself is the active end product of these sequences and has a gene regulatory function (Davidson, 1969).

The third and final DNA fraction of the chromosome is the so-called unique DNA fraction and represents about 20–25% of the genome (Davidson *et al.*, 1973). because of its unique nature, it is believed that this particular fraction of DNA contains sequences that code for the cells' structural genes.

These studies represent only a preliminary approach to the difficult task of analyzing the organization and molecular characteristics of the genetic material. Keeping in mind the fact that only a minimal part of the DNA could be deranged in neoplasia, it is easy to understand why up to now no alterations have been found in the composition of the DNA species in transformed cells (Shearer, 1971).

4. DNA Transcription in Neoplasia

Several authors have reported that neoplastic cells synthesize different species of RNA from those synthesized by normal cells. These various changes in DNA transcripts can be summarized in three groups:

1. It has been shown that some RNA species observed in normal liver are not synthesized in some hepatomas, suggesting that the genome in cancer cells is more repressed (Drews *et al.*, 1968; Mendecki *et al.*, 1969; Ono *et al.*, 1971).

2. It has also been shown that the new RNA species, not observed in normal tissues, are synthesized in various tumors such as some hepatomas, leukemias, and mammary carcinomas (Church *et al.*, 1969; Neiman and Henry, 1969; Turkington and Self, 1970), and in transformed cells in culture (Muramatsu *et al.*, 1973).

3. In some hepatomas, both the presence of new RNA species and the absence of normal RNA species have been reported (Chiarugi, 1969).

Because of the techniques of hybridization used for the above experiments, most if not all of these RNA species represent transcripts of repetitive DNA species.

In vitro, the transcription of the chromatin of neoplastic cells has been assayed in the presence of a heterologous (bacterial) RNA polymerase and variable results have been reported. Sawada *et al.* (1973) and Arnold *et al.* (1973) have shown an increase in the overall RNA transcription from chromatin of malignant cells, or, in other cases, a normal level of transcription. Grunicke *et al.* (1970) have reported that in some hepatomas the overall RNA transcription is lower than that of the normal liver chromatin. It is still quite difficult to understand whether the variability of the data indicates that some of these changes reflect alterations that

5. Histones

5.1. Histones and Cell Proliferation

A great amount of research has been carried out on histones since Stedman and
Stedman (1950) proposed that these basic nuclear proteins might be repressors of
gene activity. Today, 25 years later, it is generally accepted that histones are not
directly involved in fine regulation of gene expression and there is no evidence
that specific histones combine with specific genes (Shih and Bonner, 1970), but
still their function is not completely clear. Bonner and Garrard (1974) have
reviewed what is known about the biological function of the histones. It is
generally accepted that histones play a role in the supercoiling of DNA and are
responsible for the aspecific restriction of transcription of DNA in 80% of the
genome that is normally permanently repressed in eukaryotes. The lack of
specificity of histones as fine gene regulators is suggested from the fact that there
are only five main classes of histones in somatic cells of most eukaryotes
(Crampton *et al.*, 1955; Luck *et al.*, 1958; Johns and Butler, 1962; Dick and Johns,
1969*a*). An exception to this rule is seen in nucleated avian erythrocytes, where
there is a unique histone species (f_{2c}) which replaces the lysine-rich histones during
maturation of erythrocytes in birds (Dick and Johns, 1969*b*) at the time that the
putative nucleus becomes picnotic and genetically inactive. The lack of specificity
of histones as gene regulators is not accepted by everybody. For example, Tsanev
and Sendor (1971) have suggested that with 60 histone molecules, each occupying
only two or three turns of the DNA for five different types of histones, there would
be 5^{60} possible histone arrangements. These different arrangements could
specifically regulate the expression of practically all the structural genes of a
eukaryotic cell.

There have been a number of studies dealing with histones and cell proliferation, and it is now generally accepted that histones are synthesized during the S
phase of the cell cycle and their synthesis is tightly coupled with the synthesis of
DNA (Bloch and Godman, 1955; Takai *et al.*, 1968; Gurley and Hardin, 1970).
After they are synthesized, histones have an extremely low metabolic turnover
and are practically immortal (Hancock, 1969).

Histones undergo extensive posttranslational modifications, and these modifications have been reported to be prevalently associated with different conditions
of cell proliferation and specific phases of the cell cycle. Detailed analysis of all
these facts can be found in the review articles by Elgin *et al.* (1971) and Borun
(1974).

Three main groups of posttranslational modifications of the histones are
known. They are acetylation of lysine and *N*-terminal amino acids (Allfrey *et al.*,
1964; Gershey *et al.*, 1968), phosphorylation of serine and threonine (Kleinsmith

et al., 1966*b*; Langan, 1968), and lysine methylation (Murray, 1964; Paik and Kim, 1967). Examples of correlation of acetylation with events of the cell cycle or gene expression have been reported by Allfrey (1969). In regenerating liver and in human lymphocytes stimulated by phytohemagglutinin, the increased acetylation of arginine-rich histones precedes the increase in the synthesis of RNA that takes place a few hours after stimulation (Pogo *et al.*, 1966, 1968). It is not clear, however, whether this represents a cause-and-effect phenomenon or both events are secondary to other cellular modifications.

A large number of studies deal with the phosphorylation of histones and how the progression of a cell through the cell cycle could be controlled by phosphorylated histones. In particular, phosphorylation of histone f_1 is of importance because it is largely present in rapidly replicating tissues and essentially absent in stationary cultures. Gurley *et al.* (1973*a,b*) have shown that phosphorylation of histone f_1 is virtually absent in cultures in the stationary phase, and Tobey *et al.* (1974) have given some evidence that f_1 phosphorylation begins approximately 2 h before the onset of DNA synthesis. The process continues at an increased rate through S phase and G_2 phase and into mitosis (Balhorn *et al.*, 1972; Marks *et al.*, 1973; Tobey *et al.*, 1974). Bradbury *et al.* (1974*a,b*) have shown that f_1 histone phosphorylation activity correlates closely in the cell cycle of *Plasmodium polycephalum* with behavior of the mitotic trigger. On this basis, it has been proposed that the phosphorylation of f_1 histone is the key initiation step for mitosis.

During the cell cycle of HeLa cells (Marks *et al.*, 1973), phosphorylation of histones f_{2a1} and f_{2a2} is at slower rate than phosphorylation of histone f_1. Also, histone f_{2a2} phosphorylation occurs in G_1-arrested cells as well as in all phases of the cell cycle (Gurley *et al.*, 1973*a,b*). Histone f_3 is phosphorylated when cells cross the G_2/M boundary and is dephosphorylated as cells move out of mitosis into G_1. The function of this specific phosphorylation is not known.

In contrast to phosphorylation and acetylation reaction, methylation of histones is highest in the late phases of the cell cycle (Hardin and Cherry, 1972; Tidwell *et al.*, 1968). The f_1 histone is not methylated and f_{2a1} and f_3 are highly methylated (Borun, 1974). It has been suggested that methylation may play a role in the condensation of the chromatin prior to mitosis (Gershey *et al.*, 1969).

5.2. Histones and Neoplasia

There is no evidence that histones of cancer cells are different from histones of normal cells (Busch, 1965). The same classes of histones are present in neoplasia, but it has been reported (Kinkade, 1971; Hohman *et al.*, 1971) that lysine-rich histones show variable quantitative differences between normal tissue and corresponding neoplastic tissue. There is presently no good explanation for these differences.

Several alterations of posttranscriptional modifications of the histones have been reported in cancer cells, but these alterations do not seem to be constant or specific for neoplasia. The acetyl group of histones in Novikoff hepatomas, for

example, turns over much more slowly than in normal liver (Libby, 1970), but
does not vary appreciably in a series of Morris hepatomas and normal liver cells
(Byvoet and Morris, 1971). Rapidly dividing tumors have a much higher level of
phosphorylation of f_1 histone (Sherod *et al.*, 1970; Balhorn *et al.*, 1972), but
phosphorylation of histone f_1 in tumors is linearly correlated with their replication
rate and simply reflects the known changes of f_1 histone during cell proliferation
that have been discussed in the previous section. Methylation of histones in
tumors is also variable. Turner and Hancock (1970) have shown that fetal liver
and hepatomas contained higher histone methylase activity than control adult
liver. Desay and Foley (1970) have reported a lower rate of f_{2a1} methylation in
various tumors. Paik *et al.* (1972) have observed that in hepatomas the rate of
methylation of arginine residues in histones roughly paralleled the growth rate of
the tumor. Baxter and Byvoet (1974) found that methylation of lysine in histones
was inhibited by certain carcinogens in liver.

6. Nonhistone Chromosomal Proteins

6.1. Nonhistone Chromosomal Proteins and Cell Proliferation

Besides histones, there is another large group of proteins present in the
chromatin: the nonhistone chromosomal proteins. This is a very heterogeneous
class of proteins that so far has been poorly characterized (for review, see Busch,
1974). The interest in these proteins is due to the fact that at least some of them
have been considered specific gene regulators. The relation between nonhistone
chromosomal proteins and cell proliferation has been the subject of active
investigation in the past few years (for review, see Baserga and Stein, 1971; Stein *et
al.*, 1974; Baserga, 1974).

The synthesis and modifications at the posttranslational level, which nonhistone
chromosomal proteins undergo during cell proliferation, have been studied in
two groups of experimental models:

1. The model in which quiescent cells (G_0 cells) are stimulated to enter the cell
cycle and divide.
2. The model in which the cells are already in the cell cycle and are continuously
dividing.

It is well known that quiescent cells (G_0 cells) can be stimulated to enter the cell
cycle and divide by an appropriate stimulus. Commonly used experimental
systems *in vivo* are the liver regenerating after partial hepatectomy, the uterus
stimulated by estrogens, the prostate by androgens, the kidney after folic acid
administration, and the salivary gland by isoproterenol. In tissue culture, commonly used systems are the lymphocytes stimulated to proliferate by phytohemagglutinin and the fibroblasts after change of conditioned medium to fresh serum.

It has been observed that every time a quiescent population of cells is stimulated to proliferate, within a few hours there is an increased synthesis of particular classes of nonhistone chromosomal proteins (Stein and Baserga, 1970a; Smith *et al.*, 1970; Rovera and Baserga, 1971; Becker and Stanners, 1972; Levy *et al.*, 1973; Le Stourgeon and Rusch, 1971; Cognetti *et al.*, 1972; Le Stourgeon *et al.*, 1973; Courtois *et al.*, 1974). The significance of the observed increased synthesis of these particular classes of nonhistone chromosomal proteins is still not completely clear. It has been shown that these nonhistone chromosomal proteins bind to DNA *in vitro* (Choe and Rose, 1974) and that their synthesis is chronologically associated with an increase in the template activity of RNA synthesis of the chromatin (Barker and Warren, 1966; Thaler and Villee, 1967; Farber *et al.*, 1971; Mayfield and Bonner, 1972; Novi and Baserga, 1972; Couch and Anderson, 1973; Spelsberg *et al.*, 1971). Experiments done with inhibitors of protein synthesis (Rovera *et al.*, 1971) or experiments in which the chromatin was dissociated and then reconstituted *in vitro* (Stein *et al.*, 1972; Stein and Farber, 1973; Kostraba and Wang, 1973) suggest that these nonhistone chromosomal proteins are required for modulating the amount of transcription at the level of the genome. These experiments, however, are still open to some criticism and need further confirmation.

In continuously cycling cells like HeLa cells or Chinese hamster cells, the synthesis of nonhistone chromosomal proteins takes place, unlike that of histones, throughout the cell cycle, and the highest rate of synthesis appears to be late in G_1 phase (Stein and Baserga, 1970a; Stein and Borun, 1972; Gerner and Humphrey, 1973). Relative increases of specific classes of these proteins, as shown by polyacrylamide gel electrophoresis, have been reported (Stein and Borun, 1972; Bhorjee and Pederson, 1972; Gerner and Humphrey, 1973).

The posttranslational modification of nonhistone chromosomal proteins has been studied better in regard to phosphorylation, and it has been suggested that these phosphoproteins may play a role in gene control mechanisms in eukaryotic cells (Kleinsmith *et al.*, 1966a; Allfrey, 1970).

When resting cells are stimulated to proliferate, phosphorylation of nonhistone chromosomal protein increases rapidly and reaches a maximum in late G_1 with specific qualitative changes (De Morales *et al.*, 1974; Johnson *et al.*, 1974; Ishida and Ahmed, 1974; Brade *et al.*, 1974). In continuously cycling cells, the rate of phosphorylation of nonhistone chromosomal proteins is maximal in late G_1 and early S phases, decreases in the late S and G_2 phases, and is suppressed during mitosis when RNA synthesis is also suppressed (Platz *et al.*, 1973; Kornberg, 1974).

6.2. Nonhistone Chromosomal Proteins in Neoplasia

Several reports have appeared in the literature in the last few years showing that there are biochemical and immunological differences in the nonhistone chromosomal proteins between transformed cells and their normal counterparts both *in vivo* and in tissue culture. Similar to what has been reported for the histones, these differences are not specific or constant for every type of tumor and often can be explained in terms of changes secondary to the rate of proliferation of the neoplastic cells. Grunicke *et al.* (1970) have shown that there are no quantitative or qualitative differences in the nonhistone chromosomal proteins between minimum-deviation hepatomas and host liver. However, fast-growing Novikoff hepatomas showed an increased amount of nuclear residual proteins. Smith and Mora (1971) and Arnold *et al.* (1973) found that some slow-growing Morris hepatomas have a slightly greater content of nonhistone proteins, but one fast-growing hepatoma had an increased amount of several species of nonhistone chromosomal proteins as shown in the electrophoretic pattern. However, Yeoman *et al.* (1973) analyzed the nonhistone chromosomal protein of regenerating liver, thioacetamide-treated liver, a Morris hepatoma, and the Walker 256 carcinosarcoma on two-dimensional gel electrophoresis and reported that tumor cells had a specific increase of a few acid-soluble proteins. Sawada *et al.* (1973) reported that normal lymphocytes had an increased amount of nonhistone chromosomal proteins and less histones compared with leukemia lymphocytes. Weisenthal and Ruddon (1972, 1973) showed that in acute leukemias, in particular, lymphoid leukemia, there is a lack of higher molecular weight nuclear proteins, and cells of chronic lymphocyte leukemia had an electrophoretic pattern of nonhistone chromosomal proteins similar to that of normal lymphocytes.

Differences in synthesis and turnover have been reported between normal fibroblasts in tissue culture and fibroblasts transformed by SV40 viruses (Cholon and Studzinski, 1974; Zardi *et al.*, 1973; Lin *et al.*, 1974; Stein *et al.*, 1974).

Interaction between specific nonhistone chromosomal proteins and carcinogens has been reported. The "H protein," a nonhistone protein, can be isolated from both cytoplasm and nuclei and binds dye carcinogens, and probably carries them from cytoplasm to nucleus (Bakey and Sorof, 1969; Bakey *et al.*, 1969; Ketterer, 1971; Libby, 1970; Morey and Litwack, 1969). Other chemical carcinogens have been shown to bind *in vivo* to histone and nonhistone proteins of rat liver nuclei (Jungmann and Schweppe, 1972). It seems that the presence of specific nonhistone chromosomal proteins in the chromatin dictates the specificity of the RNA species synthesized in tumors as well as in normal cells. When Walker tumor nonhistone proteins were used to activate the synthesis of RNA from normal rat liver chromatin in experiments in which the chromatin was reconstituted *in vitro*, the RNA produced was similar to that produced by Walker tumor chromatin (Kostraba and Wang, 1971).

7. Conclusions and Remarks

It is quite obvious from the overall picture presented in the previous pages that the studies that try to approach the problem of gene regulation in neoplasia at the molecular level are still relatively few and inadequate. This inadequacy is related to the fact that too little is known about gene regulation even in normal cells.

There are some main areas of research that need further clarification in order to increase the chances of finding some lesion at the level of the genome that is responsible for the transformed state of a cancer cell. For example, it is necessary to understand better how genes are turned on and off in eukaryotes, to find which are the relevant genes that are turned on or off in cancer cells, and to devise more adequate experimental systems that will allow rigorous comparisons between "normality" and "neoplasia."

Despite the great wealth of studies on how the expression of specific genes can be controlled at the level of the transcription, the results are still too far away from the sophistication reached in prokaryotes. The isolation of specific genes or groups of genes (Brown and Stern, 1974) and the development of *in vitro* systems for the study of how gene expression is controlled are conditions *sine qua non* for further progress in this field of molecular biology. For example, these studies could give a clue to why some particular fetal antigen may appear in cancer cells (Gold and Freedman, 1965) and why hormones are produced by non-hormone-secreting cells (Lipsett, 1965; see also Chapters 2 and 4, this volume).

There are now adequate tools that give us hope for an adequate answer also to questions such as are there cancer genes? how many? and where are they?

Recent experiments utilizing cell hybridization techniques seem to put the problem in a better perspective. When a nonproliferating normal mouse macrophage is fused with a transformed human cell, the hybrid presents a transformed phenotype, and if injected into nude mice is able to produce tumors (Croce *et al.*, 1975). However, the mouse human hybrid slowly loses all those human chromosomes that are not essential for growth and will maintain only those that are essential to keep the transformed state. For example, a hybrid between a mouse macrophage and a human fibroblast transformed by SV40 virus will require the presence of only the human chromosome C7 carrying the SV40 genome in order to proliferate (Croce and Koprowski, 1974). By use of selective procedures of this type and utilizing tumors of different sources, the genes responsible for transformation can be identified and their relationship analyzed.

Experiments by Goldenberg *et al.* (1974) also suggest that not only in tissue culture but also *in vivo* in hamster pouches hybridization seems to take place between hamster cells and human malignant cells. The resulting hybrids are able to produce metastasis in the recipient hamster and will selectively lose the human chromosomes not essential for transformation. This sort of experiment will tell us a great deal about chromosomal localization of the "cancer genes" and whether they are specific for each type of cancer or are common to all types. Hybrids of this type could also prove valuable in obtaining a relative purification of human chromosomes carrying these "cancer genes" for molecular biology studies.

Another problem is which systems are better suited for biochemical and molecular biology studies of gene regulation in transformation. Obviously it is difficult to compare a transplantable tumor to a normal tissue, or different cell lines to each other, and correlate the findings to the problem of cancer. Too many changes that do not have anything to do with transformation but have to do with tumor progression can take place.

As a practical example, those studies which try to compare the various chromosomal proteins of normal cells to those of transformed cells in tissue

culture should be regarded with caution because they could simply reflect an
enrichment of particular classes of proteins normally present secondary to
changes in the Karyotype of the transformed cells. In fact, Stubblefield and Wray
(1974) have shown that different classes of chromosomes have different relative
amounts of chromosomal proteins.

For several reasons, it appears easier to carry out molecular biology studies on
the transformed state utilizing tissue culture cells rather than tumors growing in
animals. One of the reasons, for example, is that only with tissue culture cells we
can develop conditional lethal mutants for transformation, and these genetic tools
are a necessary complement for sophisticated molecular biology (Renger and
Basilco, 1972; di Mayorca *et al.*, 1973; Rutland *et al.*, 1974). Unfortunately, there
are several problems connected with what is "normal" and what is "malignant" in
tissue culture and with what their correlation is to *in vivo* conditions (for
discussion, see Pontén, 1971).

8. References

ALLFREY, V. G., 1969, The role of chromosomal proteins in gene activation, in: *Biochemistry of Cell Division* (R. Baserga, ed.), p. 179, Thomas, Springfield, Ill.

ALLFREY, V. G., 1970, Changes in chromosomal proteins at times of gene activation, *Fed. Proc.* **29**:1447.

ALLFREY, V. G., LITTAU, V. C., AND MIRSKY, A. E., 1963, On the role of histones in regulating ribonucleic acid synthesis in the cell nucleus, *Proc. Natl. Acad. Sci. U.S.A.* **49**:414.

ALLFREY, V. G., FAULKNER, R., AND MIRSKY, A. E., 1964, Acetylation and methylation of histones and their possible role in the regulation of RNA synthesis, *Proc. Natl. Acad. Sci. U.S.A.* **51**:786.

ARNOLD, E. A., BUKSAS, M. M., AND YOUNG, K. E., 1973, A comparative study of some properties of chromatin from two minimal deviation hepatomas, *Cancer res.* **33**:1169.

ATTWOOD, H. D., AND PARK, W. W., 1961, Embolism to the lungs by trophoblasts, *J. Obstet. Gynaecol. Br. Commonw.* **68**:611.

BAKEY, B., AND SOROF, S., 1969, Zonal electrophoresis of the soluble nuclear proteins of normal and preneoplastic livers, *Cancer Res.* **29**:22.

BAKEY, B., SOROF, S., AND SIEBERT, G., 1969, Azoproteins of liver nuclei isolated in an aqueous or nonaqueous medium from rats fed an azocarcinogen, *Cancer Res.* **29**:28.

BALHORN, R., BALHORN, M., MORRIS, H. P., AND CHALKLEY, R., 1972, Comparative high resolution electrophoresis of tumor histones: Variation in phosphorylation as a function of cell replication rate, *Cancer Res.* **32**:1775.

BARKER, K. L., AND WARREN, J. C., 1966, Template capacity of uterine chromatin control by estradiol, *Proc. Natl. Acad. Sci. U.S.A.* **56**:1298.

BASERGA, R., 1974, Non-histone chromosomal proteins in normal and abnormal growth, *Life Sci.* **15**:1057.

BASERGA, R., AND STEIN, G., 1971, Nuclear acidic proteins and cell proliferation, *Fed. Proc.* **30**:1752.

BAXTER, C. S., AND BYVOET, P., 1974, Effects of carcinogens and other agents on histone methylation in rat liver nuclei by endogenous histone lysine methyltransferase, *Cancer Res.* **34**:1424.

BECKER, H., AND STANNERS, C. P., 1972, Control of macromolecular synthesis in proliferating and resting Syrian hamster cells in monolayer culture, *J. Cell. Physiol.* **80**:51.

BEKHOR, I., KUNG, G. M., AND BONNER, J., 1969, Sequence-specific interaction of DNA and chromosomal protein, *J. Mol. Biol.* **39**:351.

BHORJEE, J. S., AND PEDERSON, T., 1972, Nonhistone chromosomal proteins in synchronized HeLa cells, *Proc. Natl. Acad. Sci. U.S.A.* **69**:3345.

BLOCH, D. P., AND GODMAN, G. C., 1955, A microspectrophotometric study of the synthesis of deoxyribonucleic acid and nuclear histone, *J. Biophys. Biochem. Cytol.* **1**:17.

BONNER, J., AND GARRARD, W. T., 1974, Biology of the histones, *Life Sci.* **14**:209.

BORUN, T., 1975, Histones, differentiation and the cell cycle, in: *Results and Problems in Cell Differentiation* 7:249 (J. Reinert and H. Holtzer, eds.), Springer-Verlag, Berlin.

BRADBURY, E. M., INGLIS, R. J., AND MATTHEWS, H. R., 1974a, Control of cell division by very lysine rich histone (F_1) phosphorylation, *Nature (London)* 247:257.

BRADBURY, E. M., INGLIS, R. J., MATTHEWS, H. R., AND LANGAN, T. A., 1974b, Molecular basis of control of mitotic cell division in eukaryotes, *Nature (London)* 249:553.

BRADE, W. P., THOMPSON, J. A., CHIU, J. F., AND HNILICA, L. S., 1974, Chromatin-bound kinase activity and phosphorylation of chromatin nonhistone proteins during early kidney regeneration after folic acid, *Exp. Cell Res.* 74:183.

BRITTEN, R. J., AND DAVIDSON, E. H., 1969, Gene regulation for higher cells: A theory, *Science* 165:349.

BRITTEN, R. J., AND KOHNE, D. E., 1968, Repeated sequences in DNA, *Science* 161:529.

BROWN, D. D., AND STERN, R., 1974, Methods of gene isolation, *Ann. Rev. Biochem.* 43:862.

BUSCH, H., 1965, *Histones and Other Nuclear Proteins*, Academic Press, New York.

BUSCH, H., 1974, *The Molecular Biology of Cancer* (H. Busch, ed.), Academic Press, New York.

BYVOET, P., AND MORRIS, H. P., 1971, N-Acetylation of arginine-rich hepatoma histones, *Cancer Res.* 31:468.

CHIARUGI, V. D., 1969, *Biochim. Biophys. Acta* 179:129.

CHOE, B. K., AND ROSE, N. R., 1974, Synthesis of DNA binding protein in WI-38 cells stimulated to synthesize DNA by medium replacement, *Exp. Cell Res.* 83:261.

CHOLON, J. J., AND STUDZINSKI, C. P., 1974, Effects of aminonucleoside on serum stimulation of nonhistone nuclear proteins and DNA synthesis in normal SV40 transformed human fibroblasts, *Cancer Res.* 34:588.

CHURCH, R. B., LUTHER, S. W., AND McCARTHY, B. J., 1969, RNA synthesis in taper hepatoma and mouse liver cells, *Biochim. Biophys. Acta* 179:129.

COGNETTI, G., SETTINERI, V., AND SPINELLI, C., 1972, Developmental changes of chromatin nonhistone proteins in sea urchins, *Exp. Cell. Res.* 71:465.

COMINGS, D. E., 1973, A general theory of carcinogenesis, *Proc. Natl. Acad. Sci.* 70:3324.

COUCH, R. M., AND ANDERSON, K. M., 1973, Rat ventral prostrate chromatin: Effect of androgens on the chemical composition, physical properties and template activity, *Biochemistry* 12:3114.

COURTOIS, Y., DASTOGUE, B., AND KRUH, J., 1974, Effects of lysine deprivation and serum stimulation on the synthesis of non-histone chromosomal proteins by confluent chick fibroblasts, *Exp. Cell Res.* 83:152.

CRAMPTON, C. F., MOORE, S., AND STEIN, W. H., 1955, Chromatographic fractionation of calf thymus histone, *J. Biol. Chem.* 215:787.

CRICK, F., 1971, General model for the chromosomes of higher organisms, *Nature (London)* 234:25.

CROCE, C. M., AND KOPROWSKI, H., 1974, Somatic cell hybrid between mouse peritoneal macrophage and SV_{40} transformed human cells. I. Positive control of the transformed phenotype by the human chromosome C7 carrying the SV_{40} genome, *J. Exp. Med.* 140:1221.

CROCE, C. M., ADEN, D., AND KOPROWSKI, H., 1975, Somatic cell hybrid between mouse peritoneal macrophage and SV_{40} transformed human cells. II. Presence of human chromosome C7 carrying the SV_{40} genome in tumors induced by the hybrid cells, *Proc. Natl. Acad. Sci.* 72:1397.

DAVIDSON, E. H., 1969, *Gene Activity in Early Development*, Academic Press, New York.

DAVIDSON, E. H., HOUGH, B. R., AMENSON, C. S., AND BRITTEN, R. J., 1973, General interspersion of repetitive with non-repetitive sequence elements in the DNA of *Xenopus*, *J. Mol. Biol.* 77:1.

DE MORALES, M. M., BLAT, C., AND HAREL, L., 1974, Changes in the phosphorylation of non-histone chromosomal proteins in relationship to DNA and RNA synthesis in BHK_{21} C_{13} cells, *Exp. Cell Res.* 86:111.

DENIS, H., 1966, Gene expression in amphibian development. II. Release of the genetic information in growing embryos, *J. Mol. Biol.* 22:285.

DESAY, L. S., AND FOLEY, G., 1970, Homologies in amino acid composition and structure of histone F_{2a1} isolated from human leukaemic cells, *Biochem. J.* 119:165.

DICK, C., AND JOHNS, E. W., 1969a, The biosynthesis of the five main histone fractions of rat thymus, *Biochim. Biophys. Acta* 174:380.

DICK, C., AND JOHNS, E. W., 1969b, A quantitative comparison of histones from immature and mature erythroid cells of the duck, *Biochim. Biophys. Acta* 175:414.

DI MAYORCA, G., GREENBLATT, M., TRAUTHEN, T., AND SOLLER, A., 1973, Malignant transformation of BHK_{21} clone 13 cells *in vitro* by nitrosamines—A conditional state, *Proc. Natl. Acad. Sci. U.S.A.* 70:46.

DREWS, J., BRAVERMAN, G., AND MORRIS, H. P., 1968, Nucleotide sequence homologies in nuclear and cytoplasmic ribonucleic acid from rat liver and hepatomas, *Eur. J. Biochem.* **3**:784.

ELGIN, S. C. R., FROEHNER, S. C., SMART, J. E., AND BONNER, J., 1971, The biology and chemistry of chromosomal proteins, *Adv. Cell Mol. Biol.* **1**:1.

FARBER, J., ROVERA, G., AND BASERGA, R., 1971, Template activity of chromatin during stimulation of cellular proliferation in human diploid fibroblasts, *Biochem. J.* **122**:189.

FLAMM, W. G., WALKER, P. M. B., AND McCALLUM, M., 1969, Some properties of the single strands isolated from the DNA of the nuclear satellite of the mouse (*Mus musculus*), *J. Mol. Biol.* **40**:423.

GEORGIEV, G. P., VARSHAVSKY, A. J., RYSKOV, A. P., AND CHURCH, R. B., 1973, On the structural organization of the transcriptional unit in animal chromosomes, *Cold Spring Harbor Symp. Quant. Biol.* **38**:869.

GERNER, E. W., AND HUMPHREY, R. M., 1973, The cell cycle phase synthesis of nonhistone proteins in mammalian cells, *Biochim. Biophys. Acta* **331**:117.

GERSHEY, E. L., VIDALI, G., AND ALLFREY, V. G., 1968, Chemical studies of histone acetylation: The occurrence of N-acetyl-lysine in the f_{2a1} histone, *J. Biol. Chem.* **243**:5018.

GERSHEY, E. L., HASLETT, G. W., VIDALI, G., AND ALLFREY, V. G., 1969, Evidence for the occurrence of 3-methylhistidine in avian erythrocyte histone fractions, *J. Biol. Chem.* **244**:4871.

GILMOUR, R. S., AND PAUL, J., 1969, RNA transcribed from reconstituted nucleoprotein is similar to natural RNA, *J. Mol. Biol.* **40**:137.

GILMOUR, R. S., AND PAUL, J., 1973, Tissue specific transcription of the globin gene in isolated chromatin, *Proc. Natl. Acad. Sci. U.S.A.* **70**:3440.

GOLD, P., AND FREEDMAN, S. O., 1965, Specific carcinoembryonic antigens of the human digestive system, *J. Exp. Med.* **122**:467.

GOLDENBERG, D. M., PAVIA, R. A., AND TSAO, M. C., 1974, *In vivo* hybridization of human tumour and normal hamster cells, *Nature (London)* **250**:649.

GRUNICKE, H., POTTER, V. R., AND MORRIS, H. P., 1970, Comparative studies on nuclei and chromatin of hepatoma and rat liver, *Cancer Res.* **30**:776.

GURLEY, L. R., AND HARDIN, J. M., 1970, The metabolism of histone fractions. I. Synthesis of histone fractions during the life cycle of mammalian cells, *Arch. Biochem. Biophys.* **136**:392.

GURLEY, L. R., WALTERS, R. A., AND TOBEY, R. A., 1973*a*, The metabolism of histone fractions. VI. Differences in the phosphorylation of histone fractions during the cell cycle, *Arch. Biochem. Biophys.* **154**:212.

GURLEY, L. R., WALTERS, R. A., AND TOBEY, R. A., 1973*b*, Histone phosphorylation in late interphase and mitosis, *Biochem. Biophys. Res. Commun.* **50**:744.

HAINES, M., 1955, Hydatidiform mole and vaginal nodules, *J. Obstet. Gynaecol. Br. Emp.* **62**:6.

HALPRIN, K. M., AND TAYLOR, J. R., 1971, The biochemistry of skin disease: Psoriasis, *Adv. Clin. Chem.* **14**:319.

HANCOCK, R., 1969, Conservation of histones in chromatin during growth and mitosis *in vitro*, *J. Mol. Biol.* **40**:457.

HARDIN, J. W., AND CHERRY, J. H., 1972, Solubilization and partial characterization of soybean chromatin-bound RNA polymerase, *Biochem. Biophys. Res. Commun.* **48**:299.

HEWISH, D. R., AND BURGOYNE, L. A., 1973, Chromatin sub-structure: The digestion of chromatin DNA at regularly spaced sites by a nuclear deoxyribonuclease, *Biochem. Biophys. Res. Commun.* **52**:504.

HOHMAN, P., COLE, R. D., AND BERN, H. A., 1971, Comparison of lysine-rich histones in various normal and neoplastic mouse tissues, *J. Natl. Cancer Inst.* **47**:337.

HUANG, R. C., AND BONNER, J., 1962, Histone, a suppressor of chromosomal RNA synthesis, *Proc. Natl. Acad. Sci. U.S.A.* **48**:1216.

HUANG, R. C., AND HUANG, P. C., 1969, Effect of protein-bound RNA with chick embryo chromatin on template specificity of the chromatin, *J. Mol. Biol.* **39**:365.

ISHIDA, H., AND AHMED, K., 1974, Studies on chromatin associated protein phosphokinase of submandibular gland from isoproterenol treated rats, *Exp. Cell Res.* **84**:127.

JOHNS, E. V., AND BUTLER, J. A. V., 1962, Further fractionation of histones from calf thymus, *Biochem. J.* **82**:15.

JOHNSON, E. M., KARN, J., AND ALLFREY, V. G., 1974, Early nuclear events in the induction of lymphocyte proliferation by mitogens, *J. Biol. Chem.* **249**:4990.

JUNGMANN, R. A., AND SCHWEPPE, J. S., 1972, Binding of chemical carcinogens to nuclear proteins of rat liver, *Cancer Res.* **32**:952.

KAMIYAMA, M., AND WANG, T. Y., 1971, Activated transcription from rat liver chromatin by nonhistone proteins, *Biochim. Biophys. Acta* **228:**563.

KARN, J., JOHNSON, E. M., VIDALI, G., AND ALLFREY, V. G., 1974, Differential phosphorylation and turnover of nuclear acidic proteins during the cell cycle of synchronized HeLa cells, *J. Biol. Chem.* **249:**667.

KETTERER, B., 1971, Proteins that bind carcinogen metabolites, *Biochem. J.* **126:**3P.

KINKADE, J. M., JR., 1971, Differences in the quantitative distribution of lysine rich histones in neoplastic and normal tissues, *Proc. Soc. Exp. Biol. Med.* **137:**1131.

KLEINSMITH, L. J., ALLFREY, V. G., AND MIRSKY, A. E., 1966a, Phosphoprotein metabolism in isolated lymphocyte nuclei, *Proc. Natl. Acad. Sci. U.S.A.* **55:**1182.

KLEINSMITH, L. J., ALLFREY, V. G., AND MIRSKY, A. E., 1966b, Phosphorylation of nuclear protein early in the course of gene activation in lymphocytes, *Science* **154:**780.

KORNBERG, R. D., 1974, Chromatin structure: A repeating unit of histones and DNA, *Science* **184:**868.

KOSTRABA, N. C., AND WANG, T. Y., 1971, Transcription of Walker 256 carcinosarcoma chromatin, *Cancer Res.* **31:**1663.

KOSTRABA, N. C., AND WANG, T. Y., 1973, Nonhistone proteins and gene activation in regenerating rat liver, *Exp. Cell Res.* **80:**291.

LANGAN, T., 1968, Histone phosphorylation : Stimulation by adenosine 3 : 5 monophosphate, *Science* **162:**579.

LEHMAN, J. M., SPEERS, W. C., SWARTZENDRUBER, D. E., AND PIERCE, G. B., 1974, Neoplastic differentiation: Characteristics of cell lines derived from a murine teratocarcinoma, *J. Cell Physiol.* **84:**13.

LE STOURGEON, W. M., AND RUSCH, H. P., 1971, Nuclear acidic protein changes during differentiation in *Physarum polycephalum, Science* **174:**1233.

LE STOURGEON, W. M., WRAY, W., AND RUSCH, H. P., 1973, Functional homologies of acidic chromatin proteins in higher and lower eukaryotes, *Exp. Cell Res.* **79:**487.

LEVY, R., LEVY, S., ROSENBERG, S. A., AND SIMPSON, R. T., 1973, Selective stimulation of nonhistone chromatin protein synthesis in lymphoid cells by phytohemagglutinin, *Biochemistry* **12:**224.

LIBBY, P. R., 1970, Activity of histone deacetylase in rat liver and Novikoff hepatoma, *Biochim. Biophys. Acta* **213:**234.

LIN, J. C., NICOLINI, C., AND BASERGA, R., 1974, A comparative study of some properties of chromatin from normal diploid and SV_{40} transformed human fibroblasts, *Biochemistry* **13:**4127.

LIPSETT, M. B., 1965, Humoral syndromes associated with cancer, *Cancer Res.* **25:**1068.

LUCK, J. M., RASSMUSSEN, P. S., SATAKE, K., AND TSVETIKOV, A. N., 1958, Further studies on the fractionation of calf thymus histone, *J. Biol. Chem.* **233:**1407.

MARKS, D. B., PAIK, W. K., AND BORUN, T. W., 1973, The relationship of histone phorphorylation to deoxyribonucleic acid replication and mitosis during the HeLa S-3 cell cycle, *J. Biol. Chem.* **248:**5660.

MAYFIELD, J. E., AND BONNER, J., 1972, A partial sequence of nuclear events in regenerating rat liver, *Proc. Natl. Acad. Sci. U.S.A.* **69:**7.

MENDECKI, J., MINC, B., AND CHORAZY, M., 1969, Differences in RNA from rat liver and hepatoma revealed by DNA-RNA hybridization, *Biochem. Biophys. Res. Commun.* **36:**494.

MILLER, E. C., AND MILLER, J. A., 1974, Biochemical mechanisms of chemical carcinogenesis, in: *The Molecular Biology of Cancer* (H. Busch, ed.), p. 377, Springer, New York.

MONAHAN, J. J., AND HALL, R. H., 1974, Chromatin and gene regulation in eukaryotic cells at the transcriptional level, *CRC Crit. Rev. Biochem.* **1:**67.

MOREY, K. S., AND LITWACK, G., 1969, Isolation and properties of cortisol metabolite binding proteins of rat liver cytosol, *Biochemistry* **8:**4813.

MURAMATSU, M., NEMOTO, N., INUI, N., AND TAKAYAMA, S., 1973, Change in the transcription of repetitive DNA sequences in *N*-methyl-*N*'-nitro-*N*-nitroguanidine transformed hamster cells, *Cancer Res.* **33:**739.

MURRAY, K., 1964, The occurrence of epsilon-*N*-methyl lysine in histones, *Biochemistry* **3:**10.

NEIMAN, P. E., AND HENRY, P. H., 1969, Ribonucleic acid–deoxyribonucleic acid hybridization and hybridization—Competition studies of the rapidly labeled ribonucleic, *Biochemistry* **8:**275.

NOLL, M., 1974, Subunit structure of chromatin, *Nature (London)* **251:**249.

NOVI, A. M., AND BASERGA, R., 1972, Changes in chromatin template activity and their relationship to DNA synthesis in mouse parotid glands stimulated by isoproterenol, *J. Cell Biol.* **55:**554.

ONO, T., KAWAMURA, M., HYODA, M., AND WAKABAYASHI, K., 1971, Differences of RNA population between normal liver and hepatoma AH-130, *Gann* **62:**31.

PAIK, W. K., AND KIM, S., 1967, Epsilon-N-dimethyllysine in histones, *Biochem. Biophys. Res. Commun.* **27**:479.

PAIK, W. K., LEE, H. W., AND MORRIS, H. P., 1972, Protein methylases in hepatomas, *Cancer res.* **32**:37.

PARDON, J. F., WILKINS, M. H. F., AND RICHARDS, B. M., 1967, Super-helical model for nucleohistone, *Nature (London)* **215**:508.

PAUL, J., AND GILMOUR, R. S., 1968, Organ-specific restriction of transcription in mammalian chromatin, *J. Mol. Biol.* **34**:305.

PIERCE, G. B., AND WALLACE, C., 1971, Differentiation of malignant to benign cells, *Cancer Res.* **31**:127.

PIERCE, G. B., DIXON, F. J., AND VERNEY, E. L., 1960, Teratogenic and tissue forming potentials of the cell types comprising neoplastic embryoid bodies, *Lab. Invest.* **9**:583.

PIRROTTA, V., CHADWICK, P., AND PTASHNE, M., 1970, Active form of two coliphage repressors, *Nature (London)* **227**:41.

PLATZ, R. D., STEIN, G. S., AND KLEINSMITH, L. J., 1973, Changes in the phosphorylation of nonhistone chromatin proteins during the cell cycle of HeLa S_3 cells, *Biochem. Biophys. Res. Commun.* **51**:735.

POGO, B. G. T., ALLFREY, V. G., AND MIRSKY, A. E., 1966, RNA synthesis and histone acetylation during the course of gene activation in lymphocytes, *Proc. Natl. Acad. Sci. U.S.A.* **55**:805.

POGO, B. G. T., POGO, A. O., ALLFREY, V. G., AND MIRSKY, A. E., 1968, Changing patterns of histone acetylation and RNA synthesis in regeneration of the liver, *Proc. Natl. Acad. Sci. U.S.A.* **59**:1337.

PONTÉN, J., 1971, Spontaneous and virus induced transformation in cell culture, in: *Virology Monographs*, Vol. 8 (S. Gerd, C. Hallauer, and K. F. Meyer, eds.), Springer, New York.

RENGER, H. C., AND BASILICO, C., 1972, Mutation causing temperature sensitive expression of cell transformation by a tumor virus, *Proc. Natl. Acad. Sci. U.S.A.* **69**:109.

ROVERA, G., AND BASERGA, R., 1971, Early changes in the synthesis of acidic nuclear proteins in human diploid fibroblasts stimulated to synthesize DNA by changing the medium. *J. Cell. Physiol.* **77**:201.

ROVERA, G., FARBER, J., AND BASERGA, R., 1971, Gene activation in WI-38 fibroblasts stimulated to proliferate: Requirement for protein synthesis, *Proc. Natl. Acad. Sci. U.S.A.* **68**:1725.

RUDLAND, P. S., ECKHARDT, W., GOSPODAROWICZ, D., AND SEIFERT, W., 1974, Cell transformation mutants are not susceptible to growth activation by fibroblast growth factor at permissive temperatures, *Nature (London)* **250**:337.

RUTTER, V. J., PICTET, R. L., AND MORRIS, P. W., 1973, Toward molecular mechanisms of developmental processes, *Ann. Rev. Biochem.* **42**:601.

SAWADA, H., GILMORE, V. H., AND SAUNDERS, G. F., 1973, Transcription from chromatins of human lymphocyte leukemia cells and normal lymphocytes, *Cancer Res.* **33**:478.

SHEARER, R. W., 1971, DNA of rat hepatomas: Search for gene amplification, *Biochem. Biophys. Res. Commun.* **43**:1324.

SHEARER, R. W., AND McCARTHY, B. J., 1967, Evidence for ribonucleic acid molecules restricted to the cell nucleus, *Biochemistry* **6**:283.

SHEROD, D., JOHNSON, G., AND CHALKLEY, R., 1970, Phosphorylation of mouse ascites tumor cell lysine rich histone, *Biochemistry* **9**:4611.

SHIH, T. Y., AND BONNER, J., 1970, Template properties of DNA–polypeptide complexes, *J. Mol. Biol.* **50**:333.

SIMPSON, R. T., 1973, Structure and function of chromatin, *Adv. Enzymol.* **38**:41.

SMITH, A. A., MARTIN, L., KING, R. J. B., AND VERTES, M., 1970, Effects of oestradiol 17β and progesterone on total and nuclear protein synthesis in epithelial and stromal tissue of the mouse uterus and of progesterone on the ability of these tissues to bind oestradiol 17β, *Biochem. J.* **119**:773.

SMITH, C. E., AND MORA, P. T., 1971, Properties of chromatin from liver and from a chemically induced minimal deviation hepatoma of rat, *Biochim. Biophys. Acta* **232**:643.

SOBELL, H. M., 1973, Symmetry in protein–nucleic acid interactions and its genetic implications, *Adv. Genet.* **17**:411.

SPELSBERG, T. C., HNILICA, L. S., AND ANSEVIN, A. T., 1971, Proteins of chromatin in template restriction. III. The macromolecules in specific restriction of the chromatin DNA, *Biochim. Biophys. Acta* **228**:550.

STEDMAN, E. S., AND STEDMAN, E., 1950, Cell specificity of histones, *Nature (London)* **166**:780.

STEIN, G. S., AND BASERGA, R., 1970a, Continued synthesis of nonhistone chromosomal proteins during mitosis, *Biochem. Biophys. res. Commun.* **41**:715.

STEIN, G. S., AND BASERGA, R., 1970b, The synthesis of acidic nuclear proteins in the prereplicative phase of the isoproterenol-stimulated salivary gland, *J. Biol. Chem.* **245**:6097.

STEIN, G. S., AND BORUN, T. W., 1972, The synthesis of acidic chromosomal proteins during the cell cycle of HeLa S₃ cells. I. The accelerated accumulation of acidic residual nuclear proteins before the initiation of DNA replication, *J. Cell Biol.* **52**:292.

STEIN, G., AND FARBER, J., 1973, Role of nonhistone chromosomal proteins in the restriction of mitotic chromatin template activity, *Proc. Natl. Acad. Sci. U.S.A.* **69**:2918.

STEIN, G. S., CHAUDHURI, S. C., AND BASERGA, R., 1972, Gene activation in WI-38 fibroblasts stimulated to proliferate, *J. Biol. Chem.* **247**:3918.

STEIN, G. S., SPELSBERG, T. C., AND KLEINSMITH, L. J., 1974, Nonhistone chromosomal proteins and gene regulation, *Science* **183**:817.

STUBBLEFIELD, E., AND WRAY, W., 1974, Biochemical and morphological studies of partially purified Chinese hamster chromosomes, *Cold Spring Harbor Symp. Quant. Biol.* **38**:835.

TAKAI, S., BORUN, T. W., MUCHMORE, J., AND LIEBERMAN, I., 1968, Concurrent synthesis of histone and deoxyribonucleic acid in liver after partial hepatectomy, *Nature (London)* **219**:860.

THALER, M. M., AND VILLEE, C. A., 1967, Template activities in normal regenerating and developing rat liver chromatin, *Proc. Natl. Acad. Sci. U.S.A.* **58**:2055.

THOMAS, C. A., AND LEE, C. S., 1973, Formation of rings from *Drosophila* DNA fragments, *J. Mol. Biol.* **77**:25.

THOMAS, C. A. JR., HAMKALS, B. A., MIORA, D. N., AND LEE, C. S., 1970, Cyclization of eucaryotic deoxyribonucleic acid fragments, *J. Mol. Biol.* **51**:621.

TIDWELL, T., ALLFREY, V. G., AND MIRSKY, A. E., 1968, The methylation of histones during regeneration of the liver, *J. Biol. Chem.* **243**:707.

TOBEY, R. A., GURLEY, L. R., HILDEBRAND, C. E., RATLIFF, R. L., AND WALKER, R. A., 1974, Sequential biochemical events in preparation for DNA replication and mitosis, in: *Control of Proliferation in Animal Cells* (B. Clarkson and R. Baserga, eds.), p. 665, Cold Spring Harbor Laboratory, Cold Spring Harbor, New York.

TOOZE, J., 1973, *The Molecular Biology of Tumour Viruses* (J. Tooze, ed.), Cold Spring Harbor Laboratory, Cold Spring Harbor, New York.

TSANEV, R., AND SENDOR, B., 1971, Possible molecular mechanism for cell differentiation in multicellular organisms, *J. Theor. Biol.* **30**:337.

TURKINGTON, R. W., AND SELF, D. J., 1970, New Species of hybridizable nuclear RNA in breast cancer cells, *Cancer Res.* **30**:1833.

TURNER, G., AND HANCOCK, R. L., 1970, Histone methylase activity of adult, embryonic and neoplastic liver tissues, *Life Sci.* **9**:917.

WALKER, P. M. B., 1971, Repetitive DNA in higher organisms, *Proc. Biophys. Mol. Biol.* **23**:145.

WEISENTHAL, W., AND RUDDON, R. W., 1972, Characterization of human leukemia and Burkitt lymphoma cells by their acidic nuclear protein profiles, *Cancer Res.* **32**:1009.

WEISENTHAL, L. M., AND RUDDON, R. W., 1973, Catabolism of nuclear proteins in control and phytohemagglutinin-stimulated human lymphocytes, leukemic leukocytes, and Burkitt lymphoma cells, *Cancer Res.* **33**:2923.

WHITE, H. B., III, LAUX, B. E., AND DENNIS, D., 1972, Messenger RNA structure: Compatibility of hairpin loops with protein sequence, *Science* **175**:1264.

YEOMAN, L. C., TAYLOR, C. W., AND BUSCH, H., 1973, 2-Dimensional polyacrylamide gel electrophoresis of acid extractable nuclear proteins of normal rat liver and Novikoff hepatoma ascites cells, *Biochem. Biophys. Res. Commun.* **51**:956.

YUNIS, J. J., 1970, Satellite DNA in constitutive heterochromatin of guinea pig, *Science* **168**:263.

ZARDI, L., LIN, J. C., AND BASERGA, R., 1973, Immunospecificity to nonhistone chromosomal proteins of antichromatin antibodies, *Nature New Biol.* **245**:211.

16

Protein Synthesis

A. Clark Griffin

1. Introduction

Protein synthesis in the cancer cell appears to follow very closely the general mechanism that has been established for prokaryotic cells and for the normal eukaryotic cell systems that have been studied. Thus the same major components of the polysomal system have been identified in all cells. The same events in polypeptide formation, generally grouped as chain initiation, elongation, and peptide termination and release, are operative and indeed similar in all cells that have been studied. If protein synthesis *per se* is involved in either the origin of or the subsequent behavior of cancer cells, it must be approached at a more subtle level. This may involve structural changes, not yet identified, in the ribosomes, transfer RNAs, enzymes, or related factors.

Components with even minor alterations involving substitutions of single amino acids or nucleotides may respond differently to the hormones or other regulatory factors that modulate protein synthesis. Correspondingly, the presence (or absence) of new factors or alterations in the existing hormones in the tumor may affect protein synthesis.

The possibility does exist that protein synthesis, in either qualitative or quantitative aspects, may be involved in neoplasia. Rates of protein synthesis may be affected as indicated above. Also, differential rates of synthesis of different proteins may result in imbalances of enzymes or patterns of proteins. This may involve the presence or absence of specific hormones or other factors in tumors. Another important consideration is the accuracy or fidelity of the translation of the genetic messenger RNA during protein synthesis. Alterations in the ribosomes, tRNA, or other factors in the cancer cell that are involved in polypeptide

A. Clark Griffin • Department of Biochemistry, The University of Texas System Cancer Center, M. D. Anderson Hospital and Tumor Institute, Houston, Texas.

formation may result in a misreading of the messenger RNA, with the resultant formation of proteins with amino acid deletions or substitutions.

Finally, consideration must be given to the possibility that the mechanism of protein synthesis in the cancer cell is quite normal. Specific proteins may be involved in neoplastic development and growth as indicated by the presence of tumor-specific antigens, growth regulatory factors, etc. Several prominent investigators are of the opinion that the distribution or pattern of enzymes within the cells or tissues is more important in describing the function and behavior of cancer cells. Whatever role that proteins may play in cancer is seemingly regulated at the translational levels involving the DNA and RNA.

This chapter will be directed to elucidation of the possibilities as presented above that protein synthesis may be associated with the origin and subsequent growth of cancer cells. Since the report of the isolation of an amino acid incorporating system from Ehrlich ascites cells by Littlefield and Keller (1957), numerous cell-free systems from prokaryotic cells, normal eukaryotic cells and tissues, as well as several tumors, have been isolated and studied. As indicated, the components and the general mechanism of polypeptide synthesis in all of these cells appear to be similar. However, these various cellular systems and especially those operative in tumor cells will be compared and contrasted. In addition to the cytoplasmic polysomal system, which accounts for a relatively large proportion of protein synthesis in mammalian cells, protein synthesis occurs in the mitochondria, nuclei, and even the nucleolus. Also, a mechanism has been reported for polypeptide biosynthesis that does not require ribosomes, i.e., gramicidin S, a cyclic decapeptide, and tyrocidine (Lipmann, 1971). The N-terminal addition of amino acids to existing proteins involving a relatively new class of enzymes, the aminoacyl-tRNA protein transferases, has been found in bacterial and mammalian cells (Section 5.4).

Recently, important studies have appeared on the effects of hormones on protein synthesis and, more important, the association of protein synthesis with cellular function, growth, embryogenesis, differentiation, and viral infection. It is hoped that a perusal of this important literature may provide new insight into the processes involved in the origin of and the subsequent growth of cancer cells.

The literature pertaining to proteins and protein synthesis is indeed a vast one. It is impossible to give deserved recognition to all of the worthy and pertinent investigations that have appeared in this area. References to these will be found in the many reviews and texts that have been written in recent years, and the reader is directed to the following for a more comprehensive coverage: Griffin (1974), Ochoa and Mazumder (1974), Lucas-Lenard and Beres (1974), Tate and Caskey (1974), Arnstein (1974), Haenni (1972), Haselkorn and Rothman-Denes (1973), Grossman and Moldave (1974) and Bautz et al. (1973).

2. Ribosomal Systems

The isolation of cell-free systems of protein synthesis from bacterial and mammalian cells has made it possible to elucidate the mechanism of protein synthesis.

These systems require, in addition to ribosomes, several protein factors and nucleic acids. The presence of messenger RNA (mRNA) is required for polypeptide synthesis to proceed. Translation of synthetic polynucleotides with known nucleotide sequences resulted in the deciphering of the genetic code. Peptide bond formation occurs on the ribosome, with ATP as the ultimate energy source for this reaction. There is also a requirement for the energy derived from the hydrolysis of GTP in the complete cycle of elongation of the polypeptide chain. The events of the biosynthesis of proteins center about the ribosomes. Only a modest beginning can be reported in terms of an understanding of the complete organization as well as the molecular and surface properties and reactivities of the ribosomes. The prokaryotic ribosomes (70 S, 2.8×10^6 daltons) are made up of two subunits, 30 S and 50 S. The smaller unit consists of 21 protein species and an 18 S RNA. The 50 S subunit is composed of as many as 40 protein species and 28 S and 5 S RNA species of approximately 1 million and 40,000 daltons, respectively. Eukaryotic ribosomes are larger (80 S, 4×10^6 daltons) and also consist of two subunits. The smaller 40 S subunit is composed of 40 protein species and an 18 S RNA, while the larger 60 S component contains approximately 100 protein species and two RNA species, 5 S and 28 S. Cox (1974) has recently reviewed the structure and function of the ribosomes. A comprehensive investigation of the function and role of ribosomes in mammalian protein synthesis has been carried out by Henshaw and associates (Henshaw *et al.*, 1973; Hirsch *et al.*, 1973; Ayuso-Parilla *et al.*, 1973). Busch *et al.* (1974) have studied the nucleolar rDNA templates for the synthesis of rRNA. Their findings show that 45 S nRNA contains both 18 S and 28 S nRNA. A major effort has been made to determine the oligonucleotide sequences within the 28 S nRNA and to make structural comparisons between normal rat liver and tumors. While differences are seen, a critical evaluation of the significance of these findings in terms of cancer development and growth must await further studies in this area.

2.1. Initiation of Polypeptide Synthesis

It is at the level of initiation of polypeptide synthesis that some differences are evident between prokaryotic and eukaryotic cells. However, the cell-free systems obtained from the tumors that have been investigated do appear to resemble very closely the liver, reticulocyte, and other eukaryotic cell-free systems that have been subjected to careful study. Whether the ribosomes of the cancer cell differ in the initiation or the subsequent events of protein synthesis is largely unknown. Even minor changes within the multiple protein species or changes in the nucleotide sequences of the 28 S RNA (containing 10,000 or more nucleotides) could change the molecular topography of the ribosome and affect one of the many functional binding sites that will be discussed later in the sections on protein biosynthesis. Attention is directed to proceedings of an international symposium on ribosomes and RNA metabolism: Zelinka and Balan (1973).

2.1.1. Prokaryotic Cells

Components of polypeptide chain initiation in prokaryotic cells include:

Ribosomes, 30 S and 50 S subunits
Initiator aminoacyl-tRNA
fMet-tRNA$_f$
Initiation factors
    IF-1
    IF-2
    IF-3
GTP, Mg^{2+}
AUG or GUG codons

Polypeptide chain initiation begins with the formation of a complex on the 30 S ribosomal subunit. The 30 S subunit bearing the three initiation factors binds the messenger, and in the presence of GTP and fMet-tRNA$_f$ the 30 S initiation complex is formed. fMet-tRNA$_f$ recognizes AUG or GUG codons. IF-3 is now released from the complex and subsequently binds to free 30 S subunits. The 30 S complex combines with the 50 S subunit to form the 70 S initiation complex, which also includes GTP. At this stage, it is believed that GTP hydrolysis occurs and IF-2 is released, and the complex is now ready for chain elongation, as discussed in the next section. fMet-tRNA occupies the peptidyl (donor) site on the 70 S complex. A second site, the acceptor site, binds all other incoming aminoacyl-tRNAs.

Initiation factors 2 and 3 are released for recycling according to the above mechanism and function catalytically in the initiation sequence. The IF-1 may be a dissociable ribosomal protein; however, this has not been firmly established. Extraction of *Escherichia coli* ribosomes with 0.5–2.0 M NH$_4$Cl releases the initiation factors, and their purification may be achieved on polyacrylamide gels and other procedures. IF-1 has been obtained in crystalline form and has a molecular weight of 9400 daltons. IF-2 has a molecular weight close to 80,000 daltons, and IF-3, a heat-stable single polypeptide chain, a weight of 21,000 daltons. A more comprehensive coverage of the studies leading to determination of the initiation sequences is presented in the excellent review by Ochoa and Mazumder (1974).

2.1.2. Eukaryotic Cells

There is considerable evidence that Met-tRNA$_f$ rather than fMet-tRNA$_f$ is the initiator in most eukaryotic cells. Since, however, the *N*-terminal amino acid in both globin chains is valine, it would appear that Met-tRNA is the initiator tRNA and is removed before completion of the polypeptide globin chain. The transformylase present in bacterial cells is not found in the cytoplasm of eukaryotic cells that have been studied. It is of interest to note that cell-free reticulocyte systems can utilize fMet-tRNA from *E. coli* and other sources.

The eukaryotic initiation factors are not as well defined as those in prokaryotic systems. Three initiation factors M-1, M-2, and M-3 were obtained from the 0.5 M KCl wash of reticulocyte ribosomes by Shafritz *et al.* (1970). M-1 and M-2 are required for maximal polyphenylalanine synthesis and M-3 is also required for translation of globin messenger RNA. M-3 thus resembles the prokaryotic IF-3 in that it is required only for the translation of natural messengers. Levin *et al.* (1973), utilizing ribosomes and ribosomal factors from mouse fibroblasts, have proposed the following sequence to describe the initiation of protein synthesis in eukaryotic cells:

$$\text{IF-3} + \text{Met-tRNA}_f + \text{GTP} \rightarrow [\text{IF-L3, Met-tRNA}_f, \text{GTP}]$$
$$[\text{IF-L3, Met-tRNA}_f, \text{GTP}] + 40\,\text{S} + \text{IF-L1} \rightarrow 40\,\text{S, Met-tRNA}_f$$
$$40\,\text{S, Met-tRNA}_f + \text{mRNA} + \text{IF-L2} \rightarrow 40\text{S, Met-tRNA}_f, \text{mRNA}$$
$$40\,\text{S, Met-tRNA}_f, \text{mRNA} + 60\,\text{S} \rightarrow 80\,\text{S, Met-tRNA}_f, \text{mRNA}$$

The initiation factors were extracted from the fibroblast ribosomes with 0.8 M KCl and separated on DEAE-cellulose columns. As is the case for the prokaryotic systems, there is also a requirement for GTP. GMP-PCP (β,γ-methyleneguanosine-5′-triphosphate) can replace GTP in the first two steps as shown above. However, GTP is essential for the association of the 60 S subunit and the 40 S, Met-tRNA$_f$, mRNA complex. Thus GTP hydrolysis occurs only in the final reaction of the above sequence. In accord with the prokaryotic systems, the initiator Met-tRNA$_f$ occupies the peptidyl site on the ribosome. The stepwise assembly of the eukaryotic 80 S initiation complex occurs at 1.5–3 mM MgCl$_2$.

Cashion and Stanley (1974) have isolated two initiation factors (IF-I and IF-II) of protein synthesis from 0.5 M KCl extracts of rabbit reticulocyte polysomes. IF-I mediates the GTP-dependent, template-independent binding of the initiator tRNA to the 40 S ribosomal subunit (corresponding to the first two reactions in the above sequence of Levin *et al.*, 1973). In the presence of a 60 S subunit and AUG or rabbit globulin ribonucleoproteins, the IF-II results in a transfer of the initiator tRNA to a complex involving the 80 S ribosome. The GTP requirement and function appear to be similar to those described by Levin *et al.* (1973). The molecular weights of IF-I and IF-II are 150,000 and 220,000 daltons, respectively. These authors also report it to be highly probable that complexes of IF-I and IF-II are common to all of the sources tested, which include rabbit reticulocytes, rabbit liver, chicken reticulocytes, chicken liver, and chick embryonic leg muscle. Attention should also be directed to the studies of Schreier and Staehelin (1973) involving initiation factors in reticulocytes. Eich and Drews (1974) have isolated a peptide chain initiation factor from Krebs II ascites tumor cells.

An interesting development has been reported in terms of the nucleotide sequences within the initiator tRNA$_f^{\text{Met}}$ of prokaryotic and eukaryotic cells. Dube *et al.* (1968) worked out the complete sequence of the *N*-formyl-Met-tRNA from *E. coli* and reported the sequence -G-T-ψ-C-A in loop IV (or the -G-T-ψ-C- loop). This same sequence, -G-T-ψ-C-G-(A)-, is also present in most of the elongation tRNAs that have been sequenced. In contrast, Simsek and RajBhandary (1972) reported that initiator tRNA of yeast cells contained -G-A-U-C-G-. Subsequently, Simsek *et al.* (1974) found a similar nucleotide sequence of rabbit liver and sheep initiator tRNA. Since Piper and Clark (1974) had previously determined the primary structure of mouse myeloma cell initiator tRNA and also observed the base sequence -G-A-U-C-G, this appears to be a characteristic structure that has been conserved during eukaryotic evolution. Piper and Clark (1974) suggest that the initial binding of initiator tRNA to mammalian 40 S ribosome subunits during the formation of the initiation complex may be independent of template and the initiation site on mammalian mRNA may be selected by the anticodon of tRNA^{Met} bound to the subunit as shown above. There is increasing indication that many of the tRNAs of tumor cells differ in structure from comparable tRNAs of normal cells. These findings as well as the possible regulatory role played by the tRNAs in cell development, differentiation, and neoplasia will be considered in Section 5.

2.2. Peptide Chain Elongation

The events of peptide chain elongation are reasonably well established and are depicted in Fig. 1. It may be observed that the process is cyclic, involving the binding of an incoming aminoacyl-tRNA to the acceptor site on the ribosome, peptidyl transfer from the aminoacyl-tRNA on the peptidyl site (fMet or Met in the first cycle following the initiation sequence) to the A site, peptide bond formation, peptidyl-tRNA translocation with release of the free tRNA and "clearing" of the A site, and exposure of the next triplet codon by movement of the peptidyl–ribosome complex on the messenger RNA. GTP and elongation factors are required. While this mechanism is now assumed to be generally universal, the most definitive investigations have been carried out with bacterial systems. Similar studies have been conducted on reticulocytes, liver and other mammalian systems, wheat germ, and yeast. Also, peptide synthesis has been studied in several cell-free systems derived from tumors. Comparative aspects of all the systems will be considered later.

Two elongation factors are required for polypeptide chain elongation in bacteria. These are currently designated EF-T and EF-G. Since many designations have appeared as new systems were developed, EF-T corresponds to TI, T, and S_1 and S_3. (Actually, two forms of T, Tu and Ts, have been identified in the cell fractions. When isolated from the soluble fraction of the cell, they are associated and referred to as EF-T.) EF-G corresponds to TII, FII, G, and S_2. Gordon (1970) has found that the relative amounts of EF-T and EF-G compared to the ribosomes remain relatively constant at different rates in stages of bacterial cell growth. In addition, the amounts of these factors in the cell constitute a significant percentage of the total soluble protein, i.e., almost 10% in certain growth conditions.

EF-T forms a stable ternary complex with aminoacyl-tRNA and GTP. It is possible to retain this complex by employing Millipore gel filtration (Gordon, 1968). The ternary complex interacts with the ribosome, with a resultant hydrolysis of GTP and the binding of aminoacyl-tRNA to the ribosomal A site and

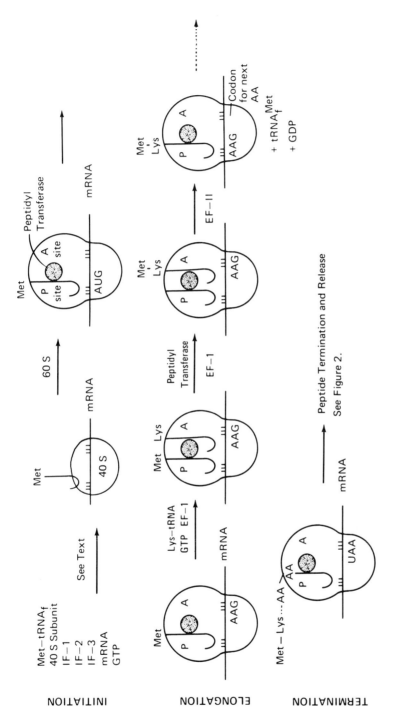

FIGURE 1. Events of polypeptide chain elongation.

the release of EF-Tu. There is a 1 : 1 stoichiometry in terms of the hydrolysis of GTP and the binding of aminoacyl-tRNA to the ribosome. Since EF-Tu functions catalytically in the above reactions, it must be disassociated from GDP, and Miller and Weissbach (1970) have suggested that this occurs through the intervention of EF-Ts.

At this stage, the P site on the ribosome is occupied by the initiator aminoacyl-tRNA (or in subsequent cycles by peptidyl-tRNA) and the A site by the oncoming aminoacyl-tRNA as described above. A new peptide bond is formed between the peptide (or initiator amino acid) from the P site and the α-amino group of the aminoacyl-tRNA on the A site. This peptide transfer is catalyzed by a ribosomal protein called peptidyltransferase. The deacylated tRNA still occupies the P site and must be ejected. Factor EF-G is involved in the translocation reactions wherein the deacylated tRNA is released, the peptidyl-tRNA is moved from the A to the P site, and the simultaneous movement of the ribosomes occurs along the messenger RNA from the 5' to the 3' direction. Mg^{2+} and K^+ are required for this translocation as well as GTP. Nishizuka and Lipmann (1966) have indicated that one molecule of GTP is hydrolyzed per peptide bond that is formed.

Puromycin and several antibiotics have played a major role in establishing ribosomal binding sites and the function of elongation factors in protein synthesis. Ribosomes charged with polyphenylalyl-tRNA and incubated in the presence of puromycin will release polyphenylalanine puromycin. Puromycin binds to the A site and competively inhibits the oncoming aminoacyl-tRNA. Peptidyltransferase transfers the nascent peptide to the puromycin and the resulting puromycin peptides are released prematurely from the ribosomes (Maden *et al.*, 1968). A more detailed discussion of ribosomal binding sites in peptide chain elongation sites is presented by Lucas-Lenard and Beres (1974). Many inhibitors at various stages of protein synthesis are known, and these have been invaluable in studying the initiation and elongation sequences (Grollman and Huang, 1973). Microbial cells deprived of an essential amino acid undergo a reduction in the accumulation of stable ribosomal and transfer RNA. This will alter the RNA–protein ratio of the cell and is referred to as the "stringent response." In this state, there is an increased rate of protein turnover (Goldberg *et al.*, 1974) and reduction of stable RNA accumulation. Among other effects are the appearance of two unusual nucleotides, guanosine-5'-diphosphate, 3' (or 2'-) diphosphate (ppGpp) and guanosine 5'-triphosphate, 3' (or 2'-) diphosphate (pppGpp) (Cashel and Kalbacher, 1970), and an inhibition in purine ribonucleoside triphosphate formation. The possible implications of these findings in terms of the effects of cellular amino acid deprivation on RNA transcription and protein translation in higher organisms must await further studies.

While the discussion of peptide chain elongation has centered largely about the studies and observations in microbial systems, there is every indication that the basic mechanism is indeed universal. *In vitro* systems capable of the synthesis of polypeptides have been obtained from a large number of mammalian systems. Perhaps the most extensively studied is the reticulocyte system obtained from phenylhydrazine-treated rabbits. The procedures employed for the isolation of ribosomes and the factors involved in polypeptide biosynthesis have been reviewed by Griffin and Black (1971). Two factors, TF-I and TF-II, corresponding to the EF-T and EF-G, have been purified to homogeneity. Liver systems have been extensively studied (see Griffin, 1974). Also, comparable systems have been isolated and partially characterized from other mammalian tissues and organs, including skeletal muscle (Florini and Breuer, 1966), chick oviduct (Means *et al.*, 1971; Palmiter *et al.*, 1970), brain (Goodwin *et al.*, 1969; Mahler and Brown, 1968), heart (Morgan *et al.*, 1971), and several human tissues (Bermek and Matthaei, 1970; see also Griffin and Black, 1971). Several tumor polypeptide-synthesizing systems have been investigated, and these will be considered in Section 3.

2.3. Polypeptide Chain Termination

In the prokaryotic and eukaryotic systems that have been investigated, peptide chain termination on the ribosome requires a soluble protein factor (RF) which recognizes the terminator codons UAA, UAG, and UGA. In *E. coli* cells, two factors have been identified, RF-1, which recognizes UAA and UAG, and RF-2, which recognizes UAA and UGA. The release factors from reticulocyte cells appear to recognize UAA, UAG, and UGA.

Peptide chain termination appears to be similar in bacterial and mammalian cells. However, the sequence of events is only tentative at this time and further extensive investigations with a larger number of cell types will be required before an overall mechanism can be finally established. There are no conclusive findings at present that would indicate that chain termination differs in cancer cells. The model of Tate and Caskey (1974) depicting the events of peptide chain termination is presented in Fig. 2.

The observations of Garen and associates (see Garen, 1968) and Brenner *et al.* (1965) of nonsense mutations in bacterial systems led to the establishment of the existence of terminator codons. Nonsense mutations of codons are now considered to be the result of a conversion of an amino acid codon to one of the terminator codons. From studies of *E. coli* mutants deficient in alkaline phosphatase and their suppressors, the *amber* codon (UAG) and *ochre* codon (UAA) were determined. Sambrook *et al.* (1967) later isolated a UGA-specific suppressor and it is now established that the occurrence of the nonsense codons UAA, UAG, or UGA in mutant positions in mRNA results in a premature peptide chain termination. Nonsense mutants and suppressors for these codons have been found in yeast but not in mammalian cells. However, mammalian cells do utilize these terminator codons. Modified tRNAs are the products of suppressor genes and will be discussed further in Section 5. Caskey *et al.* (1968) developed the widely used assay for determination of terminator codons which involves the release of labeled formylmethionine from the f[^{3}H]Met-tRNA$_f$·AUG·ribosome complex. Caskey (1970) has reviewed the RNA codon assignments and other aspects of peptide chain termination.

The protein release factors from *E. coli* have been isolated by DEAE-Sephadex chromatography (Scolnick *et al.*, 1968). RF-1, which recognizes UAA and UAG, has a molecular weight of 44,000 daltons, and RF-2, which recognizes UAA and UGA, has a molecular weight of 47,000 daltons. Two RF species have been obtained from rabbit reticulocytes, and it appears that similar components are present in other mammalian tissues (see Caskey *et al.*, 1974).

As indicated in Fig. 2, there is a requirement for GTP in the peptide termination sequence. GTP is involved in the binding of the release factors to the peptidyl–ribosome complex in response to the terminator codon. In *E. coli* this interaction involves the L-7 and L-12 proteins of the 50 S unit of the ribosome. Peptidyl-tRNA hydrolysis appears to involve a ribosomal peptidyltransferase and RF. After hydrolysis, RF is released from the ribosome, and this step appears to be dependent on the hydrolysis of GTP. While there have been some preliminary studies reported, the mechanism of dissociation of the deacylated tRNA-mRNA from ribosomes is not clearly delineated.

2.4. Protein Synthesis: Mitochondrial

Many investigators have reported the presence in mitochondria of a protein-synthesizing system that is distinct but in many aspects similar to the cytoplasmic

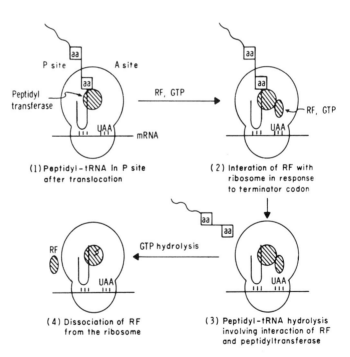

FIGURE 2. Model of peptide chain termination intermediate events. See text for description. A schematic representation of a ribosome carrying a peptidyl-tRNA is shown. From Tate and Caskey (1974). Reprinted with the permission of the authors and Academic Press, Inc.

system described above (Ashwell and Work, 1970). Mitochondrial ribosomes are relatively small (55 S) and the aminoacylsynthetases and tRNAs are present. By use of reversed-phase chromatography, it has been possible to show that the tRNAs in the mitochondrial fractions are distinct and separable from those in the cytoplasmic fraction in *Neurospora* (Epler, 1969; Borst, 1972). Mitochondrial protein synthesis requires a formylated methionine for initiation, which is analogous to the situation in the prokaryotic systems (Epler *et al.*, 1970).

Halder (1971) has reported that protein synthesis in mitochondria of rat brain and liver is inhibited by chloramphenicol and oxytetracycline but not by cycloheximide.

Little is known of the proteins synthesized by mitochondria except that they comprise a relatively small percentage (7–15% in animal tissues) of the total mitochondrial proteins and are localized in the inner membrane (Beattie, 1971). Proteins synthesized on mitochondrial ribosomes are hydrophobic and may constitute some portion of the cytochrome oxidase and the ATPase complexes. It is likely that the proteins synthesized by the mitochondrial system have a structural function. Workers in several laboratories have reported an increased number of catenated oligomers of mitochondrial DNA in tumor cells. Also, unicircular dimers of mitochondrial DNA have been found in leukocytes from human patients with chronic granulocytic leukemia, in mouse L cells, and in mouse 3T3 cells transformed by SV40 virus. However, Borst (1972) concludes that there is no evidence that tumor mitochondria can be distinguished from normal mitochondria by such specific derangements in their genetic components.

England and Attardi (1974) have conducted extensive investigations on the expression of the mitochondrial genome in HeLa cells and the synthesis of mitochondrial protein during the cell cycle. A sensitive *in vitro* protein-synthesizing system has been isolated from Ehrlich ascites mitochondria by Avadhani and Rutman (1974).

2.5. Nuclear Synthesis of Proteins

The mechanism of protein synthesis in the cell nucleus resembles very closely that already described for the ribosomal system of the cytoplasm (see Allfrey, 1970). Nuclear ribosomes have been isolated and have sedimentation coefficients of 78 S. Similar initiation and elongation factors are required as well as specific tRNAs. *In vitro* studies have also indicated the need for Mg^{2+} and GTP in amino acid incorporation.

Lamkin and Hurlbert (1972) showed that nucleoli isolated from Novikoff ascites tumor could incorporate amino acids into an acid-insoluble form. It appeared that these nucleoli contain an integrated and self-sufficient system capable of protein synthesis that involves the tRNAs and activating enzymes (Lamkin *et al.*, 1973). Liau *et al.* (1972) have also found several tRNA-methylating enzymes in the nucleoli of the Novikoff tumor cells.

Protein synthesis has been investigated in a large number of tumors. From the findings thus far, it would appear that the ribosomal system in cancer cells resembles very closely the basic mechanisms that have been described in the preceding discussion. As will be reported later, many investigators have employed ribosomes and other factors derived from tumor cells for the translation of mRNA obtained from other sources. Actually, many of the components involved in the *in vitro* synthesis of polypeptides are interchangeable from one species to another. Ribosomes and the elongation factors Ef-T and EF-G (formerly referred to as T-I and T-II) of rat liver, Novikoff tumor, and rabbit reticulocytes are completely interchangeable (see Griffin and Black, 1971; Griffin, 1974). Krisko *et al.* (1969), from studies on the *in vitro* components from liver, Novikoff tumor, and *E. coli*, showed that the microbial EF-T could be substituted for the comparable mammalian factor. The microbial EF-G could not replace the mammalian EF-G. Conversely, neither of the mammalian elongation factors would function in *E. coli* ribosomal amino acid incorporating systems. Some features of several of the tumor polypeptide-synthesizing systems will follow.

3.1. L-1210 Mouse Ascites Leukemia

The L-1210 mouse ascites leukemia cell-free system was isolated and studied by Ochoa and Weinstein (1964).

3.2. Novikoff Ascites Tumor Cells

Detailed procedures for the isolation of the components of protein synthesis in Novikoff ascites tumor cells are reviewed by Griffin and Black (1971). This is a convenient and accessible tumor cell line with which to work. The washed ribosomes require two elongation factors for polypeptide chain elongation.

3.3. Plasmacytomas

Plasmacytomas, malignant tumors in mice referred to as plasma cell tumors, are similar to multiple myeloma in humans. The tumors may be initiated in mice by several procedures and they are programmed for the synthesis of specific immunoglobulins. Potter (1974) in a review of the plasmacytomas points out that the homogeneous immunoglobulins of tumor origin appear to resemble normal immunoglobulins. The major forms of abnormal synthesis in these tumors are twofold: (1) cells that synthesize and secrete only light chains (Bence Jones protein) and (2) cells that do not synthesize any immunoglobulin. Potter (1972) has described protein-synthesizing systems obtained from plasma cell tumors.

The only transfer RNA of tumor origin that has been subjected to a complete
primary nucleotide sequencing to date is the unique methionine-accepting tRNA
isolated from the cytoplasm of P3 myeloma cells (Piper and Clark, 1974). This
structure is shown in Fig. 4C.

3.4. Krebs II Ascites Carcinoma

A very good polypeptide-synthesizing system may be obtained from Krebs II
ascites carcinoma cells (Fais et al., 1971). This system will translate mRNAs of both
mammalian and viral origin (Mathews, 1972). Bancroft et al. (1973) have derived a
protein-synthesizing system from Krebs II ascites cell. Growth hormone was
synthesized in this system under the direction of mRNA obtained from rat
pituitary tumor cells.

3.5. Other Related Systems

Koka and Nakamoto (1972) have described a protein-synthesizing system from
rat lymphosarcoma. A cell-free protein-synthesizing system from mouse sarcoma
cells with a high efficiency of translation of viral and nonviral messages has been
reported by Jenkins et al. (1973). Polyribosomes were isolated from a clonal line of
mouse neuroblastoma grown in culture by Wiche et al. (1974). In a heterologous in
vitro system containing rat brain components, the polyribosomes directed the
synthesis of neuroblastoma tubulin.

4. Regulation of Protein Synthesis

The presentation to this point has been concerned largely with the mechanistic
features of the ribosomal system of the biosynthesis of proteins. Perhaps the most
striking feature of the findings that have been reviewed is the universality of the
mechanism. Some of the comparative aspects of prokaryotic and eukaryotic cells
have been discussed. Prokaryotic ribosomes appear to differ in sedimentation
characteristics. However, McConkey (1974) has pointed out that even in this
respect there may not be as great a difference as previously recorded. It is
suggested that the composition of the 60 S mammalian subunit corresponds
closely to that of E. coli 50 S subunits. With the increasing emphasis on characterization of the multiple proteins and nucleic acids of the ribosomes, it is quite
possible that structural differences as well as alterations in the functional topography will become more apparent. The mechanism of protein synthesis in cancer
cells does not appear to differ in any fundamental aspect from that described for
many other eukaryotic cells. As noted above, this may change when the components, especially the ribosomes, have been subjected to a more extensive characterization.

Attention should be called to one additional feature of the *in vitro* studies that have been largely responsible for most of our current views of protein biosynthesis. These studies, in some aspects, are quite artificial since they have been conducted in the absence of the many regulatory factors that are present and functional in intact cells, tissues, and complete organism. It appears at this time that if the components of protein synthesis are involved in neoplasia the most likely explanation would be an alteration in the balance that must exist between these components and various regulatory factors, or a change in the fidelity or accuracy of the translational events in tumor cells. It is indeed possible that the most subtle changes in the ribosomal components or the peptide initiation, elongation, or release factors may influence the response to the regulatory factors. Such changes would not be apparent in the *in vitro* systems described in the preceding section.

Many investigators are now studying regulatory mechanisms and events in embryogenesis, differentiation, and other developmental and growth phenomena. These studies are also providing new insight into the regulatory aspects of protein synthesis. Considerable progress can be reported in the determination of the mode of action of hormones such as the hormone binding or receptor sites. In this respect, it is of interest that many investigators are studying the role of specific proteins as hormone receptors in predicting the response of breast cancer patients to hormonal or other modes of therapy. Discussion of some of the recent progress in the area of regulation of protein biosynthesis will follow, with emphasis on the cancer cell. The accuracy or fidelity of protein biosynthesis, as mentioned above, will be considered in Section 5 (see also Nirenberg, 1970; Griffin, 1974).

4.1. Hormones

The prevailing evidence at this time indicates that the hormones act at the transcriptional level to stimulate production of mRNA and subsequently of specific proteins. Many investigators have contributed to this concept, including Means and Hall (1969), Turkington and Riddle (1970), Palmiter *et al.* (1970), Palmiter (1972), and Karlson (1974). O'Malley and Means (1974) have reviewed the effects of steroid hormones in target-cell nuclei, and this excellent coverage will form the basis for this section. The biochemical events involved in hormone action on protein synthesis are depicted in Fig. 3.

The initial event involves the hormone's entry in the target cell and its binding to a specific cytoplasmic receptor. The concept of the hormone receptor has evolved from the studies of Jensen and Jacobson (1962) wherein radioactive estrogen was injected into immature rats. Since these original observations, estrogen receptors have been reported in studies with mammary gland tissues, pituitary, hypothalamus, and vagina. O'Malley *et al.* (1971) observed that when a chick treated with estrogen was subsequently injected with labeled progesterone the labeled steroid appeared in the cytoplasm and nucleus of the oviduct cells. The

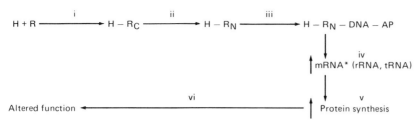

FIGURE 3. Biochemical steps in steroid hormone action. (i) Hormone (H) entering the target cell binds to a specific cytoplasmic receptor (R) and (ii) forms a hormone–receptor complex (H–R_C) which is transported to the nucleus (H–R_N), where (iii) it binds to specific acceptor sites on the genome [chromatin DNA and nonhistones (or acidic proteins, AP)]. This is followed by (iv) activation of the transcriptional apparatus that results in the appearance of new RNA species: (v) transport of the hormone-induced RNA to the cytoplasm and (vi) the steroid-mediated functional response that is characteristic of the target tissue. Among the components of such a system which may bring about functional changes in the target cell are enzymes, structural or regulatory proteins, and nuclear events that are subject to amplification. From O'Malley and Means (1974). Reprinted with the permission of the authors and *Science*. Copyright, 1974, by the American Association for the Advancement of Science.

cytoplasmic radioactivity was present in a macromolecular complex and the binding protein was subsequently shown to have a monomeric molecular weight of 90,000. Progesterone-binding proteins have been observed in the cytosol fractions of several species, including human beings.

As indicated in Fig. 3, the hormone–receptor complex is transported to the nucleus, where it binds to specific acceptor sites on the genome. This binding to DNA has been observed in target-cell nuclei and *in vitro*. The binding complex withstands centrifugation of the DNA through sucrose gradients, and it has been estimated that there are 500 receptor molecules per quantity of DNA found in a single nucleus. The acceptor sites may involve chromatin DNA and acidic proteins. The transcriptional mechanism is activated and mRNAs appear. The hormone-induced mRNAs are transported to the cytoplasm and the new proteins are synthesized by the ribosomal mechanism described in the preceding sections. O'Malley and Means (1974) have demonstrated that following treatment with estrogen up to 15,000 molecules of ovalbumin mRNA may accumulate in a single oviduct cell. When the hormone is withdrawn, there is a decrease in the ovalbumin mRNA to fewer than ten molecules per cell. As noted by these investigators, the estrogen acts in the nucleus to promote the synthesis of mRNAs, which are essential for the subsequent action of the steroid on growth and differentiation.

One of the key problems is elucidation of the mechanism by which the hormone–receptor complex regulates nuclear RNA metabolism. O'Malley and Means (1974) suggest that this might be achieved (1) by direct effects on chromatin template resulting in increased gene transcription, (2) activation of the polymerase complex, (3) inhibition of RNA breakdown, (4) intranuclear processing of large precursor molecules producing smaller biologically active sequences, and (5) transport of RNA from the nucleus to the cytoplasmic sites of cellular protein synthesis. It is possible that cancer cells may differ from normal counterparts in these events related to regulation by the hormone–receptor complex of the biosynthesis of specific proteins. There is indication from many cancer clinical centers that the steroid and other hormonal binding sites in tumor cells may have important diagnostic and prognostic implications.

4.2. Phosphorylation

Findings from several laboratories have indicated that nuclear phosphoproteins may be involved in the control of gene activity and protein biosynthesis. A number of observations have been made of the phosphorylation of nuclear acidic proteins in HeLa cells. In synchronously dividing cells, there is an increased rate of synthesis of these proteins preceding the onset of DNA synthesis (Stein and Borun, 1972). Also, more of the nuclear protein is synthesized and released in the acidic chromosomal proteins after mitosis and later in G_1 than in the S or G_2 phase. Allfrey *et al.* (1973) showed that the rate of phosphorylation of HeLa nuclear proteins is maximal in the early G_1 and S phases and decreased in the G_2 to M phases concurrent with a reduction in RNA synthesis (Karn *et al.*, 1974).

4.3. Cyclic AMP and Related Compounds

The regulatory role of cyclic AMP acting as a chemical messenger between hormones and their enzymatic effects in cells is well known. Also, there is indication that some cancer cells may have an inadequate supply of cyclic AMP (Pastan, 1972; Pastan and Johnson, 1974). Dibutyryl cyclic AMP has been shown to cause an inhibition of the growth rate and DNA synthesis and an increase in protein content in hepatoma cells in culture (H-35 and MH_1C_1). This agent also resulted in an increase in phosphoenolpyruvate carboxykinase activity in these cells (VanRijn *et al.*, 1974). The investigative approach of these workers employing hepatoma cell lines should be of value in elucidation of the mechanisms by which cAMP stimulates specific protein synthesis and tumor cell growth. Lanzani *et al.* (1974) have reported that cGMP stimulates protein synthesis in wheat germ, rat liver slices, and rat liver cell-free systems.

4.4. Chalones and Other Growth Factors

The chalones and antichalones are among the many factors that have been postulated to control cellular division and to regulate or maintain the dynamic equilibrium of cells in mammalian tissues (see also Chap. 11). Substances which inhibit mitotic activity selectively in their tissues of origin have been extracted from epidermis, kidney, liver, and granulocytes. Chalones are produced within these cells, and some authorities have speculated that they act in gene activation or repression, actually programming the patterns of protein synthesis; one program leads to mitosis and another to cell or tissue function.

An epidermal chalone has been the most extensively studied. Bullough and associates (Bullough, 1969) prepared extracts of macerated epidermis and found a mitotic inhibitor in the aqueous extract. The epidermal chalone appears to be a basic glycoprotein with an approximate molecular weight of 40,000 daltons. These investigators assumed that the highest rate of chalone production is in maturing cells and that the rate is genetically determined according to the tissue involved. Another thesis that has been presented is that cells progress toward tissue functions in the presence of sufficient chalones and that if the necessary genes are still potentially active, as in premature cells, the cells revert toward mitosis if the chalone concentration falls below a critical level. As the chalone concentration in a tissue falls, the cell's preparation for tissue function becomes less intense and their preparation for mitosis more intense.

In wounded epidermis of the ear, the whole mitotic cycle may be as short as 12 h instead of 30 days, while mitosis *per se* occupies only about 1.5 h instead of the usual 2.6–3.5 h. In the epidermis in psoriasis, decreasing the chalone concentration results in a shortening of the time recorded from mitosis to death to 4 days instead of the usual 27–30 days. This would explain why in such conditions a greatly increased mitotic rate does not result in a corresponding increase in tissue mass (Teir and Ryoma, 1967). Iversen (1970) has presented some theoretical considerations on chalones in the treatment of cancer.

Erythropoietin is a hormone that induces differentiation and mitosis in erythropoietic stem cells in the bone marrow. This factor results in induction of RNA synthesis in the bone marrow in order to provide the proteins necessary for cell growth and differentiation. Erythropoietin plays a role in leukemogenesis and its presence is essential to make bone marrow cells susceptible to chromosome aberrations with 7,12-dimethylbenz[α] anthracene and subsequent leukemic formation (Krantz and Jacobsen, 1970; Sugiyama, 1971).

Phytohemagglutinin has been shown by Ahern and Kay (1973) to increase the rate of protein synthesis in cell-free systems from human lymphocytes. Since these systems do not initiate the synthesis of new polypeptide chains in the absence of exogenous mRNA, the protein synthesis represents the completion of preexisting nascent chains. The authors conclude that the greater activity of the system may be attributed to the greater proportion of ribosomes actively engaged in protein synthesis in these cells.

5. Transfer RNAs and Neoplasia

5.1. Structural and Functional Aspects

The complete nucleotide sequences of approximately 60 tRNAs have been ascertained (see Griffin and Black, 1971). Thus far, only three of these have been obtained from mammalian tissues and their structures are shown in Figs. 4A, 4B, and 4C. One of these is the initiator $tRNA_f^{Met}$ from mouse myeloma cells, and the primary structure was worked out by Piper and Clark (1974). The difference in loop IV (the -G-T-ψ-C- loop) between the initiator tRNAs of eukaryotic and

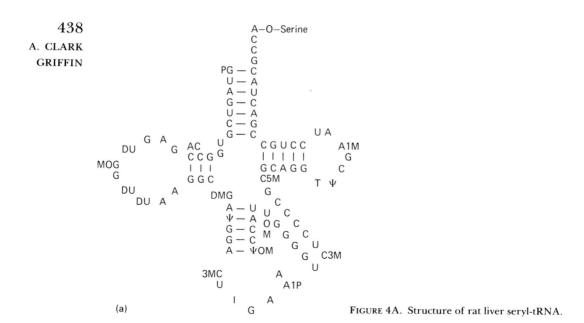

FIGURE 4A. Structure of rat liver seryl-tRNA.

(a)

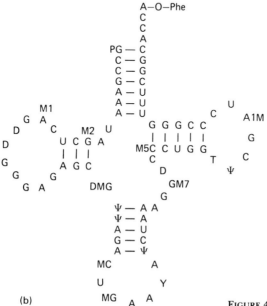

FIGURE 4B. Structure of tRNA^Phe from rabbit liver.

(b)

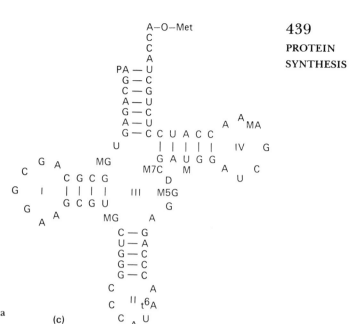

FIGURE 4C. Structure of mouse myeloma initiator tRNA$_f^{Met}$.

(c)

prokaryotic cells was discussed in Section 2.1. Simsek *et al.* (1974) found a similar nucleotide sequence for tRNA$_f^{Met}$ of rabbit liver and sheep thyroid.

Figures 5A and 5B show the primary structure of yeast phenylalanyl-tRNA as well as the resolution model of the three-dimensional structure as reported by Kim *et al.* (1972, 1974).

The major functional role of the transfer ribonucleic acids (tRNA) in protein biosynthesis has been described in Section 2. This involves the reactions with specific amino acids to form the aminoacyl-tRNA. Formation of the initiator Met-tRNA and the other aminoacyl-tRNAs involved in peptide chain elongation probably occurs by the two-stage mechanism of Norris and Berg (1964):

Aminoacylsynthetase (E) + amino acid + ATP → E-amino acid AMP + PP$_i$
E-Amino acid AMP + tRNA → aminoacyl-tRNA + E + AMP

However, Loftfield (1972), in reviewing the mechanism of aminoacylation of transfer RNA, has indicated that in many *in vivo* conditions there is a concerted reaction in which tRNA, amino acid, and the synthetase react to form aminoacyl-tRNA, AMP, PP$_i$ and free enzyme with no discrete intermediates. Other reviews on the aminoacyl-tRNA synthetase have been compiled by Jacobson (1971), Chambers (1971), Mehler (1970), Kisselev and Favorova (1974), and Söll and Schimmel (1974).

It is immediately evident that the above aminoacylation reactions are of major significance in terms of translational fidelity. This is the stage of protein synthesis wherein the nucleic acid or codon language interacts with the specific amino acids that form the building units for the many proteins required by living systems. Errors at this level could result in proteins with misplaced amino acids or altered sequences. The serial steps of aminoacylation enhance the overall accuracy of

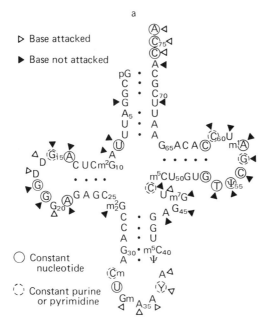

FIGURE 5A. Nucleotide sequence of yeast phenylalanyl-tRNA shown in the cloverleaf configuration. Circled bases are constant in all tRNAs, and dashed circles indicate positions which are occupied constantly by either purines or pyrimidines. From Kim *et al.* (1974). Reprinted with the permission of the authors and *Science.* Copyright, 1974, by the American Association for the Advancement of Science.

these reactions. If an error has been made in forming the initial intermediate, the aminoacyladenylate, the reaction is terminated by its hydrolysis.

Aside from the major function of the interaction of tRNAs with specific amino acids and the transport and placement of the amino acid in the specific sequence in the mRNA–polysomal systems as described in preceding sections, there is indication that the tRNAs may have other important regulatory roles. Actually, there are numerous reports in the literature that the tRNAs may have regulatory

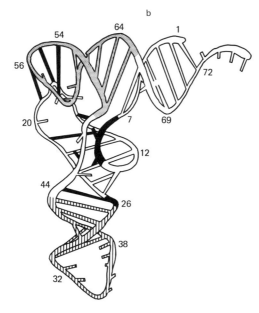

FIGURE 5B. Schematic model of yeast phenylalanyl-tRNA. The ribose phosphate backbone is drawn as a continuous cylinder with bars to indicate hydrogen-bonded base pairs. The positions of single bases are indicated by rods which are intentionally shortened. The TψC arm is heavily stippled, and the anticodon arm is marked by vertical lines. The black segments of the backbone include residues 8 and 9 as well as 26. Tertiary structure interactions are illustrated by black rods. The numbers indicate various nucleotides in accordance with the numbering system in Fig. 5A. From Kim *et al.* (1974). Reprinted with the permission of the authors and *Science.* Copyright, 1974, by the American Association for the Advancement of Science.

functions in embryogenesis, differentiation, sporulation, virus and phage infections, other growth functions, and neoplasia (Littauer and Inouye, 1973).

441
PROTEIN
SYNTHESIS

5.2. Altered tRNA Chromatographic Patterns in Tumor Cells

When the cytoplasmic tRNA is aminoacylated with a single labeled amino acid and
subjected to reversed-phase or other chromatographic procedures, several distinct peaks may be observed. For example, three or four distinct peaks are
observed when the tRNAs from liver or SV40-induced hamster kidney tumor are
aminoacylated with labeled aspartic acid and chromatographed on reversed-
phase columns. Degeneracy of the code as well as the tRNAs has been established.
However, the one codon–one tRNA relationship has not been strictly observed
because of the "wobble" hypothesized by Crick (1966). The two codons assigned to
aspartic acid are GAU and GAC and presumably would be recognized by an
aspartic acid tRNA. The above observation, that there are several chromatog-
raphically distinct tRNAs that react with aspartic acid, provides the basis for the
designation "isoaccepting tRNAs" by Novelli (1967). Many of the tumors that have
been studied have exhibited isoaccepting tRNA profiles that differ from those of
normal control tissues (Table 1). Borek and Kerr (1972) have also reviewed the
atypical tRNAs found in tumor cells. At this time, there is little concrete evidence
supporting the requirement for or the function of these isoaccepting tRNA
species. Also, little is known relative to the role of altered tRNA species in either
the origin or of the subsequent behavior of cancer cells. Since there are observable
differences in the chromatographic profiles of aminoacyl-tRNA of normal and
cancer cells, this will be discussed in some further detail.

Gallo and Pestka (1970) compared the chromatographic profiles of 20
aminoacyl-tRNAs of normal and leukemic lymphoblasts and observed small
differences for leucyl-, seryl-, threonyl-, and prolyl-tRNAs. More pronounced
differences between the two cell types were reported for tryosyl- and glutamyl-
tRNAs. A comparison between human myeloma cells and normal human
lymphoblasts revealed differences in the aspartyl-, leucyl-, seryl-, and tyrosyl-
tRNAs (Fujioka and Gallo, 1971). Concurrent findings from this laboratory and
Gallo's indicated the presence of a late-eluting aspartyl-tRNA in polyoma- and
SV40-induced tumors (Gallagher et al., 1972; Briscoe et al., 1972). A similar
late-eluting Asp-tRNA has been observed in human tumors (Fig. 6). However, at
this time we have not studied a sufficient number of human tumors to arrive at any
conclusions as to the extent or the clinical significance of this finding. Since this
late-eluting peak was first observed in DNA-virus-induced tumors, one possible
explanation is that this $tRNA^{Asp}$ was encoded in the viral genome. This does not
appear to be the case, and it would now appear that the most likely mechanism by
which this $tRNA^{Asp}_{IV}$ appears involves the repression or derepression of a gene for
the tRNA itself or for an enzyme system that modifies tRNAs.

Reversed-phase chromatography profiles of the tRNAs of mouse liver and
Ehrlich ascites cells reveal the presence of three isoaccepting $tRNA^{Phe}$ species.

TABLE 1

Alterations in Transfer RNA Chromatographic Profiles Associated with Neoplasia

Tissues or cells	Differences observed	Reference
SV40-induced tumor	New Tyr-tRNA	Holland *et al.* (1967)
Mouse tissues and tumors	Several new tRNAs	Taylor *et al.* (1967)
Rat liver and Novikoff hepatomas	His-tRNA, Tyr-tRNA	Baliga *et al.* (1969)
Plasma cell tumor	tRNA patterns differ	Yang and Novelli (1968)
Plasma cell tumor	tRNA patterns differ	Mach *et al.* (1968)
Rat liver and hepatoma	Phe-tRNA	Goldman *et al.* (1969)
Plasma cell tumor	Leu-tRNA	Mushinski and Potter (1969)
Rat liver and Morris hepatomas	Ser-tRNA, Phe-tRNA, His-tRNA	Volkers and Taylor (1971)
Ehrlich ascites tumor, drug resistant	Phe-tRNA	Richie *et al.* (1970)
Normal and leukemic lymphoblasts	Tyr-tRNA, Glu-tRNA Lys-tRNA, Leu-tRNA,	Gallo and Pestka (1970)
Livers of azo-dye-fed rats	Phe-tRNA, Tyr-tRNA	Goldman and Griffin (1970)
Rat liver and Morris hepatomas	Phe-tRNA	Gonano *et al.* (1971)
Rat liver and Novikoff hepatomas	Leu-tRNA	Ritter and Busch (1971)
Liver and Morris hepatomas	Tyr-tRNA, His-tRNA, Asn-tRNA	Srinivasan *et al.* (1971)
Human myeloma cells	Asp-tRNA, Tyr-tRNA	Fujioka and Gallo (1971)
SV40-transformed cells	Asp-tRNA, Asn-tRNA, His-tRNA	Sekiya and Oda (1972)
Polyoma- and SV40-transformed cells	Asp-tRNA	Gallagher *et al.* (1972)
SV40 tumors	Asp-tRNA	Briscoe *et al.* (1972)
Rat, mouse, hamster liver, SV40 tumors, Ehrlich ascites	Tyr-tRNA, Phe-tRNA	Hayashi *et al.* (1973)
Rous sarcoma and Rous viruses	Virus and transformed cell tRNAs	Wang, *et al.* (1973)
Morris hepatoma and liver	Increase in Phe- and other tRNAs in hepatoma	Ouellette and Taylor (1973)
Ehrlich ascites cells, drug resistant	Altered Phe-tRNA pattern	Hayashi and Griffin (1974)
Mouse plasmacytomas	Altered The- and Ser-tRNA	Bridges and Jones (1973)
Polyoma-virus-transformed cells	Extra Lys-tRNA	Jacobson *et al.* (1974)

Ehrlich tumor cells with an acquired resistance to nitrogen mustard (HN2) exhibit an altered chromatographic profile, with an almost complete absence of $tRNA_I^{Phe}$ and $tRNA_{III}^{Phe}$ and an exceptionally large $tRNA_{II}^{Phe}$ (Fig. 7). These $tRNA^{Phe}$ species have been isolated and purified to 80% or higher. The appearance of 3'-methylcytidine and an increase in 5'-methylcytidine and dihydrouracil in the predominant $tRNA_{II}^{Phe}$ of the drug-resistant tumor cells were the major structural changes observed (Hayashi and Griffin, 1974). The specific function or role of altered tRNAs in the origin or behavior of tumor cells must await further extensive investigation. Of supplemental clinical interest is the recent report of the Director of the National Cancer Program[1] that blood and urine of 63 of 65

[1] Special communication from the Director, National Cancer Program, Department of Health, Education, and Welfare, Bethesda, Maryland, October 8, 1974.

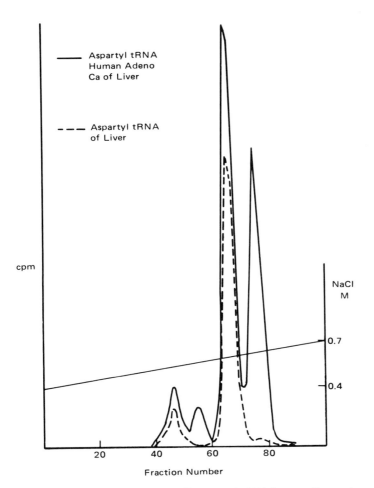

FIGURE 6. RP 5 chromatography of [^{14}C]aspartyl-tRNA from rat liver and [^{3}H]aspartyl-tRNA from a metastatic human adenocarcinoma of the liver from the lung.

breast cancer patients exhibited abnormal values for at least one of the three biological markers carcinoembryonic antigen, chorionic gonadotropin, and $N^2 N^2$-dimethylguanosine. The last component is present in many of the tRNA species that have been characterized. Determination of the significance of the reported presence of modified nucleosides in the tissues or body fluids of cancer patients must await additional observations.

5.3. Regulatory Roles of tRNA

The suppression mechanism was introduced by Yanofsky *et al.* (1961), and Benzer and Champe (1961) were the first to suggest that the tRNAs may be involved in the control of protein synthesis. Stent (1964) also postulated a regulatory role for the tRNAs in protein biosynthesis. One of the functions proposed for the isoaccepting tRNA species is an involvement in cellular regulatory activities. The modulation hypothesis was introduced by Ames and Hartman (1963) in order to explain the polarity effect in the synthesis of the histidine biosynthetic enzymes. The hypothesis is that the translation of mRNA may be limited by modulating codons corresponding to the various isoaccepting tRNAs. Anderson (1969) has suggested that regulatory codons may exist corresponding to tRNA species present in rate-limiting amounts and that the tRNA concentration could influence the rate of translation of mRNA. Infection of *E. coli* with defective transducing bacteriophage leads to the synthesis of three suppressor tRNAs that differ in the base adjacent to that codon (Gefter and Russell 1969). The findings of Vaughan and Hansen (1973) suggest that normal diploid human cells and also cells derived from cancers possess a general translational control mechanism which inhibits the initiation of protein synthesis in the presence of uncharged tRNA. Along this same approach, Ouellette and Taylor (1973) reported that the tRNA of rat hepatoma 5123 contains 5 times more molecules capable of accepting phenylalanine than liver tRNA. Bridges and Jones (1973) studied the chromatographic patterns of tRNAs from two mouse plasmacytoma tumors. Differences between the tumors were observed in the threonyl- and seryl-tRNAs. A regulatory role of seryl-tRNA is indicated in plasmacyltoma protein synthesis. The rate of estrogen-induced hepatic synthesis of phosphovitin in roosters and chicks is accompanied by a 25% increase in seryl-tRNA (Klyde and Bernfield, 1973). One

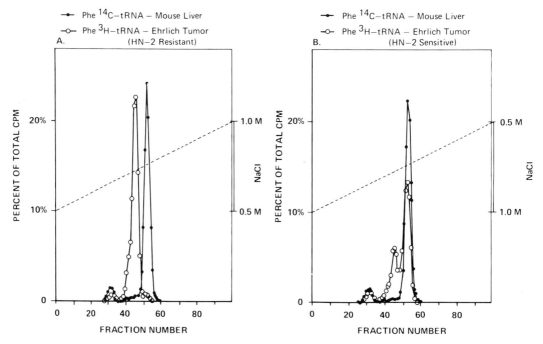

FIGURE 7. Reversed-phase chromatography profiles of phenylalanyl-tRNA. (A) Mouse liver and HN2-resistant Ehrlich tumor cells. (B) Mouse liver and HN2-sensitive Ehrlich tumor cells. From Hayashi and Griffin (1974).

of the isoaccepting species of lysyl-tRNA varies according to the proliferative rate, and it is suggested that the Lys-tRNA$_4$ may be a requirement for cell division (Ortwerth and Liu, 1973). The role of tRNA in cell differentiation, including neoplasia, has been reviewed by Sueoka and Kano-Sueoka, 1970.

5.4. Some Related Functions of tRNA

Transfer RNAs are involved in other mechanisms of polypeptide biosynthesis not involving ribosomes. Soffer and associates have reported a new group of enzymes, the aminoacyl-tRNA protein transferases, that catalyze the addition of certain aminoacyl-tRNAs to the N-terminal of acceptor proteins. Transferase enzymes have been detected for several amino acids by use of postribosomal supernatants. Kaji et al. (1963) observed a ribosome-independent incorporation of arginine employing the S100 supernatant from rat liver. This system required tRNA, ATP, and an energy-generating system. Similar activities were observed for glycine, glutamate, methionine, and tryptophane utilizing similar systems (Kaji, 1968). Significant amounts of labeled arginine and lesser quantities of glutamic acid, phenylalanine, lysine, and valine were present in a hot trichloroacetic acid insoluble form following incubation of the pH 5.0 insoluble fraction of Novikoff ascites tumor (Griffin, 1967). Weinstein and Osserman (1964) also reported an arginine transferase activity while studying protein synthesis in extracts of plasma cell tumors. Arginyl-tRNA protein transferase was obtained from the soluble fraction of sheep thyroid cytoplasm. Serum albumin was effective as the acceptor protein; however, not all proteins have this acceptor activity. Requirements for this reaction include monovalent cation. The reaction mechanism involves the transfer of arginine into a peptide bond with the N-terminal aspartic or glutamic acid residues of the acceptor proteins (Soffer et al., 1969). Soffer and Savage (1974) have reported the isolation of a mutant strain of E. coli which lacked the leucine and phenylalanine transferase activity. When grown into stationary phase and resuspended in minimal medium, the mutant exhibited a marked lag before resuming growth. This was interpreted to implicate the transferase enzymes in the regulation of growth.

Wood (1975) has investigated the incorporation of arginine into hot trichloroacetic acid insoluble material in the absence of ribosomes in a fraction isolated from rabbit reticulocytes. Arginine incorporation was dependent on an arginyl-tRNA intermediate and required the presence of a sulfhydryl reagent and either monovalent or divalent cations. In these studies, the arginine transferase activity was stimulated only by exogenous acceptor proteins. The absence of detectable physiological acceptors in rabbit reticulocyte whole cell and untreated postribosomal supernatant fractions makes it difficult to ascertain the physiological significance of this type of reaction.

The cell-free synthesis of amino-terminal L-pyroglutamic acid was demonstrated by Jones (1974) employing a microsomal protein-synthesizing system prepared from plasma cell tumor. Glutamic acid is the precursor of pyroglutamic acid, which is the amino-terminal amino acid of several naturally occurring proteins and peptides including the light and heavy chains of immunoglubulins. Two isoaccepting glutamyl-tRNA species were detected in this plasma cell tumor and both participate in the synthesis of L-pyroglutamic acid.

In microbial systems, there is evidence that aminoacyl-tRNA is involved in the nonribosomal synthesis of the peptidoglycan of the cell walls. Stewart *et al.* (1971) have found two forms of glycyl-tRNA that function in the nonribosomal synthesis of cell wall peptidoglycans. These two tRNA^{Gly}'s have only one modified base, have the usual anticodon sequences, UCC, for glycine, and lack the Tψ of the GTψ region (Roberts, 1973).

Modifications in the tRNA patterns are common in virus-transformed cells. Some of these are indicated in Table 1. In several of these transformed lines, there is evidence suggesting that the altered tRNAs are the result of derepressed or modified host tRNA rather than a viral genome product. However, there is also evidence for viruses that carry their own tRNA or gene for tRNA into the host. Erikson and Erikson (1970) have isolated 4 S RNA from avian myeloblastosis virus that has amino acid acceptor activity for valine, proline, methionine, glycine, aspartic acid, and arginine when incubated with the host (chick) aminoacyl-tRNA synthetases. Rous sarcoma virus carries its own 4 S RNA that has a different base composition than host tRNA (Bishop *et al.*, 1970). Finally, mention should be made of the interesting observations of Haenni and associates that the RNA of turnip yellow mosaic virus possesses valine acceptor activity. The entire molecule, 23–25 S, will react with *E. coli* valyl-tRNA synthetase and ATP to form an aminoacyl bond between valine and the 3'-end of the RNA. When placed in a protein-synthesizing system, the virus valyl-RNA can donate its valine into a polypeptide chain. It was also shown that the 23 S RNA is broken down into a 4.5 S RNA when it engages in protein synthesis (Haenni *et al.*, 1973; Prochiantz and Haenni, 1973).

6. Further Observations Related to Protein Synthesis and Metabolism

6.1. Metabolic Effects

Pitot and coworkers (Pitot *et al.*, 1974; Pitot, Chap. 6) have made extensive studies relative to phenotypic variability and translational control mechanisms. They have proposed that the stable template consists of a combination of a functioning polysome and an intracellular membrane. This unit has been termed the "membron." Other aspects of the polysome–membrane complex and the biosynthesis of proteins have been investigated by this group.

This chapter has been concerned largely with the intracellular aspects of protein biosynthesis, which include the ribosomes and other factors that are involved on the translation of the genetic messages. Many of these observations have been obtained under essentially *in vitro* conditions. Even at these levels it is quite apparent that the essential biosynthetic reactions are influenced by many conditions, including the relative concentrations of free amino acids, tRNAs, inhibitors, ATP, and GTP. In the intact organism or animal, these factors are compounded. The influence of the quality and quantity of diet, transport processes, degradative processes, as well as the large number of regulatory mechanisms in general must also be considered. Finally, the overall aspects of protein biosynthesis may be further complicated both in tumors and in the tumor-bearing patient or animal.

The familiar cachexia of patients with advanced neoplastic disease is well recognized. This has been attributed or related to malnutrition, toxemia, infection, and psychic depression. Several authorities believe that these symptoms are the result of systemic changes produced by the tumor. The concept has emerged that the tumor may act as a "nitrogen trap"; i.e., nitrogen is transferred from the body tissues to the tumor accompanied by a progressive loss in body weight. Specific substances (toxins) elaborated by tumors have been reported that alter the levels of liver, kidney, and erythrocyte catalase as well as certain other enzymes. The most studied of these toxins is a substance termed "toxohormone" (Nakahara and Fukuoka, 1961). However, the toxohormone concept requires further extensive investigation (Aoki et al., 1969). Many studies have been recorded relative to the generalized anemia observed in many cancer patients. An excellent compilation of the early studies of tumor-host effects was carried out by Greenstein (1954).

Attention is directed to an area of investigation that, in the writer's opinion, provides new impetus and potential for metabolic study, especially amino acid and protein requirements and metabolism, in the cancer patient. Dudrick and associates have developed procedures of parenteral hyperalimentation so that patients can receive their total nutritional requirements by this means for an indefinite period of time. These procedures have been used in approximately 5000 patients with a spectrum of disorders and with a minimum of complications (Dudrick and Copeland, 1973). Approximately 600 cancer patients are included in this series (Copeland et al., 1974). Each of the patients had lost at least 10 lb of his usual body weight. The nutrient solution is hypertonic, consisting of 4–5% protein hydrolysates or crystalline amino acids in 20–25% dextrose. Electrolyte additives are included just prior to infusion in order to satisfy the metabolic requirements of each patient. The solutions are delivered employing long-term subclavian vein catheterization. In one study, the average duration of a single catheterization was 24 days and the longest a single catheter remained in place was approximately 100 days. The general consensus now prevails that cancer patients may be maintained in weight and positive nitrogen balance. Since the dietary imput is under rigid control, this approach provides new opportunity to study amino acid and protein metabolism in the cancer patient. The effect of amino acid levels, amino acid imbalances, specific amino acid antagonists, etc., on protein synthesis in the tumor and host may be studied as well as the metabolism and excretion of the metabolites. This investigative approach should make it possible to obtain new insight into many of the tumor-host phenomena that have been observed for many years.

The literature relative to amino acid and protein metabolism in neoplastic tissues is extensive. Only a few recent studies will be included in this presentation. The reader is directed to the many reviews in *Advances in Cancer Research, Progress in Experimental Cancer Research,* and *Advances in Enzyme Regulation* for a more comprehensive coverage of this aspect of protein metabolism. Weinhouse (1973) has provided a review of the profound alterations in the isozyme patterns that occur in experimental hepatomas. Weinhouse states in this article that "there is a common thread, interwoven throughout a large body of recent literature, pointing to a common biochemical lesion in cancer; namely, a misprogramming of genetic expression, manifested by aberrations of protein synthesis."

Goldberg *et al.* (1974) point out that cell proteins within organelles or bound to membranes may be synthesized and degraded many times during the life span of the cell. They discuss the factors that regulate protein catabolism and the reasons why different proteins have distinct half-lives. Christensen *et al.* (1973) have investigated the transport systems of amino acids in Ehrlich ascites cells. Protein and RNA metabolism in single-cell suspensions from Morris hepatoma 5123 to and from normal rat liver has been studied. A few of the observations from this experimental system are included (Schreiber *et al.,* 1974). The hepatoma cells synthesized 1.4 μg protein/h/mg cellular protein compared to 0.54 μg in the liver cells. Incorporation of L-leucine into protein of the hepatoma cells was independent of the concentration of K^+, Mg^{2+}, and Ca^{2+} in the medium, whereas distinct maxima of incorporation rates were observed in liver cells at 65 mM K^+, 3.5 mM Mg^{2+}, and 2.5 mM Ca^{2+}. Mitochondrial protein synthesis contributed a minor portion to protein synthesis in both cell types. Radioactivity was transferred into the medium by hepatoma or liver cells incubated with labeled leucine with kinetics similar to that found for liver in the intact animal. This is in contrast to the lack of secretion of proteins by the hepatoma as observed *in vivo*. Olivotto and Paoletti (1974) have found the Yoshida ascites hepatoma to be a useful model for studying protein metabolism in relation to the growth of these cells.

6.2. *Production of Abnormal Proteins in Cancer Patients*

Several proteins, including those related to the antigenic potential of tumor cells, have been described or related to growing cancer masses. The presence of certain of these proteins in body fluids provides the basis for the detection and prognosis of tumors in humans and experimental animals. Of these methods, the detection of α-fetoprotein (αFP) by precipitation reactions in gel, for the diagnosis of primary liver cancer, was originally thought to be the most reliable (see Chap. 2). αFP is an α-globulin and has been obtained in a crystalline form. At this time, it would appear that αFP assay procedures, including a radioimmunoassay, are positive in approximately 75% of patients with hepatomas. A monograph appeared in 1973 covering many aspects of αFP and hepatomas (Hirai and Miyaji, 1973). Becker and Sell (1974) detected an increase in circulating αFP in rats immediately following the administration of extremely small quantities of

N-2-fluorenylacetamide. They suggested that this increase may be attributable to a highly selective derepression of protein synthesis that occurs after the formation of a complex between the metabolites of this carcinogen and the specific chromatin loci. The synthesis of αFP by membrane-bound polysomes of ascites hepatoma cells has been reported by Kanai *et al.* (1974).

There is a growing interest in the utilization of procedures, biological and biochemical, that may be of diagnostic and prognostic significance in cancer in man. As mentioned previously, a recent report from the Director of the National Cancer Program stated that 63 of a group of 65 breast cancer patients (97.7%) showed abnormal levels in the blood and urine of at least one of the three markers carcinoembryonic antigen, human chorionic gonadotropin, N^2, N^2-dimethylguanosine (see Section 5.2). The extension of this approach employing multiple biological markers which include unique or abnormal proteins from tumors for the detection of other cancer types will be followed with interest.

Myeloma patients successfully treated by chemotherapy later developed monocyctic leukemia and began to excrete abnormally large quantities of the enzyme lysozyme. This aspect of a possible relation between these tumors as well as the regulatory mechanism and conditions directing the synthesis of large quantities of specific proteins such as lysozyme in cancer cells are discussed in a reference work on lysozyme research by Osserman *et al.* (1974).

The tumor angiogenesis factor which is elaborated by solid tumors is discussed by Folkman in Chapter 13 of this volume. This factor, which is mitogenic to capillary endothelial cells, appears to be a RNA–protein complex. Reich (1973) has advanced the concept that fibrinolysis has a definite association with tumor development and growth. He indicates that fibrinolysis is observed in primary cultures of chemically induced mammary carcinomas, hepatomas, and skin cancers. It is found in human and animal tumor cell lines and is associated with the transformation of avain and mammalian cells in culture by DNA and RNA viruses. Reich has shown that the mechanism by which neoplastic cells initiate fibrinolysis depends on two protein factors, one present in all vertebrate sera, the other released by cells following transformation. The serum factor has been identified as the known zymogen plasminogen. The cell factor is an arginine-specific protease of molecular weight 38,000 daltons. It is a serine protease that is inhibited by diisopropylfluorophosphate and it hydrolyzes a single peptide bond in plasminogen, thereby forming the active fibrinolytic protease, plasmin. Further characterization of the fibrinolysis mechanism and its association with oncogenic transformation are presented in three publications by Reich and associates: Unkeless *et al.* (1974), Quigley *et al.* (1974), and Ossowski *et al.* (1974).

A transplantable mouse fibrosarcoma, HSDM, produces a potent bone-resorption-stimulating factor. These cells synthesize and secrete large quantities of prostaglandin E_2. Mice bearing the HSDM tumor have elevated concentrations of calcium and PGE_2 in the serum. The authors (Tashjian *et al.*, 1974) conclude that the bone-resorption-stimulating factor is PGE_2 and that the secretion of this prostaglandin by the tumor produces a hypercalcemic syndrome in the mouse which is similar in many respects to the unexplained ectopic humoral hypercalcemias in some cancer patients.

7. Conclusion

The mechanisms involved in protein synthesis in a wide range of organisms have been reviewed in some detail. It appears that the components as well as the reaction sequences of the polypeptide initiation, chain elongation, and release events are indeed similar in the prokaryotic and eukaryotic cellular systems that have been investigated. The universality of this ribosomal mechanism of protein synthesis is well established. Comparable studies in several types of cancer cells have revealed that, within the limitations of the investigative procedures employed, protein synthesis in the cancer cell does not differ in any fundamental aspect from that found in normal eukaryotic cells. In other words, ribosomes and the requisite initiation, elongation, and release factors obtained from the Krebs or Ehrlich tumor cells, as well as other tumors, will efficiently translate mRNAs from many viruses and prokaryotic and eukaryotic cells. These observations suggest that if protein biosynthesis is involved in neoplasia it cannot be detected in the rather artificial conditions that are characteristic of the *in vitro* amino acid incorporating systems.

Most of the studies on the mechanism of protein biosynthesis have been carried out in the absence of regulatory influences that are operative in the intact cell or in more complex organisms. Actually, it is at these regulatory levels that we may reasonably expect that differences may exist between normal and cancer cells. Such differences may be the result of subtle molecular changes in the ribosomes or polypeptide initiation, elongation, or release factors in the cancer cell. These components would fail to respond normally to the regulatory factors that control protein synthesis. The extensive studies now in progress to characterize the multiple proteins and the classes of RNA within the large and small ribosomal subunits will undoubtedly provide new insight into the molecular topography and the multiple binding sites on ribosomes that are operative in protein synthesis. Correspondingly, the possibility also exists that new or altered hormones or other regulatory factors that influence protein synthesis are present in cancer cells.

The tRNA profiles obtained from several chromatographic procedures suggest that many tumors differ in this respect from the most appropriate normal control tissues. In view of the role now ascribed to the tRNAs in embryogenesis, differentiation, virus infection, and other regulatory activities, including rates of protein biosynthesis, there is reason to believe that the tRNAs may be associated with the development of neoplastic cells.

It would still appear that the basic events resulting in the development of tumor cells occur within the deoxyribonucleoproteins and at transcriptional levels. Altered genes may result in abnormal proteins with altered functional properties. However, the consensus at present is that, qualitatively, the enzymes and other proteins of normal and cancer cells are indeed similar. Perhaps the repression or derepression patterns present in the cells are even more important considerations. Weinhouse (1973) states: "An anomaly of gene expression in cancer in which genes normally coding for proteins of adult differentiated tissue are switched off, and genes expressed during the fetal stage but inactivated during normal embryonic development are reactivated." Dr. Clement L. Markert has expressed the view that there are no unique properties of cancer cells. He believes that there is only an aggregation of properties not normally found in normal cells. Markert also suggests that cancer represents the activity of normal genes functioning in an abnormal manner.

Considerable progress has been achieved in the elucidation of the mechanisms by which hormones and their cellular receptors regulate nuclear RNA metabolism and subsequent protein synthesis. The biochemical events involved are shown in Fig. 3. Continued progress in this important area will contribute to a better understanding of many regulatory mechanisms involved in embryogenesis and differentiation and very likely to a better understanding of many aspects of neoplasia.

Some of the unique proteins elaborated by tumor cells are mentioned in this chapter. These include α-fetoprotein, carcinoembryonic antigen, tumor angiogenesis factor, which is mitogenic to capillary endothelial cells, and fibrinolytic factor. In addition to any direct or indirect roles these factors may play in the origin and function of cancer cells, their presence in body fluids may be of value in the detection and prognosis of human tumors. In this same connection, the application of combinations of "biological markers," which include, in addition to the above, isozymes, dimethylguanosine, and hormones, may prove to be a useful adjunct to tumor diagnosis.

Finally, it is of interest to point out the remarkable progress that has been recorded in the understanding of the biosynthesis of proteins during the past 10–15 years. The genetic code has been elucidated during this period, as has the development of most of the *in vitro* amino acid incorporating systems. Holley and associates reported the first complete nucleotide sequence of a transfer RNA in 1965. During this time span, the ribosomal mechanism which accounts for almost all protein synthesis in all living cells has been elucidated. Recently, a 500-page volume entitled *Normal and Pathological Protein Synthesis in Higher Organisms* has been published (Schapira *et al.*, 1973). The next decade will undoubtedly produce major progress in the characterization of the structural components of protein biosynthesis as well as structure–function interrelationships that exist in terms of regulatory mechanisms. This will provide new opportunity to study the precise role of protein synthesis, whether primary or secondary, in the origin and the subsequent behavior of the cancer cell.

ACKNOWLEDGMENTS

The author is an American Cancer Society Professor of Biochemistry. Studies included in this chapter were supported by grants from the American Cancer Society and The Robert A. Welch Foundation.

A. CLARK
GRIFFIN

AHERN, T., AND KAY, J. E., 1973, The control of protein synthesis during the stimulation of lymphocytes by phytohaemagglutin. II. Studies with cell-free systems, *Biochim. Biophys. Acta* **331**:91.

ALLFREY, V. G., 1970, in: *Aspects of Protein Synthesis* (C. B. Anfinsen, Jr., ed.), Part A, pp. 247–365, Academic Press, New York.

ALLFREY, V. G., JOHNSON, E. M., KARN, J., AND VIDALI, G., 1973, in: *Protein Phosphorylation in Control Mechanisms* (J. Huijing and E. Y. C. Lee, eds.), pp. 217–249, Academic Press, New York.

AMES, B. N., AND HARTMAN, P. E., 1963, The histidine operon, *Cold Spring Harbor Symp. Quant. Biol.* **28**:349.

ANDERSON, W. F., 1969, The effect of tRNA concentration in the rate of protein synthesis, *Proc. Natl. Acad. Sci. U.S.A.* **62**:566.

AOKI, T., HNILICA, L. S., AND GRIFFIN, A. C., 1969, The effect of histone fractions on liver catalase and tryptophan pyrrolase activities, *Arch. Biochem. Biophys.* **131**:538.

ARNSTEIN, H. R. V., 1974, *Synthesis of Amino Acids and Proteins*, University Park Press, Baltimore.

ASHWELL, M., AND WORK, T. S., 1970, The biogenesis of mitochondria, *Ann. Rev. Biochem.* **39**:251.

AVADHANI, N. G., AND RUTMAN, R. J., 1974, A sensitive *in vitro* protein synthesizing system from Ehrlich ascites mitochondria, *Biochem. Biophys. Res. Commun.* **58**:42.

AYUSO-PARILLA, M., HENSHAW, E. C., AND HIRSCH, C. A., 1973, The ribosome cycle in mammalian protein synthesis. III. Evidence that the nonribosomal proteins bound to the native smaller subunits are initiation factors, *J. Biol. Chem.* **248**:4386.

BALIGA, B. S., BOREK, E., WEINSTEIN, I. B., AND SRINIVASAN, P. R., 1969, Differences in the transfer RNA's of normal liver and Novikoff hepatoma, *Proc. Natl. Acad. Sci. U.S.A.* **62**:899.

BANCROFT, F. C., WU, G.-J., AND ZUBAY, G., 1973, Cell-free synthesis of rat growth hormone, *Proc. Natl. Acad. Sci. U.S.A.* **70**:3646.

BAUTZ, E. K. F., KARLSON, P., AND KERSTEN, H., 1973, *Regulation of Transcription and Translation in Eukaryotes*, Springer, New York.

BEATTIE, D. S., 1971, The synthesis of mitochondrial proteins, *Sub-Cell. Biochem.* **1**:1.

BECKER, F. F., AND SELL, S., 1974, Early elevation of α_1-fetoprotein in N-2-fluorenylacetamide hepatocarcinogenesis, *Cancer Res.* **34**:2489.

BENZER, S., AND CHAMPE, S. P., 1961, Ambivalent *r II* mutants of phage T4, *Proc. Natl. Acad. Sci. U.S.A.* **47**:1025.

BERMEK, E., AND MATTHAEI, H., 1970, The effect of antibiotics on an optimized polyphenylalanine synthesizing cell-free system from human lymphatic tissue, *Hoppe-Seylers Z. Physiol. Chem.* **351**:1377.

BISHOP, J. M., LEVINSON, W. E., QUINTRELL, N., SULLIVAN, D., FANSHIER, L., AND JACKSON, J., 1970, The low molecular weight RNAs of Rous sarcoma virus, *Virology* **42**:182.

BOREK, E., AND KERR, S. J., 1972, Atypical transfer RNA's and their origin in neoplastic cells, *Adv. Cancer Res.* **15**:163.

BORST, P., 1972, Mitochondrial nucleic acids, *Ann. Rev. Biochem.* **41**:333.

BRENNER, S., STRETTON, A. O. W., AND KAPLAN, S., 1965, Genetic code: The "nonsense" triplets for chain termination and their suppression, *Nature (London)* **206**:994.

BRIDGES, K. R., AND JONES, G. H., 1973, Tumor ribonucleic acids from mouse plasmacytoma tumors producing κ and λ immunoglobulin chains, *Biochemistry* **12**:1208.

BRISCOE, W. T., 1974, Studies on a unique aspartyl-transfer ribonucleic acid appearing in SV40-induced and other tumors, dissertation, University of Texas Health Science Center at Houston, Graduate School of Biomedical Sciences.

BRISCOE, W. T., TAYLOR, W., GRIFFIN, A. C., DUFF, R., AND RAPP, F., 1972, Aspartyl transfer RNA profiles in normal and cancer cells, *Cancer Res.* **32**:1753.

BULLOUGH, W. S., 1969, The chalones, *Sci. J.* **5**:71.

BUSCH, H., 1974, Messenger RNA and other high molecular weight RNA, in: *The Molecular Biology of Cancer* (H. Busch, ed.), pp. 187–239, Academic Press, New York.

CASHEL, M., AND KALBACHER, B., 1970, The control of ribonucleic acid synthesis in *Escherichia coli*. V. Characterization of a nucleotide associated with the stringent response, *J. Biol. Chem.* **245**:2309.

CASHION, L. M., AND STANLEY, W. M., JR., 1974, Two eukaryotic initiation factors (IF-I and IF-II) of protein synthesis that are required to form an initiation complex with rabbit reticultoyte ribosomes, *Proc. Natl. Acad. Sci. U.S.A.* **71**:436.

CASKEY, C. T., 1970, The universal RNA genetic code, *Quant. Rev. Biophys.* **3**:295.

CASKEY, C. T., BEAUDET, A. L., AND TATE, W. P., 1974, Mammalian release factor; *in vitro* assay and purification, *Methods Enzymol.* **30**:293.

CASKEY, T., SCOLNICK, E., CARYK, T., AND NIRENBERG, M., 1968, Sequential translation of trinucleotide codons for the initiation and termination of protein synthesis, *Science* **162**:135.

CHAMBERS, R. W., 1971, On the recognition of tRNA by its aminoacyl-tRNA ligase, in: *Progress in Nucleic Acid Research and Molecular Biology*, Vol 11, (J. N. Davidson and W. E. Cohn, eds.), pp. 489–525, Academic Press, New York.

CHRISTENSEN, H. N., DECESPEDES, C., HANDLOGTEN, M. E., AND RONQUIST, G., 1973, Energization of amino acid transport, studied for the Ehrlich ascites tumor cell, *Biochim. Biophys. Acta* **300**:487.

COPELAND, E. M., MACFAYDEN, B. V., AND DUDRICK, S. J., 1974, Intravenous hyperalimentation in cancer patients, *J. Surg. Res.* **16**:241.

COX, R. A., 1974, Ribosome structure and function, in: *Synthesis of Amino Acids and Proteins* (H. Arnstein, ed.), University Park Press, Baltimore.

CRICK, F. H. C., 1966, Codon-anticodon pairing: The wobble hypothesis, *J. Mol. Biol.* **19**:548.

DUBE, S. K., MARCKER, K. A., CLARK, B. F. C., AND CORY, S., 1968, Nucleotide sequence of N-formyl-methionyl-transfer RNA, *Nature (London)* **218**:232.

DUDRICK, S. J., AND COPELAND, E. M., 1973, *Parenteral Hyperalimentation* (L. M. Nyhus, ed.), pp. 69–95, Appleton-Century-Crofts, New York.

EICH, F., AND DREWS, J., 1974, Isolation and characterization of a peptide chain initiation factor from Krebs II ascites tumor cells, *Biochim. Biophys. Acta* **340**:334.

ENGLAND, J. M., AND ATTARDI, G., 1974, Expression of the mitochondrial genome in HeLa cells. XXI. Mitochondrial protein synthesis during the cell cycle, *J. Mol. Biol.* **85**:433.

EPLER, J. L., 1969, The mitochondrial and cytoplasmic transfer ribonucleic acids of *Neurospora crassa*, *Biochemistry* **8**:2285.

EPLER, J. L., SHUGART, L. R., AND BARNETT, W. E., 1970, N-Formylmethionyl transfer ribonucleic acid in mitochondria from *Neurospora*, *Biochemistry* **9**:3575.

ERIKSON, E., AND ERIKSON, R. L., 1970, Isolation of amino acid acceptor tRNA from purified avian myeloblastosis virus, *J. Mol. Biol.* **52**:387.

FAIS, D., SHAKULOV, R. C., AND KLYACHKO, E. V., 1971, Protein content and biological activity of ribosomal particles from ascites carcinoma Krebs II cells, *Biochim. Biophys. Acta* **246**:530.

FLORINI, J. R., AND BREUER, C. B., 1966, Amino acid incorporation into protein by cell-free systems from rat skeletal muscle. V. Effects of pituitary growth hormone on activity of ribosomes and ribonucleic acid polymerases in hypophysectomized rats, *Biochemistry* **5**:1870.

FUJIOKA, S., AND GALLO, R. C., 1971, Aminoacyl transfer RNA profiles in human myeloma cells, *Blood* **38**:246.

GALLAGHER, R. E., TING, R. C., AND GALLO, R. C., 1972, A common change of aspartyl tRNA in polyoma- and SV-40-transformed cells, *Biochim. Biophys. Acta* **272**:568.

GALLO, R. C., AND PESTKA, S., 1970, Transfer RNA species in normal and leukemic human lymphoblasts, *J. Mol. Biol.* **52**:195.

GAREN, A., 1968, Sense and nonsense in the genetic code, *Science* **160**:149.

GEFTER, M. L., AND RUSSELL, R. L., 1969, Role of modifications in tyrosine transfer RNA: A modified base affecting ribosome binding, *J. Mol. Biol* **39**:145.

GOLDBERG, A. L., HOWELL, E. M., LI, J. B., MARTEL, S. B., AND PROUTY, W. F., 1974, Physiological significance of protein degradation in animal and bacterial cells, *Fed. Proc.* **33**:1112.

GOLDMAN, M., AND GRIFFIN, A. C., 1970, Transfer RNA patterns in livers of rats fed diets containing 3'-methyl-4-dimethylaminoazobenzene, *Cancer Res.* **30**:1677.

GOLDMAN, M., JOHNSTON, W. M., AND GRIFFIN, A. C., 1969, Comparison of transfer ribonucleic acids and aminoacyl synthetases of liver and ascites tumor cells, *Cancer Res.* **29**:1051.

GONANO, F., CHIARUGI, V. P., PIRRO, G., AND MARINI, M., 1971, Transfer ribonucleic acids in rat liver and Morris 5123 minimal deviation hepatoma, *Biochemistry* **10**:900.

GOODWIN, F., SHAFRITZ, D., AND WEISSBACH, H., 1969, *In vitro* polypeptide synthesis in brain, *Arch. Biochem. Biophys.* **130**: 183.

GORDON, J., 1968, A stepwise reaction yielding a complex between a supernatant fraction from *E. coli*, guanosine 5'-triphosphate and aminoacyl-SRNA, *Proc. Natl. Acad. Sci. U.S.A.* **59**:179.

GORDON, J., 1970, Regulation of the *in vivo* synthesis of the polypeptide chain elongation factors in *Escherichia coli*, *Biochemistry* **9**:912.

GREENSTEIN, J. P., 1954, *Biochemistry of Cancer*, 2nd ed., Academic Press, New York.

GRIFFIN, A. C., 1967, *In vitro* studies on protein synthesis by malignant cells, *Adv. Cancer Res.* **10**:83.

GRIFFIN, A. C., 1974, Protein synthesis, in: *The Molecular Biology of Cancer* (H. Busch, ed.), pp. 355–375, Academic Press, New York.

GRIFFIN, A. C., AND BLACK, D. D., 1971, Protein biosynthesis, in: *Methods in Cancer Research* (H. Busch, ed.), pp. 189–251, Academic Press, New York.

GROLLMAN, A. P., AND HUANG, M. T., 1973, Inhibitors of protein synthesis in eukaryotes: Tools in cell research, *Fed. Proc.* **32**:1673.

GROSSMAN, L., AND MOLDAVE, K., 1974, Nucleic acids and protein synthesis, *Methods Enzymol.* **30**:1.

HAENNI, A. L., 1972, in: *The Mechanism of Protein Synthesis and Its Regulation* (L. Bosch, ed.), pp. 36–51, North-Holland, Amsterdam.

HAENNI, A. L., PROCHIANTZ, A., BERNARD, O., AND CHAPEVILLE, F., 1973, TYMV valyl-RNA as an amino acid donor in protein biosynthesis, *Nature New Biol.* **241**:166.

HALDER, D., 1971, Protein synthesis in isolated rat brain mitochondria, *Biochim. Biophys. Acta* **42**:899.

HASELKORN, R., AND ROTHMAN-DENES, L. B., 1973, Protein synthesis, *Ann. Rev. Biochem.* **42**:397.

HAYASHI, M., AND GRIFFIN, A. C., 1974, Purification and properties of the major phenylalanyl transfer RNA species in drug-resistant Ehrlich tumor cells, *Cancer Research* **34**:331.

HENSHAW, E. C., GUINEY, D. G., AND HIRSCH, C. A., 1973, The ribosome cycle in mammalian protein synthesis. I. The place of monomeric ribosomes and ribosomal subunits in the cycle, *J. Biol. Chem.* **248**:4367.

HIRAI, H., AND MIYAJI, T. (eds.), 1973, *Alpha Fetoprotein and Hepatoma*, Monograph on Cancer Research, No. 14, University Park Press, Baltimore.

HIRSCH, C. A., COX, M. A., VANVENROOIJ, J. W., AND HENSHAW, E. C., 1973, The ribosome cycle in mammalian protein synthesis. II. Association of the native smaller ribosomal subunit with protein factors, *J. Biol. Chem.* **248**:4377.

HOLLAND, J. J., TAYLOR, M. W., AND BUCK, C. A., 1967, Chromatographic differences between tyrosyl transfer RNA from different mammalian cells, *Proc. Natl. Acad. Sci. U.S.A.* **58**:2437.

HOLLEY, R. W., APGAR, J., EVERETT, G. A., MADISON, J. T., MARQUISEE, M., MERRILL, S. H., PENSWICK, J. R., AND ZAMIR, A., 1965, Structure of a ribonucleic acid, *Science* **147**:1462.

IVERSEN, O. H., 1970, Some theoretical considerations on chalones and the treatment of cancer, *Cancer Res.* **30**:1481.

JACOBSON, E. L., JUAREZ, H., HEDGOOTH, C., AND CONSIGLI, R. A., 1974, An extra species of lysine transfer ribonucleic acid in polyoma virus-transformed cells in tissue culture, *Arch. Biochem.* **163**:666.

JACOBSON, K. B., 1971, Reaction of aminoacyl-tRNA synthetases with heterologous tRNA's, in: *Progress in Nucleic Acid Research and Molecular Biology* Vol. 11 (J. N. Davidson and W. E. Cohn, eds.), pp. 461–481, Academic Press, New York.

JENKINS, N., TAYLOR, M. W., AND RAFF, R. A., 1973, In vitro translation of oogenetic messenger RNA of sea urchin eggs and picornavirus RNA with a cell-free system from sarcoma 180, *Proc. Natl. Acad. Sci. U.S.A.* **70**:3287.

JENSEN, E. V., AND JACOBSON, H. I., 1962, Basic guides to the mechanism of estrogen action, *Recent Prog. Hormone Res.* **18**:387.

JONES, G. H., 1974, Cell-free synthesis of amino-terminal L-pyroglutamic acid, *Biochemistry* **13**:858.

KAJI, H., 1968, Further studies on the soluble amino acid incorporating systems from rat liver, *Biochemistry* **7**:3844.

KAJI, H., NOVELLI, G. D., AND KAJI, A., 1963, A soluble amino acid-incorporating system from rat liver, *Biochim. Biophys. Acta* **76**:474.

KANAI, K., ENDO, Y., ODA, T., AND TANAKA, N., 1974, Synthesis of alpha-fetoprotein by membrane-bound polysomes of rats ascites hepatoma cells, *Cancer Res.* **34**:1813.

KARLSON, P., 1974, Mode of action of Ecdysones, in: *Invertebrate Endocrinology and Hormonal Heterophylly* (W. Burdette, ed.), pp. 43–54, Springer, New York.

KARN, J., JOHNSON, E. M., VIDALI, G., AND ALLFREY, V. G., 1974, Differential phosphorylation and turnover of nuclear acidic protein during the cell cycle of synchronized HeLa cells, *J. Biol. Chem.* **249**:667.

KEITH, G., PICAUD, P., WEISSENBACH, J., EBEL, J. P., PETRISSANT, G., AND DIRHEIMER, G., 1973, The primary structure of rabbit liver tRNA[Phe] and its comparison with known tRNA[Phe] sequences, *FEBS Lett.* **31**:345.

KIM, S. H., QUIGLEY, G., SUDDATH, F. L., MCPHERSON, A., SNEDEN, D., KIM, J. J., WEINZIERL, J., BLATTMANN, P., AND RICH, A., 1972, The three-dimensional structure of yeast phenylalanine transfer RNA: Shape of the molecule at 5.5-A resolution, *Proc. Natl. Acad. Sci. U.S.A.* **69**:3746.

KIM, S. H., SUDDATH, F. L., QUIGLEY, G. S., MCPHERSON, A., SUSSMAN, J. L., WANG, A. H. J., SEEMAN, N. E., AND RICH, A., 1974, Three-dimensional tertiary structure of yeast phenylalanine transfer RNA, *Science* **185**:435.

KISSELEV, L. L., ANDFAVOROVA, O. O., 1974, Aminoacyl-tRNA synthetases: Some recent results and achievements, *Adv. Enzymol.* **40**:141.

KLYDE, B. J., AND BERNFIELD, M. R., 1973, Rate of serine transfer ribonucleic acid synthesis during estrogen-induced phosphoprotein synthesis in chick liver, *Biochemistry* **12**:3758.

KOKA, M., AND NAKAMOTO, T., 1972, Studies on polyphenylalanine synthesis with a cell-free system of rat lymphosarcoma, *Biochim. Biophys. Acta* **262**:381.

KRANTZ, S. B., AND JACOBSEN, L. O., 1970, *Erythropoietin and the Regulation of Erythropoiesis*, University of Chicago Press, Chicago.

KRISKO, I., GORDON, J., AND LIPMANN, F., 1969, Studies on the interchangeability of one of the mammalian and bacterial supernatant factors in protein synthesis, *J. Biol. Chem.* **244**:6117.

LAMKIN, A. F., AND HURLBERT, R. B., 1972, Amino acid activation by nucleoli isolated from the Novikoff ascites tumor, *Biochim. Biophys. Acta* **272**:321.

LAMKIN, A. F., SMITH, D. W., AND HURLBERT, R. B., 1973, Independent protein synthesis in isolated rat tumor nucleoli, aminoacylation of endogenous transfer ribonucleic acid, *Biochemistry* **12**:4137.

LANZANI, G. A., GIANNATTASIO, M., MANZOCCHI, L. A., BOLLINI, R., SOFFIENTINI, A. N., AND MACCHIA, V., 1974, The influence of cyclic GMP on polypeptide synthesis in a cell-free system derived from wheat embryos, *Biochem. Biophys. Res. Commun.* **58**:172.

LEVIN, D. H., KYNER, D., AND ACS, G., 1973, Protein synthesis initiation in eukaryotes: Characterization of ribosomal factors from mouse fibroblasts, *J. Biol. Chem.* **248**:6416.

LIAU, M. C., O'ROURKE, C. M., AND HURLBERT, R. B., 1972, Transfer ribonucleic acid methylases of nucleoli isolated from a rat tumor, *Biochemistry* **11**:629.

LIPMANN, F., 1971, Attempts to map a process evolution of peptide biosynthesis, *Science* **173**:875.

LITTAUER, U. Z., AND INOUYE, H., 1973, Regulation of tRNA, *Ann. Rev. Biochem.* **42**:439.

LITTLEFIELD, J. W., AND KELLER, E. B., 1957, Incorporation of C^{14}-amino acids into ribonucleoprotein particles from the Ehrlich mouse ascites tumor, *J. Biol. Chem.* **224**:13.

LOFTFIELD, R. B., 1972, The mechanism of amino acylation of transfer RNA, *Prog. Nucleic Acid Res. Mol. Biol.* **12**:87.

LUCAS-LENARD, J., AND BERES, L., 1974, Protein synthesis—Peptide chain elongation, in: *The Enzymes* (P. Boyer, ed.), pp. 53–86, Academic Press, New York.

MACH, B., KOBLET, H., AND GROS, D., 1968, Chemical identification of specific immunoglobulins as the product of a cell-free system from plasmacytoma tumors, *Proc. Natl. Acad. Sci. U.S.A.* **59**:445.

MADEN, B. E. H., TRAUT, R. R., AND MONRO, R. E., 1968, Ribosome-catalyzed peptidyl transfer: The polyphenylalanine system, *J. Mol. Biol.* **35**:333.

MAHLER, H. R., AND BROWN, B. J., 1968, Protein synthesis by cerebral cortex polysomes: Characterization of the System, *Arch. Biochem. Biophys.* **125**:387.

MATHEWS, M. B., 1972, Further studies on the translation of globin mRNA and encephalomyocarditis virus RNA in a cell-free system from Krebs II ascites cells, *Biochim. Biophys. Acta* **272**:108.

MCCONKEY, E. H., 1974, Composition of mammalian ribosomal subunits: A reevaluation, *Proc. Natl. Acad. Sci. U.S.A.* **71**:1379.

MEANS, A. R., AND HALL, P. F., 1969, Protein biosynthesis in the testis. V. Concerning the mechanism of stimulation by follicle stimulating hormone, *Biochemistry* **8**:4293.

MEANS, A. R., ABRASS, I. B., AND O'MALLEY, B. W., 1971, Proteins biosynthesis on chick oviduct polyribosomes. I. Changes during estrogen-mediated tissue differentiation, *Biochemistry* **10**:1561.

MEHLER, A. H., 1970, Induced activation of amino acid activating enzymes by amino acid and tRNA, *Prog. Nucleic Acid Res. Mol. Biol.* **10**:1.

MILLER, D. L., AND WEISSBACH, H., 1970, Interactions between the elongation factors: The displacement of GDP from the Tu-GDP complex by factor Ts, *Biochem. Biophys. Res. Commun.* **38**:1016.

MORGAN, H. E., JEFFERSON, L. S., WOLPERT, E. B., AND RANNELS, D. E., 1971, Regulation of protein synthesis in heart muscle. II. Effect of amino acid levels and insulin on ribosomal aggregation, *J. Biol. Chem.* **246**:2163.

MUSHINSKI, J. F., AND POTTER, M., 1969, Variations in leucine transfer ribonucleic acid in mouse plasma cell tumors producing κ-type immunoglobin light chains, *Biochemistry* **8**:1684.

NAKAHARA, W., AND FUKUOKA, F., 1961, *Chemistry of Cancer Toxin Toxohormone*, Thomas, Springfield, Ill.

NIRENBERG, M., 1970, The Flow of Information from Gene to Protein, in: *Aspects of Protein Biosynthesis* (C. B. Anfinsen, ed.), pp. 215–246, Academic Press, New York.

NISHIZUKA, Y., AND LIPMANN, F., 1966, Comparison of guanosine triphosphate split and polypeptide synthesis with a purified *E. coli* system, *Proc. Natl. Acad. Sci. U.S.A.* **55**:212.

NORRIS, A. T., AND BERG, P., 1964, Mechanism of aminoacyl RNA synthesis: Studies with isolated aminoacyl adenylate complexes of isoleucyl RNA synthetase, *Proc. Natl. Acad. Sci. U.S.A.* **52**:330.

NOVELLI, G. D., 1967, Amino acid activation for protein synthesis, *Ann. Rev. Biochem.* **36**:449.

OCHOA, M., JR., AND WEINSTEIN, I. B., 1964, Polypeptide synthesis in a subcellular system derived from the L1210 mouse ascites leukemia, *J. Biol. Chem.* **239**:3834.

OCHOA, S., AND MAZUMDER, R., 1974, Polypeptide chain initiation, in: *The Enzymes* (P. Boyer, ed.), pp. 1–51, Academic Press, New York.

OLIVOTTO, M., AND PAOLETTI, F., 1974, Protein metabolism in tumor cells at various stages of growth *in vivo*, *J. Cell Biol.* **62**:585.

O'MALLEY, B. W., AND MEANS, A. R., 1974, Female steroid hormones and target cell nuclei, *Science* **183**:610.

O'MALLEY, B. W., TOFT, D. O., AND SHERMAN, M. R., 1971, Progesterone-binding components of chick oviduct. II. Nuclear components, *J. Biol. Chem.* **246**:1117.

ORTWERTH, B. J., AND LIU, L. P., 1973, Correlation between a specific isoaccepting lysyl transfer ribonucleic acid and cell division in mammalian tissues, *Biochemistry* **12**:3978.

OSSERMAN, E. F., CANFIELD, R. E., AND BEYCHOK, S., 1974, *Lysozyme*, Academic Press, New York.

OSSOWSKI, L., QUIGLEY, J. P., AND REICH, E., 1974, Fibrinolysis associated with oncogenic transformation, *J. Biol. Chem.* **249**:4312.

OUELLETTE, A. J., AND TAYLOR, M. W., 1973, Elevated levels of acceptor activity of hepatoma transfer ribonucleic acid, *Biochemistry* **12**:3542.

PALMITER, R. D., 1972, Regulation of protein synthesis in chick oviduct. I. Independent regulation of ovalbumin, conalbumin, ovomucoid and lysozyme induction, *J. Biol. Chem.* **247**:6450.

PALMITER, R. D., CHRISTENSEN, A. K., AND SCHIMKE, R. T., 1970, Organization of polysomes from pre-existing ribosomes in chick oviduct by a secondary administration of either estradiol or progesterone, *J. Biol. Chem.* **245**:833.

PASTAN, I., 1972, Cyclic AMP, *Sci. Am.* **227**:97.

PASTAN, I., AND JOHNSON, G. S., 1974, Cyclic AMP and the transformation of fibroblasts, *Adv. Cancer Res.* **19**:303.

PIPER, P. W., AND CLARK, B. F. C., 1974, Primary structure of a mouse myeloma cell initiator transfer RNA, *Nature (London)* **247**:516.

PITOT, H. C., SHIRES, T. K., MOYER, G., AND GARRETT, C. T., 1974, Phenotypic variability as a manifestation of translational control, in: *The Molecular Biology of Cancer* (H. Busch, ed.), pp. 523–534, Academic Press, New York.

POTTER, M., 1972, Immunoglobulin-producing tumors and myeloma proteins of mice, *Physiol. Rev.* **52**:631.

POTTER, M., 1974, Plasmacytomas, in: *The Molecular Biology of Cancer* (H. Busch, ed.), pp. 535–567, Academic Press, New York.

PROCHIANTZ, A., AND HAENNI, A. L., 1973, TYMV-RNA as a substrate of the tRNA maturation endonuclease, *Nature New Biol.* **241**:168.

QUIGLEY, J. P., OSSOWSKI, L., AND REICH, E., 1974, Plasminogen, the serum proenzyme activated by factors from cells transformed by oncogenic viruses, *J. Biol. Chem.* **249**:4306.

REICH, E., 1973, Tumor-associated fibrinolysis, *Fed. Proc.* **32**:2174.

RICHIE, R. C., ENGLISH, M. G., AND GRIFFIN, A. C., 1970, Phenylalanyl transfer RNA alteration in drug resistant Ehrlich ascites tumor cells, *Proc. Soc. Exp. Biol. Med.* **134**:1156.

RITTER, P. O., AND BUSCH, H., 1971, Chromatographic comparison of cytoplasm, nuclear and nucleolar valine and leucine tRNAs from Novikoff hepatoma cells and cytoplasm tRNAs from rat liver cells, *Physiol. Chem. Phys.* **3**:411.

ROBERTS, R. J., 1973, Glycyl-tRNA—Two structures from *Staphylococcus epidermidis*, *Nature New Biol.* **237**:44.

SAMBROOK, J. F., FAN, D. P., AND BRENNER, S., 1967, A strong suppressor specific for UGA, *Nature (London)* **214**:452.

SCHAPIRA, G., DREYFUS, J. C., KRUH, J., AND LABIE, D., 1973, *Normal and Pathological Protein Synthesis in Higher Organisms*, Institut National de la Sante' et de la Recherche Medicale, Paris.

SCHREIBER, M., SCHREIBER, G., AND KARTENBECK, J., 1974, Protein and ribonucleic metabolism in single-cell suspensions from Morris hepatoma 5123 tc and from normal rat liver, *Cancer Res.* **34**:2143.

SCHREIER, M. H., AND STAEHELIN, T., 1973, Initiation of eukaryotic protein synthesis: [Met-tRNA$_f$·40S ribosome] initiation complex catalyzed by purified initiation factors in the absence of mRNA, *Nature New Biol.* **242**:35.

SCOLNICK, R., TOMPKINS, R., CASKEY, T., AND NIRENBERG, M., 1968, Release factors differing in specificity for terminator codons, *Proc. Natl. Acad. Sci. U.S.A.* **61**:768.

SEKIYA, T., AND ODA, K., 1972, The altered patterns of transformed RNA in SV40-infected and transformed cells, *Virology* **47**:168.

SHAFRITZ, D. A., PRICHARD, P. M., GILBERT, J. M., AND ANDERSON, W. F., 1970, Separation of two factors, M$_1$ and M$_{21}$, required for poly U dependent polypeptide synthesis by rabbit reticulocyte ribosomes at low magnesium ion concentration, *Biochem. Biophys. Res. Commun.* **38**:721.

SIMSEK, M., AND RAJBHANDARY, U. L., 1972, The primary structure of yeast initiator transfer ribonucleic acid, *Biochem. Biophys. Res. Commun.* **49**:508.

SIMSEK, M., RAJBHANDARY, U. L., BOISNARD, M., AND PETRISSANT, G., 1974, Nucleotide sequence of rabbit liver and sheep mammary gland cytoplasmic initiator transfer RNAs, *Nature (London)* **247**:518.

SOFFER, R. L., AND SAVAGE, M., 1974, A mutant of *Escherichia coli* defective in leucyl, phenylalanyl tRNA–protein transferase, *Proc. Natl. Acad. Sci. U.S.A.* **71**:1004.

SOFFER, R. L., HORINISHI, H., AND LEIBOWITZ, M. J., 1969, The aminoacyl tRNA–protein transferases, *Cold Spring Harbor Symp. Quant. Biol.* **34**:529.

SÖLL, D., AND SCHIMMEL, P. R., 1974, Aminoacyl-tRNA synthetases, in: *The Enzymes* 3rd Ed., Vol. 10 (P. Boyer, ed.), pp. 489–538, Academic Press, New York.

SRINIVASAN, D., SRINIVASAN, P. R., GRUNBERGER, D., WEINSTEIN, I. B., AND MORRIS, H. P., 1971, Alterations in specific transfer ribonucleic acids in a spectrum of hepatomas, *Biochemistry* **10**:1966.

STAEHELIN, M., ROGG, H., BAGULEY, B. C., GINSBERG, T., AND WEHRLI, W., 1968, Structure of a mammalian serine tRNA, *Nature (London)* **219**:1363.

STEIN, G. S., AND BORUN, T. W., 1972, The synthesis of acidic chromosomal proteins during the cell cycle of HeLa S-3 cells. I. The accelerated accumulation of acidic residual nuclear protein before the initiation of DNA replication, *J. Cell Biol.* **52**:292.

STENT, G. S., 1964, The operon: On its third anniversary, *Science* **144**:816.

STEWART, T. S., ROBERTS, R. J., AND STROMINGER, J. L., 1971, Novel species of tRNA, *Nature (London)* **230**:36.

SUEOKA, N., AND KANO-SUEOKA, T., 1970, Transfer RNA and cell differentiation, *Prog. Nucleic Acid Res. Mol. Biol.* **10**:23.

SUGIYAMA, T., 1971, Role of erythropoietin in 7,12-Dimethylbenz(*a*)anthracene induction of acute chromosome aberration and leukemia in the rat, *Proc. Natl. Acad. Sci. U.S.A.* **68**:2761.

TASHJIAN, A. H., JR., VOELKEL, E. F., GOLDHABER, P., AND LEVINE, L., 1974, Prostaglandins, calcium metabolism and cancer, *Fed. Proc.* **33**:81.

TATE, W. P., AND CASKEY, C. T., 1974, Polypeptide chain termination, in: *The Enzymes* (P. Boyer, ed.), pp. 87–118, Academic Press, New York.

TEIR, H., AND RYTOMAA, T., 1967, *Control of Cellular Growth in Adult Organisms*, A Sigrid Juselius Foundation Symposium, Academic Press, New York.

TAYLOR, M. W., GRANGER, G. A., BUCK, C. A., AND HOLLAND, J. J., 1967, Similarities and differences among specific tRNA's in mammalian tissues, *Proc. Natl. Acad. Sci. U.S.A.* **57**:1712.

TURKINGTON, R. W., AND RIDDLE, M., 1970, Hormone-dependent formation of polysomes in mammary cells *in vitro*, *J. Biol. Chem.* **245**:5145.

UNKELESS, J., DANØ, K., KELLERMAN, G. M., AND REICH, E., 1974, Fibrinolysis associated with oncogenic transformation: Partial purification and characterization of the cell factor, a plasminogen activator, *J. Biol. Chem.* **249**:4295.

VANRIJN, H., BEVERS, M. M., VANWIJK, R., AND HICKS, W. D., 1974, Regulation of phosphoenolpyruvate carboxykinase and tyrosine transaminase in hepatoma cell cultures. III. Comparative studies on H35, HTC, MH$_1$C$_1$ and RLC cells, *J. Cell Biol.* **60**:181.

VAUGHAN, M. H., AND HANSEN, B. S., 1973, Control of initiation of protein synthesis in human cells: Evidence for a role of unchanged transfer ribonucleic acid, *J. Biol. Chem.* **248**:7087.

VOLKERS, S. A. S., AND TAYLOR, M. W., 1971, Chromatographic comparison of the transfer ribonucleic acids of rat livers and Morris hepatomas, *Biochemistry* **10**:488.

WEINHOUSE, S., 1973, Metabolism and isozyme alterations in experimental hepatomas, *Fed. Proc.* **32**:2162.

WEINSTEIN, I. B., AND OSSERMAN, E. F., 1964, Amino acid incorporation into protein by a cell-free system from plasma cell tumors, *Acta Int. Contra Cancrum* **20**:932.

WICHE, G., ZOMZELY-NEURATH, C., AND BLUME, A. J., 1974, *in vitro* synthesis of mouse neuroblastoma tubulin, *Proc. Natl. Acad. Sci. U.S.A.* **71:**1446.

WOOD, T. G., 1975, An arginine transferase activity in enzyme preparation from rabbit reticulocytes, dissertation, University of Texas Health Science Center at Houston, Graduate School of Biomedical Science.

YANG, W. K., AND NOVELLI, G. D., 1968, Multiple isoaccepting transfer RNA's in a mouse plasma cell tumor, *Proc. Natl. Acad. Sci. U.S.A.* **59:**208.

YANOFSKY, C., HELINSKI, D. R., AND MALING, B. D., 1961, The effects of mutation with composition and properties of the A protein of *Escherichia coli* tryptophan synthetase, *Cold Spring Harbor Symp. Quant. Biol.* **26:**11.

ZELINKA, J., AND BALAN, J., 1973, *Ribosomes and RNA Metabolism*, Publishing House of the Slovak Academy of Sciences, Bratislava, Czechoslovakia.

Index